# Biological Response Modifiers
## and
# Cancer Therapy

# IMMUNOLOGY SERIES

*Editor-in-Chief*
**NOEL R. ROSE**
*Professor and Chairman*
*Department of Immunology and*
*Infectious Diseases*
*The Johns Hopkins University*
*School of Hygiene and Public Health*
*Baltimore, Maryland*

*European Editor*
**ZDENEK TRNKA**
*Basel Institute for*
*Immunology*
*Basel, Switzerland*

1. Mechanisms in Allergy: Reagin-Mediated Hypersensitivity
   *Edited by Lawrence Goodfriend, Alec Sehon and Robert P. Orange*

2. Immunopathology: Methods and Techniques
   *Edited by Theodore P. Zacharia and Sidney S. Breese, Jr.*

3. Immunity and Cancer in Man: An Introduction
   *Edited by Arnold E. Reif*

4. *Bordetella pertussis:* Immunological and Other Biological Activities
   *J.J. Munoz and R.K. Bergman*

5. The Lymphocyte: Structure and Function (in two parts)
   *Edited by John J. Marchalonis*

6. Immunology of Receptors
   *Edited by B. Cinader*

7. Immediate Hypersensitivity: Modern Concepts and Development
   *Edited by Michael K. Bach*

8. Theoretical Immunology
   *Edited by George I. Bell, Alan S. Perelson, and George H. Pimbley, Jr.*

9. Immunodiagnosis of Cancer (in two parts)
   *Edited by Ronald B. Herberman and K. Robert McIntire*

10. Immunologically Mediated Renal Diseases: Criteria for Diagnosis and Treatment
    *Edited by Robert T. McCluskey and Giuseppe A. Andres*

11. Clinical Immunotherapy
    *Edited by Albert F. LoBuglio*

12. Mechanisms of Immunity to Virus-Induced Tumors
    *Edited by John W. Blasecki*

13. Manual of Macrophage Methodology: Collection, Characterization, and Function
    *Edited by Herbert B. Herscowitz, Howard T. Holden, Joseph A. Bellanti, and Abdul Ghaffar*

14. Suppressor Cells in Human Disease
    *Edited by James S. Goodwin*

15. Immunological Aspects of Aging
    *Edited by Diego Segre and Lester Smith*

16. Cellular and Molecular Mechanisms of Immunologic Tolerance
    *Edited by Tomáš Hraba and Milan Hašek*

*Additional Volumes in Preparation*

# Biological Response Modifiers and Cancer Therapy

edited by

## J.W. Chiao

*New York Medical College*
*Valhalla, New York*

MARCEL DEKKER, Inc.          New York and Basel

Library of Congress Cataloging-in-Publication Data

Biological response modifiers and cancer therapy

(Immunology series ; v. 40)
Includes index.
1. Biological response modifiers--Testing.
2. Cancer--Immunotherapy--Evaluation. I. Chiao,
J. W. II. Series. [DNLM: 1. Antibodies,
Monoclonal--therapeutic use. 2. Antineoplastic Agents--
therapeutic use. 3. Interleukins--therapeutic use.
4. Lymphokines--therapeutic use. 5. Neoplasms--
immunology. W1 IM53K v.40 / QZ 267 B6156]
RC271.B53B56 1988          616.99'4061          88-11802
ISBN 0-8247-7860-X

MARCEL DEKKER, INC.
270 Madison Avenue, New York, New York 10016

Current printing (last digit):
10 9 8 7 6 5 4 3 2 1

PRINTED IN THE UNITED STATES OF AMERICA

# Series Introduction

In the saga of modern immunology, nothing is more remarkable than the rapid transference of fundamental discoveries in the research laboratory into new tools for the clinic. Such laboratory-to-clinic transference is not exclusively a property of immunology, but the rate at which it happens is particularly striking for this discipline. Perhaps the explanation for this is that immunologists have never erected a barrier between basic research and clinical applications. As a science, immunology is as much at home in medicine, pediatrics, and surgery as it is in molecular and cellular biology. Fortunately, even though immunologists are often dispersed in different academic departments, lines of communication have been established and are kept open.

Research on biological response modifiers exemplifies particularly well this state of affairs. Originally, monoclonal antibodies were developed as a tool to learn about the mechanisms of antibody formation. The first of the lymphokines, macrophage migration inhibition factor, emerged from experiments on the mechanisms of cell-mediated immunity. Therapeutic applications followed, after basic investigators and clinician-colleagues became aware that changes induced in the immune system could be of great benefit in treating human disease. Conversely, the opportunity for clinical usefulness greatly stimulated basic investigation. The present volume dramatically illustrates the advantages of maintaining strong links between fundamental research and its applications.

*Noel R. Rose*
Professor and Chairman
Department of Immunology and
Infectious Diseases
The Johns Hopkins University
School of Hygiene and Public Health
Baltimore, Maryland

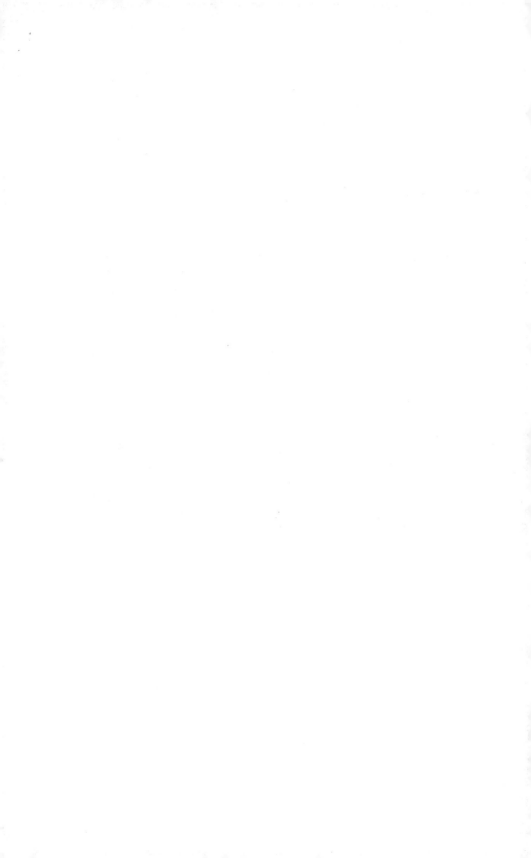

# Foreword

When, independently but at about the same time, Lewis Thomas and Sir McFarlane Burnet restated for the modern era an earlier postulate of Paul Ehrlich that immunological resistance to cancer must exist, it seemed a near certainty that it was but a matter of time—perhaps but a very brief time—until the body's immune defenses would be harnessed to prevent and treat human cancer. The concept of immunosurveillance, derived from this postulate, became a rallying cry for many who enthusiastically accepted the challenge to bring the body's powerful immunological systems to bear on cancer. The task did not prove easy; indeed, most efforts failed.

There is now little doubt that immunosurveillance exists and provides a remarkable survival advantage by inhibiting development of virus-associated neoplasia. One example of the failure of immunosurveillance (opening the door to cancer) is the occurrence of numerous cancers in patients subjected to long-term immunosuppression to make possible allotransplantation of organs and tissues. Other examples involve congenital immunodeficiencies such as severe combined immunodeficiency disease, Wiskott-Aldrich syndrome, common variable immunodeficiencies, IgA deficiencies, and ataxia telangiectasia. Perhaps most threatened are patients with acquired immunodeficiencies (such as AIDS). These patients develop many opportunistic cancers—lymphomas, Kaposi's sarcoma, etc. However, the common cancers of modern civilization (colon, lung, breast, and prostate cancers) pose another question. All of these have remained impressively aloof to immunological attack and have been difficult to address in terms of immunological resistance as conventionally conceived.

From the ashes of the attempted immunological conquest of cancer has arisen a new and exciting hope. In large part, this hope derives from an evolving understanding of the body's methods of developing, organizing, and controlling its own complex cellular systems and essential cellular interactions, coupled with biotechnology rooted in modern molecular biology. These developing disciplines have led to the definition of a new and rapidly expanding discipline—the study of biological response modifiers.

We are learning a new language, the language by which the body's cells and molecules initiate, promote, stop, and start cellular proliferation and differentiation, and promote or permit cell termination. Many of the peptides, receptors

for these peptides, autocrines, lymphokines, cytokines, growth factors, differentiation factors, hormones and biological modifiers of the immunological systems,
hematopoiesis, and other host responses may soon become efficacious drugs.
These molecules, originally responsible for the control of body functions, cell
populations, and cell-cell interactions, may provide a basis for a new kind of
pharmacology that may ultimately be developed into prophylactically or therapeutically useful new approaches to cancer and immunoregulation.

Recently, we found it possible to correct profound immunodeficiencies by
treating children who lack the ability to produce interleukin-2 with interleukin-2.
We were also able to probe the otherwise mysterious controls of immunological
processes by looking to the peptide hormone prolactin, only recently recognized
as a powerful immunomodulator.

The exciting approaches reflected and promised in the series of scientific
and clinical analyses that make up the current volume reveal important aspects
of this potentially powerful new biology. The scientists represented here are at
the leading edge of this new field. They have much to teach us all and also still
have much to learn as they explore the great new vistas of this exciting line of
inquiry.

*Robert A. Good, Ph.D., M.D.*
Chairman, Department of Pediatrics
University of South Florida/St. Petersburg
Physician-in-Chief
All Children's Hospital
St. Petersburg, Florida

# Preface

Historically, modification of the functions of the immune system has been a prime area of research involving the biological response modifiers (BRMs). There have been many attempts to stimulate or regulate the various types of immune responses and to manipulate the immunological processes and diseases. These modulators for the immune system include products of bacteria and viruses and a multitude of chemicals, antigens, antibodies, other cellular and natural products, and cells. In the beginning, almost all of the BRMs were classified as nonspecific compounds acting on specific immune mechanisms. More recently, we have seen the discovery and identification of physiological regulators that are the natural molecules mediating cellular development and functions.

The regulator molecules produced by lymphocytes of the immune system or by cells in general are referred to as lymphokines or cytokines. These substances may act directly on target cells or systems by influencing their growth, development, functions, and termination. BRMs may also act indirectly on other cells, as part of a cascade of processes eventually affecting the target cells. Investigation of these cytokines has been extensive since they are believed to be specific molecules that interact with particular targets resulting in a defined physiological or biochemical response. With the advent of molecular biology and genetic engineering techniques, large quantities of the natural protein molecules have become available. This has led to detailed characterization of many of the physiological regulators. Research laboratories and industrial sectors have been involved in research development, and applications of BRMs including the various forms of interferons, the interleukins, lymphocyte activated killer cells, and monoclonal antibodies.

The advance in this area has had a revolutionary impact on the thinking and practice of cancer research and treatment. Conventionally, surgery, radiation, and chemotherapy have been the methods of eliminating cancers. Biological therapy employing various BRMs has become a new area of cancer detection and therapy. This new method works by mobilizing and utilizing the body's natural factors and processes; ultimately, to restore the normal states. Since many biological agents are natural materials and specific for certain processes, they may, therefore, be better than conventional drugs in leaving the normal cells untouched and far more effective in eliminating the defects. Many biological agents have already been used in clinical trials and have been approved for clinical use. Already researchers are investigating new approaches to minimize the side effects and to maximize the benefits by using more than one BRM. They also have used BRMs in combination with chemotherapeutic drugs, radiation, or other treatment protocols. This book documents advances in some representative areas, illustrating historical developments and principles and opening vistas to the future.

*J. W. Chiao*

# Contents

# Contributors

*Ken-ichi Arai, M.D., Ph.D.* DNAX Research Institute of Molecular and Cellular Biology, Palo Alto, California

*Naoko Arai, M.D., Ph.D.* DNAX Research Institute of Molecular and Cellular Biology, Palo Alto, California

*Bruce J. Averbook, M.D.\** University of California at Irvine, Irvine, California

*W. Borkowsky, M.D.* New York University Medical Center, New York, New York

*J. W. Chiao, Ph.D.* New York Medical College, Valhalla, New York

*Robert M. Crawford* Walter Reed Army Institute of Research, Washington, D.C.

*Charles A. Dinarello, M.D.* Tufts University School of Medicine and New England Medical Center Hospital, Boston, Massachusetts

*David S. Finbloom, M.D.* Walter Reed Army Institute of Research, Washington, D.C.

*Allan L. Goldstein* George Washington University Medical Center, Washington, D.C.

*Gale A. Granger* University of California at Irvine, Irvine, California

*David Greenblatt, M.D.* George Washington University, Washington, D.C.

*Hajime Hagiwara, M.D.†* DNAX Research Institute of Molecular and Cellular Biology, Palo Alto, California

*Maureen Howard, Ph.D.* DNAX Research Institute of Molecular and Cellular Biology, Palo Alto, California

*René I. Jahiel, M.D., Ph.D.* New York University Medical Center, New York, New York

*Kozo Kaibuchi, M.D., Ph.D.* DNAX Research Institute of Molecular and Cellular Biology, Palo Alto, California

---

*\*Present affiliation*: University of California at Irvine Medical Center, Orange, California
† Deceased

*Mathilde Krim, Ph.D.* St. Luke's-Roosevelt Hospital Center, New York, New York

*Kathleen Last-Barney, M.S.* Boehringer Ingelheim Pharmaceuticals, Inc., Ridgefield, Connecticut

*Frank Lee, Ph.D.* DNAX Research Institute of Molecular and Cellular Biology, Palo Alto, California

*John Lutton, Ph.D.* New York Medical College, Valhalla, New York

*I. Masunaka* University of California at Irvine, Irvine, California

*Monte S. Meltzer* Walter Reed Army Institute of Research, Washington, D.C.

*Vincent J. Merluzzi, Ph.D.* Boehringer Ingelheim Pharmaceuticals, Inc., Ridgefield, Connecticut

*James W. Mier, M.D.* Tufts University School of Medicine and New England Medical Center Hospital, Boston, Massachusetts

*Abraham Mittelman, M.D.* New York Medical College, Valhalla, New York

*Atsushi Miyajima, Ph.D.* DNAX Research Institute of Molecular and Cellular Biology, Palo Alto, California

*Schoichiro Miyatake, M.D.* DNAX Research Institute of Molecular and Cellular Biology, Palo Alto, California

*Tim Mosmann, Ph.D.* DNAX Research Institute of Molecular and Cellular Biology, Palo Alto, California

*Carol A. Nacy, Ph.D.* Walter Reed Army Institute of Research, Washington, D.C.

*Robert Kenneth Oldham, M.D.* The Biological Therapy Institute, Franklin, Tennessee

*S. Orr* University of California at Irvine, Irvine, California

*Takeshi Otsuka, M.D., Ph.D.* DNAX Research Institute of Molecular and Cellular Biology, Palo Alto, California

*Jolanda Schreurs, Ph.D.* DNAX Research Institute of Molecular and Cellular Biology, Palo Alto, California

*Richard S. Schulof, M.D., Ph.D.* George Washington University Medical Center, Washington, D.C.

*Marcelo B. Sztein, M.D.* George Washington University Medical Center, Washington, D.C.

*Yutaka Takebe, M.D., Ph.D.* DNAX Research Institute of Molecular and Cellular Biology, Palo Alto, California

*Gary B. Thurman, Ph.D.* Biotherapeutics Inc., Franklin, Tennessee

*Fatih M. Uckun, M.D., Ph.D.* University of Minnesota, Minneapolis, Minnesota

*Thomas R. Ulich, M.D.*   University of California at Irvine, Irvine, California

*Daniel A. Vallera, Ph.D.*   University of Minnesota, Minneapolis, Minnesota

*Robert S. Yamamoto*   University of California at Irvine, Irvine, California

*Takashi Yokota, Ph.D.*   DNAX Research Institute of Molecular and Cellular Biology, Palo Alto, California

**Biological Response Modifiers
and
Cancer Therapy**

# Part I

**Monoclonal Antibodies
as Agents for Cancer Therapy**

# 1

# Monoclonal Antibody Therapy

Robert Kenneth Oldham / The Biological Therapy Institute, Franklin, Tennessee

## I. INTRODUCTION

Monoclonal antibodies (MoAb) are now being tested with increasing frequency in the treatment of human cancer (1). Initial trials focused on typical phase I parameters of toxicity and tolerance. Then defined localization of the antibody in tumor deposits and the distribution of antibody in normal and neoplastic tissues (2-4). There is now a considerable body of evidence that murine monoclonal antibodies are initially well tolerated by patients. Although clinical responses to unconjugated antibody have generally not been striking, there is unequivocal evidence that antibody binds to individual tumor cells after intravenous injection (5).

Biodistribution studies utilizing antibody conjugated to isotopes have demonstrated considerable antibody in the liver, spleen, and other organs of the reticuloendothelial system (6) and antibody/isotope conjugates are retained selectively and considerably longer in the tumor than in normal tissues where binding may be less specific.

These findings support the strategy of diagnosing, staging, and treating human malignancies with monoclonal antibodies conjugated to isotopes, drugs, toxins, and biologics (1,7-9). This chapter will review recent data on antibody in the treatment of human solid tumors and evaluate the potential clinical uses of antibody conjugates.

## II. DEVELOPMENTAL THERAPEUTICS OF MONOCLONAL ANTIBODIES

Multiple murine monoclonal antibodies have been assessed in clinical trials in cancer patients (10,11). For cancers such as melanoma, lung, breast, and colon

3

cancer multiple antibodies have been described and characterized. Thus, clinical use of monoclonal antibodies will not be limited by a shortage of antibody preparations (1). With the possible exception of anti-idiotype antibodies in lymphoma, the ideal antibody (i.e., *absolute* specificity for cell surface antigens of a particular tumor) has not been identified for any human solid tumor; however, a number have sufficient selectivity to warrant clinical testing (11).

Selection criteria of monoclonal antibodies appropriate for clinical trials have been widely debated. It seems reasonable to consider the following in selecting antibodies for in vivo application.

1. Antibody binds to an antigen on the cell surface.
2. Antigen highly expressed on cell surface and found on most or, preferably, all cells in a tumor.
3. Antibody binds with high affinity.
4. Antigen expressed at very low levels on a very limited number of normal tissues and/or found only on occasional cells in normal tissues.
5. Antigen-antibody complexes internalize.
6. Biodistribution studies reveal localization in tumor far in excess of uptake by the reticuloendothelial system.
7. Antibody mediates antibody-dependent cellular cytotoxicity (unconjugated antibody).

Antibodies that satisfy most of these criteria are to be preferred until more clinical data are available. There may be reasons why certain antibodies that bind to few cells could be of clinical interest if, for example, binding to "tumor stem cells" could be demonstrated. However, the burden of proof is on the proponent of an antibody that does not meet these criteria to show it is worthy of clinical interest.

Antibody, conjugated or not, must reach the tumor bed to be effective. Smaller antibodies (IgG rather than IgM) or antibody fragments may be more likely to diffuse from the vascular compartment into the tumor bed. The greater the amount of whole IgG antibody infused into the vascular compartment, the more antibody that is delivered to the tumor cell bed. Doses of 200-500 mg of antibody can saturate all sites on the tumor cell in cutaneous melanoma metastases (5).

While entry into the tumor mass is clearly critical, retention within that tumor bed may be equally or more important. Thus, fragments may diffuse more quickly into the nodule, but whole antibody may be retained for a longer time within that same nodule. Only clinical studies with a range of antibody preparations will clarify this issue (11).

## III.  CLINICAL TRIALS WITH UNCONJUGATED ANTIBODIES

The design and execution of clinical trials using monoclonal antibodies for the treatment of cancer patients differ considerably from those used to test anti-

Table 1  Critical Parameters in Phase I Trials of Monoclonal Antibodies in Patients with Cancer

---

A. Pretherapy
   1. Tumor sample for antigen expression
   2. Serum for circulating antigen
   3. Serum for antiglobulin and idiotype (where applicable)
B. During and/or after therapy
   1. Antibody localization: Immunohistochemistry on fresh frozen tumor sample
   2. Antigenic saturation: Flow cytometry on fresh tumor cell suspension
   3. Pharmacokinetics
   4. Immune complexes
   5. Idiotype levels (leukemia/lymphoma)
   6. Antiglobulin and/or anti-idiotype responses

---

cancer drugs (1,12). A competent laboratory must be available to select antibodies and monitor their fate and distribution (see Table 1). To demonstrate that antibody reached the tumor cells and binds to antigen in vivo, requires biopsy specimens subsequent to infusion using immunohistochemistry and/or flow cytometry (5,13,14). Immunohistochemistry helps define the distribution of antibody within the tumor nodule and surrounding normal tissues and flow cytometry allows accurate quantitative assessment of the percentage of cells binding antibody and the degree of saturation. Additional monitoring should include antibody pharmacokinetics, circulating antigen, determining the presence of immune complexes, and antiglobulin and anti-idiotypic responses to murine antibody. The latter responses will be critical in determining the dose and timing of conjugate therapy since significant levels of either may alter biodistribution of the infused antibody. Finally, careful clinical observations are critical to the ongoing success of these laboratory-based studies.

Monoclonal antibodies, being biologic substances, require both laboratory and clinical expertise to carry out meaningful investigations. These preparations should not be considered as just another class of drugs to be given by individuals or groups expert in the use of chemotherapy. Biological substances have clinical and biological activities very different from the chemicals used in chemotherapy, and expertise in biotherapy is needed to pursue these studies (15).

## A. Leukemia/Lymphoma

The treatment of leukemia and lymphoma has often involved monoclonal antibodies directed at the idiotype on the cell membrane (16). These anti-idiotypic

Table 2    Anti-Idiotypic Antibody Therapy of Lymphoma

| No. of patients | Pretherapy serum (mg/ml) | Highest single/total dose | Duration of therapy (days) | Responses | Toxicity |
|---|---|---|---|---|---|
| 11 | 0.01-400 | 120-900/ 400-3183 | 7-57 | 1 Complete remission 5 Partial remission 5 No remission | Fever, chills, rash, dyspnea, thrombocytopenia |

antibodies are as close to a specific antibody to a specific tumor-associated antigen as currently exists. Worldwide, few patients have been treated with anti-idiotypic antibodies. the bulk of the data currently available is from the studies of Levy and Miller of Stanford University (16,17). Levy and Miller have treated a series of leukemia and lymphoma patients using murine monoclonal antibodies they have raised against the rescued idiotype from the membranes of the patient's tumor cells. Through a heterohybrid fusion technique, idiotype production has been selected, leading to the isolation of the immunoglobulin as the immunogen with the production of specific antibodies to the idiotype.

Initial studies were reported in 1982 with the first patient being treated with up to 150 mg of antibody followed by disappearance of the circulating idiotype and a complete remission. This patient remains in continuous disease-free remission for more than 5 years. Levy and Miller have reported on more than 10 other patients with advanced B-cell malignancies, and while many of these patients were resistant to other forms of treatment, they showed interesting partial responses (Table 2). While critics of this technique have focused on the lack of further complete and durable responses using monoclonal antibody to the idiotype, the resistant nature of the lymphoma in these patients must encourage us to continue with these responses. In all cases, unconjugated antibody was used because of the evidence Levy and Miller have garnered that the mechanism of action involves T cells in the tumor bed which become more active with the influx of anti-idiotypic antibody. However, one must speculate that an immunoconjugate may strengthen the signal and perhaps produce more complete responses in such patients. To date, immunoconjugate therapy using anti-idiotypic antibody conjugated to toxic substances has not been reported. Several laboratories are moving in this direction, and it is anticipated that such trials will soon be underway.

In addition to studies using anti-idiotypic antibody, there have been a series of studies using T101, an antibody to the 65 kD antigen on the surface of T cells. These studies have been reviewed extensively (18). Briefly, they have demonstrated the feasibility of infusing an antibody reactive with normal and neoplastic T cells in patients with chronic lymphocytic leukemia and T-cell leukemia/lymphoma. Because the antibody reacts with circulating cells, there appear to be aggregation of cells in the lung with resultant dyspnea as a toxicity over and above the fever, chills, and fatigue seen with other monoclonal antibody trials. Transient reduction of circulating T-cell numbers, lymph nodes, and skin lesions were seen. However, the use of unconjugated monoclonal antibody did not produce prolonged, partial, or complete responses in these patients. Targeting of the antibody to the leukemia/lymphoma cell was effectively demonstrated, leading investigators to suggest that immunoconjugates of these antibodies would likely be useful. Antigenic modulation was noted in these hematological malignancies and the early impression is that modulation is a more frequent and more extensive process with these neoplasms when compared to nonhematopoietic solid tumors (19,20). Current trials are focusing on immunoconjugates of isotopes using T101 antibody preparations. Initial studies with radioimmunoconjugates of indium-111 ($^{111}$In) and T101 demonstrated excellent localization of the labeled antibody in afflicted bone marrow, lymph nodes, and skin. Significant localization was seen also in the liver and spleen, tissues containing both T cells and components of the reticuloendothelial system which naturally remove circulating antibody and immunoconjugates (21). These studies have indicated the feasibility of pursuing immunoconjugate therapy, a subject which is covered elsewhere in this book.

## B. Solid Tumors

At the Biological Response Modifiers Program, National Cancer Institute, a series of melanoma patients was treated with the 9.2.27, an $IgG_{2a}$-murine monoclonal antibody developed by Morgan and co-workers (22). This antibody recognizes a 250 kD glycoprotein/proteoglycan antigen on the surface of melanoma cells and meets most of the criteria listed here. It binds to more than 90% of melanomas freshly removed from patients, exhibits both high affinity and quantiatively high binding to melanomas, and does not appear to bind to normal tissues with the exception of occasional basal cells, blood vessel endothelium, and sebaceous glands in the skin. After intravenous administration of antibody, we used flow cytometry to assess binding and saturation and immunohistochemistry on frozen freshly removed tumor to determine distribution. As shown in Table 3, antibody staining of tumor cells was seen at doses above 10 mg, with greater staining at higher doses. The immunoperoxidase studies indicated that areas of tumor near blood vessels or lymphatic spaces stained first (at the 50 mg level) and only with higher doses did the antibody diffuse well out into the tumor nodule. At doses of 200 mg and higher, binding to all tumor cells and then saturation of available binding sites was seen using flow cytometry. The latter finding is important for several reasons:

1. It defines the maximum useful dose for a single injection.
2. It determines the dose range expected for immunoconjugate delivery.
3. It shows that maximum doses of immunoconjugate can reach every cell lessening the chance of selecting resistant cells due to suboptimal delivery.
4. It ensures that hypoxic cells furthest from blood vessel access receive the maximum deliverable dose.

Pharmacokinetic studies defined the peak antibody concentration and the half-life. Peak levels and half-life were affected by antiglobulin levels but localization occurred in spite of circulating antiglobulin (5).

Table 3   In Vitro[a] and In Vivo[b] Reactivity of 9.2.27 Antibody with Melanoma Cells in Skin Lesions

| | | | 9.2.27 Reactivity | | | |
|---|---|---|---|---|---|---|
| Patient | Dose 9.2.27 (mg) | Days post-treatment | Flow cytometry % positive cells in vitro/in vivo | | Immunoperoxidase[c] score in vitro/in vivo | |
| D.F. | Pretreat | | 83 | ND | ++ | − |
| | 1 | 1 | 0 | 0 | + | − |
| | 50 | 1 | 72 | 0 | ++ | + |
| | 200 | 1 | ND | ND | ++ | + |
| M.F. | Pretreat | | 97 | ND | ++ | + |
| | 10 | 1 | 98 | 2 | + | − |
| | 100 | 1 | 72 | 50 | + | + |
| | 200 | 4 | 98 | 91 | + | + |
| B.C. | Pretreat | | 90 | ND | ++ | − |
| | 200 | 1 | 73 | 71 | + | |
| C.S. | Pretreat | | 76 | ND | ++ | − |
| | 1 | 1 | 91 | 0 | ++ | − |
| | 200 | 1 | 41 | 35 | ++ | + |
| A.T. | Pretreat | | 0 | ND | + | − |
| | 50 | 1 | ND | ND | ++ | ++ |
| | 200 | 1 | 14 | 50 | ++ | ++ |

[a]In vitro reactivity refers to binding when excess 9.2.27 was added during the staining procedure.

[b]In vivo reactivity refers to endogenously bound 9.2.27 after i.v. antibody therapy.

[c]Staining of melanoma cells with 9.2.27 was graded on a + to ++ scale which represents a combination of both percent positive cells and intensity of staining.

ND, not done.

No antitumor responses were seen with this unconjugated antibody which prompted further studies using immunoconjugates. Radioimmunolocalization using 9.2.27 conjugated to indium-111 was done to study the biodistribution of the antibody. Labeled antibody localized in the reticuloendothelial system and the tumors (23). The hepatic uptake was especially significant, but studies with [131]I-labeled 9.2.27 by another group have shown much less in that organ (O. Fodstad, personal communication). It is likely that hepatic halogenases remove [131]I, which is then excreted as iodide, whereas the free [111]In is protein bound and remains in liver cells. These studies raise critical issues concerning immunoconjugates and illustrate the need to test after the conjugation procedure to determine immunoreactivity and biodistribution (11).

Phase I studies with antibody to a 97 kD antigen (p97) and with antibody 48.7 directed at the same antigen recognized by 9.2.27 confirmed the results discussed above (13). Houghton and co-workers have reported major tumor regressions in 3 of 12 patients with melanoma using a monoclonal antibody that binds to the sialoganglioside GD3. This antibody is lytic with human complement and mediates ADCC (23). Tumor biopsies during and after treatment demonstrated lymphocyte and mast cell infiltration, mast cell degranulation, and complement deposition.

Larson and co-workers have gone one step further and administered an anti-p97 antibody labeled with *therapeutic* doses of [131]I to show therapeutic activity for isotope conjugates in patients with melanoma. Localization of the labeled antibody has been seen and evidence of minor tumor regression was noted (24). Thus, these early clinical trials have progressed rapidly from antibody alone to therapeutic attempts with immunoconjugates. Recently, an antimelanoma antibody/toxin conjugate has been reported to have some antimelanoma activity (25).

The other major solid tumor system studied with in vivo monoclonal antibody has been gastrointestinal cancer. Sears and co-workers treated more than 20 patients with gastrointestinal malignancies using antibody 17-1A ($IgG_{2a}$) and demonstrated localization of the antibody in the tumor (4,14). Single doses of 15-1000 mg per patient have been given without severe side effects. Circulating immunoglobulin has been seen for as long as 50 days, compared to 9.2.27 which has a half-life of approximately 30 hours, and disappears from the serum within days. This may be due to the low affinity of 17-1A and its shedding from the tumor cell surface. In addition, 17-1A has a much wider normal tissue reactivity than 9.2.27 and thus the "sink" for antibody deposition and subsequent shedding is much larger.

Antiglobulin responses to 17-1A initially were reported to be dependent on the dose of antibody. Doses above 366 mg produced less antimouse immunoglobulin. These data were not confirmed in later studies (26). They reported but did not definitely document clinical antitumor responses in three of these patients, and postulated that this salutory effect may be due to antibody-macrophage interactions within the tumor bed. On the other hand, they have attempted to correlate these clinical responses with development of anti-idiotype antibodies to 17-1A, but have not documented that nonresponders did not develop anti-idiotypes. They suggested that a combination of high doses of antibody to reduce the antiglobulin response and the use of $IgG_{2a}$ subclass might be a reasonable approach in studying further patients with unconjugated antibody with gastrointestinal carcinoma.

Dillman and co-workers have given infusions of anticarcinoembryonic antigen (anti-CEA) monoclonal antibody to several patients with evidence of clinical localization but no antitumor responses (27). A brief report on the use of an $IgG_3$ monoclonal antibody which had in vitro cytotoxicity against human gastrointestinal carcinoma was reported by Lemkin and co-workers (28). In 8 patients treated with infusion of this antibody, complement consumption and fever were noted and murine antiglobulins appeared to give a syndrome consistent with serum sickness. Immunohistologic evidence of antibody localization was seen but no clinical responses were observed.

Melino and co-workers produced antibodies by allogeneic immunization in 12 volunteers. These heterologous antibodies were used to target daunorubicin and chlorambucil in 12 neuroblastoma patients over the age of 2. These preparations were well tolerated and no antiglobulin, allergic, or toxic effects were noted. Marked antitumor responses were reported in 9 or 12 patients and all responding patients are said to be disease free after more than 3 years (29). Careful analysis of a complete report on these findings is awaited unexpectantly.

A summary of recent serotherapy trials using monoclonal antibody for solid tumors is shown in Table 4. Older data with heteroantisera have previously been reviewed (8). Approaches using heteroantisera are of interest but they lack the essential features of reproducibility, high titer, unlimited quantity, and molecular purity needed to proceed with large-scale clinical trials. Emerging evidence on the use of antibodies derived by in vitro or in vivo immunizations of humans for the purpose of producing human monoclonal antibody are of interest, but no clinical trials have yet been reported with human monoclonal antibodies. These preparations possess certain potential advantages but may also have inherent disadvantages (1). The use of conjugated preparations in vitro and in animal tumor models is discussed elsewhere in this book. Conclusions from monoclonal antibody serotherapy trials are summarized in Table 5.

The monoclonal antibodies used to date have been of murine origin and are thus foreign proteins in humans. Factors other than reaction to an infused foreign protein that could provoke toxicity include circulating antigen, that may form immune complexes and the serum sickness syndromes associated with them, and the presence of antigen on circulating cells that has been noted to provoke severe bronchospasm and skin rash without other associated allergic

Table 4   Monoclonal Antibody Serotherapy Trials in Patients with Solid Tumors

| Institution | Disease | MoAb | References |
|---|---|---|---|
| U. of Pennsylvania (Wistar) | GI cancer | 17-1A | (4,14) |
| UCLA | GI cancer | CCOLI | (28) |
| U. California San Diego | Colon cancer | 065 | (27) |
| U. California San Diego | Melanoma | Ab to p97 Ab to p240 | (3) |
| Fred Hutchinson Cancer Center | Melanoma | Ab to p97 | (24) |
| Swedish Hospital Med. Center, Seattle | Melanoma | 48.7 and Ab to p97 | (13) |
| National Cancer Institute | Melanoma | 9.2.27 | (5) |
| Sloan-Kettering, New York City | Melanoma | Anti-GD3 | (23) |

Table 5   Summary: Monoclonal Antibody Serotherapy Trials

1. Intravenous murine-derived MoAb can be given safely by prolonged infusion (more than 1 hr) without immediate side effects.
2. Bronchospasm and hypotension have followed rapid infusion (more than 5 mg/hr) with antibodies that bind to circulating cells.
3. Antigenic modulation occurs following treatment with some but not all MoAbs. Most evident in hematologic cancer.
4. Free antigen may be detected in the serum before and following MoAb treatment.
5. Clear evidence of selective localization of infused antibody in solid tumors is available.
6. Antibodies to mouse cells develop following MoAb therapy.
7. There is considerable variation with respect to toxicity, bioavailability, and activity of MoAb related to immunoglobulin class, antigen, and distribution in tumor.
8. Immunoconjugates will be more effective in cancer treatment than unconjugated MoAb.

symptoms. The likely explanation for the latter is leukoagglutination and/or release of vasoactive substances in small bronchial arterioles (21). Recognition of the problems and their causes has led to strategies to ameliorate these toxicities (21), thereby enhancing the potential therapeutic activity of these preparations.

Based on the information available unconjugated antibodies are not likely to have an important therapeutic use. Minor clinical therapeutic effects with unconjugated antibody have been seen mainly in leukemia and certain lymphomas. In the area of solid tumors, only the report of Houghton and co-workers on the clinical effects of unconjugated anti-GD3 antibody in melanoma is encouraging (23). The major conclusions to be drawn from these studies in solid tumors are that monoclonal antibodies are reasonably safe, target to tumor, and that strategies can be designed to bind to all available antigenic sites on all tumor cells.

The in vitro selectivity and activity, as well as some preclinical in vivo activity without severe toxicity in animal models achieved with immunoconjugates are encouraging. Very early studies with the use of immunoconjugates of antibody and isotopes in human solid tumors have shown encouraging localization and even some evidence of therapeutic effects (11,24,25). These data, together with historical data on the use of heteroantisera, drug, and isotope conjugates suggest that immunoconjugates are likely to be very useful in improving the selectivity and efficacy of cancer treatments in the near future (30-40).

Prospectively it is worth commenting on the likely ultimate outcome of this area of research. All of our current data suggest antibody will traffic to the reticuloendothelial system so that even the most highly specific antibody by in vitro assessment will exhibit substantial in vivo normal organ distribution. Thus, the immunoconjugates will most likely improve the therapeutic index (tumor response vs. toxicity) by targeting toxic agents selectively to tumor thereby decreasing, but not eliminating, normal organ exposure. If this, rather than an elusive search for absolute tumor specificity in vivo, is accepted as an appropriate goal, then immunoconjugates with monoclonal antibodies should have a rapid and wide use in the armamentarium of weapons against cancer. The lack of selectivity of systemic chemotherapy means that any substantial improvement in the selective delivery of toxic substances to tumor cells through monoclonal antibody technology will be a step in the right direction. Attempts to find the perfect antibody (absolute specificity for cancer) and perfect immunoconjugate (toxic only to cancer) will only slow the translation of an effective new approach to cancer treatment to our patients (11).

One factor that could potentially dampen this enthusiasm is the known heterogeneity of cancer and the ability of cancer cells to mutate. If one uses a single antibody or a set combination of a few antibodies that together bind only to a portion of the tumor cells, or if the small percentage of the true replicating cell (tumor stem cell) is not eliminated, eventual recurrence of the tumor, perhaps with resistant cells, will result. It seems logical, therefore, to "type" human tumors with a panel of antibodies and to deliver toxic substances utilizing "cocktails" of antibodies sufficient to bind strongly to all the tumor cells for each patient. This approach requires a considerable amount of laboratory testing for each patient and a "typing" of one or more tumors from each patient.

Such approaches may need to be more individually specified than is easily achievable through the product development paradigm that has been used with some success in the development of new cancer drugs. Clinical investigators have heretofore been satisfied with statistical analysis of empirically selected therapies. Indeed, reputations flowered on a particular alphabet of anticancer drugs which actually worked in certain cancers. Immunoconjugates will place added burdens on investigators: selecting correct combinations for individual patients and explaining the nonresponses on the basis of biology, not statistics.

## REFERENCES

1. Oldham, R.K. Monoclonal antibody in cancer therapy. J. Clin. Oncol. 1: 582-590, 1983.
2. Larson, S.M., Brown, J.P., Wright, P.W., Carrasquillo, J.A., Hellstrom, I., and Hellstrom, K. E. Imaging of melanoma with Il-131-labeled monoclonal antibodies. J. Nucl. Med. 24: 123-129, 1983.
3. Sobol, R.E., Dillman, R.O., and Smith, J. D. In *Hybridomas in Cancer Diagnosis and Treatment.* Edited by M.S. Mitchell and H.F. Oettgen. Raven Press, New York, 1981, pp. 199-206.
4. Sears, H. F., Atkinson, B., Mattis, J., Ernst, C., Herlyn, D., Steplewski, Z., Hayry, P., and Koprowski, H. Phase I clinical trial of monoclonal antibody in treatment of gastrointestinal tumors. Lancet 1: 762-765, 1982.
5. Oldham, R.K., Foon, K.A., Morgan, A.C., Woodhouse, C.S., Schroff, R.W., Abrams, P.G., Fer, M., Schroenberger, C.S., Farrell, M., Kimball, E., and Sherwin, S.A. Monoclonal antibody therapy of malignant melanoma: *In vivo* localization in cutaneous metastasis after intravenous administration. J. Clin. Oncol. 2: 1235-1242, 1984.
6. Goldenberg, D.M., and DeLand, F.H. History and status of tumor imaging with radiolabeled antibodies. J. Biol. Response Modif. 1: 121-136, 1982.
7. Foon, K.A., Bernhard, M.I., and Oldham, R.K. Monoclonal antibody therapy: assessment by animal tumor models. J. Biol. Resp. Modif. 1: 277-304, 1983.
8. Rosenberg, S.A., and Terry, W.D. Passive immunotherapy of cancer in animals and man. Adv. Cancer Res. 25: 323-388, 1977.
9. Dillman, R.O. Monoclonal antibodies in the treatment of cancer. CRC Crit. Rev. Oncol./Hematol. 1: 357-385, 1984.
10. Abrams, P.G., and Oldham, R.K. Monoclonal antibody therapy of solid tumors. In *Monoclonal Antibody Therapy of Human Cancer.* Edited by K.A. Foon and A.C. Morgan, Jr. Martinus Nijhoff, Boston, 1985, pp. 103-120.
11. Oldham, R.K. Antibody-drug and antibody toxin conjugates. In *Immunity to Cancer.* Edited by A.E. Reif and M.S. Mitchell. Academic Press, New York, 1985, pp. 575-586.

12. Oldham, R.K. Biologicals and biological response modifiers: New strategies for clinical trials. In *Interferons*, IV. Edited by N.B. Finter and R.K. Oldham. Elsevier Science Publishers, Amsterdam, 1985, pp. 235-249.

13. Goodman, G.E., Beaumier, P., Hellstrom, I., Fernyhough, B., and Hellstrom, K.E. Pilot trial of murine monoclonal antibodies in patients with advanced melanoma. J. Clin. Oncol. 3: 340-352, 1985.

14. Sears, H.F., Herlyn, D., Steplewski, Z., and Koprowski, H. Effects of monoclonal antibody immunotherapy on patients with gastrointestinal adenocarcinoma. J. Biol. Response Modif. 3: 138-150, 1984.

15. Oldham, R.K. Biotherapy: The fourth modality of cancer treatment. Cancer: Perspective for Control Symposium, J. Cell. Physiol. Supplement 4: 91-99, 1986.

16. Miller, R.A., et al. Treatment of B-cell lymphoma with monoclonal anti-idiotype antibody. N. Engl. J. Med. 306: 517, 1982.

17. Meeker, T.C., et al. A clinical trial of anti-idiotype therapy for B-cell malignancy. Blood 65: 1349, 1985.

18. Dillman, R.O., Beauregard, J., Shawler, D.L., Halpern, S.E., Markman, M., Ryan, K.P., Baird, S.M., and Clutter, M. Continuous infusion of T101 monoclonal antibody in chronic lymphocytic leukemia and cutaneous T-cell lymphoma. J. Biol. Resp. Modif. 5: 394-410, 1986.

19. Foon, K.A., Schroff, R., Bunn, P.A., Mayer, D., Abrams, P.G., Fer, M.F., Ochs, J., Bottino, G., Sherwin, S.A., Carlo, D.J., Herberman, R.B., and Oldham, R.K. Effects of monoclonal antibody therapy in patients with chronic lymphocytic leukemia. Blood 64: 1085-1093, 1984.

20. Schroff, R.W., Farrell, M.M., Klein, R.A., Oldham, R.K., Sherwin, S.A., and Foon, K.A. Recombinant alpha interferon in retreatment of two patients with pulmonary lymphoma, Dramatic responses with resolution of pulmonary complications. Am. J. Med. 77: 355-358, 1984.

21. Carrasquillo, J.A., Bunn, P.A., Jr., Kennan, A.M., Reynolds, J.C., Schroff, R.W., Foon, K.A., Ming-Hsu, S., Gazdar, A.F., Mulshine, J.L., Oldham, R.K., Perentsis, P., Horowitz, M., Eddy, J., James, P., and Larson, S.M. Radioimmunodetection of cutaneous T-cell lymphoma with 111In-T101 monoclonal antibody. New Engl. J. Med. 315: 673-680, 1986.

22. Morgan, A.C. Jr., Galloway, D.R., and Reisfeld, R.A. Production and characterization of monoclonal antibody to a melanoma specific glycoprotein. Hybridoma 1: 27-36, 1981.

23. Houghton, A.N., Mintzer, D., Cordon-Cardo, C., Welt, S., Fliegel, B., Vadhan, S., Carswell, E., Melamed, M.R., Oettgen, H.F., and Old, L.J. Mouse monoclonal IgG3 antibody detecting GD3 ganglioside: A phase I trial in patients with malignant melanoma. Proc. Natl. Acad. Sci. USA 82: 1242-1246, 1985.

24. Larson, S.M., Carrasquillo, J.A., and Krohn, K.A. In *Proceedings of the Third World Congress of Nuclear Medicine and Biology*, vol. 4. Pergamon Press, New York, 1982, pp. 3666-3669.

25. Spitler, L.E. Clinical trials with Ricin-A chain conjugates in solid tumors. (Abstr.) Monoclonal antibody immunoconjugates for cancer. March 6-8, 1986.

26. Wistar Symposium on Immunodiagnosis and Immunotherapy with CO17-1A MAb in Gastrointestinal Cancer. Mary Ann Liebert, Inc. Publishers, New York. Hybridoma 5: 1-187, 1986.

27. Dillman, R.O., Beauregard, J.C., Shawler, D.L., et al. In *Protides of the Biological Fluids*. Edited by H. Peeters. Pergamon Press, New York, 1983, pp. 353-358.

28. Lemkin, S., Tokita, K., Sherman, G., Simko, T., Schwartz, L., Ciccirilli, J., Drew, S., and Terasaki, P. Phase I-II study of monoclonal antibodies (MCA) in gastrointestinal cancer. Proc. Am. Soc. Clin. Oncol. 3: 47, 1984.

29. Melino, G., Elliott, P., Cooke, K.B., Evans, A., and Hobbs, J.R. Allogeneic antibodies (Abs) for drug targeting to human neuroblastoma (Nb). Proc. Am. Soc. Clin. Oncol. 3: 47, 1984.

30. Oldham, R.K. Biologicals and biological response modifiers: The fourth modality of cancer treatment. Cancer Treat. Rep. 68: 221-232, 1984.

31. Foon, K.A., Schroff, R., Bunn, P.A., Mayer, D., Abrams, P.G., Fer, M.F., Ochs, J., Bottino, G., Sherwin, S.A., Carlo, D.J., Herberman, R.B., and Oldham, R.K. Effects of monoclonal antibody therapy in patients with chronic lymphocytic leukemia. Blood 64: 1085-1093, 1984.

32. Key, M.E., Bernhard, M.I., Hoyer, L.C., Foon, K.A., Oldham, R.K., and Hanna, M.G., Jr. Guinea pig 10 hepatocarcinoma model of monoclonal antibody serotherapy: *In vivo* localization of a monoclonal antibody in normal malignant tissues. J. Immunol. 139: 1451-1457, 1983.

33. Bernhard, M.I., Foon, K.A., Oeltmann, T.N., Key, M.E., Hwang, K.M., Clarke, G.C., Christensen, W.L., Hoyer, L.C., Hanna, Jr., M.G., and Oldham, R.K. Guinea pig line 10 hepatocarcinoma model: Characterization of monoclonal antibody and *in vivo* effect of unconjugated antibody and antibody conjugated to diptheria toxin A chain. Cancer Res. 43: 4420-4428, 1983.

34. Bernhard, M.I., Hwang, K.M., Foon, K.A., Keenan, M., Kessler, R.M., Frincke, J.M., Tallam, D.J., Hanna, M.G., Jr., Peters, L., Oldham, R.K. Localization of 111In- and 125I-labeled monoclonal antibodies in guinea pigs bearing line 10 hepatocarcinoma tumors. Cancer Res. 43: 4429-4433, 1983.

35. Hwang, K.M., Foon, K.A., Cheung, P.H., Pearson, J.W., and Oldham, R.K. Selective antitumor effect on L-10 hepatocarcinoma cells of a potent immunoconjugate composed of the A-chain of abrin and a monoclonal antibody to a hepatoma-associated antigen. Cancer Res. 44: 4578-4586, 1984.

36. Hwang, K.M., Fodstad, O., Oldham, R.K., and Morgan, A.C. Radiolocalization of xenografted human malignant melanoma by a monoclonal antibody (9.2.27) to a melanoma associated antigen. Cancer Res. 45: 4150-4155, 1984.

37. Hwang, K.M., Keenan, A.M., Frincke, J., David, G., Pearson, J., Oldham, R.K., and Morgan, A.C. Jr. Dynamic interaction of 111 indium-labeled monoclonal antibodies with surface of solid tumors visualized in vivo by external scintigraphy. J. Nat. Cancer Inst. 76: 849-855, 1986.

38. Oldham, R.K. Perspectives on the use of immunotoxins in clinical medicine. In *Immunoconjugates: The Current Status of Antibody Conjugates for Radioimaging and Therapy of Cancer*. Edited by C.-W. Vogel. Oxford University Press, 1986.

39. Oldham, R.K. Monoclonal antibodies: Does sufficient selectivity to cancer cells exist for therapeutic application? J. Biol. Response Modif. 6: 227-234, 1987.

40. Oldham, R.K. Therapeutic monoclonal antibodies: Effects of tumor cell heterogeneity. In *Therapeutic Monoclonal Antibodies: Effects of Tumor Cell Heterogeneity*. S. Karger Ag. Cancer Treatment Symposium, München, West Germany, 1988.

41. Oldham, R.K. Biologicals: New horizons in pharmaceutical development. J. Biol. Resp. Modif. 2: 199-206, 1983.

# 2

# Immunoconjugates

Daniel A. Vallera and Fatih M. Uckun / University of Minnesota, Minneapolis, Minnesota

The investigation of immunoconjugates as antitumor agents and biological response modifiers has gained momentum from the discovery of hybridoma technology (1). Unlimited quantities of monoclonal antibodies (MoAb) can be harvested from hybridomas grown in tissue culture or ascites fluid. Monoclonal antibodies are homogeneous, stable, and exquisitely specific to different antigenic epitopes. Unmodified MoAb are useful tools in cancer research for diagnostics; however, their therapeutic utility against cancer has been limited. Researchers have employed various methods to enhance the performance of MoAb against target cancer cell populations. Toxins and conventional chemotherapeutic agents have been conjugated to antibodies to produce cytotoxic and potentially therapeutic reagents. Antibodies have also been labeled with radionuclides for purposes of diagnostic imaging and therapy. This is not a comprehensive review, but a highlight of the primary accomplishments, obstacles, and prospects of these immunoconjugates, specifically referred to as immunotoxins, drug conjugates, and radiolabeled antibodies. Although all three strategies have disadvantages, the expansion of laboratory and clinical investigations, as well as the quantity of published reports, emphasizes their current utility and future possibilities against a variety of cancers.

## I. IMMUNOTOXINS

Cell type-specific MoAb are linked to catalytic toxins to form immunotoxins (IT) (reviewed in Refs. 2-5). New advances in hybridoma technology, crosslinking procedures, and protein purification have promoted the interest in IT for a variety of clinical purposes including cancer therapy, treatment of autoimmune disease, immunoregulation, and bone marrow transplantation (BMT).

## A. Toxins

The variety of toxins that have been employed by investigators can be broadly categorized into two groups. The first group consists of intact toxins, such as intact ricin and abrin, composed of A plus B chains. The second group includes A chain proteins only, which may be produced by reducing the bond between A and B chains, or they can occur naturally, as in the case of hemitoxins such as pokeweed antiviral protein (PAP), momordin, saporin, or gelonin. Although A chains are toxic enzymes, they do not have receptors on human cells and thus cannot penetrate cell membranes.

Numerous studies have focused on the potent toxin ricin extracted from the seeds of the Castor bean plant *Ricinis communis.* Ricin consists of two 30 kD subunits. The A chain is a potent catalytic enzyme that inhibits ribosomal protein synthesis, following simple enzyme kinetics. One ricin A chain molecule may inactivate as many as 1500 ribosomes per minute, and a single molecule in the cytosol can kill a cell (6). The B chain of ricin recognizes nonreducing terminal galactose receptors on cell surfaces and thus represents the moiety by which native ricin attaches to cells. B chain also facilitates A chain entry through an undefined mechanism. Internalization is assumed to occur through receptor-mediated endocytosis and coated pits. Once inside the cytoplasm, A chain binds to the 60S subunit, and ribosomal inactivation occurs (7). The nonselectivity of B chain is typically blocked or inhibited by galactose to prevent binding to cell surface carbohydrates.

## A Plus B Chain Immunotoxins

Kinetic studies of protein synthesis inhibition in a murine tumor cell line model demonstrated that the inactivation rate of an A chain IT was augmented fivefold when excess purified B chain was added (8). In the human system, peripheral blood mononuclear cells (PBMC) were pretreated with a MoAb reacting with a determinant (CD11a) of the LFA-1 family (9) called TA1 (10). TA1 conjugated to intact ricin or ricin A chain was tested for inhibition of mitogenic response. TA1-intact ricin was 39-fold more inhibitory than TA1-ricin A chain (11). Thus, the primary advantage of B chain was its ability to facilitate A chain entry. Other advantages for intact ricin include (i) reliability, (ii) potency, (iii) stability, (iv) availability, and (v) established clinical use. The primary disadvantage relates to the absolute requirement for the presence of lactose. A failure to block the galactose gal binding site of B chain would result in indiscriminate toxicity to all human cells coming in contact with the reagent. Lactose blockade of intact ricin IT results in highly selective reagents; however, because of the difficulty in maintaining high lactose levels in vivo, other strategies employing B chain are under investigation. These strategies include the chemical modification of the gal binding site of B chain and the use of separate IT carrying A chains and B chains (12).

Some other A plus B chain toxins used as IT include diptheria toxin (13,14), abrin (15), and pseudomonas exotoxin (16).

A Chain Immunotoxins

A chain ricin is approximately $10^3$-$10^5$ less toxic than the whole polypeptide toxin (17) because the binding and entry mechanisms of B chain are absent. However, the potency of ricin A chain IT can be enhanced. The addition of A chain potentiators such as ammonium chloride or carboxylic ionophores may increase lysosomal and endosomal pH, which in turn inhibits IT proteolysis and facilitates A chain entry through the endosomal membrane and into the cytosol (18). Researchers have demonstrated an increase of 3 logs inhibition of colony formation for MoAb T101-ricin A chain in the presence of 10 mM ammonium chloride (19). Although the in vitro toxicity of ricin A chain IT can be increased by the addition of potentiators, these factors have not been effective in increasing the activity of ricin A chain IT in vivo. This is perhaps attributed to the rapid uptake and degradation of lysosomotropic factors in vivo. More imaginative strategies for potentiator delivery, such as the use of high molecular weight carriers, are under investigation (20) and may be necessary for effective potency against established clinical tumors.

Another possible way of improving A chain potency is the use of recombinant ricin A chain. Recombinant DNA techniques provide an opportunity to engineer one's own toxin. The ricin gene (21) and the diphtheria toxin gene (22) have been cloned. When successfully expressed in bacteria, the gene produces modified toxin. The potential for this technique is realized in the case of ricin where the presence of B chain augments efficacy but renders toxin unsafe for in vivo use. Gene manipulation may enable identification and preservation of fragments encoding the enzymatic and hydrophobic regions of the gene, while identifying and deleting regions encoding the gal binding site by site-specific mutagenesis. Transcription and translation would result in the possibility of a new toxin devoid of nontarget binding, but with the facilitory roles of B chain intact.

Several naturally occurring A chains have been described (23). These ribosome-inhibitory proteins have potential for in vivo use as IT (24,25). Some, like PAP, do not undergo posttranslational modifications and are thus carbohydrate free. This may decrease nonspecific localization and organ toxicity, as well as prolong in vivo half-life. Investigators initially demonstrated that PAP conjugated to anti-Thy-1 MoAb caused the selective suppression of a spontaneous AKR leukemia when injected intraperitoneally into tumor-bearing mice (26). Although any additional effect of IT over antibody could not be ascertained, since antibody alone could protect in this model, no nonspecific IT toxicity was observed.

Other researchers have shown that a single intravenous injection of saporin IT into nu-nu mice bearing a peritoneal AKR lymphoma selectively prolonged survival (27). The extent of survival corresponded to that which would be expected if 99.999% of tumor cells had been eliminated by IT. The toxicity of saporin to mice was unexpectedly elevated 8-16-fold by conjugation to antibody, implying that careful dose analysis is mandatory. Our laboratory has examined the efficacy of another hemitoxin IT, B43-PAP (28). This human B-cell-directed IT, which contains the hemitoxin PAP, reacts with leukemia progenitor cells from common B-lineage acute lymphoblastic leukemia (ALL) patients. B43-PAP was able to selectively eliminate 99.96% of blast progenitor cells with minimal inhibition of stem cells. These studies are important because B43-PAP is effective in selectively killing common B-lineage ALL blasts and their progenitors, and B43-PAP may have utility for systemic use.

## B.  Antibodies and Antigens

The activity of IT depends on several variables. The role of antibody affinity has been investigated in a murine model (8). An IT made with a high affinity anti-Thy MoAb was $10^5$ times more toxic than an IT made with a low affinity anti-Thy MoAb. Other variables that may significantly affect IT activity are antibody subclass, isotype, and the use of antibody fragments instead of whole antibody molecules. The nature of the antigenic determinant recognized by the IT may also have a major role in IT activity. We have studied the internalization of IT directed against a highly modulated antigenic cluster (CD5) on T cells and found that IT are internalized better than unconjugated antibody (29). Factors such as the state of differentiation of a given cell population or the various phases of the cell cycle may influence antigens expressed on tumor cell surfaces (30). Significantly, investigators have been able to produce MoAb to unique antigens on human leukemia cells raised by immunizing mice with soluble preparations of leukemia antigen (31). These monoclonals conjugated to ricin A chain have made effective A chain IT.

Since the reactivity of an individual MoAb involves recognition of a single epitope, mixtures of MoAb have been evaluated. The activity of IT mixtures against homogeneous populations as represented by T-leukemia cell lines was examined by our group (32). Four anti-human T-cell MoAb against different antigenic clusters on T cells (CD5, CD7, CD2, and CD11a) were conjugated to intact ricin using thioether linkage. These four unrelated determinants are expressed in varying intensities on the surface of Molt 3 T-ALL cells (CD5 > CD7 > CD11a > CD2 by FACS analysis). Of the four IT, anti-CD5-ricin inactivated protein synthesis at the greatest rate. At high concentrations, an equimolar mixture of the four IT exhibited protein synthesis kinetics at a rate equal to or greater than the rate for anti-CD5 IT. Despite fast kinetics, the four-IT mixture was not as potent as anti-CD5-ricin alone as measured in clonogenic leukemia cell assays. These results suggest that the efficacy of an individual IT depends in part on surface antigen density, since the CD5 determinant was expressed more intensely than the other three determinants; therefore, mixtures of IT may not be as effective against homogeneous cell populations as certain individual IT. Different results were obtained when mixtures of IT were tested against mitogen-stimulated human T lymphocytes. Mitogenic response is dependent on a variety of cells including monocytes and subpopulations of T cells. In an earlier study, we found that a mixture of IT more efficiently inhibited mitogenesis in a heterogeneous cell population than any of the individual IT (33). Thus, the superior efficacy of IT mixtures over individual IT may depend on the cellular nature of the disease. In the case of ALL, the clonality of the disease remains controversial. A leukemia progenitor cell assay has recently been developed for the cultivation of fresh leukemia cells from T-ALL patients (34). Studies utilizing this assay will substantially improve our understanding of the clonal nature of leukemia and the efficacy of IT mixtures.

As suggested by the Molt 3 T-ALL cell line study, antigen density may significantly affect IT reactivity. A threshold density probably exists below which antibody localization does not occur. Studies on melanoma cells indicate that IT are ineffective below a certain level of surface antigen expression (35). However, MoAb have been produced that demonstrate an ability to recognize low density antigens. For example, an anti-CD10 IT has shown excellent recognition of the low density common acute lymphoblastic leukemia antigen (CALLA) (36).

Nonspecific uptake of antibody by the reticuloendothelial system (RES) or undesirable uptake by organs such as liver and spleen may further complicate antibody targeting. Nontarget tissue or organ involvement has encouraged biodistribution studies, exploration of alternative routes of IT administration, and the possible use of antibody fragments. These issues are discussed in greater detail in the sections on radionuclide and drug conjugates.

## C. Conjugation

MoAb and toxins have been conjugated by numerous methods. In the case of intact ricin IT, we have employed a heterobifunctional crosslinking reagent m-maleimidobenzoyl-N-hydroxysuccinimide ester (MBS) (37). Antibody and toxin are linked by a selective two-step process. N-hydroxysuccinimide ester reacts with the toxin amino groups and maleimide combines with thiol groups of the MoAb via double bond. MBS offers the advantages of simplicity, ease of purification, and a stable, covalent bond that is not easily reduced in a biological system. Conjugates generated in our laboratory have remained active greater than 6-12 months at 4°C and greater than 2 years at −70°C. Ricin A chain conjugates may be synthesized by derivatizing antibody with the crosslinker N-succinimidyl-3-(2-pyridyldithio)-propionate (SPDP) followed by conjugation to available sulfhydryl groups on the reduced toxin A chain. SPDP conjugation, which finally results in a disulfide bond between the antibody and toxin moiety, is primarily used for preparing A chain conjugates. Other linkage procedures include the use of 2-imino-thiolane, which may potentiate cytotoxicity by increasing the ratio of ricin mole-cules per immunoglobulin (141). The appropriate conjugation procedure is an im-portant issue. For example, recent studies with the hemitoxin gelonin conjugated to MoAb by a disulfide bond demonstrated significantly greater in vitro cytotoxi-city than when conjugated by a thioether bond (38). Perhaps obstruction or in-activation of certain functional groups affected IT activity, or perhaps thioether linkage does not permit the release of A chain from antibody in the cell, as does SPDP (disulfide) linkage. Failure of A chain to react properly with the ribosome would hinder toxicity. Specific linkages may also be preferred because the par-ticular bond may possibly affect the exposure of critical IT cleavage sites to pro-teases during circulation. In vivo studies in nonhuman primates were conducted utilizing gelonin and saporin conjugated individually to an anti-T-lymphocyte MoAb by disulfide bond (39). Of particular concern for the in vivo administra-tion of IT is stability during circulation and target-specific binding. Both gelonin and saporin conjugates remained intact and attached in substantial quantities to target T cells with minimal toxic side effects in rhesus monkeys. Conjugation methods continue to be investigated and compared in an attempt to increase yield and quality of IT for preparation of optimal patient batches.

## D. Problems

Some researchers have reported that, when compared to unconjugated antibody, conjugates experience a reduced half-life that adversely affects tumor site locali-zation. For example, one ricin-MoAb conjugate had a reported 15-fold decrease in localization (30). This could be attributed to the increased size and carbohy-drate content of the IT. The presence of certain carbohydrates such as mannose has been associated with increased reactivity with the liver and the RES. Chemical "deglycosylation" (42,142), which removes mannose residues from ricin molecules by oxidative cleavage, may produce IT that are less prone to elimination by the liver and the RES. Strategies for reducing carbohydrate, in addition to deglyco-sylation, include the use of recombinant toxins (22) and hemitoxins (23) that do not undergo posttranslational glycosylation. Large tumor burdens present a significant obstacle, and compensatory strategies are under consideration in-cluding increasing conjugate dosages, inhibiting nonspecific uptake, and targeting metastases that could control subsequent tumor development. Therapeutic regi-mens involving chemotherapy (41,42) or radiation (43) in addition to IT admin-istration are being evaluated. Particularly advantageous synergistic results might be obtained when the drawbacks associated with one agent, such as low inter-nalization or low cytotoxicity, would be remedied by the attributes of another agent. Our group has investigated the use of intact ricin IT combined with cyclo-phosphamide congeners both in vitro (41) and in vivo (42). Whereas toxins in-hibit protein synthesis, cyclophosphamide inhibits DNA synthesis. In one study, the drug enhanced the target cell toxicity of IT 2-3 logs (41). Data show that IT in combination with cyclophosphamide congener results in a maximum elimination of 6.2 logs of neoplastic CEM T cells with minimal toxicity to normal bone marrow progenitors.

Risk of a host immune response to either toxin or antibody exists, which jeopardizes the delivery and cytotoxic activity of an immunoconjugate. Antitoxin antibodies have been reported in mice receiving ricin A chain or PAP conjugates (26). However, antibodies produced against ricin A were not reactive against PAP, suggesting that alternate toxins in conjugate therapy may avoid or delay an immune response. Also, toxins such as PAP have different immunological forms depending on whether they are extracted from seeds or leaves. Furthermore, less immunogenic toxins may become available through genetically engineered antibody and/or toxin. It may be possible to selectively target and suppress cells responsible for host immunoreactivity. Anti-Ig response to murine monoclonals may be eliminated with the advent of chimeric antibodies or human-human hybridomas.

## E.  Ex Vivo Use of IT

The first clinical application of IT has come in the field of bone marrow transplantation (BMT). Bone marrow transplantation has become the optimal treatment for a variety of life-threatening hematological disorders including aplastic anemia, leukemia, immunodeficiency disease, and lymphoma (reviewed in Refs. 44-46). Lymphohematopoietic cells arise from progenitors that share common origin in bone marrow. Because of the developmental and regenerative capabilities of bone marrow, its transplantation has provided a useful therapy for diseases arising from abnormalities in this complex developmental process. As the number of international centers utilizing BMT increases, so does our awareness of complications and the need for more sophisticated strategies. One of the most pressing problems in BMT involves graft-versus-host disease (GVHD).

Prior to allogeneic BMT, the abnormal hematopoietic cells of the patient are ablated by aggressive chemoradiotherapy. A bone marrow graft from a human leukocyte antigen (HLA)-matched sibling donor is infused into the immunosuppressed recipient to reintroduce stem cells that provide a basis for normal lymphohematopoietic recovery. Differences in HLA and non-HLA antigens may cause immunocompetent T cells from the donor graft to respond against recipient antigens, resulting in a serious, and sometimes fatal, pathological syndrome known as GVHD. Unfortunately, only a minority of patients have HLA-matched siblings (47). Even in HLA-matched siblings, differences in non-HLA antigens may cause GVHD with a 30-70% incidence (44). IT can be used to deplete GVHD-causing cells in the donor bone marrow.

We have transplanted over 40 patients in the University of Minnesota Bone Marrow Transplantation Program using this approach. In our first clinical trial, 17 patients ranging from 7 to 53 years received HLA-mixed lymphocyte culture (MLC)-matched allogeneic BMT (48). Twelve patients with high risk acute leukemia and five with chronic myelogenous leukemia were conditioned with fractionated total body irradiation (TBI) plus cyclophosphamide. Donor bone marrow was depleted of T lymphocytes using an intact ricin IT mixture of TA1 (anti-CD11a)-ricin, UCHT1 (anti-CD3)-ricin, and T101 (anti-CD5)-ricin. No other GVHD prophylaxis was used. Twelve of 17 patients demonstrated full donor engraftment by posttransplant day 28. Bone marrow from five other patients showed mixed chimerism, and four patients eventually experienced either autologous marrow recovery or graft rejection. Compared with an historical group of patients who received GVHD prophylaxis with methotrexate, antithymocyte globulin, and prednisone, engrafted patients experienced faster recovery of leukocytes and shorter posttransplant hospitalizations. Recovery of total lymphocytes, B- and T-cell subsets, and T-cell function by day 28 was similar to patients in both the IT-treated group and historical controls. Five patients developed grade 2 skin GVHD, but none had severe grade 3 or 4 GVHD. IT treatment of donor marrow was evaluated in another clinical trial using non-HLA identical one haplotype-matched (haploidentical) donors and nine patients with diseases including Wiskott-Aldrich syndrome, Wolman disease, or leukemias such as chronic myelocytic or acute nonlymphocytic leukemia. Patients ranged in age from 1 to 29 years. Conditioning regimens included TBI. Depletion of T lymphocytes from donor marrow was very effective, as determined by phytohemagglutinin (PHA) and cytotoxic T lymphocyte (CTL) assays, and only one patient developed GVHD. However, six patients experienced graft rejection/failure and one patient developed posttransplant lymphoma. Thus, in both HLA and non-HLA matched transplants, depletion of donor T lymphocytes reduced the incidence of GVHD but increased the risk of graft failure/rejection.

A high incidence of graft failure/rejection has been noted in other centers utilizing matched and mismatched T-cell-depleted donor bone marrow (49-52). A variety of factors might contribute. The most notable are: (1) the elimination of T cells that secrete factors such as GM-CSF, IL-2, or IL-3 that directly affect hematopoiesis. The effect of recombinant growth factors on hematopoietic reconstitution and sustained donor engraftment has been evaluated in murine models (143); (2) suboptimal recipient conditioning that spares graft-rejecting cells in the host. In murine experiments, T-cell depletion combined with less aggressive conditioning regimens, such as total lymphoid irradiation (TLI), resulted in graft failure/rejection (53,54). However, engraftment did occur when mice were more aggressively conditioned, with single high dose TBI for example, and given T-cell depleted marrow; (3) elimination of graft-promoting cells in the donor. Certain subpopulations of T cells in the donor may play a role in engraftment, which would make the choice of anti-T-cell IT an important consideration in reversing graft failure/rejection. Donor natural killer (NK) cells may contribute to recipient immunosuppression, offer defense against viral antigens such as cytomegalovirus (CMV), and increase the graft-vs.-leukemia (GVL) potential of the allogeneic graft (58,144). Another IT mixture has been synthesized that is potent in anti-T cell activity but spares NK effectors (56).

T101-ricin A chain IT in the presence of 10 mM $NH_4Cl$ has been reported to demonstrate cytoreduction of nearly 99-99.9% against normal T lymphocytes (57). These IT have been used clinically (58).

Autologous BMT is a critical alternative for patients without HLA-MLC compatible sibling donors. By prior removal and preservation of remission bone marrow, supralethal doses of radio- and chemotherapy may be given to eradicate leukemia cells in the patient's body. Cryopreserved remission bone marrow is purged ex vivo with IT to eliminate occult leukemia cells prior to reinfusion. In animal experiments. IT have purged four logs or more of leukemia cells and prolonged survival (59,60). In humans, the number of leukemia cells in remission grafts that will cause relapse is unknown. Researchers have reported that less than 5% residual leukemia cells remaining in IT-treated bone marrow that was initially harvested in complete remission is sufficient to cause leukemic relapse (17). Therefore, it is imperative to employ highly efficient bone marrow purging strategies prior to reinfusion. Reports indicate that at least five logs of leukemia cells can be eliminated in human bone marrow with IT (61). Using combined immunochemotherapy and IT, even greater levels of kill have been demonstrated (41). A leukemia model system has been used in which human T-ALL cells from a clonogenic cell line were mixed with irradiated bone marrow cells (61). Cells were treated with a selective anti-CD5-reactive intact ricin IT. When cells were evaluated for clonogenic growth, IT specifically eliminated greater than 99.99% of leukemia cells from human bone marrow with minimal effect on human multipotent stem cells. Others have demonstrated similar levels of tumor inhibition in mouse models (59,60).

In a pilot study at the University of Minnesota, seven patients with T-lineage ALL/lymphoma and ranging in age from 5 to 23 years received IT-treated autologous bone marrow transplantations (62). Indications from these preliminary studies are that IT represents a safe, specific, and simple method for purgation of autologous bone marrow. The value of the procedure remains to be proven in randomized clinical trials.

Researchers have also studied the ex vivo purgation of autologous bone marrow utilizing A chain IT in the presence of $NH_4Cl$ (63). T101-ricin A chain demonstrated more than four log kill on uncloned CEM cells and more than 6 log kill on recloned CEM cells mixed with normal bone marrow. The anti-T lineage MoAb WT1 conjugated to ricin A chain demonstrated selective potency against two T-ALL cell lines (18). This IT was used to treat an autologous graft. The patient experienced hematopoietic reconstitution, which demonstrates that WT1-ricin A chain was not toxic to normal bone marrow progenitor cells (64). Despite encouraging results in ex vivo autologous bone marrow purging, the residual cells that are resistant to radiation and chemotherapy and survive in the leukemia patient emphasize the need for safe and effective in vivo strategies.

## F.  In Vivo Use of IT

The systemic use of IT may potentially solve three major problems in BMT involving (1) treatment of residual leukemia since incomplete recipient conditioning and subsequent leukemic relapse persist in both allogeneic and autologous BMT. Relapse occurs in 79% of autologous transplants (65); (2) treatment of severe GVHD. Conventional treatment involves administration of nonselective immunosuppressive agents such as steroids, ATG, and methotrexate. A phase I study is underway to evaluate a pan-T lymphocyte ricin A chain IT for systemic GVHD therapy (145). To date, patients have tolerated infusions well, and a reduction in the symptoms of severe acute GVHD has been noted. Another problem is (3) treatment of graft rejection. Studies have suggested that recipient cells may respond against donor grafts (66). In vivo IT treatment could perhaps selectively eliminate these cells, increase immunosuppression, and significantly promote recipient engraftment of donor bone marrow. Systemic therapy may also reduce the need for highly aggressive TBI and drug-induced immunosuppression that may cause myocardial and neural complications (67) as well as reduce patient susceptibility to viral infections and bacteria during the 2-3 week period of neutropenia following autologous BMT (18).

Immunotoxins have shown potential for in vivo treatment in several models of hematopoietic malignancy. When rodents were injected with tumor cells and then given ricin A chain IT, cancer was delayed and the survival rate was improved (68-70). Nonspecific cytoreductive therapy (TLI) and splenectomy, followed by treatment with an anti-Ig IT, was used against large tumor burdens induced by a murine B-cell leukemia ($BCL_1$) (71). Although mice experienced long-term remission, latent tumor cells that were identified in transferred tissue induced recurrent leukemia. This study suggests the possible utility of combined therapy in order to reduce tumor burden and permit immunological tumor management by the host. Since contaminating ricin B chain may have contributed to the therapeutic efficacy of these putative A chain IT, B chain continues to be considered in the construction of clinical reagents.

Clinical studies for systemic treatment of leukemia with ricin A chain IT are in the initial stages; however, results are encouraging. For example, target cell binding without IT-treatment associated complications was observed in two leukemia patients who received in vivo-administered T101-ricin A chain (72). A significant decrease in lymphocytes was sustained by one patient. The feasibility of in vivo applications for potentiators or alternatives such as modified B chains could result in extremely effective ricin A chain reagents for systemic therapy. The recent phase I clinical trial for melanoma therapy also is of interest in regard to ricin A chain IT (73). Nonspecific ricin A chain toxicity was of primary concern to these investigators; however, patient toxocity was observed as primarily mild, transient, and reversible. Hypoalbuminemia did arise as an unexpected and currently unexplained complication.

Intact ricin IT with an intravenous lactose bolus may be useful in the treatment of localized treatment of inoperable cancers (42,74). We have investigated the intratumoral use of intact ricin IT in a nude mouse model in which human tumors were grown subcutaneously (42,74). Intact ricin IT was tested for anti-tumor activity against an established human T leukemia cell line. We found that (1) intact ricin IT caused regression of small (0.3-0.5 cm$^2$) tumors in the presence of lactose, (2) regression was selective, however, selectivity was not absolute, (3) A chain IT, in the presence of potentiators, did not inhibit tumor growth, (4) a combinative regimen of intact ricin IT plus cyclophosphamide congener was able to cause regression of large (3-6 cm$^3$) tumors, and (5) intact ricin IT, as a new class of potential in vivo antitumor reagent, may be useful for treatment of local-ized tumors or inoperable solid tumors.

The systemic and localized use of IT is considerably more complex than ex vivo purging strategies. The suitability of IT in vivo must be examined relative to $LD_{50}$, biodistribution, pharmacokinetics, and damage to nontarget tissue. Basic research and clinical trials must be coordinated to address the specific problems and prospects associated with the safety and efficacy of in vivo IT reagents. The accomplishments of researchers have been significant when we consider that (1) localized and systemic therapy with IT is a relatively new and rapidly expanding field, and (2) preliminary clinical trials have already been conducted with favor-able results.

## II.  RADIOLABELED ANTIBODIES

Antibodies conjugated to radionuclides may be used for either cancer detection or therapy. For radioimmunodetection, the antibody moiety specifically binds tumor and external imaging methods detect the emissions of the radiolabeled moiety. Radioimmunodetection may offer advantages over conventional diag-nostic procedures by reducing the risks associated with biopsy and providing greater specificity as a result of antibody-directed binding to tumor cells. Radio-active labels need to stay attached to antibody until delivered to tumor, be re-tained in tumor tissue for many half-lives, have a high linear energy transfer to specifically irradiate target tissue, and not create radiation risks to patients and technicians. For cancer therapy, a clinically effective dose of radiation must be delivered to targeted malignancies. Radiolabeled antibodies offer potential im-provement in the treatment of solid and hematopoietic malignancies by deliver-ing therapeutic doses of radionuclides to places unobtainable by other methods. Another potential advantage is a higher tumor/whole body dose if the proper radionuclide can be chosen, resulting in less toxicity to normal tissue, particularly bone marrow.

### A.  Radioiodine Labels

Chloramine T was initially used for labeling with iodine radionuclides (75), and later, lactoperoxidase was employed (76). Iodine monochloride and iodogen or iodobeads have also been used by investigators (77,78). Although the radionuclide $^{131}$iodine ($^{131}$I) has been widely used for diagnostic imaging and therapy, alternatives are being enthusiastically explored. Iodine-131 is readily available, relatively inexpensive, and its iodination activities are fairly well established. The considerably rapid dehalogenation of $^{131}$I can be beneficial in normal tissues and organs by lowering nonspecific background activity. However, dehalogenation can result in greater accumulation in tissues that metabolize iodine such as thyroid, stomach, small intestine, and bladder. In vivo deiodination can shorten the iodine radiolabel's duration at the tumor site and thereby limit efficacy. The extent of dehalogenation or deiodination appears to depend on what antibody is used, the size of the antibody molecule, the method of radioiodination, and the radionuclide used. The rate of dehalogenation varies in different organ systems. In order to reduce nonspecific radioactivity and false positive results, background subtraction methods with technetium-99m- ($^{99m}$TC) labeled human serum albumin and free $^{99m}$TcO-$_4$ have been utilized (79).

Considering the current capabilities of diagnostic imaging equipment, radiolabels would ideally have a range of 120-250 KeV gamma emissions that are also highly abundant, with isomeric transmission or electron capture mode of decay, and a sustained (up to several days) physical half-life compatible with the pharmacokinetics of the labeled antibody (80). Iodine-131 has a high energy gamma emission of 364 KeV and a relatively long half-life of 8.04 days. However, its use in diagnostic imaging is limited because the energy is too high for efficient detection by external imaging devices. Among the alternatives, another iodine radionuclide, $^{123}$I, has a preferable gamma energy emission of 159 KeV (83% abundance) for detection by external detectors and a half-life of 13.3 hours, but like $^{131}$I, may be handicapped by deiodination in vivo. The short half-life of $^{123}$I may limit its usefulness unless the antibody or fragment localizes in tumor in this time period.

The potential of $^{131}$I-labeled antibodies for cancer therapy has also been investigated. In animal studies, treatment of established murine AKR T-cell lymphomas with $^{131}$I-labeled anti-Thy 1.1 caused tumor regression in nearly half of treated mice, and in some cases, resulted in cures or prolonged survival (81). $^{131}$I-MoAb have also been able to substantially inhibit tumor development in mice transplanted with human colon tumor xenografts (82). Clinical trials utilizing $^{131}$I-labeled antibodies for therapy against human cancers have had some favorable results, which are discussed briefly below in the context of antibodies and routes of administration.

## B. Radiometal Labels

Dehalogenation of iodine radiolabels from antibody has prompted the investigation of radioactive metals such as $^{111}$indium ($^{111}$In), $^{90}$yttrium ($^{90}$Y), and $^{99m}$technetium ($^{99m}$Tc). Metal ions attached by chelation techniques may be preferred because they are less likely to be detached during delivery and do not interfere with biodistribution and kinetics (78,83,84). For purposes of detection, the radiometal $^{111}$In has a favorable gamma emission of 171 and 245 KeV (88 and 94% abundance), a half-life of 2.8 days, and electron capture mode of decay. Melanoma patient studies utilizing MoAb labeled with $^{111}$In resulted in over half (60-70%) of lesions greater than 1.5 cm being detected and detection of at least one tumor site in all patients with metastatic disease (84). In 18 patients with carcinoembryonic antigen (CEA)-producing tumors, primarily colorectal, the lesion detection rate was greater than 70% (83). Successful localization of metastatic sites occurred in patients when other methods had failed. In vivo and in vitro studies utilizing a MoAb recognizing CEA labeled with $^{111}$In demonstrated that the antibody could retain target antigen binding (85). Furthermore, when the $^{111}$In-MoAb to CEA was compared to MoAb radioiodinated with $^{125}$I in nude mice with human colorectal tumor implants, the radiometal-labeled antibody demonstrated superior localization.

The physical and chemical properties of the radiometal $^{90}$Y, such as insignificant gamma radiation, intermediate beta energy, suitable half-life, and stability (86), have generated much interest in $^{90}$Y for radiolabeled antibody therapy. A clinical trial utilizing an antiferritin antibody labeled with $^{90}$Y for treatment of hepatoma resulted in low hematologic toxicity, and 3 of 6 patients experienced partial or complete remission (87).

Advantages for detection utilizing the radiometal $^{99m}$Tc include availability, low cost, and good physical characteristics. However, to overcome the relatively short half-life of 6 hours, some researchers have utilized MoAb fragments to accelerate blood clearance and expedite localization and tumor uptake. Indications from localization studies in nude mice with human tumor xenografts are that MoAb fragments [F(ab')$_2$] labeled with $^{99m}$Tc form a stable bond, retain immunoreactivity, and could be useful clinical tools for diagnostic imaging (88).

## C. Polyclonal Antibodies

In the early 1950s, researchers demonstrated successful localization utilizing a $^{131}$I-labeled polyclonal antibody in a murine sarcoma tumor model (89). Radiolabeled polyclonal antibodies have subsequently been used to locate tumors in patients. Encouraging results have been obtained in radioimmunodetection with polyclonal anti-CEA. A majority of primary and metastatic sites were detected with radiolabeled goat and sheep anti-CEA (90,91). Other favorable studies have used polyclonal antialphafetoprotein (AFP) for tumor imaging (92,93), and $^{131}$I-labeled antihuman chorionic gonadotrophin, which had remarkable, nearly 100% successful tumor detection sensitivity in patients with trophoblastic and germinal tumors (94).

Radiolabeled polyclonal antibodies for cancer therapy have had limited success. Although in 1951, the first clinical application of radiolabeled antibody in a patient with widely metastatic melanoblastoma using a rabbit immunoglobulin labeled with [131]I resulted in complete tumor regression as confirmed by autopsy nine years later, subsequent treatment of 13 melanoma patients did not result in tumor regression nor did [131]I localize tumors (95). Antifibrin animal-derived antibodies labeled with [131]I were useful for tumor localization in animal studies, but were ineffective in therapy of terminal cancer patients (96,97). Another clinical trial involved rabbit [131]I-labeled antiferritin or anti-CEA antibody in addition to other therapeutic modalities (98). [131]I antibody did not demonstrate significant toxicity, yet therapeutic outcome cannot be entirely attributed to radiolabeled antibody treatment. More recently, clinical trials have had encouraging results: A remission rate of 50% was achieved in 81 hepatoma patients and 14 intrahepatic biliary cancer patients treated with [131]I-labeled antiferritin and [131]I-labeled anti-CEA, respectively (99,100). A phase 1-2 trial of 105 hepatoma patients utilized an innovative combination of chemotherapy and [131]I-labeled antiferritin (101). Although toxicity (thrombocytopenia) was noted with the integrated administration of doxorubicin and 5-fluorouracil, an amplified clinical response rate could be attributed to the increased cytotoxicity of drug and low dose rate radiation.

### D.  Monoclonal Antibodies and Fragments

Monoclonal antibodies offer the advantage of homogeneity and availability over polyclonal antibodies. One of the first in vivo clinical applications of radiolabeled MoAb for diagnostic tumor imaging involved colorectal cancer. Moderate improvement with anti-CEA monoclonal over a goat polyclonal was observed (102). Subsequent diagnostic imaging studies for colorectal cancer had successful radioimmunodetection of well over half (60-70%) of colon cancer sites using whole MoAb and MoAb fragments labeled with [131]I (77,103). A combined approach utilizing two MoAb, 17-1A and 19-9, identified 77% of tumor sites (104). More recently, MoAb fragments labeled with [123]I have demonstrated exceptionally high sensitivity and specificity for colon carcinoma as detected by immunoscintigraphy (105). In a study of 23 patients [123]I-labeled F(ab)$_2$ fragments and Fab fragments of MoAb 35, respectively, located 23 of 28 tumor sites and 30 of 31 tumor sites that included primary or recurrent carcinomas and metastases (105). Melanoma imaging studies have employed [131]I-labeled MoAb and their Fab fragments specific for p97 antigen (106,107). For metastasized tumors greater than 1.5 cm, detection of melanoma was 88% using [131]I-Fab. A strong correlation between tumor uptake and retention of radiolabeled antibody fragment and concentration of p97 antigen was reported (107).

These studies highlight the efficacy of MoAb fragments. In vivo nude mouse studies with human solid tumors have also demonstrated a preference for use of fragments over intact antibody molecules because they are less prone to induce immunogenicity and therefore, successive injections over an extended period of time are feasible for radioimmunotherapy (107,108). Furthermore, fragments have not been retained in the circulatory system as long as whole antibody. This reduces background activity by rendering fragments less prone to demonstrate nonselective binding to macrophages, monocytes, neutrophils, and other cells, in contrast to the Fc-mediated binding properties shown by whole antibody (109). Fab fragments have also demonstrated superior localization (110). Additional detailed comparisons of whole MoAb and their fragments are needed. One complication is that two similar MoAb, such as ones having the same isotype, may display different pharmacokinetics in vivo, and when radiolabeled for example, may exhibit different tendencies toward nontarget tissue localization. The extent that radiolabeling procedures reduce or modify antibody activity may vary. In order to optimize radioimmunodetection and therapy, every MoAb must be examined individually for in vivo activity.

Therapy with radiolabeled MoAb has been initiated with some encouraging results. For example, [131]I-labeled MoAb UJ13A was used against neuroblastoma in diagnostic studies of 12 children and 4 of these patients also received therapeutic doses of the radiolabeled MoAb (111). Mild transient toxicity (pyrexia, vomiting) occurred in 2 of 4 patients receiving the therapeutic doses. Two of 4 had more serious marrow aplasia; 1 case was intractable, the other recovered quickly even though this patient had a higher dose/unit body weight and also had marrow related tumors. Furthermore, this patient's marrow was tumor-free posttreatment for eight months. One patient with mild anaphylaxis experienced a 95% loss of therapeutic dose by excretion within 24 hours. This study again demonstrates the therapeutic potential of radiolabeled MoAb but also emphasizes the great variability of patient response and the need to evaluate each diagnosis individually. Also, these researchers warned against using a murine Ig for diagnostic imaging, if the patient is also a candidate for therapy, in order to avoid an antimurine response prior to treatment.

A therapeutic strategy under investigation is the radiolabeling of MoAb conjugated to potent toxins (i.e., immunotoxins) (43). We have evaluated the anti-human T-leukemia MoAb T101 (anti-CD5) linked to intact ricin and labeled with $^{90}$Y. When this radioimmunotoxin (RIT) was tested against the human T-leukemia cell line CEM, $^{90}$Y-labeled T101-ricin at a concentration of 10 $\mu$g/ml demonstrated the ability to eliminate over 3.5 logs of T-leukemia cells. Interestingly, the RIT retained immunoreactivity and cytotoxicity. Such reagents may potentially benefit antitumor therapy because the same anticancer reagent could simultaneously deliver two independent cytotoxic signals.

## E. Immunogenicity

The production of anti-immunoglobulin (anti-Ig) in recipients of radiolabeled antibodies has been observed repeatedly, yet the problem of immunogenicity persists in both diagnostic imaging and radiotherapy. How many doses and how frequently they may be given before patients develop an anti-Ig response is under investigation. Patient immune response to foreign antibody is a major concern because therapeutic protocols involve serial treatments with varying frequency. Anti-Ig are responsible for a lower incidence of tumor-specific targeting, a reduced, less efficient half-life, and therefore, decreased therapeutic efficacy. Use of murine-derived monoclonals is particularly susceptible to an anti-mouse response. One way this problem is avoided is by a "cycling method" using antibodies derived from different species of animals and thus circumventing a patient's immune response to one particular species (112). However, as improved protocols increase patient survival time, reinjection or "recycling" of the original species-specific radiolabeled antibody may be necessary. Considering that clinical studies utilizing radiolabeled antibodies for both diagnostic imaging and treatment continue to have promising results, there is a need to determine the frequency and amount of radiolabeled antibody allowed before an immune response develops.

Other factors that may influence the outcome of treatment with radiolabeled antibody are the concentrations of antibody, pharmacokinetics, half-life, and blood supply to tumor. Also, the state of the patient's immune system is a factor, for example, disease-associated immunosuppression or the development of anti-Ig responses by previous unrelated exposure to immunoglobulin. As radioactive labeling technology progresses, combined radionuclides and larger doses of radiation may influence immunogenic response (112). Perhaps the further development and use of human-human hybridomas, antibody fragments, chimeric antibodies, or genetically engineered antibodies will eventually eliminate this obstacle.

## F.  Antigens

Expression of antigen on the tumor cell surface may not be uniform. Antigens may localize in a specific area, may be scattered over the cell surface (113), or may even be present during one phase of tumor cell activity and absent in another. Antigen expression typically reaches a maximum during the S phase of the cell cycle (114). Furthermore, the antibody itself may induce antigen modulation and decrease the expression of a specific antigen on the tumor surface. Use of radiolabeled antibody mixtures may help overcome this problem. A mixture of two anticolon carcinoma antibodies has demonstrated improved results over use of an individual antibody (104).

Tumor antigens are commonly shared by normal tissue as well as other tumors. Cross-reactivity with normal tissue presents problems, as documented in the study of six patients injected with $^{111}$In-labeled anti-CEA MoAb (115). Cross-reactivity with and subsequent substantial decrease in circulating granulocytes, in addition to systemic toxicity, was observed in five patients. This also points out that animal studies, although useful, still have limitations since destruction of granulocytes was not observed when the same antibody was utilized in preliminary animal studies. An absence of antigen specificity also complicates diagnostic imaging and produces nonrelevant tissue reactivity as a result of nonspecific, nontumor binding by the MoAb. Circulating antigens or cross-reactive antigens originating from normal tissue may result in nonspecific uptake of radiolabeled MoAb. Saturation of nontarget antigens by antibodies may be necessary to overcome this problem.

## G. Route of Administration

One significant limitation of radiolabeled antibody therapy is that the amount of radioactivity that actually reaches the tumor is too small to render it therapeutically effective for many cancers, including those of the epithelial tissues. The processes of dilution, dissociation, and catabolism occurring after intravenous injection and during antibody delivery to the tumor area are partially responsible for the reduced efficacy of the radionuclide. Thus, the route of injection is extremely important. Both therapy and imaging studies have primarily used intravenous injections, as opposed to subcutaneous, intracavitary, intraperitoneal, or arterial injection. As an alternative to intravenous administration of therapeutic quantities of radiolabeled MoAb, regional administration for tumors confined to a specific area is being evaluated. Intraperitoneal injections of four MoAb labeled with $^{131}$I were given either as single antibody or mixtures for ovarian cancer to 15 patients (116). Doses over 100 mCi resulted in reversible toxicity (diarrhea, leukopenia, thrombocytopenia). Six of 6 patients in stage 3 with minimal residual disease sustained a complete remission for up to a year and a half (3-18 months). In another phase 1 clinical trial of 12 ovarian cancer patients receiving intraperitoneal injection of $^{131}$I-labeled MoAb, the therapeutic outcome varied with the stage of disease (117). A total of eight patients in stage 3 responded favorably to radiolabeled antibody therapy, two having the disease stabilized at 6-8 months, four experiencing complete remission for 3-24 months posttreatment, and two remaining in remission for over two years. Toxicity was noted in some patients, which may in part be attributed to previous radiotherapy. A larger phase 2 study has been undertaken to supplement these results and to further understand the physical properties and pharmacokinetics behind MoAb-directed radioimmunotherapy.

In summary, radiolabeled antibodies have potential that is still under evaluation for diagnostic imaging and therapy of human malignancies. Antibody-directed radionuclides must combine optimal radiotoxicity and safety for clinical therapy, as well as perform efficiently and reliably for diagnostic purposes. Although human studies are in the early stages, the results are often highly favorable, and researchers are investigating a large number of radiolabeled monoclonal antibodies directed against various types of cancer.

## III.  DRUG CONJUGATES

Chemotherapy has had a dramatic impact on the history of cancer treatment. However, as more sophisticated cytotoxic drugs and their congeners are developed, the problem of high toxicity combined with low selectivity persists. A more selective delivery system is desirable to overcome the adverse side effects that have occurred during clinical chemotherapy. Antibodies may provide a useful vector for a more selective means of drug delivery.

### A.  Antibodies

The antibody moiety of a drug conjugate improves drug localization. As in other targeting strategies, antibodies are chosen that react with certain determinants on the surface of malignant cells. These determinants are often found on normal cells, but at lower densities. MoAb that demonstrate highly specific binding affinity and avidity to the predominant cancer cell antigen are thus chosen to direct and attach therapeutic drugs to targeted malignancies. Although the homogeneity of MoAb represents a tremendous advantage, a major difficulty in all forms of antibody therapy is cross-reactivity with normal tissues sharing the same antigenic determinants with target cancer cells. An example of a shared antigen is CEA, which has been found in colorectal tumors and normal granulocytes. Studies have shown that treatment with anti-CEA MoAb induced fever, vomiting, and rigors caused by reactivity with and subsequent destruction of circulating granulocytes (115). Conjugation of anti-CEA MoAb to cytotoxic agents could very well increase the severity of side effects. However, cross-reactivity might be circumvented by the use of a different MoAb. For example, the MoAb 11.285.14 is considered highly tumor-specific, with notable reactivity being limited to normal epithelial cells of the gastrointestinal tract (118,119). Significantly, the adverse effect upon granulocytes observed in other studies (115) was not apparent when this MoAb was administered to a group of advanced colorectal carcinoma patients (120). Such results emphasize the need to test normal cell reactivity with each antibody. The nature of an antibody's binding site must also be considered; in particular, properties involving mobility, uptake, and internalization appear to have a significant impact on an antibody's effectiveness as a drug carrier (121).

### B.  Drugs

Cytotoxic drugs may destroy cancer cells by several mechanisms, including direct inhibition of DNA synthesis, cell surface modification, protein synthesis inhibition, and enzyme inhibition. However, the precise mechanism is not always easily determined. The cytotoxic actions of anthracyclines, for example, have been attributed to DNA intercalation, pinocytosis, or possibly interaction with cell surface receptors (125).

The ultimate goal of drug targeting with antibodies is to improve drug potency while reducing toxicity to normal human tissue. Drugs vary widely in their efficacy as either a single modality or a conjugate. Among the major categories of drugs that have been used in clinical cancer treatment are antimetabolites, alkylators, vinca alkaloids, anthracyclines, and antibiotics. From these groups, a variety of drugs have been investigated as possible conjugates to individual antibodies. Within the scope of this review, only a few of the extensively studied and promising approaches to drug targeting are discussed.

The antimetabolite methotrexate (MTX), frequently used for treatment of human cancers including leukemias and lymphomas (122), has been examined as a conjugate (123). Studies have shown that MTX conjugated to a rabbit polyclonal against a mouse lymphoma and a MoAb directed against human melanoma cells are superior to free MTX as tumor inhibitors (124). In in vivo murine and in vitro human tumor cell line experiments, these conjugates demonstrated greater tumor cell localization than did unconjugated MTX, and therefore greater efficacy. In further studies, conjugated MTX was retained in circulation and ascites fluid for longer periods of time and persisted in larger quantites for longer periods in lymphoma cells. Pharmacokinetics, catabolism, and uptake were examined with favorable results. Both the conjugate and catabolized fragments of MTX withstood effluxion and retained toxic activity once inside the target cell with greater success than did unconjugated MTX. Other studies have reported similarly promising results with conjugated MTX being retained longer by melanoma cells and maintained in higher concentrations (121).

Anthracyclines such as adriamycin and daunomycin have also performed more effectively as conjugates. Adriamycin attached to a monoclonal antialphafetoprotein (AFP) experienced improved protein synthesis inhibition against human hepatoma cell lines (125). In previous studies, both drug and antibody activities were retained when adriamycin was directed against neuroblastoma cell lines by the MoAb Thy-1 (126). Recent results of studies with doxorubicin and the anti-T-cell MoAb, T101, showed an antitumor effect when drug and antibody were combined as a mixture and as a conjugate (127). Intravenous injections of a daunomycin anti-AFP conjugate prevented tumor development and prolonged survival in rat hepatoma models (128). Intraperitoneal treatment of a B lymphoma with a daunomycin conjugate resulted in cures for the majority of treated mice (129). Tests indicated that both antibody binding and drug cytotoxicity were maintained; furthermore, conjugation permitted the use of high doses of daunomycin that would be too toxic if the drug was administered separately.

The glycopeptide antibiotic, bleomycin, when attached to anti-HLA antibodies, has demonstrated specificity and increased potency (13). The protein antibiotic neocarzinostatin conjugated to an antileukemia immunoglobulin (Ig) has retained drug activity and target cell binding (131).

In vitro selectivity studies have had encouraging results employing MoAb and the vinca alkaloid, vindesine (VDS). For example, VDS was conjugated to the anti-T lymphocyte MoAb, RFT-11 (132). RFT-11-VDS was highly cytotoxic against the human T cell line, MOLT-3, and ineffective against control cell lines. Tumor suppression has also been achieved utilizing antimelanoma, antiosteogenic sarcoma, and anti-CEA MoAb-VDS conjugates in immunosuppressed mice (133). Although some decrease in drug activity was observable, nonspecific toxicity was also favorably reduced.

Chlorambucil, an alkylating agent, directed against IgM-secreting lympho- blastoid cell lines by a noncovalent bond to antibody, was selectively toxic to target cells and minimally potent against control cell lines (134). Furthermore, this conjugate could successfully target secreted proteins rather than membrane antigens.

## C. Conjugates

The precise mechanism of conjugate activity is currently undefined. Conjugate may specifically locate, bind, and destroy target cancer cells by the following methods: (1) cytotoxic agent is released after conjugate is internalized or may remain bioactive as the conjugate; (2) the drug moiety is released at the cell sur- face (extracellularly) after delivery by the MoAb and subsequently, the drug acts on its own; or (3) drug and MoAb may work together on the cell surface to inhibit cellular function without ever being internalized.

Antibodies are linked to anticancer drugs utilizing a variety of chemical reac- tions induced by, for example, active ester formation of carboxyl groups, perio- date oxidation of sugar residues, diazotization, glutaraldehyde coupling between amino groups, or carbodiimide condensation between carboxyl and amino groups (132). The drug moiety is conjugated directly to Ig or indirectly by linking Ig to drug-laden carriers such as polymeric derivatives of dextran, polyglutamic acid, *cis* aconityl, or albumin. Indirect conjugation procedures employ amplification techniques that allow a greater amount of cytotoxic agent to be delivered to the target cell. The increased distance between drug and antibody may also decrease adverse interaction between the two moieties. One amplification technique is to link the drug to a carrier such as human serum albumin (HSA), prior to linkage to MoAb. A drug-antibody ratio of 30:1 has been reported for MTX attached to MoAb via HSA (135). Drug-antibody ratios by direct methods have a maximum of 10:1 without risking a decrease in MoAb reactivity (132). The preparation of MTX-HSA-MoAb conjugates has recently been improved, facilitating the synthe- sis of larger, purified quantities of useful conjugate with greater cytotoxicity by the elimination of competing free antibody (136). Cytotoxicity may potentially be achieved against cells resistant to MTX due to a poor transport system. An- other possible advantage of the HSA carrier is greater efficiency for drugs that have demonstrated low uptake by target cells.

*Cis* aconityl has been utilized as a carrier between daunomycin and a MoAb against osteogenic sarcoma and carcinoma cell lines (137). In vitro results dem- onstrated favorable stability, retention of drug toxicity, and antigen-specific bind- ing. Dextran derivatives that form Schiff bases have also been extensively used with anthracyclines (125). Adriamycin linked to antibody via a dextran bridge was extremely stable, and studies routinely demonstrated greater efficacy for daunomycin or adriamycin-dextran-antibody conjugates over free drug, antibody, and mixtures. Poly-L-glutamic acid has allowed the linkage of 10-20 moles of daunomycin to anti-AFP antibody (138). Substantial inhibition of tumor development and prolongation of survival was achieved in rat hepatoma models in vivo.

From the research reported to date, conjugation procedures with MoAb and spacer molecules that act as carriers apparently increase the toxicity of less potent drug conjugates (136). However, conjugation to antibody may also significantly modify and reduce drug cytotoxicity. This can be advantageous by allowing drugs that are too toxic by themselves to be used therapeutically as a conjugate (137). Daunomycin is an example of a drug that is ineffective at low dosages, yet too toxic when administered as a free drug at high dosages. Although reduction of MoAb activity by conjugation procedures is an occasionally problematic phenomenon, it has been reported that even after a loss of 50-70% of original activity, MoAb often retain sufficient ability to recognize target antigens (139). Investigators have extensively studied the MoAb 791T/36 conjugated to daunomycin, VDS, and MTX (140). Although in most instances conjugation of drug to MoAb significantly reduces cytotoxicity, these researchers found that drug activity could be maintained after conjugation to 791T/36. Conjugation to this particular antibody also proved advantageous in that specificity to the target antigen was realized. The three drugs studied varied in their effect upon antibody reactivity. Only 4 mol of MTX could be attached to 1 mol of 791T/36 without adverse effects upon antibody, whereas 6 mol or more of VDS has no impact upon the antibody moiety. As these researchers point out, such results encourage the use of carrier molecules such as HSA to exploit the maximum cytotoxic potential of the drug conjugate. Yet, carrier strategies have limitations in that increased quantities of drug, and thus the larger size of the conjugate, may impede binding and entry into target cells, in vivo clearance, and bonding stability (137). This possibility suggests one advantage for utilizing powerful, highly potent drugs such as vinca alkaloids and relying on direct conjugation procedures. Another alternative, as mentioned in the context of immunotoxin strategies, is the use of chemical activators that may improve immunoconjugate potency. In one study, the lysosomotropic amine, chloroquine, was added to an MTX-antibody conjugate. Intracellular degradation of MTX was inhibited, thereby enhancing cytotoxic potential (121).

In conclusion, other variables that may affect the efficacy of drug conjugates should be given brief mention. As in alternate forms of immunoconjugate therapy, the recipient's defense system may produce its own antibodies against the conjugate's specific antibody. In such cases, the drug may never reach the target tumor cells. The prospective employment of human-human hybridomas may eliminate this complication. The utilization of antibody fragments that lack the

Fc portion of the Ig may also result in less immunogenicity. Another advantage for antibody fragments is a reduced half-life, which would mean that conjugate not attached to target antigen would have a shorter duration in the circulatory system. Furthermore, since binding to nontarget tissue may be complement mediated, removal of the Fc portion could reduce nonspecific toxicity to normal tissue (125). One other major consideration in drug targeting is the great variety of tumor types and the vast range of characteristics that could facilitate or avert an antibody delivery system. Thus, the utility of conjugate therapy could vary considerably among specific types of cancer, and caution is advised when making generalizations about potential therapeutic benefits.

## D. Closing Remarks

Three major approaches to antibody-directed cell targeting for the treatment of cancer have been discussed in this review. Based on our current knowledge, an objective statement as to the superiority of one particular immunoconjugate is neither possible nor practical. To favor one approach may be no more realistic than trying to identify a single chemotherapeutic agent as most efficacious for cancer therapy. One immunoconjugate may be useful against a particular cancer, but perhaps more importantly, combining strategies that destroy tumors by different mechanisms may prove advantageous. One general conclusion is possible: More information must be generated by continued academic and fiscal support. Intensive research is mandatory to overcome the major difficulties concerning potency, selectivity, immunogenicity, stability, and cross-reactivity with normal tissue. Maximum specificity combined with sufficient cytotoxicity to eliminate all tumor cells is the ultimate requirement for an effective in vivo anticancer conjugate. Each of the strategies described in this review share some problems and also suggest solutions for others. For example, IT have proven highly selective and potent when used clinically for ex vivo purging of bone marrow; however, their utility for in vivo therapy is a complex issue. The same attributes that render IT effective ex vivo, dramatic potency and catalytic nature, may result in unacceptable in vivo risks. Yet, the use of highly toxic radionuclides or drugs may also be hazardous. Furthermore, toxin conjugates may have an advantage over radiolabeled antibodies in that optimal crosslinking procedures render IT extremely stable. Radionuclide conjugates may be limited by in vivo dehalogenation or the short half-lives of certain radionuclides. Some drug conjugates undergo alterations that significantly reduce drug cytotoxicity and influence their efficacy. Undoubtedly, the variable successes reported in this review may be attributed in part to differences in antibody choice. Development of higher quality MoAb with greater affinity/avidity and identification of the correct subclass or isotype for maximum localization to target tissue will represent significant achievements in the area of cross-reactivity. The implementation of antibody fragments, human-human MoAb, and chimeric antibodies genetically engineered from manipulated immunoglobulin genes may eliminate immunogenicity and promote in vivo half-life. Finally, immunoconjugates will perhaps be combined with other forms of biological response modifiers in order to produce a more complete antitumor response. Because of problems related to expression of tumor-associated antigens on normal tissue, more selective targeting of either growth factor receptors or oncogene products that are expressed on tumor cells may play a significant role. Despite obstacles, the interrelated areas of immunoconjugate research will continue to expand as a result of impressive preliminary clinical findings and progress toward selective destruction of highly invasive tumors.

## ACKNOWLEDGMENTS

Supported in part by National Institutes of Health Grants Nos. R01 CA-31618 and R01 CA-36725, and the Minnesota Medical Foundation. D.A.V. is a Scholar of the Leukemia Society of America. F.M.U. is a recipient of New Investigator Award No. I R23 CA-42111-01 from the National Institutes of Health, and is a Special Fellow of the Leukemia Society of America. This is Center for Experimental Transplantation and Cancer Research paper #32.

The authors wish to acknowledge the dedication and productivity of the University of Minnesota Bone Marrow Transplantation Team. Drs. D.J. Buchsbaum and J.A. Sinkule provided critical reading of the manuscript and helpful comments. The exceptional editorial skills of M. J. Hildreth are greatly appreciated. We thank Jo Ann Mattson for excellent secretarial services.

## REFERENCES

1. Kohler, G., and Milstein, C. Continuous cultures of fused cells secreting antibody of a predefined specificity. Nature, 256: 495-497, 1975.
2. Vallera, D.A. The use of immunotoxins in bone marrow transplantation: Eradication of T cells and leukemic cells. In *Immunoconjugates: Antibodies in Radioimaging and Therapy of Cancer.* Edited by C.-W. Vogel. Oxford University Press, New York, 1987, pp. 217-240.
3. Vitetta, E.S., Krolick, K.A., Miyama-Inaba, M., Cushley, W., and Uhr, J.W. Immunotoxins: A new approach to cancer therapy. Science 219: 644-650, 1983.
4. Thorpe, P.E. Antibody carriers of cytotoxic agents in cancer therapy: a review. In *Monoclonal Antibodies 1985: Biological and Clinical Applications.* Edited by A. Pinchera, G. Doria, F. Dammacco, and A. Bargellesi. Editrice Kurtis s.r.l., Milan, 1985, pp. 475-512.
5. Neville, D.M., Jr. Immunotoxins: Current use and future prospects in bone marrow transplantation and cancer treatment. In *CRC Critical Reviews in Therapeutic Drug Carrier Systems.* Edited by D. Seligson. CRC Press, Inc., Boca Raton, Florida, 1985.
6. Olsnes, S., Pihl, A. Abrin, ricin, and their associated immunoglobulins. In *Receptors and Recognition,* Series B. *The Specificity and Action of Animal,*

*Bacterial, and Plant Toxins.* Edited by P. Cuatrecasas. Chapman and Hall, London, 1976, pp. 129-173.

7. Olsnes, S., and Pihl, A. Toxin lectins and related proteins. In *Molecular Actions of Toxins and Viruses.* Edited by P.L. Cohen and S. van Heyningen. Elsevier, Amsterdam, 1982, pp. 51-105.

8. Youle, R.J., and Neville, D.M. Jr. Kinetics of protein synthesis inactivation by ricin-anti-Thy 1.1 monoclonal antibody hybrids. J. Biol. Chem. 257: 1598-1601, 1982.

9. Sanchez-Madrid, F., Krensky, A.M., Ware, C.F., Robbins, E., Strominger, J.L., Burakoff, S.J., and Springer, T.A. Three distinct antigens associated with human T-lymphocyte-mediated cytolysis: LFA-1, LFA-2, and LFA-3. Proc. Natl. Acad. Sci. USA 79: 7489-7493, 1982.

10. LeBien, T.W., and Kersey, J.H. A monoclonal antibody (TA-1) reactive with human T lymphocytes and monocytes. J. Immunol. 125: 2208-2214, 1980.

11. Vallera, D.A., Quinones, R.R., Azemove, S.M., and Soderling, C.C.B. Monoclonal antibody toxin conjugates reactive against human T lymphocytes: A comparison of antibody linked to intact ricin toxin and antibody linked to ricin A chain. Transplantation 37: 387-392, 1984.

12. Vitetta, E.S. Synergy between immunotoxins prepared with native ricin A chains and chemically modified ricin B chains. J. Immunol. 136: 1880-1887, 1986.

13. Gilliland, D.G., Steplewski, Z., Collier, R.J., Mitchell, K.F., Chang, T.H., and Koprowski, H. Antibody-directed cytotoxic agents: Use of monoclonal antibody to direct the action of toxin A chains to colorectal carcinoma cells. Proc. Natl. Acad. Sci. USA 77: 4539-4543, 1980.

14. Moolten, F.L., and Cooperband, S.R. Selective destruction of target cells by diphtheria toxin conjugated to antibody directed against antigens on the cells. Science 169: 68-70, 1970.

15. Thorpe, P.E., Cumber, A.J., Williams, N., Edwards, D.C., Ross, W.C.J., and Davies, A.J.S. Abrogation of the non-specific toxicity of abrin conjugated to anti-lymphocyte globulin. Clin. Exp. Immunol. 43: 195-200, 1981.

16. FitzGerald, D.J.P., Waldmann, T.A., Willingham, M.C., and Pastan, I. Pseudomonas exotoxin-Anti-TAC. Cell-specific immunotoxin active against cells expressing the human T cell growth factor receptor. J. Clin. Invest. 74: 966-971, 1984.

17. Jansen, F.K., Laurent, G., Liance, M.C., Blythman, H.E., Berthe, J., Canat, X., Carayon, P., Carriere, D., Cassellas, P., Derocq, J.M., Dussossoy, D., Fauser, A.A., Gorin, N.C., Gros, O., Gros, P., Laurent, J. C., Poncelet, P., Remandet, B., Richer, G., and Vidal, H. Efficiency and tolerance of the treatment with immuno-A-chain-toxins in human bone marrow transplantations. In *Monoclonal Antibodies for Cancer Detection and Therapy.* Edited by R.W. Baldwin and V.S. Byers. Academic Press; Harcourt Brace Jovanovich, New York, 1985, pp. 223-248.

18. Myers, C. The use of immunotoxins to eliminate tumor cells from human leukaemic marrow autografts. In *Monoclonal Antibodies for Cancer Detection and Therapy.* Edited by R.W. Baldwin and V.S. Byers. Academic Press; Harcourt Brace Jovanovich, New York, 1985, pp. 249-267.

19. Jansen, F.K., Blythman, H.E., Carriere, D., Cassellas, P., Gros, O., Laurent, J.C., Paolucci, F., Pau, B., Poncelet, P., Richer, G., Vidal, H., and Voisin, G.A. Immunotoxins: Hybrid molecules combining high specificity and potent cytotoxicity. Immunol. Rev. 62: 185-216, 1982.

20. Jansen, F.K., Casellas, P., Blythman, H.E., Bourrie, B., Derocq, J-M., Dussossoy, D., and Laurent, G. Ricin-A-chain immunotoxins in hematologic malignancies. Intl. Conf. on Monoclonal Antibody Immunoconjugates for Cancer, San Diego, March, 1986, p. 22.

21. Lamb, F.I., Roberts. L.M., and Lord, J.M. Nucleotide sequence of cloned cDNA coding for preproricin. Eur. J. Biochem. 148: 265-270, 1985.

22. Greenfield, L., Bjorn, M.J., Horn, G., Fong, D., Buck, G.A., Collier, R.J., and Kaplan, D.A. Nucleotide sequence of the structural gene for diphtheria toxin carried by corynebacteriophage beta. Proc. Natl. Acad. Sci. USA 80: 6853-6857, 1983.

23. Barbieri, L., and Stripe, F. Ribosome-inactivating proteins from plants: properties and possible uses. Cancer Surveys 1: 489-520, 1982.

24. Uckun, F.M., Ramakrishnan, S., and Houston, L.L. Immunotoxin-mediated elimination of clonogenic tumor cells in the presence of human bone marrow. J. Immunol. 134: 2010-2016, 1985.

25. Uckun, F.M., Houston, L.L., Vallera, D.A. Pokeweed antiviral protein immunotoxins and their clinical potential for systemic prophylaxis/treatment of major complications of bone marrow transplantation in acute lymphoblastic leukemia. In *Membrane-Mediated Cytotoxicity*, New Series, Vol. 45. Edited by B. Bonavida and R.J. Collier. Alan R. Liss, New York, 1987, pp. 243-256.

26. Ramakrishnan, S., and Houston, L.L. Prevention of growth of leukemia cells in mice by monoclonal antibodies directed against Thy 1.1 antigen disulfide linked to two ribosomal inhibitors: pokeweed antiviral protein and ricin A chain. Cancer Res. 44: 1398-1404, 1984.

27. Thorpe, P.E., Brown, A.N.F., Bremmer, J.A.G., Jr., Foxwell, B.M.J., and Stirpe, F. An immunotoxin composed of monoclonal anti-Thy 1.1 antibody and a ribosome-inactivating protein from *Saponaria officinalis*: potent antitumor effects in vitro and in vivo. JNCI 75: 151-159, 1985.

28. Uckun, F.M., Gajl-Peczalska, K.G., Kersey, J.H., Houston, L.L., and Vallera, D.A. Use of a novel colony assay to evaluate the cytotoxicity of an immunotoxin containing pokeweed antiviral protein against blast progenitor cells freshly obtained from patients with common B-lineage acute lymphoblastic leukemia. J. Exp. Med. 163: 347-368, 1986.

29. Manske, J.M., Buchsbaum, D.J., Azemove, S.M., Hanna, D.E., and Vallera, D.A. Antigenic modulation by anti-CD5 immunotoxins. J. Immunol. 136: 4721-4728, 1986.

30. Morgan, A.C. Jr., Schroff, R.W., Hwang, K.M., and Pavanasasivam, G. Monoclonal antibody therapy of cancer: Parameters which affect the efficacy of immunotoxins. In *Monoclonal Antibody Therapy of Human Cancer*. Edited by K.A. Foon and A.C. Morgan, Jr. Martinus Nijhoff Publishing, Boston, 1985, pp. 1-22.

31. Seon, B.K. Specific killing of human T-leukemia cells by immunotoxins prepared with ricin A chain and monoclonal anti-human T-cell leukemia antibodies. Cancer Res. 44: 259-264, 1984.

32. Stong, R.C., Uckun, F.M., Youle, R.J., Kersey, J.H., and Vallera, D.A. Use of multiple T-cell directed intact ricin immunotoxins for autologous bone marrow transplantation. Blood 66: 627-635, 1985.

33. Vallera, D.A., Ash, R.C., Zanjani, E.D., Kersey, J.H., LeBien, T.L., Beverley, P.C.L., Neville, D.M. Jr., and Youle, R.J. Anti-T cell reagents for human bone marrow transplantation: Ricin linked to three monoclonal antibodies. Science 222: 8512-8515, 1983.

34. Uckun, F.M., Gajl-Peczalska, K., Myers, D.E., Kersey, J.H., Colvin, M., and Vallera, D.A. Marrow purging in autologous bone marrow transplantation for T-lineage acute lymphoblastic leukemia: Efficacy of ex vivo treatment with immunotoxins and 4-hydroperoxycyclophosphamide against fresh leukemia marrow progenitor cells. Blood 69: 361-366, 1987.

35. Casellas, P., Brown, J.P., Gros, O., Gros, P., Hellstrom, I., Jansen, F.K., Poncelet, P., Roncucci, R., Vidal, H., and Hellstrom, K.E. Human melanoma cells can be killed in vitro by an immunotoxin specific for melanoma-associated antigen p97. Int. J. Cancer 30: 437-443, 1982.

36. Raso, V., Ritz, J., Busala, M., and Schlossman, S. Monoclonal antibody-ricin A chain conjugate selectively cytotoxic for cells bearing the common acute lymphoblastic leukemia antigen. Cancer Res. 42: 457-464, 1982.

37. Youle, R.J., and Neville, D.M. Jr. Anti-Thy 1.2 monoclonal antibody linked to ricin is a potent cell type specific toxin. Proc. Natl. Acad. Sci. USA 77: 5483-5486, 1980.

38. Lambert, J.M., Senter, P.D., Yau-Young, A., Blattler, W.A., and Goldmacher, V.S. Purified immunotoxins that are reactive with human lymphoid cells: Monoclonal antibodies conjugated to the ribosome-inactivating proteins gelonin and the pokeweed antiviral proteins. J. Biol. Chem. 260: 12035-12041, 1985.

39. Letvin, N.L., Goldmacher, V.S., Ritz, J., Yetz, J.M., Schlossman, S.F., and Lambert, J.M. In vivo administration of lymphocyte-specific monoclonal antibodies in nonhuman primates. In vivo stability of disulfide-linked immunotoxin conjugates. J. Clin. Invest. 77: 977-984, 1986.

40. Blakey, D.C., and Thorpe, P.E. Effect of chemical deglycosylation on the in vivo fate of ricin A-chain. Cancer Drug Delivery 3: 189-196, 1986.

41. Uckun, F.M., Stong, R.C., Youle, R.J., and Vallera, D.A. Combined ex vivo treatment with immunotoxins and mafosfamid: A novel immunochemotherapeutic approach for elimination of neoplastic T cells from autologous marrow grafts. J. Immunol. 134: 3504-3515, 1985.

42. Weil-Hillman, G., Uckun, F.M., and Vallera, D.A. Combined immunochemotherapy of human solid tumors in nude mice. Cancer Res. 47: 579-585, 1987.

43. Buchsbaum, D.J., Nelson, L.A., Hanna, D.E., and Vallera, D.A. Human leukemia cell binding and killing by anti-CD5 radioimmunotoxins. Int. J. Radiation Oncology Biol. Phys. 13: 1701-1712, 1987.

44. O'Reilly, R.J. Allogeneic bone marrow transplantation, current status and future directions. Blood 62: 941-964, 1983.

45. Gale, R.P., Kersey, J.H., Bortin, M.M., Dicke, K.A., Good, R.A., Zwaan, F.E., and Rimm, A.A. Bone marrow transplantation for acute lymphoblastic leukemia. Lancet 2: 663-667, 1983.

46. Thomas, E.D. Bone marrow transplantation: A lifesaving applied art. JAMA 249: 2528-2536, 1983.

47. Glucksberg, H., Storb, R., Fefer, A., Buckner, C.D., Neimer, P.E., Clift, R.A., Lerner, K.G., and Thomas, E.D. Clinical manifestations of graft-versus-host disease in human recipients of marrow from HLA-matched sibling donors. Transplantation 18: 295-304, 1974.

48. Filipovich, A.H., Vallera, D.A., Youle, R.J., Haake, R., Blazar, B.R., Neville, D.M., Jr., Ramsay, N.K.C., McGlave, P., and Kersey, J.H. Graft-versus-host disease prevention in allogeneic bone marrow transplantation. A pilot study using immunotoxins for T cell depletion in donor bone marrow. Transplantation 44: 62-69, 1987.

49. Martin, P.J., Hansen, J.A., Storb, R., and Thomas, E.D. A clinical trial of in vitro depletion of T cells in donor marrow for prevention of acute graft-versus-host disease. Transplant. Proc. 17: 486, 1985.

50. O'Reilly, R.J., Collins, N., Brochstein, J., Dinsmore, R., Kirkpatrick, D., Kernan, N., Siena, S., Shank, B., Wolf, L., Dupont, B., and Reisner, Y. Transplantation of marrow-depleted T cells by soybean lectin agglutination and E-rosette depletion: major histocompatibility complex-related graft resistance in leukemia transplant recipients. Transplant. Proc. 17: 455, 1985.

51. Sondel, P.M., Bozdech, M.J., Trigg, M.E., Hong, R., Finlay, J.L., Kohler, P.C., Longo, W., Hank, J.A., Billing, R., Steeves, R., and Flynn, B. Additional immunosuppression allows engraftment following HLA-mismatched T cell-depleted bone marrow transplantation for leukemia. Transplant. Proc. 17: 460, 1985.

52. Kapoor, N., Filler, J., Engelhard, D., Jung, L., Larson, G., DeBault, L., and Good, R.A. Role of T cells in marrow transplantation for aplastic anemia. Exp. Hematol. 12: 473, 1984.

53. Vallera, D.A., Soderling, C.C.B., Carlson, G., and Kersey, J.H. Bone marrow transplantation across major histocompatibility barriers in mice. II. T cell requirement for engraftment in TLI-conditioned recipients. Transplantation 33: 243-248, 1982.

54. Soderling, C.C.B., Song, C.W., Blazar, B.R., and Vallera, D.A. A correlation between conditioning and engraftment in recipients of MHC mismatched T cell depleted murine bone marrow transplants. J. Immunol. 135: 941-946, 1985.

55. Weiden, P., Sullivan, K.M., Flournay, N., Storb, R., and Thomas, E.D. Anti-leukemic effect of chronic graft-versus-host disease. Contribution to improved survival after allogeneic transplantation. N. Engl. J. Med. 304: 1529-1533, 1981.

56. Uckun, F.M., Azemove, S.M., Myers, D.E., and Vallera, D.A. Anti-CD2 (T, p50) intact ricin immunotoxins for GVHD-prophylaxis in allogeneic bone marrow transplantation. Leukemia Res. 10: 145-153, 1985.

57. Poncelet, P., and Carayon, P. Cytofluorometric quantification of cell-surface antigens by indirect immunofluorescence using monoclonal antibodies. J. Immunol. Methods 85: 65-74, 1985.

58. Gorin, N.C., Douay, L., Laporte, J.P., Lopez, M., Zittoum, R., Rio, B., David, R., Stachowiak, J., Jansen, F.K., Casellas, P., Poncelet, P., Liance, M.C., Vioson, G.A., Salmon, C., LeBlanc, G., Deloux, J., Najma, A., and Duhamel, G. Autologous bone marrow transplantation with marrow decontaminated by immunotoxin T101 in the treatment of leukemia and lymphoma: first clinical observations. Cancer Treat. Rep. 69: 953-959, 1985.

59. Thorpe, P.E., Mason, D.W., Brown, A.N.F., Simmonds, S.J., Ross, W.C., Cumber, A.J., and Forrester, J.A. Selective killing of malignant cells in a leukaemic rat bone marrow using an antibody-ricin conjugate. Nature 297: 594-596, 1982.

60. Krolick, K.A., Uhr, J.W., and Vitetta, E.S. Selective killing of leukaemia cells by antibody-toxin conjugates: Implications for autologous bone marrow transplantation. Nature 295: 604-605, 1982.

61. Stong, R.C., Youle, R.J., and Vallera, D.A. Elimination of clonogenic T-leukemic cells from human bone marrow using anti-M 65,000 protein immunotoxins. Cancer Res. 44: 3000-3006, 1984.

62. Filipovich, A.H., Ramsay, N.K.C., Hurd, D., Stong, R., Youle, R., Vallera, D.A., and Kersey, J.H. Autologous bone marrow transplantation (BMT) for T cell leukemia and lymphoma using marrow cleaning with anti-T cell immunotoxins. Autologous BMT Meeting, University degli Studi di Parma, Parma, Italy, 1985.

63. Casellas, P., Canat, X., Fauser, A.A., Gros, O., Laurent, G., Poncelet, P., and Jansen, F.K. Optimal elimination of leukemia T cells from human bone marrow with T101-ricin A-chain immunotoxin. Blood 65: 289-297, 1985.

64. Medical Oncology Unit, St. Bartholomew's Hospital, London (Drs. T.A. Lister, A.Z.S. Rohatiner, M.J. Barnett, et al.). Myers, C. The use of immunotoxins to eliminate tumor cells from human leukaemic marrow autografts. In *Monoclonal Antibodies for Cancer Detection and Therapy*. Edited by R.W. Baldwin and V.S. Byers. Academic Press; Harcourt Brace Jovanovich, New York, 1985, pp. 249-267.

65. Kersey, J.H., Weisdorf, D., Nesbit, M.E., et al. Comparison of autologous and allogeneic bone marrow transplantation for treatment of high-risk refractory acute lymphoblastic leukemia. N. Engl. J. Med. 317: 461-467, 1987.

66. Cudkowicz, G., and Bennett, M. Peculiar immunobiology of bone marrow allografts. I: Graft rejection by irradiated responder mice. J. Exp. Med. 134: 83-100, 1971.

67. Rubin, P. The Franz Buschke lecture: late effects of chemotherapy and radiation therapy: a new hypothesis. Int. J. Radiat. Oncol. Biol. Phys. 10: 5-34, 1984.

68. Blythman, H.E., Casellas, P., Gros, O., Gros, P., Jansen, F.K., Paolucci, F., Paul, B., and Vidal, H. Immunotoxins: Hybrid molecules of monoclonal antibodies and a toxin subunit specifically kill tumour cells. Nature 290: 145-146, 1981.

69. Neville, D.M., Jr., and Youle, R.J. Monoclonal antibody-ricin or ricin A chain

hybrids: Kinetic analysis of cell killing for tumor therapy. Immunol. Rev. 62: 75-91, 1982.

70. Thorpe, P.E., and Ross, W.C.J. The preparation and cytotoxic properties of antibody-toxin conjugates. Immunol. Rev. 62: 119-158, 1982.

71. Vitetta, E.S., Krolick, K.A., and Uhr, J.W. Neoplastic B cells as targets for antibody-ricin A chain. Immunol. Rev. 62: 159-183, 1982.

72. Laurent, G., Pris, J., Farcet, J-P., Carayon, P., Blythman, H., Casellas, P., Poncelet, P., and Jansen, F.K. Effects of therapy with T101 ricin A-chain immunotoxin in two leukemia patients. Blood 67: 1680-1687, 1986.

73. Spitler, L.E., del Rio, M., Khentigan, A., et al. Therapy of patients with malignant melanoma using a monoclonal antimelanoma antibody-ricin A chain immunotoxin. Cancer Res. 47: 1717-1723, 1987.

74. Weil-Hillman, G., Runge, W., Jansen, F.K., and Vallera, D.A. Cytotoxic effect of anti-M, 67,000 protein immunotoxins on human tumors in a nude mouse model. Cancer Res. 45: 1328-1336, 1985.

75. Pressman, D., Day, E.D., and Blau, M. The use of paired labeling in the determination of tumor-localizing antibodies. Cancer Res. 17: 845-850, 1957.

76. Marchalonis, J.J. An enzyme method for the trace iodination of immunoglobulins and other proteins. Biochem. J. 113: 299-305, 1969.

77. Mach, J.P., Chatal, J.F., Lumbroso, J-D., Buchegger, F., Forni, M., Ritschard, J., Berche, C., Douillard, J-Y., Stephan, C., Heryln, M., Steplewzki, Z., and Koprowski, H. Tumor localization in patients by radiolabeled monoclonal antibodies against colon carcinoma. Cancer Res. 43: 5593-5600, 1983.

78. Buchsbaum, D.J., Randall, B., Hanna, D., Chandler, R., Loken, M., and Johnson, E. Comparison of the distribution and binding of monoclonal antibodies labeled with [131]Iodine or [111]Indium. Eur. J. Nucl. Med. 10: 398-402, 1985.

79. Deland, F.H., Kim, E.E., Simmons, G., and Goldenberg, D.M. Imaging approach in radioimmunodetection. Cancer Res. 40: 3046-3049, 1980.

80. Woolfenden, J.M., and Larson, S.M. Radiolabeled monoclonal antibodies for imaging and therapy. In *Monoclonal Antibody Therapy of Human Cancer*. Edited by K.A. Foon and A.C. Morgan, Jr. Martinus Nijhoff, Boston, 1985, pp. 139-160.

81. Badger, C.C., Krohn, K.A., Peterson, A.V., Shulman, H., and Bernstein, I.D. Experimental radiotherapy of murine lymphoma with [131]I-labeled anti-Thy 1.1 monoclonal antibody. Cancer Res. 45: 1536-1544, 1985.

82. Zalcberg, J.R., Thompson, C.H., Lichtenstein, M., and McKenzie, I.F.C. Tumor immunotherapy in the mouse with the use of [131]I-labeled monoclonal antibodies. JNCI 72: 697-704, 1984.

83. Halpern, S.E., and Dillman, R.O. Human studies with radiometal conjugates. Int'l Conf. on MoAb Immunoconjugates for Cancer, San Diego, March 1986, p. 19.

84. Halpern, S.E., Dillman, R.O., Witztum, K.F., Shega, J.F., Hagan, P.L., Burrows, W.M., Dillman, J.B., Clutter, M.L., Sobol, R.E., Frincke, J.M., Bartholomew, R. M., David, G.S., and Carlo, D.J. Radioimmunodetection of melanoma utilizing

[111]In-96.5 monoclonal antibody: a preliminary report. Radiology 155: 493-499, 1985.

85. Hnatowich, D.J., Layne, W.W., Childs, R.L., Lanteigne, D., and Davis, M.A. Radioactive labeling on antibody: a simple and efficient method. Science 220: 613-615, 1983.

86. Wessels, B.W., and Rogus, R.D. Radionuclide selection and model absorbed dose calculations for radiolabeled tumor associated antibodies. Med. Phys. 11: 638-645, 1984.

87. Order, S.E., Klein, J.L., Leichner, P.K., Frincke, J., Lollo, C., and Carlo, D.J. [90]Yttrium-antiferritin—A new therapeutic radiolabeled antibody. Int. J. Radiat. Oncol. Biol. Phys. 12: 277-281, 1986.

88. Rhodes, B.A., Zamora, P.O., Newell, K.D., and Valdez, E.F. [99m]Technetium-labeling of murine monoclonal antibody fragments. J. Nuc. Med. 27: 685-693, 1986.

89. Pressman, D., and Korngold, L. In vivo localization of anti-Wagner-osteogenic-sarcoma antibodies. Cancer 6: 619-623, 1953.

90. Goldenberg, D.M., Deland, F.H., Kim, E., Bennett, S., Primus, F.J., van Nagell, J.R.I., Estes, N., DeSimone, P., and Rayburn, P. Use of radiolabeled antibodies to carcinoembryonic antigen for the detection and localization of diverse cancers by external photoscanning. New Engl. J. Med. 298: 1384-1388, 1978.

91. Dykes, P.W., Hine, K.R., Bradwell, A.R., Blackburn, J.C., Reeder, T.A., Drok, Z., and Booth, S.N. Localization of tumor deposits by external scanning after injection of radiolabeled anti-carcinoembryonic antigen. Br. Med. J. 280: 220-222, 1980.

92. Goldenberg, D.M., Kim, E.E., Deland, F.H., Spremulli, E., Nelson, M.O., Gockerman, J.P., Primus, F.J., Corgan, R.L., and Alpert. E. Clinical studies on the radioimmunodetection of tumors containing alpha-fetoprotein. Cancer 45: 2500-2505, 1980.

93. Halsall, A.K., Fairweather, D.S., Bradwell, A.R., Blackburn, J.C., Dykes, P.W., Howell, A., Reeder, A., and Hine, K.R. Localization of malignant germ-cell tumours by external scanning after injection of radiolabeled anti-alpha-feto-protein. Br. Med. J. 283: 942-944, 1981.

94. Goldenberg, D.M., Kim, E.E., and Deland, F.H. Human chorionic gonado-tropin radioantibodies in the radioimmunodetection of cancer and for the disclosure of occult metastases. Proc. Natl. Acad. Sci. USA 78: 7754-7758, 1981.

95. Beierwaltes, W.H., and Khazaeli, M.B. Radioimmunotherapy of cancer: Historical perspectives and prospects for the future. In *Radioimmunoimaging and Radioimmunotherapy*. Edited by S.W. Burchiel and B.A. Rhodes. Elsevier, New York, 1983, pp. 419-435.

96. Bale, W.F., Spar, I.L., and Goodland, R.L. Experimental radiation therapy of tumors with [131]I-carrying antibodies to fibrin. Cancer Res. 20: 1488-1494, 1960.

97. Spar, I.L., Bale, W.F., Marrack, D., Dewey, W.C., McCardle, R.J., and Harper, P.V. [131]I-labeled antibodies to human fibrinogen. Diagnostic studies and therapeutic trials. Cancer 20: 865-870, 1967.

98. Order, S.E., Klein, J.L., Ettinger, D., Alderson, P., Siegelman, S., and Leichner, P. Phase I-II study of radiolabeled antibody integrated in the treatment of primary hepatic malignancies. Int. J. Rad. Oncol. Biol. Phys. 6: 703-710, 1980.

99. Order, S.E., Klein, J.L., Leichner, P.K., Self, S., Leibel, S., and Ettinger, D. $^{131}$I-radiolabeled antibody (antiferritin) in the treatment of hepatoma—an update. Proc. Am. Soc. Clin. Oncol. 3: 138, 1984.

100. Order, S.E., and Leibel, S.A. Radiolabeled antibodies in the treatment of primary liver cancer. Appl. Radiol. 13: 67-73, 1984.

101. Order, S.E., Stillwagon, G.B., Klein, J.L., Leichner, P.K., Siegelman, S.S., Fishman, E.K., Ettinger, D.K., Haulk, T., Kopher, K., Finney, K., Surdyke, M., Self, S., and Leibel, S. $^{131}$Iodine-antiferritin, a new treatment modality in hepatoma: a radiation therapy oncology group study. J. Clin. Oncol. 3: 1573-1582, 1985.

102. Mach, J-P., Buchegger, F., Forni, M., Ritschar, J., Berche, C., Lumbroso, J.D., Schreyer, M., Girardet, C., Accolla, R.S., and Carrel, S. Use of radiolabeled monoclonal anti-CEA antibodies for the detection of human carcinomas by external photoscanning and tomoscintigraphy. Immunol. Today 2: 239-249, 1981.

103. Moldofsky, P.J., Powe, J., Mulhern, C.B., Jr., Hammond, N., Sears, H.F., Gatenby, R.A., Steplewski, Z., and Loprowski, H. Metastatic colon carcinoma detected with radiolabeled F(ab')$_2$ monoclonal antibody fragments. Radiology 149: 549-555, 1983.

104. Chatal, J-F., Saccavini, J-C., Fumoleau, P., Douillard, J.V., Curtet, C., Kremer, M., Le Mevel, B., and Koprowski, H. Immunoscintigraphy of colon carcinoma. J. Nucl. Med. 25: 307-314, 1984.

105. March, J-P., Buchegger, F., Grob, J-Ph., vonFliedner, V., Carrel, S., Barrelet, L., Bishof-Delaloye, A., and Delaloye, B. Improvement of colon carcinoma imaging: from polyclonal anti-CEA antibodies and static photoscanning to monoclonal Fab fragments and ECT. In *Monoclonal Antibodies for Cancer Detection and Therapy*. Edited by R.W. Baldwin and V.S. Byers. Academic Press, London, 1985, pp. 53-64.

106. Larson, S.M., Brown, J.P., Wright, P.W., Carrasquillo, J.A., Hellstrom, I., and Hellstrom, K.E. Imaging of melanoma with $^{131}$I-labeled monoclonal antibodies. J. Nucl. Med. 24: 123-129, 1983.

107. Larson, S.M., Carrasquillo, J.A., Krohn, K.A., Brown, J.P., McGuffin, P.W., Ferens, J.M., Graham, M.M., Hill, L.D., Beaumier, P.L., Hellstrom, K.E., and Hellstrom, I. Localization of $^{131}$I-labeled p97-specific Fab fragments in human melanoma as a basis for radiotherapy. J. Clin. Invest. 72: 2101-2114, 1983.

108. Delaloye, B., Bischof-Delaloye, A., Buchegger, F., vonFliedner, V., Grob, J.P., Volant, J.C., Pettavel, J., and Mach, J-P. Detection of colorectal carcinoma by emission computerized tomography after injection of $^{123}$I-labeled Fab or F(ab')$_2$ fragments from monoclonal anti-CEA antibodies. J. Clin. Invest. 77: 301-311, 1986.

109. Dorrington, K.J., and Painter, R.H. Biological activities of the constant region of immunoglobulin G. In *Progress in Immunology III*. Edited by T.E. Mandel. North Holland, New York, 1977, pp. 298-305.

110. Buchegger, F., Mach, J-P., Leonnard, P., and Carrel, S. Selective tumor localization of radiolabeled anti-human melanoma monoclonal antibody fragment demonstrated in the nude mouse model. Cancer 58: 655-662, 1986.

111. Lashford, L., Jones, D., Pritchard, J., Gordon, I., Breatnach, F., and Kem-
stead, J.T. Therapeutic application of radiolabeled MoAb UJ13A in children with disseminated neuroblastoma. Cancer Drug. Del. 2: 233, 1985.

112. Klein, J.L., Sandoz, J.W., Kopher, K.A., Leichner, P.K., and Order, S.E.
Detection of specific anti-antibodies in patients treated with radiolabeled
antibody. Int. J. Rad. Oncol. Biol. Phys. 12: 939-943, 1986.

113. Horan Hand P., Nuti, M., Colcher, D., and Schlom, J. Definition of antigenic heterogeneity and modulation among human mammary carcinoma
cell populations using monoclonal antibodies to tumor-associated antigens.
Cancer Res. 43: 728-735, 1983.

114. Kufe, D.W., Nadler, L., Sargent, L., Shapiro, H., Hand, P., Austin, F., Colcher, D., and Schlom, J. Biological behavior of human breast carcinoma-
associated antigens expressed during cellular proliferation. Cancer Res. 43:
851-857, 1983.

115. Dillman, R.O., Beauregard, J.C., Sobol, R.E., Royston, I., Bartholomew,
R.M., Hagan, P.S., and Halpern, S.E. Lack of radioimmunodetection and
complications associated with monoclonal anti-carcinoembryonic antigen
antibody cross-reactivity with an antigen on circulating cells. Cancer Res.
44: 2213-2218, 1984.

116. Epentos, A.A. (on behalf of the Hammersmith Oncology Group). Clinical
results with regional antibody-guided irradiation. Cancer Drug. Del. 2: 233,
1985.

117. Epentos, A.A. Intraperitoneal therapy of ovarian cancer. Int'l Conf on
Monoclonal Antibody Immunoconjugates for Cancer. San Diego, March
1986, p. 17.

118. Gatter, K.C., Abdulaziz, Z., Beverley, P., Corvalan, J.R.F., Ford, C., Lane,
E.B., Mota, M., Nash, J.R.G., Pulford, K., Stein, H., Taylor-Papadimitriou,
J., Woodhouse, C., and Mason, D.Y. Use of monoclonal antibodies for the
histopathological diagnosis of human malignancy. J. Clin. Pathol. 35: 1253-
1267, 1982.

119. Corvalan, J.R.F., Axton, C.A., Brandon, D.R., Smith, W., and Woodhouse,
C. Classification of anti-CEA monoclonal antibodies. Protides Biol. Fluids
31: 921-924, 1984.

120. Hockey, M.S., Ford, C.H.J., Newman, C., Corvalan, J.R.F., Rowland, G.F.,
Stokes, H.J., Thompson, H., and Fielding, J.W.L. The immunohistochemical localization of carcinoembryonic antigen (CEA) with monoclonal antibody in gastric adenocarcinomas. Br. J. Surg. 70: 300, 1983.

121. Uadia, P., Blair, A.H., Ghose, T., and Ferrone, S. Uptake of methotrexate
linked to polyclonal and monoclonal antimelanoma antibodies by a human
melanoma cell line. JNCI 74: 29-35, 1985.

122. Johns, D.G., and Bertino, J.R. Folate antagonists. In Cancer Medicine, 2nd
ed. Edited by J.F. Holland and E. Frei, III. Lea and Febiger, Philadelphia,
1982, pp. 775-790.

123. Mathé, G., Loc, T.B., and Bernard, J. Effect sur la leucemie 1210 de la souris, d'une combinaison par diazotation d'amethopterine et de γ-globulines de hamsters porteurs de cette leucemie par heterographe. C.R. Acad. Sci. 246: 1626-1628, 1958.

124. Ghose, T., Blair, A.H., Uadia, P., Kulkarni, P.N., Goundalkar, A., Mezei, M., and Ferrone, S. Antibodies as carriers of cancer chemotherapeutic agents. Ann. NY Acad. Sci. 446: 213-227, 1985.

125. Sela, M., and Hurwitz, E. Conjugates of antibodies with cytotoxic drugs. In *Immunoconjugates: Antibody Conjugates in Radioimaging and Therapy of Cancer.* Edited by C-W. Vogel. Oxford University Press, New York, 1987 pp. 189-216.

126. Hurwitz, E., Arnon, R., Sahar, E., and Danon, Y. A conjugate of adriamycin and monoclonal antibodies to Thy-1 antigen inhibits human neuroblastoma cells in vitro. Ann. NY Acad. Sci. 417: 125-136, 1983.

127. Dillman, R.O., Shawler, D.L., Johnson, D.E., Meyer, D.L., Koziol, J.A., and Frincke, J.M. Preclinical trials with combinations and conjugates of T101 monoclonal antibody and doxorubicin. Cancer Res. 46: 4886-4891, 1986.

128. Tsukada, Y., Hurwitz, E., Kashi, R., Sela, M., Hibi, N., Hara, A., and Hirai, H. Chemotherapy by intravenous administration of conjugates of daunomycin with monoclonal and conventional anti-rat alphafetoprotein antibodies. Proc. Natl. Acad. Sci. USA 79: 7896-7899, 1982.

129. Hurwitz, E., Kashi, R., Burowsky, D., Arnon, R., and Haimovich, J. Site-directed chemotherapy with a drug bound to anti-idiotypic antibody to a lymphoma cell-surface IgM. Int. J. Cancer 31: 745-748, 1983.

130. Manabe, Y., Tsubota, T., Haruta, Y., Okazaki, M., Haisa, S., Nakamura, K., and Kimura, I. Production of a monoclonal antibody-bleomycin conjugate utilizing dextran T40 and the antigen-targeting cytotoxicity of the conjugate. Biochem. Biophys. Res. Commun. 115: 1009-1014, 1983.

131. Kimura, I., Ohnoshi, T., Tsubota, T., Sato, Y., Kobayashi, T., and Abe, S. Production of tumor antibody-neocarzinostatin (NCS) conjugate and its biological activities. Cancer Immunol. Immunother. 7: 235-242, 1980.

132. Rowland, G.F., and Simmonds, R.G. Effects of monoclonal antibody-drug conjugates on human tumour cell cultures and xenografts. In *Monoclonal Antibodies for Cancer Detection and Therapy.* Edited by R.W. Baldwin and V.S. Byers. Academic Press, London, 1985, pp. 345-364.

133. Rowland, G.F., Axton, C.A., Baldwin, R.W., Brown, J.P., Corvalan, J.R.F., Embleton, M.J., Gore, V.A., Hellstrom, I., Hellstrom, K.E., Jacobs, E., Marsden, C.H., Pimm, M.V., Simmonds, R.G., and Smith, W. Anti-tumor properties of vindisine-monoclonal antibody conjugates. Cancer Immunol. Immunother. 19: 1-7, 1985.

134. Tung, E., Goust, J.M., Chen, W.Y., Kang, S.S., Wang, I.Y., and Wang, A.C. Cytotoxic effect of anti-idiotype antibody-chlorambucil conjugates against human lymphoblastoid cells. Immunology 50: 57-64, 1983.

135. Garnett, M.C., Embleton, M.J., Jacobs, E., and Baldwin, R.W. Preparation and properties of a drug-carrier-antibody conjugate showing selective antibody directed cytotoxicity in vitro. Int. J. Cancer 31: 661-670, 1983.

136. Garnett, M.C., and Baldwin, R.W. An improved synthesis of a methotrexate-albumin-791T/36 monoclonal antibody conjugate cytotoxic to human osteogenic sarcoma cell lines. Cancer Res. 46: 2407-2412, 1986.

137. Gallego, J., Price, M.R., and Baldwin, R.W. Preparation of four daunomycin-monoclonal antibody 791T/36 conjugates with anti-tumour activity. Int. J. Cancer 33: 734-744, 1984.

138. Tsukada, Y., Kato, Y., Umemoto, N., Takeda, Y., Hara, T., and Hirai, H. An anti-alphafetoprotein-daunomycin conjugate with a novel poly-L-glutamic acid derivative as intermediate drug carrier. JNCI 73: 721-729, 1984.

139. Arnon, R., and Hurwitz, E. Monoclonal antibodies as carriers for immunotargeting of drugs. In *Monoclonal Antibodies for Cancer Detection and Therapy*. Edited by R.W. Baldwin and V.S. Byers. Academic Press, London, 1985, pp. 365-383.

140. Baldwin, R.W. Design and development of drug-monoclonal antibody 791T/36 conjugate for cancer therapy. In *Monoclonal Antibody Therapy of Human Cancer*. Edited by K.A. Foon and A.C. Morgan, Jr. Martinus Nijhoff, Boston, 1985, pp. 23-56.

141. Marsh, J.W., and Neville, D.M., Jr. Kinetic comparison of ricin immunotoxins: Biricin conjugate has potentiated cytotoxicity. Biochemistry 25: 4461-4467, 1986.

142. Thorpe, P.E., Detre, S.I., Foxwell, B.M., et al. Modification of the carbohydrate in ricin with metaperiodate-cyanoborohydride mixtures. Effects on toxicity and in vivo distribution. Eur. J. Biochem. 147: 197-206, 1985.

143. Blazar, B.R., Widmer, M.B., Soderling, C.C.B., et al. Augmentation of donor bone marrow engraftment in histoincompatible murine recipients by granulocyte/macrophage colony-stimulating factor. Blood 71 (Feb.): 1988.

144. Blazar, B.R., Soderling, C.C.B., Koo, G.C., and Vallera, D.A. Absence of a facilitory role for NK 1.1 positive donor cells in engraftment across a major histocompatibility barrier in mice. Transplantation 1988 (in press).

145. Byers, V., Kernan, N., Henslee, J., et al. A phase I study using pan T lymphocyte-ricin A chain immunotoxin to treat graft-versus-host disease. Second International Conference on Monoclonal Antibody Immunoconjugates for Cancer, San Diego, 1987, p. 40.

# Part II

**Interleukins and Cells as Regulators for Immune Functions and Cancer Therapy**

# 3

## Interleukin-1 and Host Defense Against Malignant Cells

James W. Mier and Charles A. Dinarello / Tufts University School of Medicine and New England Medical Center Hospital, Boston, Massachusetts

### I. INTRODUCTION

Throughout the animal kindgom, one observes the elaborate measures and strategies which various species have developed in order to combat life-threatening microbial invasion. Clearly, before the antibiotic era, the outcome of this struggle between host and microbe was determined by the ability of each to develop evasive action. Mammals, in particular, have developed a wide variety of responses which both signal the onset of microbial invasion and trigger host defense mechanisms. Some of the defenses include behavioral changes. For example, animals when injured or ill, often will stop eating, reduce activity, conserve energy output, and increase sleeptime. Despite these and substantial metabolic and hematological defense responses, the host is still highly vulnerable to infection. A similar case can be made for malignant disease.

Since recorded time, efforts have been targeted at augmentation of various defense mechanisms in order to shift the balance in favor of the host. Interleukin-1 (IL-1), a polypeptide produced by several different tissues is one of the body's key mediators of responses to microbial invasion, inflammation, immunological reaction, injury, and malignant disease. IL-1 is one of the first and most prominent molecules synthesized by the body in response to infection and injury and its biological effects are manifested in nearly every tissue and organ system. The various biological activities of IL-1 fall into two patterns of augmenting host responses: the late components of host defenses are associated with activation of immunocompetent cells and take several days whereas the acute phase responses are not associated with immunocompetent cells and are manifested within hours following a microbial challenge. For example, fever and hepatic acute phase protein synthesis are initiated within hours of the onset of infection or trauma. Slowly evolving diseases such as growth of a tumor are less likely to involve IL-1 until the tumors reach sufficient size to trigger tissue damage. In the present chapter, we will review the biological properties of IL-1 with particular reference as to how this cytokine may play role in defense against malignant cells.

## II.  IMMUNOREGULATORY EFFECTS OF INTERLEUKIN-1

Interleukin-1 (IL-1) mediates virtually every aspect of acute and chronic inflammation. In addition to its inflammatory properties, IL-1 exerts profound effects on the cells of the immune system, amplifying immunoglobulin synthesis as well as various T-cell functions, thereby enhancing the ability of the host to eliminate invading microorganisms. Several investigators have conjectured that these IL-1-mediated effects may also influence the immune response to malignant cells. Evidence supporting an association between host resistance to malignancy and the acute phase response, is, however, highly controversial and is reviewed in detail in subsequent sections. Recently IL-1 has been shown to share several biological properties with tumor necrosis factor (TNF), including the ability to directly suppress the growth of certain tumor cells in vitro and, in some instances, to lyse neoplastic cells. Furthermore, elevated body temperature, one of the major biological effects mediated by IL-1, has inhibitory as well as augmenting effects on various cellular immune functions relevant to the control of tumor metastases. Thus, IL-1 is capable of both directly and indirectly modulating several components of the immune response to infection and neoplasia.

### A.  Effects on B-Cell Differentiation and Immunoglobulin Synthesis

The prospect that a monocyte-derived pyrogen might enhance immunoglobulin synthesis was long suspected because of the well-known association of hypergammaglobulinemia with chronic febrile illness. Interleukin-1 is known to influence immunoglobulin synthesis both through its effects on helper and suppressor T cells and by directly interacting with B lymphocytes. Wood et al. first demonstrated that an endotoxin-inducible macrophage product augmented the production of antisheep erythrocyte antibodies by the splenocytes of nude and T-cell-depleted C57BL/6 mice (1,2). Although this factor was originally termed B-cell-activating factor (BAF), subsequent biochemical analysis demonstrated that it had a molecular weight (15 kD), isoelectric point, and other physical properties similar to those reported for a monocyte-derived factor that enhanced thymocyte proliferation, now known to be IL-1 (3,4). As early as 1979, several investigators had conjectured that the multiple biological effects of endotoxin-primed macrophage supernatants on B-cell differentiation and thymocyte proliferation were mediated by a single polypeptide, a contention now amply verified with the advent of recombinant IL-1 (5,6).

Although IL-1 does not induce the proliferation of resting B cells, it is similar to B-cell growth factor (BCGF) in its ability to induce [$^3$H]thymidine incorporation in B-cell preparations minimally activated by low concentrations of antisurface immunoglobulin antibody (7). The strongest argument supporting a role for IL-1 in B-cell activation stems from a series of experiments with an anti-IL-1 antiserum in which the antibody was shown to markedly inhibit pokeweed mitogen (PWM)-induced B-cell proliferation and the generation of immunoglobulin-secreting cells, as assessed in reverse hemolytic plaque assays (8). The anti-IL-1 antibody was able to abort immunoglobulin synthesis only if added with the PWM and not later, implying that IL-1 was necessary for a B-cell triggering event induced by the lectin. The results of these experiments could be duplicated with isolated Fab fragments. Moreover, the inhibitory effect of the antibody could be overridden by adding purified IL-1 to the peripheral blood mononuclear cells (PBMC) cultures. Repeated absorption of the antiserum with PBMC failed to reduce its suppressive effects, implying that it did not interact directly with the immunoglobulin-secreting cells. These experiments demonstrate that IL-1 directly enhances the proliferation of B cells previously activated by a crosslinking antibody (and presumably by an appropriate antigen) and their subsequent maturation into immunoglobulin-secreting plasma cells by a mechanism that is not entirely dependent upon its interaction with helper T lymphocytes.

Recently, Kurt-Jones et al. described a membrane-associated form of IL-1 present on activated macrophages (9). Although this polypeptide can be solublized with detergent, it appears to be an integral part of the membrane and is both functionally and antigenically identical to the secreted form. Whether such a molecule is merely a biosynthetic intermediate between the cytoplasmic precursor and the secreted form of IL-1 or whether it plays a unique role in the facilitation of antigen presentation by activated macrophages remains to be determined.

## B.  Effects on T Lymphocytes

The factor produced by endotoxin-primed macrophages that induces fever in rabbits (leukocytic pyrogen) copurifies with a similarly derived factor that enhances the proliferation of murine thymocytes to submitogenic concentrations of phytohemagglutinin (PHA) (lymphocyte-activating factor), suggesting that these apparently unrelated phenomena are mediated by the same peptide. The advent of recombinant IL-1 has eliminated all doubt regarding the identity of these factors (6). IL-1 is known to induce both fever and the proliferation of murine thymocytes, the latter of which is due to the induction of the synthesis of IL-2, a T-cell-derived lymphokine easily detected in the supernatant media of thymocytes stimulated with both IL-1 and lectin (10,11). Recombinant IL-1 is likewise able to substitute for macrophages in assays measuring the synthesis of IL-2 by PHA-activated, macrophage-depleted human T lymphocytes (12). IL-1 can also replace macrophages in the induction of murine cytotoxic T lymphocytes (CTL) against allogeneic cells (13). These results suggest that, although IL-1 alone may have little effect on T-cell proliferation, it augments the effects of other stimulatory agents including antigens and mitogenic lectins, causing T-cell proliferation by inducing the synthesis of IL-2, a factor critical for T-cell growth.

## C.  Role in Host Defense Against Neoplasia

### Effects of IL-1 on Natural and IL-2-Induced Cell-Mediated Cytotoxicity

Although human PBMC are generally unable to kill fresh autologous tumor cells, they readily lyse a variety of immortalized cell lines, in particular those of leukemic or lymphoid derivation. The cells responsible for this spontaneous cytolytic activity are natural killer (NK) cells, a distinct lymphocyte subpopulation that constitutes approximately 3% of circulating mononuclear cells (see Ref. 14 for a detailed review). These cells have a characteristic morphology with abundant cytoplasm, a reniform nucleus, and prominent azurophilic cytoplasmic granules. They are highly bouyant and easily isolated from other PBMC with Percoll density gradient centrifugation (15). They have a unique hybrid surface phenotype in that they express membrane antigens otherwise peculiar to monocytes such as M1 as well as T-cell antigens such as T11 (the sheep erythrocyte receptor), but not the T-cell antigen receptor (16). They also have membrane receptors for the Fc portion of IgG.

Natural killer cells are thought to play a major role in the immune surveillance against spontaneously arising malignancies. In support of this view is the fact that NK-deficient strains of mice are extremely prone to develop lymphomas (17), as are humans with the Chediak-Higashi syndrome, a disorder associated with impaired NK function (18). The direct injection of highly purified murine splenic large granular lymphocytes (LGL, or NK cells) into animals previously injected with radiolabelled tumor cells has been shown to markedly reduce the radioactivity of excised lungs, implying that NK cells are able to inhibit the establishment of pulmonary micrometastases (19) and further confirming the critical importance of NK cells in the resistance against malignancy.

One of the more interesting attributes of the NK cell is its sensitivity to immunoregulatory cytokines. Exposure of these cells to interferon, for example, markedly amplifies their tumoricidal activity (20). More recently, the T-cell-derived lymphokine interleukin-2 (IL-2) has been shown to increase the cytolytic activity of both murine and human NK cells against sensitive cell lines and to induce these cells to lyse tumor cell lines resistant to unstimulated NK cells (21,22). The effects of IL-1 on NK cells are somewhat controversial. Dempsey et al. have shown that the incubation of either unfractionated human PBMC or NK cell-enriched lymphocyte populations with monocyte-derived IL-1 has a minimal effect on the cytolytic activity of these cells against any of several target cell lines (22). Similar results have been obtained more recently with recombinant IL-1. However, despite the fact that IL-1 alone appears to be inert in these assays, it has profound effects on NK cells exposed to other immunomodulatory cytokines. The stimulatory effects of both alpha and gamma interferon are markedly enhanced by the addition of IL-1 to the incubating culture medium. This apparent synergy is also evident with interleukin-2 in that lymphocyte preparations exposed to IL-1 and IL-2 in combination are much more active in cytolysis assays than cells exposed only to IL-2. Thus, consistent with its effects on other cellular immune functions, IL-1 acts primarily as an amplifier of the effects of other stimulatory cytokines in the activation of NK cells.

Others have suggested that IL-1 may exert a direct effect on NK cells, which is masked by the IL-1 generated in situ in response to the endotoxin present in most culture media. This argument is supported by experiments with neutralizing anti-IL-1 heteroantisera, which markedly inhibit baseline NK activity, suggesting that small quantities of IL-1 are vital to the function of large granular lymphocytes (LGL) and presumably to host defense against neoplasia (Dinarello et al., unpublished data). The significance of these results is, however, difficult to determine, as even a gross excess of exogenous IL-1 does not override the inhibitory effects of the neutralizing antibody, suggesting that the mechanism of the inhibition of NK activity is independent of the neutralization of IL-1. One possible explanation of these conflicting data is that membrane-associated IL-1, which is thought to play a critical role in cytotoxic T lymphocytes (CTL) induction, may be similarly important in natural cell-mediated cytotoxicity. If this hypothesis is correct, an anti-IL-1 antibody would be expected to have an adverse effect on NK activity that would not necessarily be overcome by the addition of IL-1 to the culture media. Experiments to verify this interpretation are currently underway.

Natural killer activity is frequently depressed in patients with advanced carcinoma. Herman et al. have shown that the monocytes of some of these patients produce reduced amounts of IL-1 in response to endotoxin (23). Furthermore, the NK defect of some of these cancer patients can be restored by preincubating the target cells with IL-1 (24). The ability of purified NK cells to synthesize IL-1 (25), which at least in some circumstances may render the target cell more vulnerable to lysis, suggests that modest amounts of this cytokine are critical for optimal NK cell function and confirms the results of the aforementioned experiments with the anti-IL-1 antiserum.

Natural killer cells comprise but one example of major histocompatibility complex (MHC) unrestricted cytotoxic cells capable of lysing a target cell in the absence of antibody. Grimm et al. have recently demonstrated a population of phenotypically null cells which, although functionally inert prior to activation, acquire tumoricidal activity after a protracted exposure to IL-2 (26). These lymphokine-activated killer (LAK) cells are similar to NK cells in that they are able to lyse target cells that are not antibody coated (antibody-dependent cellular cytotoxicity independent) and to kill tumor cells independent of their expression of Class I histocompatibility antigens (MHC unrestricted). They differ from

NK cells in that they are derived from inert precursors which differentiate into tumoricidal cells only after exposure to high concentrations of IL-2. They have a distinct surface phenotype (27) and are able to lyse fresh autologous tumor cells, which are consistently ignored by NK cells. Furthermore, in contrast to NK cells, which respond within hours to low concentrations (10 units/ml) of IL-2, LAK precursors require extremely high concentrations (1000 units/ml), which are probably never achieved in vivo and prolonged exposure (3-4 days) to develop into tumoricidal effector cells. These important differences suggest that, although LAK cells are readily produced in vitro, they rarely arise in vivo and therefore may not play a role in host defense against neoplasia. In contrast to what has been consistently observed with NK cells, the inclusion of other cytokines in the IL-2-containing culture medium employed to activate LAK cell precursors does not augment the tumoricidal activity of the resultant LAK cells beyond the level achieved with IL-2 alone. In particular, IL-1 does not exert a synergistic effect with IL-2 on LAK cell precursors, which is easily demonstrable with NK cells. However, as was the case with NK cells, anti-IL-1 antisera markedly inhibit the induction of LAK cells, suggesting that modest amounts of IL-1 are critical for IL-2-dependent differentiation of LAK cell precursors into effectors capable of lysing fresh tumor cells (Mier et al., unpublished data).

These experiments and others demonstrate that IL-1 has variable effects on the cells that mediate MHC-unrestricted cytolysis. Exogenous IL-1 has little effect on IL-2-dependent LAK cell induction, although minimal amounts, possibly generated in situ may be essential. IL-1 may be similarly necessary for NK cells to recognize and lyse tumor cells, although, as with LAK cells, the amount of

Table 1  Immunologic Effects of IL-1

---

*T-cell activation*
  IL-2 production, increased IL-2 receptor number or binding

*B-cell activation*
  Synergism with B-cell growth factor (BSF-1/IL-4)
  Induction of interferon-beta-2/hybridoma growth factor/BSF-2

*Natural killer cells*
  Synergism with IL-2 and IFN for tumor killing
  Increased natural killer cell-tumor binding
  Production of IL-1 from NK cells

*Increased lymphokine production*
  IL-2, IL-3, GM-CSF, interferon-beta-1, interferon-beta-2
  interferon-gamma, leukocyte inhibitory migration factor

*Macrophage cytotoxicity*
  Increased IL-1 production

---

IL-1 necessary for optimal NK activity appears to be a quantity easily produced in situ by the involved cells, except in cases of advanced malignancy. In contrast to IL-2-dependent LAK cell induction, which is not influenced by exogenous IL-1, the amplification of NK activity with IL-2 is markedly enhanced by IL-1. Since the concentration of immunomodulatory cytokines achieved locally at the site of a lymphocyte-tumor cell interaction is likely to be extremely small, the amplifying effect of IL-1 on the response of natural killer cells to other cytokines may be important in the immune response to transformed cells. Table 1 summarizes the immunologic effects of IL-1.

## D.  Cytolytic Effects on Neoplastic Cells

In addition to its modulating effects on immunocompetent cells, IL-1 interacts with tumor cells, influencing their sensitivity to lysis by NK and other cytolytic cells. Herman et al. have shown that the incubation of K562 leukemia cells with IL-1 increases the formation of LGL-K562 cell conjugates and corrects the impaired lysis of these cells by LGL from patients with advanced carcinoma (24). This observation suggests the effects of IL-1 on NK activity may be partly mediated through the tumor target cell rather than the effector. IL-1 has also been shown to exert a direct toxic effect on certain tumor cells independent of lymphocyte-mediated cytotoxicity (28). In this respect, the monokine resembles other products of activated lymphocytes and monocytes such as lymphotoxin (LT) and tumor necrosis factor (TNF). The observation that IL-1 shares direct tumoricidal effects with TNF, a cytokine defined primarily in terms of its ability to kill tumor cells, is not surprising as TNF has been shown to induce fever, fibroblast proliferation, and other phenomena otherwise attributed to IL-1 (29). Indeed, the multiple biological effects mediated by these pyrogenic cytokines extensively overlap, and there are only a few properties that are absolutely unique to one or the other.

Onozaki et al. demonstrated that the melanoma cell line A375 responds to highly purified monocyte-derived IL-1 as it does to LT with a prompt cessation of growth as measured by the incorporation of [$^3$H]thymidine and the formation of colonies in agarose (28). This is followed by a marked decline in cell viability as assessed by trypan blue staining and by the release of previously incorporated $^{125}$IUdR. The addition of antibodies that neutralize TNF and LT to the IL-1 preparation failed to attenuate the cytostatic and cytocidal properties of IL-1 in these assays, eliminating the possibility that the tumoricidal effects of IL-1 were mediated by residual TNF or LT contaminating the IL-1 preparation. Lachman et al. have reported similar results with recombinant IL-1 (30).

These results demonstrate an unexpected property of IL-1, which was until recently regarded exclusively as mediator of the acute phase response. The direct toxic effect of IL-1 on certain tumor cells may be as important as its ability to enhance the sensitivity of tumor cells to cytolytic lymphocytes and its synergy

with IL-2 and interferon in the activation of NK cells in mediating host defense
against neoplasia.

## E.  Indirect Effects on Cellular Immune Function: Effects of Hyperthermia

Implicit in its early designation, leukocytic pyrogen (31), one of the most prominent physiological effects of IL-1 is the elevation of body temperature. The development of fever in response to infection is known to favorably influence several
immunologic parameters, such as immunoglobulin synthesis, which are critical to
the elimination of invading microorganisms. At the turn of the century, Dr. William
Coley, a leading New York surgeon, noted the regression of malignant tumors in
some of his cancer patients who developed postoperative infections. He conjectured that the fever and other aspects of the acute phase response resulting from
this surgical complication not only facilitated the clearance of the infection but
stimulated the body to eradicate the tumor as well. So convinced was he of the
association between dever and tumor regression that he deliberately injected cancer patients with filtrates from *Erysipelas* strains of streptococci and endotoxin-
producing *Serratia marcescens* in an effort to induce tumor shrinkage (32). There
is little doubt that this approach was occasionally successful as recent trials with
pyrogenic toxins conducted primarily in Japan and the United States have shown
some positive results (33-35).

Whether the benefit accruing to toxin recipients is a consequence of the induction of immunomodulatory cytokines such as IL-1 or of elevated body temperature is controversial. The effects of IL-1 on neoplastic cells and on tumoricidal
lymphocytes have been reviewed in the preceding sections. Fever itself is known
to affect most cellular immune functions relevant to the control of tumor metastases and it is conceivable that the pyrogenic effects of IL-1 are as important as
its immunomodulatory effects in the containment and possible eradication of
transformed cells.

The effects of elevated temperature on cellular immune function in vitro are
variable. In general, T-lymphocyte proliferative responses are augmented at higher
temperatures. Duff et al. have shown that minimal degrees of hyperthermia ($39°C$)
enhance 4- to 10-fold murine thymocyte proliferative responses to both IL-2 and
IL-1 whereas the response of splenic B cells to endotoxin is relatively independent of temperature (36,37). A more quantitative analysis of T-cell proliferation
carried out by Hanson et al. yielded similar results (38). In these studies, the effects of temperature on thymocyte responses to IL-1 and IL-2 in the presence of
phytohemagglutinin were examined. The increase in [3H] thymidine incorporation per $10°$ temperature change ($Q_{10}$) was determined by extrapolation from a
curve in which isotope incorporation was plotted as a function of temperature.
The $Q_{10}$ for the response to IL-2 was approximately 9, whereas that for IL-1
was as high as 300 in some experiments. These results suggest an exquisite sensitivity of cytokine-activated T cells to temperature that is grossly disproportionate

to that observed in most biological reactions, in which the $Q_{10}$ is usually approximately 2. These results also demonstrate that the temperature increase necessary to significantly influence T-cell proliferative responses to mitogenic cytokines in vitro is well within the range achieved in the course of a febrile illness.

The incubation of human PBMC with allogeneic cells gives rise to a lymphocyte population capable of lysing the stimulator cells. When these incubations are carried out at 39°C, the resultant cytotoxic T lymphocytes (CTL) are able to kill the target cells more readily than when the incubations are carried out at 37°C. Likewise, when CTL generated at 37°C were assayed in conventional 4-hr $^{51}$Cr-release assays at various temperatures, the lysis of the target cells was greater at the higher temperature; thus both CTL induction and target cell lysis are enhanced by elevated temperatures (39). Similar results were obtained by Muellbacher et al. who demonstrated that murine CTL induction against cells infected with influenza virus was more efficient at 39°C than at 37°C (40). The actual lysis of the infected targets was, however, unaffected by temperature in these experiments. The incubation of human macrophages at 40°C markedly enhances their cytolytic activity against U937 lymphoma cells (41). The tumoricidal activity of macrophages activated by exposure to PHA-stimulated lymphocyte-conditioned media was similarly enhanced at higher temperatures.

Hyperthermia has been shown to retard the growth of certain tumor cell lines in vitro and established tumors in vivo (42,43). The inhibitory effects of elevated temperature on tumor cell growth as well as its enhancing effects on T-lymphocyte proliferation, CTL induction, and the lysis of neoplastic cells by CTL and macrophages suggest that elevated temperatures may be beneficial to a tumor-bearing animal or cancer patient. Hyperthermia has in fact become an important adjunct to chemotherapy and radiation therapy in the management of patients with metastatic malignancies. However, it is unclear whether tumor shrinkage induced by heat treatment is due to the enhancement of cellular immunity as outlined above or another mechanism such as ischemic infarction resulting from the increased oxygen requirements at higher temperatures. Although certain immunologic functions are definitely enhanced at higher temperatures, others, including several parameters intimately associated with host defense against malignancy, are adversely affected. This observation has led several investigators to conclude that the beneficial effects of fever are not due to the hyperthermia per se but rather to circulating pyrogenic cytokines which, in addition to producing fever, directly stimulate tumoricidal effector cells.

Of the various cytolytic cells tested, natural killer cells appear to be the most sensitive to elevated temperature (39). In complete contrast to CTL, an overnight incubation of NK cells at 39°C markedly reduces their tumoricidal activity. In experiments with microwave-induced hyperthermia, hamster splenic NK activity was markedly depressed for several hours after a brief period of hyperthermia (44). A 1-hr incubation at 40°C markedly suppressed the NK activity of human PBMC, and this decrement was shown to be irreversible by exposure to alpha

interferon (45). Although NK cells remain sensitive to the stimulatory effects
of IL-2 and interferon at higher temperatures, the enhancing effects of these
cytokines are almost completely negated by the inhibitory effects of temperatures that are easily achieved during fever (39). The adverse effects of elevated
temperature on NK activity in vitro have raised questions regarding the potentially deleterious effects of fever on cellular immunity. These results have suggested that the fever associated with the administration of pyrogenic biological
response modifiers such as interferon and IL-2 may partially offset the direct
stimulatory effects of these cytokines on NK activity and other cellular immune
functions.

The production of immunomodulatory cytokines such as interferon, IL-1,
and IL-2 is impaired at higher temperatures (39,46). Human monocytes exposed
to endotoxin generate considerably less IL-1 at 39°C than at 37°C. Similarly, the
production of IL-2, burst-promoting activity, and colony-stimulating factors by
PHA-stimulated nonadherent PBMC supplied with exogenous IL-1 is reduced at
higher incubation temperatures (39). This reduction in protein synthesis is not a
general phenomenon as heat shock proteins are specifically induced in lymphocytes at elevated temperatures (47,48). Furthermore, the decrement in the synthesis of inducible cytokines does not appear to be secondary to prostaglandin
synthesis, which is increased at higher temperatures, as cyclo-oxygenase inhibitors such as indomethacin fail to modify the temperature dependency (39).

The adverse effect of increased temperature on baseline and cytokine-enhanced
NK activity and on inducible cytokine synthesis suggests that increased temperature may actually hinder host defense against malignancy. Despite the enhancing
effects of IL-1 on several immune parameters in vitro and the beneficial effects
of elevated temperature induced by IL-1 on certain immune functions, other
parameters are profoundly suppressed by even a modest degree of hyperthermia,
suggesting that IL-1 may play a dual role in modulating the host response to neoplastic cells.

## III.  THE ROLE OF INTERLEUKIN-1 IN MEDIATING THE
ACUTE PHASE RESPONSE

Beginning in the 1940s, researchers had described a substance from acute inflammatory tissue which when injected into rabbits or humans would produce fever
(reviewed in Ref. 49). This material was a small protein (m.w. 10-20,000) and
was called endogenous pyrogen. Endogenous pyrogens are polypeptides produced
by the host and cause fever by their ability to stimulate hypothalamic prostaglandins. The first endogenous pyrogen was described by Beeson in 1948 and in 1953
Atkins and Wood showed that it circulated during fever. Endogenous pyrogens
are potent inducers of prostaglandins in the brain and the mechanisms include
the following steps: (i) endogenous pyrogens produced as a result of infection,

injury, or other response to tissue damage reach the anterior hypothalmic area via the arterial circulation; (ii) there they stimulate the endothelium of vascular organs to begin synthesizing prostaglandins; (iii) the newly synthesized prostaglandins enter the brain substance through large spaces between the endothelial cells; and (iv) these prostaglandins activate thermoregulatory neurons via increased cyclic AMP levels. The preoptic area of the hypothalamus is thought to contain the highest concentration of thermosensitive neurons and the proximity of the vascular organs to these neurons probably accounts for their responses to the prostaglandins. Lesions near these neurons, in particular hemorrhagic events or neoplasic involvement, may produce prostaglandins which independently activate the thermosensitive neurons.

It was later shown that endogenous pyrogen was not preformed in cells but rather was synthesized de novo when phagocytic cells, primarily macrophages, were stimulated with small (pg/ml) concentrations of endotoxins or by phagocytosis of a few (3-5) bacteria. Attempts to purify the endogenous pyrogen activity in inflammatory fluids or stimulated macrophage culture supernates proved difficult. Subnanogram amounts of protein seemingly possessed potent biological activity and, during multiple purification steps, loss of activity was common. Nevertheless, purification procedures were published in the 1970s (50,51) and it was established that 30-50 ng/kg of homogeneous endogenous pyrogen produced monophasic fever in rabbits. No amino acid sequence for endogenous pyrogen activity was known at that time.

An important consequence of the development of purification methods was the demonstration that endogenous pyrogen did more than cause fever. Kampschmidt and co-workers showed that endogenous pyrogen activity copurified with a substance called leukocytic endogenous mediator and that this material induced hepatic acute phase protein synthesis, caused a decrease in plasma iron and zinc levels, and produced a neutrophilia (52). Immunologists had also become interested in macrophage products, and in 1972, lymphocyte-activating factor was described as a 10-20,000 dalton protein which augmented T-cell responses to mitogens and antigens (53). The early reports on the chemical characteristics of lymphocyte-activating factor suggested several similarities to endogenous pyrogen and in 1979 and 1980, the first reports were published on the ability of purified endogenous pyrogens to act as lymphocyte activating factor (reviewed in Ref. 49). The name lymphocyte-activating factor was changed to interleukin-1 (IL-1) and included the originally described endogenous pyrogen and leukocytic endogenous mediator activities.

This concept that a molecule which acted on the brain to produce fever or the liver to induce acute phase protein synthesis was the same molecule which stimulated T cells and B cells was not easily accepted by immunologists. However, preparations of endogenous pyrogens which were homogeneous by SDS-PAGE induced T-cell proliferation (54,55). The dilemma was resolved by the molecular cloning of IL-1. Two IL-1 forms have been cloned, IL-1-beta from human monocytes (5) and IL-1-alpha from a murine macrophage line (56). The two forms had originally been identified as pI 7 (beta) and pI 5 (alpha) on isoelectric focusing. Homologues of IL-1-beta and -alpha have been found in other species. The cDNAs for IL-1 resulted in two important advances: (i) the entire amino acid sequences were deduced from the nucleotide sequence, and (ii) expression of the cDNAs resulted in ample quantities of recombinant IL-1s for biological experimentation.

Both forms of IL-1 are initially synthesized as 31,000 precursor polypeptides and share only small stretches of amino acid homology (26% in the case of human IL-1). Neither form contains a signal peptide sequence which would indicate a cleavage site for the N-terminus. But amino acid sequence analysis of IL-1 which was purified as a 17,500 dalton molecule from human blood mononuclear cells revealed that the mature peptide N-terminus was at position 117 (alanine) of the 269 amino acid precursor (57). The N-terminus of the IL-1-alpha was in a similar position. There is now evidence that elastase is one of the enzymes which cleaves the IL-1 precursor at the alanine position yielding the mature peptide.

For the most part, both forms of recombinant IL-1 have confirmed the previous studies (reviewed in Ref. 58). Both recombinant human IL-1-beta and -alpha augment T-cell responses to antigens or mitogens and cause fever in rabbits and other species (59). Both forms induce hepatic acute phase protein synthesis and cause sleep. However, some biological properties claimed to be due to natural IL-1 have not been demonstrated with either recominant form. These are the ability of IL-1 to cause neutrophil enzyme degranulation and muscle proteolysis in vitro. It appears that these apparent biological properties of IL-1 may have been due to contaminating protein(s) or to the ability of IL-1 to augment the biological property of another protein. One likely candidate for contaminating protein is cachectin (also known as tumor necrosis factor) (discussed below).

Although recombinant IL-1 forms do not induce neutrophil degranulation, they do induce histamine release from human blood basophils and eosinophil degranulation. In addition to confirming the biological activities of natural IL-1, the recombinant molecules have been used to demonstrate new biological properties. These include increases in adrenocorticotropic hormone (ACTH) and corticosteroid release, increased sodium excretion, inhibition of lipoprotein lipase, increased neutrophil and monocyte thromboxane $A_2$ synthesis, and IL-1-induced hemodynamic shock (60).

## A.  Systemic vs. Local Effects

Interleukin-1 induces a variety of changes when injected into the host (Table 2). These types of studies are carried out by injecting either intravenously or intraperitoneally recombinant or purified IL-1 into experimental animals, and in many cases, these changes mimic the animal's response to an injection of endotoxins or

Table 2  Systemic Effects of Recombinant Human IL-1

| *Central nervous system* | *Metabolic* |
|---|---|
| Fever | Hypozincemia, hypoferremia |
| Brain PGE-2 synthesis | Decreased cytochrome P450 enzyme |
| Increased ACTH | Increased acute phase proteins |
| Increased corticosteroid | Decreased albumin synthesis |
| Increased slow-wave sleep | Increased survival rate in mice |
| Decreased appetite | Increased bacterial clearance |
| | Increased (high dose decreased) insulin |
| *Hematologic* | Lipoprotein lipase inhibition |
| Neutrophilia | Increased sodium excretion |
| Lymphopenia | |
| Neutrophil TxA | *Vascular wall* |
| Tumor necrosis | Increased leukocyte adherence |
| Bone marrow release | Increased PGI and PGE synthesis |
| | Increased platelet-activating factor |
| *Hemodynamic effects* | Increased procoagulant activity |
| Hypotension | Increased plasminogen-activator inhibitor |
| Decreased systemic vascular resistance | |
| Decreased central venous pressure | |
| Increased cardiac output | |
| Increased heart rate | |
| Decreased blood pH | |

other microbial toxin or product. To date, these include fever, increased ACTH, corticosterone, slow-wave sleep, insulin, copper levels, hepatic acute phase protein synthesis, and blood neutrophils (late). In vivo IL-1 decreases circulating neutrophils (early), lymphocytes and monocytes (early), systemic arterial pressure, systemic vascular resistance, serum albumin, iron, zinc, and cytochrome P-450 enzyme activity. When injected intradermally, IL-1 induces an intense neutrophilic infiltration and can substitute for endotoxin in the local Swartzman response. These systemic effects are probably the "tip of the iceberg" in that systematic study has yet to be made on the metabolic, endocrinologic, hematologic, and nervous system changes induced by a systemic injection of IL-1. However, those changes that have been reported are not due to "industrial" doses of IL-1. In fact, the half-life of IL-1 in rabbits after an intravenous injection is 5 minutes. The plasma level of IL-1 45 minutes after an intravenous injection which results in a 1°C fever is approximately 100 pg/ml and this concentration is similar to the in vitro concentration for one-half maximal lymphocyte-activating unit/ml (59).

When compared to whole animal studies, there have been considerably more studies on the in vitro effects of IL-1. However, some of the in vitro effects are probably relevant to systemic responses. For example, the effects of IL-1 on endothelial cell arachidonic acid metabolism and procoagulant activity in vitro likely explain the shocklike state that IL-1 produces in vivo. In addition, the ability of IL-1 to induce various lymphokines in vitro likely occurs in vivo, but it is difficult to demonstrate circulating levels of interferons (beta or gamma) and interleukins (2 and 3) unless large doses are given. Some human studies, however, have employed large amounts of recombinant IL-2 and interferon-gamma and some of the systemic effects of these therapies may be due to IL-1 production.

However, one approach to interpreting the large body of evidence for the multiple biological effects of IL-1 is to view local production and action as the "autocrine" action of IL-1 and the systemic effect as the "hormonal" property. At present, it seems that autocrine effects of IL-1 predominate in some diseases, whereas systemic effects are characteristic of IL-1 produced as a result of toxemia, septicemia, widespread tissue damage, or intravenous antigenic challenge. What seems increasingly clear is that tissues that produce IL-1 are either themselves the targets of local IL-1 effects or are capable of acting on adjoining tissue. For example, IL-1 produced by macrophages in the lymph nodes likely induces IL-2, IL-2 receptors, IL-3, hybridoma growth factor, and IFN-gamma which exert their effects on nearby T, B, and NK cells. In addition, in a dense cellular response, even low doses of IL-1 probably synergize with IL-2 and IL-4 for enhancement of lymphocyte responses. Table 1 summarizes some immunologic properties of IL-1.

Interleukin-1 produced by microglia and astrocytes in the brain affects local gliosis, but may induce no systemic responses. A similar case can be made for the ability of IL-1 to stimulate fibroblast granulocyte-macrophage colony-stimulating factor, interferon-beta (57), and hybridoma growth factor (61). IL-1 produced by keratinocytes in the skin is another example. However, local production and biological activity of IL-1 in the joint space has attracted considerable attention as a factor in the pathogenesis of various joint diseases, such as rheumatoid and osteoarthritis.

The joint macrophage has been shown to produce IL-1, and IL-1 has been measured in a variety of human arthritides. Special dendritic fibroblasts cultured from human arthritis synovia produce large amounts of collagenase and $PGE_2$ in response to IL-1 (62) and this local property of IL-1 likely contributes to pain and destructive disease. In addition, IL-1 production is directly stimulated by de novo collagen synthesis and induces fibroblast proliferation. Thus, it also has a role in the process of thickening synovial membrane. IL-1 has been shown to stimulate chondrocyte metalloproteinases and $PGE_2$ production, and, in its role as an osteoclast activating factor, induces the resorption of bone. Thus, the autocrime effects of IL-1 may play a major role in the pathogenesis of several disease processes in addition to being a prominent response to local infection and injury. Table 3 lists some possible autocrine effects of IL-1.

Table 3  Autocrine Effects of Interleukin-1

Attraction of neutrophils, lymphocytes, monocytes (in vivo)

Basophil histamine release

Eosinophil degranulation

Proliferation of dermal fibroblasts

Increased collagen synthesis

Increased collagenase production

Chondrocyte protease release

Induction of fibroblast and endothelial GM-CSF activity

Production of PGE-2 in dermal and synovial fibroblasts

Increased neutrophil and monocyte thromboxane synthesis

Cytotoxic for human melanoma cells

Cytotoxic for human beta islet cells (insulin producing)

Cytotoxic for thymocytes

Increased bone resorption (osteoclast-activating factor)

Stimulation of fibroblast interferon-beta synthesis

Stimulation of fibroblast hybridoma growth factor synthesis

Keratinocyte proliferation

Mesangial cell proliferation

Gliosis

From the preceding discussion, it seems clear that IL-1 affects many tissues and organ systems. Are these effects beneficial to the host in the struggle to overcome microbial invasion or malignant disease? IL-1-mediated responses appear to fall into two categories: (i) acute phase changes such as fever, sleep, ACTH release, effects on vascular tissue, hepatic acute phase protein synthesis, decreased plasma Fe and Zn, increased neutrophil levels, and increased interferon and colony-stimulating factor production, and (ii) general immunologic stimulation leading to the development of specific antibodies or specific cytotoxic T cells which are involved with the ultimate eradication of the invader.

The acute phase changes are produced within hours of the onset of infection. IL-1 increases synthesis of several proteins in isolated hepatocytes and, at the same time, decreases synthesis of albumin. Some of the hepatic proteins are synthesized normally and include various antiproteases, several complement components, fibrinogen, haptoglobin, ceruloplasmin, and others. In these cases, the action of IL-1 on the hepatocyte is to increase the rate of synthesis of the proteins at the transcriptional level. However, IL-1 also initiates gene expression of new products, generally proteins not synthesized in health but in association with infection or injury or other pathological processes. The IL-1-induced increases in normal hepatic proteins is usually 2-3-fold, but the IL-1-initiated synthesis of pathological proteins can be 100-1000-fold. Two such proteins, serum amyloid A (SAA) protein and C-reactive protein (CRP) are classical "acute phase reactants," and disease markers. SAA contributes to the development of secondary amyloidosis. Other pathological acute phase proteins include, alpha macroglobulin and acid-1-glycoprotein.

Do these hepatic proteins play a role in host defense mechanisms? The strongest implication that they serve an important function comes from data which show the presence of acute phase reactants such as the pentaxins SAA and CRP in the invertebrate *Limulus* horseshoe crab. Not only is their presence for 400 million years of evolution an indication of their importance to the host, but, in addition, their structure has been amazingly preserved in that primary structure of the *Limulus* pentaxin is nearly identical to that of the human. Moreover, the starfish coelomocyte, which behaves like a macrophage, synthesizes large amounts of a protein called sea star factor (63), which shares certain similarities with IL-1.

The overwhelming physical property of CRP and SAA is their ability to bind to lipids. In addition, other proteins such as alpha-1-macroglobulin and ceruloplasmin act as oxygen scavengers. Because many of the acute phase proteins are large glycoproteins, they bind to bacterial surfaces, physical property which allows them to act as all-purpose, nonspecific opsonins. Acute phase proteins also include a series of antiproteases and these may play a role in offsetting the action of some bacterial proteases. Finally, the liver is the source of other proteins which bind divalent cations such as iron and zinc. These metalloproteins are usually not secreted, but bind plasma iron and zinc and localize these in the liver, spleen, and bone marrow. Of major benefit to the host is that the lowered tissue levels of iron and zinc result in reduced microbial replication, particularly at febrile temperatures. It appears that the acute phase proteins served evolution and host defense well enough that many species survive without T cells, B cells, or the ability to make specific antibody.

The clinical association of increased sleepiness with infectious disease has received clarification and new information from studies on IL-1. The so-called "sleep factor," isolated from the urine of sleep-deprived humans and the cerebrospinal fluid of animals, has been chemically identified as an N-acetylated muramic acid linked to a tetrapeptide structure, similar to the peptidoglycan units of muramic acid-tetrapeptide found in all bacterial cell walls (64). Sleep factor purified from either human urine or peritoneal dialysis fluid is, like other muramyl peptides, an inducer of IL-1 (19). Like sleep factor, both natural and recombinant IL-1 induce increased slow-wave sleep when injected either intravenously or intracerebroventricularly. The onset of IL-1-mediated increases in slow-wave sleep is considerably faster than that of sleep factor, and there is evidence that sleep factor induces slow-wave sleep via the production of IL-1 either peripherally or from astrocytes and microglia within the central nervous system. The benefit to the host of increased sleep may be one of conserved energy and metabolic resources at a time when these are needed to fight infection. Therefore, sleep and decreased appetite, also an IL-1-induced change associated with acute phase responses, may be considered part of the behavioral alterations serving a host defense machanism. The decrease in appetite would reduce the desire to seek food, an activity with numerous attendant dangers for much of the animal world. It is unclear how effective reduced food intake would be to specific host defense mechanisms. Nevertheless, we are reminded of Pasteur's comment that during infection, the host attempts to "starve out" the microbe as a mechanism of resistance.

Recent evidence demonstrates that IL-1 induces the production of a B-cell-stimulating factor from fibroblasts. This factor was originally described as a 26 kD protein from IL-1-stimulated fibroblasts which had hybridoma growth factor activity. The 26 kD protein also had the ability to stimulate plasmacytoma cell growth. The N-terminal sequence of the homogeneous 26 kD factor matches that of an IFN-beta-2 (61). Others have also reported a B-cell-stimulating factor (BSF-2) which is the same molecule as the 26 K IFN-beta-2 (65). Thus, it seems that the role of IL-1 in augmenting B-cell function ultimately leading to the production of protective or antimicrobial antibodies may be through its ability to induce B-cell-stimulating factors. However, this does not rule out a role for IL-1 augmenting BSF or upregulating their receptors.

The ability of IL-1 to activate the vascular endothelium may explain several host responses to disease processes. We have recently shown that rabbits injected with recombinant IL-1-alpha or -beta manifest the typical hemodynamic changes characteristic of septic shock (60). IL-1 (5 $\mu$g/kg) induces a sudden and dramatic fall in arterial blood pressure, systemic vascular resistance, and central venous pressure, but a compensatory increase in cardiac output and heart rate. Concomitantly, there is also massive leukopenia (70% reduction) and thrombocytopenia (40% reduction). The IL-1-induced shocklike state is averted by a previous intravenous injection of a cyclooxygenase inhibitor and is reversed by a similar injection given during the hypotension. These observations are consistent with a fundamental property of IL-1: its ability to induce rapid increases in cyclooxygenase products, particularly prostaglandin $E_2$. In fact, the onset and maximum effect of an intravenous bolus injection of IL-1 on hemodynamic parameters is nearly identical with that observed for fever (59) and neutropenia (66).

## B.  Comparison Between IL-1 and Cachectin/Tumor Necrosis Factor

Another monocyte/macrophage product, synthesized and released as a consequence of microbial stimulation, is tumor necrosis factor (TNF). TNF is identical to a substance described as cachectin which is a key mediator of the "cachexin" observed in animals with parasitic disease. The subject of TNF/cachectin has recently been reviewed (67). The biological properties of TNF/cachectin share remarkable similarities to those of IL-1 with the notable exception that TNF/ cachectin, at concentrations which induce acute phase changes in many tissues, has no immunostimulatory effects. However, nearly every biological property of IL-1 has been observed with TNF/cachectin. These include fever, the induction of $PGE_2$ and collagenase from a variety of tissues, bone resorption, inhibition of lipoprotein lipase, increases in hepatic acute phase reactants, and a decrease in albumin synthesis. Slow-wave sleep is also observed following the injection of TNF or IL-1. Both molecules also induce fibroblast proliferation and new collagen synthesis. The cytotoxic activity of TNF/cachectin differs from that of IL-1. For example, IL-1 is cytotoxic for the beta cells of the pancreatic islets of Langerhans and also for human melanoma cells; but, in the same assays, TNF/cachectin has no effect. Likewise, IL-1 is inactive on a variety of tumor targets for which TNF is a potent cytotoxin. In fact, the cell line most often used in cytotoxic assay for TNF, L929 fibroblasts, is unaffected by IL-1.

In vivo, IL-1 and TNF/cachectin induce fever by their direct ability to induce hypothalamic $PGE_2$. In addition to fever, these cytokines will result in hypotension, leukopenia, and local tissue necrosis. On a weight basis, rabbits are equally sensitive to the shock-inducing properties of IL-1 and TNF/cachectin. These responses likely reflect the effects of these two cytokines on the vascular endothelium. Both IL-1 and TNF/cachectin stimulate $PGI_2$, $PGE_2$, and platelet-activating factor production from cultured endothelium. In addition, both cytokines stimu-

Table 4  Comparison of Biological Properties Between IL-1 and TNF/Cachectin

| Biological property | IL-1 | TNF/cachectin |
|---|---|---|
| Endogenous pyrogen fever | + | + |
| Slow-wave sleep | + | + |
| Hemodynamic shock | + | + |
| Increased hepatic acute phase protein synthesis | + | + |
| Decreased albumin synthesis | + | + |
| Activation of endothelium | + | + |
| Decreased lipoprotein lipase | + | + |
| Decreased cytochrome p450 | + | + |
| Decreased plasma Fe/Zn | + | + |
| Increased fibroblast proliferation | + | + |
| Increased synovial cell collagenase and PGE | + | + |
| Induction of IL-1 | + | + |
| T/B-cell activation | + | − |

late procoagulant activity, leukocyte adherence and plasminogen activator inhibitor on these cells. Despite these similarities, receptors for TNF/cachectin have been shown to be specific and distinct, and receptor binding is unaffected by IL-1. Thus, the most likely explanation is that TNF/cachectin and IL-1 stimulate similar intracellular messages and alter cellular metabolism in a similar way. Table 4 lists the biological similarities between TNF/cachectin and IL-1. As noted, both TNF/cachectin and IL-1 stimulate the production of more IL-1. This can be shown in vivo and in vitro from human monocytes and human endothelium. Substances that activate macrophage cytotoxicity are thought to accomplish this through TNF/cachectin. Furthermore, animal models of in vivo tumor necrosis are clearly observed following injection of TNF/cachectin and less so following comparable doses of IL-1.

At present, there are no data to suggest that IL-1 (alpha or beta) and TNF are related at the amino acid level or even secondary or tertiary structural level. However, it does seem clear that the cytokines are biologically related molecules. One can only speculate that acute phase responses such as fever, hepatic protein synthesis, decreases in plasma Fe/Zn, et al., were of such importance to host survival that nature imparted these responses to more than a single molecule.

## C. Production of IL-1

It has been proposed that IL-1 is important to the host's ability to fight an invading microbe. This concept is supported by findings of considerable amounts of polyadenylated RNA in macrophages following stimulation codes for IL-1. As much as 2-5% of the total poly A is IL-1-beta. The predominance of the IL-1 suggests that the host requires a significant amount of IL-1 at a critical time following the onset of infection.

Recently, we have developed a radioimmunoassay specific for human IL-1-beta. We have determined the levels of IL-1 produced by human blood monocytes stimulated with heat-killed *Staphylococcus albus* or endotoxin using this specific assay. The IL-1 activity as measured by this method is free of interfering substances (both enhancing as well as inhibiting) and hence reflects the amount of IL-1 as antigen. In general, we have found that human blood monocytes produce approximately 5-10 ng/million monocytes over an 8-hr period. The intracellular IL-1 levels are high after 4 hr but these are reduced as the extracellular levels increase with time. The amount of IL-1-alpha has not been determined. Thus these results are consistent with the prominence of IL-1-beta mRNA in a stimulated monocyte and suggests that IL-1 is a major product of these cells. The conclusion is that IL-1 production and function are linked to host defense mechanisms not only because of its multiple biological activities but also because the amount made is hardly an epiphenomenon of cell activation but rather a major product of the cell.

Fixed Macrophagic Cells

These cells are often located in strategic blood-filtering organs and are involved
in primary phagocytic defense mechanisms for invading microorganisms. For example, there are fixed macrophages lining the alveolar space, in the lamina propria
and in the dermis. Fixed macrophagic cells also make up the lining of blood-filtering organs, for example, the Kuppfer cells of the liver, the splenic sinusoidal cells,
and lymph node macrophages. Peritoneal macrophages are also part of the primary phagocytic defense mechanism since these cells would be involved with
microorganisms derived from intestinal perforations. Several studies have shown
that peritoneal, splenic, and alveolar cells produce IL-1 when stimulated in vitro.
The different methods used to remove and purify these cells from other tissue
cells may affect IL-1 production. Most studies involving IL-1 production from
peritoneal cells employ agents such as oil or thioglycollate and these agents may
raise not only the total number of peritoneal macrophages in the peritoneal cav-
ity, but also may "prime" the macrophage for subsequent stimulation in vitro.
Several biologically active molecules such as tuftsin, while not an IL-1 inducer,
lower the threshold of peritoneal macrophages to exogenous stimuli like endotoxin. Such "priming" may also be part of the mechanism by which pretreatment
of blood monocytes with interferons increases endotoxin-induced IL-1 production.
        Langerhans' cells isolated from the skin can be separated from keratinocytes
by adherence techniques and when stimulated, these cells produce IL-1 (68). Using a similar method, dendritic cells from human synovium can also be separated
from other synovial cells and produce IL-1 upon stimulation.

Keratinocytes

Several keratinocyte lines of human or mouse origin produce IL-1 without any
apparent stimulant but increase production when incubated with endotoxin or
toxic shock syndrome toxin-1. Keratinocyte-derived IL-1 exists in multiple weight
species (50-15,000) and three different isoelectric points of 7.4, 6.1, and 5.1,
chracteristic of human blood monocytes. Keratinocyte IL-1 also shares with
monocyte-derived IL-1 such multiple biological activities as fever induction. Keratinocyte-derived IL-1 is the source of IL-1 found in the cornified epidermis. Rabbits irradiated with ultraviolet lights have circulating levels of IL-1 and it seems
probable that this may be keratinocyte-derived. It is also speculated that keratinocyte IL-1 production may be involved in a variety of skin lesions, including acute
sunburn or as a result of treatment with ultraviolet B-wave phototherapy for certain skin diseases.

B-cell IL-1

Scala and co-workers were the first to demonstrate that Epstein-Barr-infected
human B-cell lines produce IL-1 (69). Circulating B cells isolated from the blood

of apparently healthy humans can be stimulated by a variety of agents to produce IL-1. Many of these agents, such as *Staphylococcus auerus* Cowan's strain, anti-mu, and endotoxin are used as stimulators of B-cell activity and part of their stimulation may be mediated via IL-1 induction. A considerable amount of the B-cell-derived IL-1 may be membrane bound (70) and this finding is consistent with several studies implicating B cells as antigen-resenting cells in which IL-1 could not be detected. An explanation for this may be that the IL-1 is bound and stimulates T cell in its bound form.

Large Granular Lymphocytes

These cells are also known as natural killer cells and have been purified from human blood and shown to release IL-1 upon stimulation with endotoxin or tumor cell targets (25,71). Patients with large tumor burdens have circulating NK cells which produce little IL-1 and have markedly reduced ability to bind and lysis tumor targets.

Mesangial Cells

Rat mesangial cell lines produce IL-1 and this IL-1 is active in both the thymocyte and fever assay. The rat IL-1 derived from mesangial cells has been subjected to several purification procedures and this mesangial cell IL-1 has multiple molecular weight and charged forms. In addition to stimulating thymocytes and the thermoregulatory center, mesangial cell IL-1 has also been shown to act as a growth factor for itself.

Astroglia and Microglia

Brain astrocytes present antigen and express major histocompatibility complex (MHC) class II antigens on their cell surface. In addition, these neural cells produce IL-1. Human glioma cell lines produce an IL-1 which is antigenically related to human monocyte IL-1. Mice injected with endotoxin intraperitoneally develop fever for several hours and astrocytes separated from other neural tissue contain large amounts of intracellular IL-1 (72). In fact, astrocyte IL-1 may play an important role in fever induction. IL-1 also stimulates glial cell proliferation and locally produced IL-1 may be involved with central nervous system tissue scarring, also known as gliosis (73). Recent studies have also focused on another central nervous system cell, the microglia, as a potent source of IL-1. The relative production of IL-1 from microglia seems 10-50 times greater than that from astrocytes. This is not surprising since microglia are considered brain tissue macrophages.

IL-1 Production from Blood Vessel Cells

The two major blood vessel cells, endothelium and smooth muscle, both produce IL-1. Endothelial cell IL-1 has been reported by several groups to produce IL-1 and recently has been shown at the level of gene expression (74). In general, IL-1 production from endothelial cells is inducible and endotoxin is particularly effective

Table 5  Cells Sources of IL-1

---

Monocyte/macrophage

Skin keratinocyte/Langerhans cells

Renal mesangial cells

Vascular endothelial and smooth muscle cells

Gingival and corneal epithelial cells

Brain astrocytes and microglial cells

Normal and EBV-infected B cells

Natural killer cells

---

when compared to other well-known inducers of monocyte IL-1. Freshly isolated adult human saphenous vein endothelium or newborn umbilical artery endothelium and cell lines derived from these cells have been used.

Smooth muscle cell lines of human origin produce IL-1 which is similar to monocyte IL-1 by immunoprecipitation and mRNA hybridization (75). The findings that both blood vessel-derived cells produce IL-1 is important to the understanding of pathological processes in vasculitis since endothelial cells are activated by IL-1 to increase their adhesiveness for leukocytes and procoagulant activity (reviewed in Ref. 76). Therefore, in disease processes such as antigen-antibody complex-mediated diseases or tissue injury and vessel disruption, endothelial and/or smooth muscle IL-1 likely acts as an autocoid and contributes to the progression of the lesion.

Epithelial Cells

Epithelial cell IL-1 production has been reported in two studies: (i) IL-1 from the gingival epithelial cell and (ii) IL-1 produced by corneal epithelium. In the gingiva, local IL-1 production clearly plays an important role since IL-1 stimulates bone resorption and osteoclast-activating factor has been shown to be the same polypeptide sequence as IL-1-beta. IL-1 production by corneal epithelium is also of considerable clinical significance since IL-1 is chemotactic for neutrophils, monocytes, and lymphocytes. Table 5 depicts the cells which produce IL-1.

## ACKNOWLEDGMENTS

These studies are supported by NIH Grant AI 15614 to C. A. D. and funds from Cistron Biotechnology, Inc., Pine Brook, NJ. The authors wish to thank Dr. Sheldon M. Wolff for his support in these studies.

## REFERENCES

1. Wood, D.D., Cameron, P.M., Poe, M.T., and Morris, C.A. Resolution of factor that enhances the antibody response of T cell-depleted murine splenocytes from several other monocyte products. Cell Immunol. 21: 88-95, 1976.
2. Wood, D.D., and Cameron, P.M. Stimulation of the release of a B cell-activating factor from human monocytes. Cell Immunol. 21: 133-145, 1976.
3. Wood, D.D. Purification and properties of human B cell-activating factor. I. Comparison of the plaque-stimulating factivity with thymocyte-stimulating activity. J. Immunol. 123: 2395-2399, 1979.
4. Wood, D.D. Mechanism of action of human B cell-activating factor. J. Immunol. 123: 2400-2407, 1979.
5. Auron, P.E., Webb, A.C., Rosenwasser, L.J., Mucci, S.F., Rich, A., Wolff, S.M., and Dinarello, C.A. Nucleotide sequence of human monocyte interleukin-1 precursor cDNA. Proc. Natl. Acad. Sci. USA 81: 7907-7911, 1984.
6. Dinarello, C.A., Cannon, J.G., Mier, J.W., Bernheim, H.A., LoPreste, G., Lynn, D.L., Love, R., Webb, A.C., Auron, P.E., Reuben, R., Rich, A., Wolff, S.M., and Putney, S. Multiple biological activities of human recombinant interleukin-1. J. Clin. Invest. 77: 1734-1739, 1986.
7. Falkoff, R.J.M., Muraguchi, A., Hong, J-X., Butler, J.L., Dinarello, C.A., and Fauci, A.S. The effects of interleukin-1 on human B cell activation and proliferation. J. Immunol. 131: 801-805, 1983.
8. Lipsky, P.E., Thompson, P.A., Rosenwasser, L.J., and Dinarello, C.A. The role of interleukin-1 in human B cell activation: inhibition of B cell proliferation and the generation of immunoglobulin secreting cells by an antibody against huma leukocytic pyrogen. J. Immunol. 130: 2709-2714, 1983.
9. Kurt-Jones, E.A., Beller, D.I., Mizel, S.B., and Unanue, E.R. Identification of a membrane-associated interleukin-1 in macrophages. Proc. Natl. Acad. Sci. USA 82: 1204-1208, 1985.
10. Smith, K.A., Lachman, L.B., Oppenheim, J.J., and Favata, M.F. The functional relationship of the interleukins. J. Exp. Med. 151: 1551-1556, 1980.
11. Rao, A., Mizel, S.B., and Cantor, H. Disparate functional properties of two interleukin-1-responsive Ly-1+2- T cell clones: distinction of T cell growth factor and T cell-replacing factor activities. J. Immunol. 130: 1743-1748, 1983.
12. Maizel, A.L., Mehta, S.R., Ford, R.J., Lachman, L.B. Effect of interleukin-1 on human thymocytes and purified human T cells. J. Exp. Med. 153: 470-475, 1981.
13. Farrar, W.L., Mizel, S.B., and Farrar, J.J. Participation of lymphocyte activating factor (Interleukin-1) in the induction of cytotoxic T cell responses. Immunology 124: 1371-1377, 1980.
14. Herberman, R.B. Natural killer cells and their possible roles in resistance against disease. Clin. Immunol. Rev. 1: 1-65, 1981.
15. Timonen, T., Reynolds, C.W., Ortaldo, J.R., and Herberman, R.B. Isolation of human and rat natural killer cells. J. Immunol. Meth. 51: 269, 1982.

16. Ritz, J., Campen, T.J., Schmidt, R.E., Royer, H.D., Hercend, T., Hussey, R.E., and Reinherz, E.L. Analysis of T-cell receptor gene rearrangement and expression in human natural killer clones. Science 228: 1540, 1985.

17. Roder, J.C. The beige mutation in the mouse. I. A stem cell predetermined impairment in natural killer cell function. J. Immunol. 123: 2168-2173, 1979.

18. Katz, P., Zaytoun, A.M., and Fauci, A.S. Deficiency of active natural killer cells in the Chediak-Higashi syndrome. Localization of the defect using a single cell cytotoxicity assay. J. Clin. Invest. 69: 1231-1236, 1982.

19. Barlozzari, T., Reynolds, C.W., and Herberman, R.B. In vivo role of natural killer cells: Involvement of large granular lymphocytes in the clearance of tumor cells in anti-asialo GM-treated mice. J. Immunol. 131: 1024-1028, 1983.

20. Herberman, R.B., and Ortaldo, J.R. Augmentation by interferon of human natural and antibody-dependent cell-mediated cytotoxicity. Nature 277: 221, 1979.

21. Henney, C., Kurobayashi, K., Kern, D., and Gillis, S. Interleukin-2 augments natural killer activity. Nature 291: 357-359, 1981.

22. Dempsey, R.A., Dinarello, C.A., Mier, J.W., Rosenwasser, L.J., Allegretta, M., Brown, T.E., and Parkinson, D.L. The differential effects of human leukocytic pyrogen/lymphocyte activating factor, T cell growth factor and interferon on human natural killer cell activity. J. Immunol. 129: 2504-2510, 1982.

23. Herman, J., Kew, M.C., and Rabson, A.R. Defective Interleukin-1 production by monocytes from patients with malignant diseases: interferon increases IL-1 production. Cancer Immunol. Immunother. 16: 182-185, 1984.

24. Herman, J., Dinarello, C.A., Kew, M.C., and Rabson, A.R. The role of Interleukin-1 (IL-1) in tumor-NK cell interactions: correction of defective NK cell activity in cancer patients by treating targets with IL-1. J. Immunol. 135: 2882-2886, 1985.

25. Scala, G., Allavena, P., Djeu, J., Kasahara, T., Ortaldo, J.R., Herberman, R.B., and Oppenheim, J.J. Human large granular lymphocytes are potent producers of Interleukin-1. Nature 309: 56-59, 1984.

26. Grimm, E., Mazumder, A., Zhang, Z., and Rosenberg, S. Lymphokine-activated killer cell phenomenon. I. Lysis of natural killer-resistant fresh solid tumor cells by Interleukin-2-activated autologous human peripheral blood lymphocytes. J. Exp. Med. 155: 1823-1835, 1982.

27. Grimm, E., Ramsey, K., Mazumder, A., Wilson, D., Djeu, J., and Rosenberg, S. Lymphokine-activated killer cell phenomenon. II. Precursor phenotype is serologically distinct from peripheral T-lymphocytes, memory cytotoxic thymus-derived lymphocytes, and natural killer cells. J. Exp. Med. 157: 884-896, 1983.

28. Onozaki, K., Matsushima, K., Aggarwal, B.B., and Oppenheim, J.J. Interleukin-1 as a cytocidal factor for several tumor cell lines. J. Immunol. 135: 3962-3968, 1985.

29. Dinarello, C.A., Cannon, J.G., Wolff, S.M., Berheim, H.A., Beutler, B., Cerami, A., Figari, I.S., Palladino, M.A., and O'Connor, J.V. Tumor necrosis factor (cachectin) is an endogenous pyrogen and induces production of Interleukin-1. J. Exp. Med. 163: 1433-1451, 1986.

30. Lachman, L.B., Dinarello, C.A., Llanska, N.D., and Fidler, I.J. Natural and recombinant human Interleukin-1B is cytotoxic for human melanoma cells. J. Immunol. 136: 3098-3103, 1986.

31. Aarden, L.A., et al. Revised nomenclature for antigen-nonspecific T cell proliferation and helper factors letter. J. Immunol. 123: 2938-2929, 1979.

32. Nauts, H.C. Bacterial products in the treatment of cancer: past, present and future. In Bacteria and Cancer. Edited by J. Jeljaszewicz, G. Pulverer, and W. Roskowski. Academic Press, New York, 1982, pp. 1-27.

33. Coley, W.B. Further observations on the conservative treatment of sarcoma of the long bones. Ann. Surg. 60: 633-660, 1919.

34. Miller, T.R., and Nicholson, J.T. End results in reticulum cell sarcoma of bones treated by bacterial toxin therapy alone or combined with surgery and/or radiotherapy (47 cases) or with concurrent infection (5 cases). Cancer 27: 524-548, 1971.

35. Uchida, A., and Hoshimo, T. Reduction of suppressor cells in cancer patients treated with OK-432 immunotherapy. Int. J. Cancer 26: 401-412, 1980.

36. Duff, G.W., and Durum, S.K. Fever and immunoregulation: hyperthermia, interleukin-1 and -2 and T-cell proliferation. Yale J. Biol. Med. 55: 437-442, 1982.

37. Duff, G.W., and Durum, S.K. The pyrogenic and mitogenic actions of interleukin-1 are related. Nature 304: 449-451, 1983.

38. Hanson, D.F., Murphy, P.A., Silicano, R., and Shin, H.S. The effect of temperature on the activation of thymocytes by interleukins 1 and 2. J. Immunol. 130: 216-221, 1983.

39. Dinarello, C.A., Dempsey, R.A., Allegretta, M., LoPreste, G., Dainiak, N., Parkinson, D.R., and Mier, J.W. Inhibitory effects of elevated temperature on human cytokine production and natural killer activity. Cancer Res. in press.

40. Muellbacher, A. Hyperthermia and the generation of and activity of murine influenza-immune cytotoxic T cells in vitro. J. Virol. 52: 928-931, 1984.

41. Andreesen, R., Osterholtz, J., and Schultz, A. Enhancement of spontaneous and lymphokine activated human macrophage cytotoxicity by hyperthermia. Blut 47: 225-229, 1983.

42. Hall, E.J., and Roizin-Towle, L. Biological effects of heat. Cancer Res. 44: 4708s-4713sw, 1984.

43. Li, D.J., and Hahn, G.M. Responses of RIF tumors to heat and drugs: dependence on tumor size. Cancer Treat. Rep. 68: 1149-1151, 1984.

44. Yang, H.K., Cain, C.A., Lockwood, J., and Tompkins, W.A. Effects of microwave exposure on the hamster immune system. I. Natural killer cell activity. Bioelectromagnetics 4: 123-139, 1983.

45. Kalland, T., and Dahlquist, I. Effects of in vitro hyperthermia on natural killer cells. Cancer Res. 42: 1842-1846, 1983.

46. Girard, D.J., Fleischaker, R.J., and Sinskey, A.J. Kinetics of human beta interferon production under different temperature conditions. Interferon Res. 2: 471-477, 1982.

47. Maytin, E.V., and Young, D.A. Separate glucocorticoid, heavy metal, and heat shock domains in thymic lymphocytes. J. Biol. Chem. 258: 12718-12722, 1983.

48. Morimoto, R., and Fodor, E. Cell-specific expression of heat shock proteins in chicken reticulocytes and lymphocytes. J. Cell. Biol. 99: 1316-1323, 1984.

49. Dinarello, C.A. Interleukin-1. Rev. Infect. Dis. 6: 51-95, 1984.

50. Murphy, P.A., Chesney, J., and Wood, W.B., Jr. Further purification of rabbit leukocyte pyrogen. J. Lab. Clin. Med. 83: 310-322, 1974.

51. Dinarello, C.A., Renfer, L., and Wolff, S.M. Human leukocytic pyrogen: purification and development of a radioimmunoassay. Proc. Natl. Acad. Sci. USA 74: 4624-4627, 1977.

52. Kampschmidt, R.F. Leukocytic endogenous mediator/endogenous pyrogen. In *Physiology & Metabolic Responses of the Host.* Edited by M.C. Powanda and P.G. Canonico. Elsevier/North-Holland, Amsterdam, 1981, pp. 55-74.

53. Gery, I., and Waksman, B.H. Potentiation of the T-lymphocyte response to mitogens. II. The cellular source of potentiating mediator(s). J. Exp. Med. 136: 143-155, 1972.

54. Dinarello, C.A., Bernheim, H.A., Cannon, J.G., LoPreste, G., Warner, S.J.C., Webb, A.C., and Auron, P.E. Purified, [35]S-met,[3]H-leu-labeled human monocyte interleukin-1 with endogenous pyrogen activity. Br. J. Rheumatol. 24 (suppl): 59-64, 1985.

55. Hanson, D.F., and Murphy, P.A. Demonstration of interleukin-1 activity in apparently homogeneous specimens of the pI 5 form of rabbit endogenous pyrogen. Infect. Immun. 45: 483-490, 1984.

56. Lomedico, P.T., Gubler, U., Hellman, C.P., Dukovich, M., Giri, J.G., Pan, Y.E., Collier, K., Semionow, R., Chua, A.O., and Mizel, S.B. Cloning and expression of murine interleukin-1 in *Escherichia coli.* Nature 312: 458-462, 1984.

57. Van Damme, J., De Ley, M., Opdenakker, G., Billiau, A., and De Somer, P. Homogeneous interferon-inducing 22K factor is related to endogenous pyrogen and interleukin-1. Nature 314: 266-268, 1985.

58. Dinarello, C.A. Interleukin-1: amino acid sequences, multiple biological activities and comparison with tumor necrosis factor (cachectin). Year Immunol. 2: 68-89, 1986.

59. Dinarello, C.A., Cannon, J.G., Mier, J.W., Bernheim, H.A., LoPreste, G., Lynn, D.L., Love, R.N., Webb, A.C., Auron, P.E., and Putney, S.D. Multiple biological activities of human recombinant interleukin-1. J. Clin. Invest. 77: 1734-1739, 1986.

60. Okusawa S., Gelfand J.A., Ikejima, T., Connolly, R.A., Dinarello, C.A. Interleukin-1 induces a shock-like state in rabbits: Synergism with tumor necrosis factor and the effect of cyclooxygenase inhibition. J. Clin. Invest., in press.

61. van Damme, J., Opdenakker, G., Simpson, R.J., et al. Identification of the human 26-kD protein, interferon $\beta_2$ (IFN-$\beta_2$), as a B cell hybridoma/plasmacytoma growth factor induced by interleukin 1 and tumor necrosis factor. J. Exp. Med. 165: 914-919, 1987.

62. Dayer, J-M., de Rochemonteix, B., Burrus, B., Demczuk, S., and Dinarello, C.A. Human recombinant interleukin-1 stimulates collagenase and prostaglandin $E_2$ synthesis by human synovial cells. J. Clin. Invest. 77: 1734-1739, 1986.

63. Marcum, J.A., Levein, J., and Prendergast, R.A. Clotting enzyme activity derived from coelomocytes of the sea star *Asterias forbesi*. Thromb. Haemost. 62: 1-3, 1984.

64. Krueger, J.M., Karaszewski, J.W., Davenne, D., and Shoham, S. Somnogenic muramyl peptides. Fed. Proc. 45: 2552-2555, 1986.

65. Hirano, T., Yasukawa, K., Harada, H., Taga, T., Wantanabe, Y., Matsuda, T., Kashiwamura, S., Nakajima, K., Koyama, K., Iwasmatsu, A., Tsunasawa, S., Sakiyama, F., Matsui, H., Takahara, Y., Taniguchi, T., and Kishimoto, T. Complementary DNA for a novel human interleukin (BSF-2) that induces B lymphocytes to produce immunoglobulin. Nature 324: 73-76, 1986.

66. Van Damme, J., Opdenakker, G., LeLey, M., Heremans, H., and Billiau, A. Pyrogenic and haematological effects of the interferon-inducing 22K factor (interleukin-1 beta) from human leukocytes. Clin. Exp. Immunol. 66: 303-311, 1986.

67. Beutler, B., and Cerami, A. Cachectin and tumor necrosis factor as two sides of the same biological coin. Nature 320: 584-588, 1986.

68. Sauder, D.N. Epidermal-derived cytokines: Properties of epidermal-derived thymocyte activating factor. Lymphokine Res. 3: 145-151, 1985.

69. Scala, G., Kaung, Y.D., Hall, R.E., Muchmore, A.V., and Oppenheim, J.J. Accessory cell function of human B cells. Production of both interleukin-1-like activity and an interleukin-1 inhibitory factor by an EBV-transformed human B cell line. J. Exp. Med. 159: 1637-1652, 1984.

70. Kurt-Jones, E.A., Kiely, J.M., and Unanue, E.R. Conditions required for expression of membrane IL-1 on B-cells. J. Immunol. 135: 1548-1550, 1985.

71. Numerof, R., Dinarello, C.A., and Mier, J.W. Interleukin-2 induces interleukin-1 from large granular lymphocytes. Lymphokine Res. 6: 1207, 1987.

72. Fontana, A., and Grob, P.J. Astrocyte-derived interleukin-1-like factors. Lymphokine Res. 3: 11-16, 1984.

73. Giulian, D., and Lachman, L.B. Interleukin-1 stimulation of astroglial proliferation after brain injury. Science 228: 497-499, 1985.

74. Libby, R., Ordovas, J.M., Auger, K.R., Robbins, A.H., Birinyi, L.K., and Dinarello, C.A. Endotoxin and tumor necrosis factor induce interleukin-1 gene expression in adult human vascular endothelial cells. Am. J. Pathol. 124: 179-186, 1986.

75. Libby, P., Ordovas, J.M., Auger, K.R., Robbins, A.H., Birinyi, L.K., and Dinarello, C.A. Inducible interleukin-1 gene expression in vascular smooth muscle cells. J. Clin. Invest. 78: 1432-1438, 1986.

# 4

# Interleukin-2-Activated Cytotoxic Cells

Kathleen Last-Barney and Vincent J. Merluzzi / Boehringer Ingelheim
Pharmaceuticals, Inc., Ridgefield, Connecticut

## I. BACKGROUND

Much of our current understanding of classic cytotoxic T lymphocyte (CTL)
function came from early studies utilizing in vitro cytotoxic assays. These assays
provided a means of studying the details of activation, differentiation, and target
specificity. The specificity of the response was believed to be the result of receptors present on the effector T cell which recognized the stimulating antigen in
the context of the determinants of the major histocompatibility complex (MHC)
(1). The necessity for specificity, though accepted as rule, was not always observed in experimental systems. Many investigators observed nonspecific lysis in
addition to specific lysis. The nonspecific responses were often elicited from effector cells generated in a mixed lymphocyte reaction (MLR), in conditioned
media derived from MLR cultures or from cultures of lymphocytes stimulated
with mitogens, such as phytohemagglutinin (PHA) or concanavalin A (ConA).

In early studies, this phenomenon was seen in human culture systems in
which allogeneic and xenogeneic killing of targets occurred by lymphocytes transformed with purified protein derivative (2,3). It was suggested that lymphocytes
could be recruited nonspecifically to become cytotoxic by a mitogen-like factor
produced in the cell cultures. This nonspecific cytotoxicity developed early,
around 3 days, prior to the development of CTL activity. The nonspecific cytotoxicity occurred regardless of whether the stimulating factors were nonspecific
(mitogen) or specific (antigen). It was proposed that nonspecific stimulation represented a mechanism present in the animal for amplifying an antigen-specific
response (3). This response may also be involved in delayed-type hypersensitivity and tumor/graft rejection (3). A low degree of spontaneous cytotoxicity was

observed when normal human T cells were grown in culture with conditioned media for 5-7 days (4). Serological examination of the effectors revealed that a significant number of cells did not have Fc receptors and no detectable antibody-dependent cellular cytotoxic (ADCC) activity occurred. These results suggested that a population different from natural killer (NK) cells was involved. It was believed that the effectors might represent a population enriched in polyclonally activated T cells having a low spontaneous activity against a variety of targets (4). A different study examined the specificity of Fc+ cells generated during the culture of human peripheral blood lymphocytes (PBL). After 7 days in culture, these effectors lysed NK-sensitive targets. NK-insensitive targets were not tested. One explanation suggested that NK-like activity, arising after 7 days of culture, was due to factors present in conditioned media. The effector population was thought to consist of both NK and polyclonally activated T cells (5).

Seeley and others in several reports (6-8), described another type of non-specific cytotoxicity by effectors generated in a MLR. This "anomalous killing" (AK) activity was clearly distinguishable by kinetics and range of susceptible targets from specific classic CTL activity. AK occurred 1-2 days prior to the expected CTL activity and declined sooner. AK activity was not limited to target cells bearing cross-reactive antigens and this cytotoxicity was exhibited against a wide range of cell lines. These AK cells however, could be generated from populations enriched in T cells, and AK activity could be derived from NK-depleted populations. AK populations were proposed to be (1) CTL precursors (CTLp), (2) a T-helper (Th) cell subset, or (3) the result of a polyclonal activation of T cells. It was suggested that AK activity was mediated by a soluble factor produced during the MLR because a stronger reaction was seen from MLR cultured cells than from control cells (8).

In another study AK activity was shown to develop from human PBL cultured with the Daudi lymphoblastoid cell line (9). Serological analysis showed that the generation of AK was dependent upon thymus-derived cells and the effectors displayed T-cell antigens. The precursor frequency of AK from normal peripheral blood lymphocytes (PBL) ranged from 1/166-1/689. This precursor frequency dropped after treatment with fractionated irradiation or cytoreductive therapy. Interestingly, lymphokine-containing supernatants partially restored AK activity after irradiation (9).

Nonspecific cytotoxic activity (murine and human) in cultures containing only fetal calf serum (FCS), MLR culture supernatants, or mitogenic factor (MF, derived from PHA-stimulated cultures) was examined by several investigators (10-13). The lymphocytes were activated by each one of these culture conditions. The human effector cells, after 6 days of culture, lysed both the NK-sensitive target, K562, and the NK-insensitive target, Daudi (10). It was concluded that the "activated lymphocyte killing" (ALK) was a property of activated T cells generated in vitro and was not due to the survival of NK. Supernatants from AK cultures enhanced the lytic activity of fresh lymphocytes and gamma-interferon (IFN-γ) was suspected to be involved in this enhancement (10).

Nonspecific cytotoxicity from murine splenocytes cultured in FCS alone was also observed. After one week in culture a T-killer cell arose spontaneously which was capable of lysing a variety of lymphohematopoietic tumor cells (11). The cytolytic activity peaked between day 3 and day 6 of culture. The cytotoxic effector population was derived from an NK population capable of lysing solid tumors and whose activity increases in culture. Another cytotoxic effector was also present in culture concomitant with this NK-like killer. This second population was described as a Thy1+, Ly1+, and Ly2+ T-killer cell (11).

Murine lymphocytes cultured without stimulators in mouse serum and media supplemented with MLR supernatants also gave rise to nonspecific cytotoxic cells (12). These effectors mediated high levels of cytotoxicity against all targets tested, except for syngeneic or allogeneic Con A blasts. The activation of the effectors in this system was suggested to involve lymphokines produced during the MLR. The murine effectors in many of these systems phenotypically were $Ly2^+$. Depletion of the $Ly2^+$ cell population prior to the $^{51}$chromium release assay (CRA) reduced lysis by 75% (12). Similar effectors were generated from human MLR cultures. These lymphocytes gave rise to an NK-like effector as well as the expected CTL effector (13). The NK-like cells, generated after 7 days, lacked the OKT3+, OKT8+ markers and these effectors were not removed by pretreatment with anti-OKM1 and complement (C). It was unclear however, if this effector population was derived from NK precursors (NKp). The effectors displaying nonspecific cytotoxicity in all these studies were distinguishable from classic CTL or NK. Strassmann et al. (13) suggested that their activation was due to IFN or interleukin-2 (IL-2).

Some laboratories have described a "spontaneously" arising cytotoxic cell (SCTL) (14,15) which had characteristics of both CTL and NK. This cell may represent a subset stage in the T-cell lineage. Through the use of depletion studies (murine) it was demonstrated that the precursors bear low levels of the Thy1 antigen which increased in density as the cells differentiated into cytotoxic effectors. The appearance of SCTL was markedly enhanced by the addition of IL-2 or conditioned media.

It was not clear whether these effectors represented a population of polyclonally activated T cells or whether the observed nonspecific cytotoxicity (directed against different determinants expressed on the targets) was accomplished by several NK effector cell types. Results from independent laboratories supported the idea that the effectors were derived from heterogeneous populations (16,17). In one study, normal human T cells were grown in vitro with conditioned media as colonies on semisolid agar. The derived effectors demonstrated a spontaneous cytotoxicity after 5-7 days in culture. In this study, cells arising from different colonies preferentially lysed different tumor targets. The specificity of the initially heterogeneous population was proposed to have segregated independently into individual colonies. This data implied that the effectors were specifically restricted. Serological analyses of the effector populations showed that they were unlikely to be NK cells because they lacked an Fc receptor (16). In related experiments, limiting dilution assays were used to generate T-cell clones from murine splenocytes (17). Mature Ly2+ T cells gave rise to clones after 8 days which were able to lyse a wide range of targets. The initially heterogeneous population, once cultured in limiting dilution and cloned were cytotoxic for several targets. The clones were described morphologically as large granular lymphocytes (LGL) and their action was not blocked by anti-Ly2 treatment. It was suggested that these activated killer cells may be differentiated elements of the $Ly2^+$ T-cell lineage. A subsequent report indicated that the development of nonspecific cytotoxicity from specific CTLs was a normal feature of most CTL clones (18).

Cells exhibiting nonspecific cytotoxic potential were shown to arise from normal as well as tumor-bearing animals. Lymphocytes isolated from tumors acquired this nonspecific potential when grown in cultures containing T-cell growth factor (TCGF). This phenomenon was observed with murine lymphocytes isolated from methylcholanthrene- (MCA) induced tumors and from normal spleens (19). In Winn-type neutralization assays, inhibition of tumor growth occurred when Thy1+ cells, derived from small MCA-induced sarcomas were incubated with TCGF (20). A similar phenomenon in human culture models was reported. Peripheral blood lymphocytes from cancer patients lysed autologous fresh or cultured tumor cells. This occurred when the PBL were expanded in culture in media containing TCGF (21). In addition, lymphocytes from normal and tumor-bearing patients cultured, expanded, and maintained in IL-2 were shown to lyse isolated tumors grown as single-cell suspensions (22).

In other investigations, the generation of both human and murine effectors displaying nonspecific cytotoxicity seemed to correlate with the generation of IL-2 within the culture systems. Nonspecific lytic activation of normal human PBL following stimulation by allo-PBL, or PHA was described (23,24). Con A-induced nonspecific activation of murine lymphocytes (25) and IL-2 enhanced all of these in vitro reactions. The cytotoxic effectors generated in these systems had a broad range of activity and did not require antigen for activation. The cells were categorized serologically as $Ly2^+$, asialo $GM_1$- (murine) or $OKT8^+$, $OKM1^-$ (human). All of the nonspecific killers were suggested to share a common pathway for activation and the lymphokine, IL-2, was implicated as having a central role.

Several investigators have looked at the effects of purified IL-2, free of other factors, in various cytotoxic systems. Many observed that culturing lymphocytes with IL-2 alone resulted in the production of killers with nonspecific cytotoxicity. Using preparations of IL-2 lacking IFN activity, it was shown that IL-2 caused a rapid increase in NK activity (26). NK regulation was studied by using purified

NK populations and monoclonal antibodies to IL-2 (27). In these systems the addition of an anti-IL-2 antibody to a 4 hr CRA resulted in a significant decrease in NK activity. The data suggested that the spontaneous activity of NK cells depended upon their continual exposure to IL-2.

A previously unappreciated effector system was described as distinct from the NK and CTL systems (28). The effectors were called "lymphokine-activated killers" (LAK) and were generated from unstimulated normal PBL in a 2-3 day culture period by purified IL-2. These cells lysed NK-sensitive and -insensitive targets. Other investigators cultured murine lymphocytes isolated from several tissue sources with IL-2 (29). The resultant effectors all exhibited strong cytotoxic activity in vitro toward a variety of fresh, cultured, syngeneic, allogeneic, and xenogeneic tumors. Extensive lysis was also observed against NK-resistant targets. This data suggested that these "cultured lymphoid cells" (CLC), were selected or activated because they were propagated in IL-2. The CLC exhibited characteristics of both NK and classic CTL. Supplement-induced cytotoxic cells (SICC) were also described (30). In this system, a similar activity developed from normal murine splenocytes or thymocytes. Cytotoxicity occurred after the cells were cultured with various factors: IFN, mitogens, heterologous sera, MLR supernatants, some nucleic acid polymers, and IL-2. The effectors were generated without a stimulating antigen and they displayed a broad reactivity against various targets including syngeneic, allogeneic, and xenogeneic tumor targets as well as fibroblasts. Mitogen-induced lymphoblasts were resistant to this lytic activity (30). Recombinant IL-2 (rIL-2) when added to cell cultures induced the expression of spontaneous cytotoxicity from normal resting PBL (31). This effect occurred after a very brief (18 hr) incubation period.

Gronvik and Andersson (32) suggested that highly purified TCGF preparations at high concentrations were mitogenic for a small number of resting T cells. To explain this action of IL-2, they speculated that the IL-2 receptor molecule might occur in more than one conformation. The predominant form of this molecule found on resting populations may possibly prevent IL-2 binding. They suggested that this inhibitory state was unstable and transitions to the receptor state might occur at a certain rate. High IL-2 concentrations however, might stabilize the receptor state and this stabilized form would allow the cell to bind sufficient IL-2 to become activated and therefore proliferate.

The results described suggest that resting cells do respond to IL-2 and that IL-2 augments both classic CTL and NK responses. Central to the activation of the classical CTLp is the release of IL-2 by the activated Th cell. Probably in the normal milieu, this lymphokine is released in minute amounts, has a short half life (33,34), but would still be potent for neighboring CTLp. It has been shown that in conjunction with a stimulating antigen, IL-2 activates specific CTLp to differentiate and divide (35).

In a study by Vohr and Hunig (36), CTLp were shown to require only the presence of IL-2 for proliferation and differentiation. When this activation system is circumvented by high concentrations of IL-2, then IL-2 may activate CTLp in a polyclonal manner.

## II. GENERATION OF IL-2-DRIVEN NONSPECIFIC CYTOTOXIC T LYMPHOCYTES (LYMPHOKINE-ACTIVATED KILLER CELLS)

It could be stated that the generation of nonspecific killers in vitro from fresh murine or human lymphocytes requires only IL-2 (14,15,19,21,28,30,37-39, 41,42). In fact, IL-2 was shown to be the sole factor responsible for LAK activation. It was shown that the LAK activating factor was directly and consistently associated with IL-2 activity (39). The generation of cells with nonspecific cytotoxicity was also demonstrated to be due to IL-2 utilizing IL-2 absorption techniques. When IL-2 was removed from culture systems, cells with nonspecific cytotoxicity could no longer be generated (43). Fetal calf serum was ruled out as the source of activation because murine LAK could be generated using 1% normal mouse serum (44).

The induction process of LAK was shown to be sensitive to gamma irradiation (28,40,43). Grimm and Wilson (42) examined the effects of mitomycin C treatment or gamma irradiation on LAKp. They found that PBL treated with mitomycin C and subsequently incubated with IL-2 could not develop into LAK effectors. It was concluded from this study that proliferation was required for LAK generation.

Several investigators suggest that other lymphokines/factors as well as IL-2 are required for the generation of LAK effector cells (45-49). Yang et al. (49) described a novel lymphokine, "cytotoxic cell differentiation factor" (CCDF). In their study both CCDF and IL-2 together induced higher levels of cytotoxicity than either lymphokine alone. The nonspecific killing they observed arose early in their culture system and they suggest that these two lymphokines are required for the generation of LAK under physiological conditions. Burns et al. (47) developed a monoclonal antibody (MoAb) to what they believe is a human T-lineage-specific activation antigen (TLiSA). The presence of this MoAb during the generation of CTL or LAK in a MLR inhibited the induction of effectors but not their proliferation. Limiting dilution confirmed this inhibitory effect. They suggested that this TLiSA antigen may represent a receptor for a differentiation factor that is separate from the IL-2 receptor. This study suggests that other factors may be involved in the activation of CTLp and LAKp. Several investigators suggested that IFN-$\gamma$ is implicated in LAK generation (45,46,48), while others have observed that gamma IFN is probably not necessary (40).

It has been suggested that the generation of LAK involved a re-expression of cytolytic activity from inactive memory CTL (43,50,51). This process of reactivation seems to require only IL-2. This proposal is based in part on the belief that fresh nonactivated T cells did not respond to the growth-promoting effects of IL-2 until IL-2 receptors were expressed following antigen or mitogen stimulation (51). It was suggested that IL-2 may activate these memory CTL by a process that depended on the cell proliferation (43). These superactivated CTL may then be able to lyse targets bearing antigens to which they have low affinity binding.

Interestingly, LAK cells can be generated in vivo in mice (33,52,53). Chang et al. (33) accomplished this by the continuous administration of rIL-2 over a 4-day period, through the use of osmotic mini pumps implanted into the animals. This procedure resulted in the generation of LAK from splenocytes and peritoneal exudate cells. A similar system was utilized by an independent laboratory. LAK effectors and the therapeutic effects of adoptively transferred LAK cells were enhanced in EL-4 lymphoma-bearing mice by the slow continuous release of rIL-2 in the animals (53). The slow release of IL-2 seemed to be more advantageous than one single bolus injection (53). Rosenberg et al. (53) induced LAK in vivo by the systemic administration of rIL-2. The protocol included several doses of rIL-2 given in intraperitoneal injections every 8 hr for 5 days. LAK activity was observed from the spleens of treated mice. They observed that increasing doses of rIL-2 resulted in enhanced lytic activity.

## III. CELLULAR REQUIREMENTS FOR LAK GENERATION

There seems to be no accessory cell requirement for the generation of LAK cells. Teh and Yu (43) described this process as being partially dependent upon adherent cells, while others (48,51,54) showed that the removal of either the adherent or Ly1$^+$ (Th cell) populations did not inhibit LAK generation. The expansion and maintenance of human cultured LAK over long periods (> 80 days), however, seems to require feeder cells (fresh irradiated PBL) and PHA to maintain the extended activity of the LAK cells (55). Simultaneous activation of various cells in a LAK cell culture may lead to a significant cooperation between distinct cell populations (56). It would be plausible then, that even within a purified population of T cells there may be an interaction of several subsets, each at different levels of maturation.

## IV. GENETIC RESTRICTION AND TARGET SPECIFICITY OF LAK CELLS

Monoclonal antibodies were generated to the LAK cell surface which recognized a structure common on both the LAK and NK populations but not on CTL (57). This antigen, called lymphokine-activated cell-associated antigen (LAA), seems to be involved in the binding of LAK or NK to their targets. This property was illustrated in a CRA in which the anti-LAA antibody would inhibit lysis by either NK and LAK but not CTL effectors in a dose-dependent manner. LAA is on all lymphocytes, but there seems to be a greater concentration on LAK cells. This observation implies that IL-2 treatment induces a greater expression of LAA. This

LAA antigen appears to be associated with the binding molecules of nonspecific cytotoxic cells (NK, LAK). The anti-LAA antibody also inhibits the T-cell response to Con A. This observation suggests that this antigen may play a role in T-cell activation mechanisms involving IL-2 (57). The lack of target specificity suggests that genetic restriction does not occur in this system. While the mechanism of cytotoxicity is similar to that described for both CTL and NK (58), the target structures recognized by LAK effector cells is still very unclear.

## V.  PRECURSOR AND EFFECTOR PHENOTYPE(S) OF LAK CELLS

The effector phenotype of LAK cells in humans has been defined by some as a classic CTL. For example in humans it has been defined as $OKT3^+$, $OKT8^+$, $OKM1^-$, $OKT4^-$, $LEU1^-$, and $4F2^+$ (55,59). Some studies argue that the effector cells are composed of at least two cytotoxic populations, T cells and non-T cells (60,61) and perhaps NK cells. One study suggested that the LAK effector cells are a population of NK cells and are responsible for the majority of "LAK" activity (62). In murine studies the effector cell has been described as $Thy1^+$, $Ly2^+$, and $Ly1^-$ (15,40,44). Some investigators would describe the phenotype of murine effectors differently. Nonspecific murine effectors generated early in culture with IL-2 and conditioned media were typed as $Thy1^+$, $Ly2^-$, asialo $GM_1^-$ (49). Other studies suggest that LAK effector cells are asialo $GM_1^\pm$, NK.1.1+, Qa 5+, and Ly2+ (63). It is generally agreed that the effector cells have both NK- and CTL-like characteristics and the differences in monitoring certain cell surface markers on the LAK effector cells may be due to the length and types of culture conditions used. For example, the phenotypes of cytotoxic cells are different depending upon when the serological analyses are done. There is a difference between the phenotypes of IL–2-activated cells on days 1, 3, and 7 (64-66) and this may represent different stages of activation. It is possible that the LAK effector cells are indeed a heterogeneous population of cells including both NK-like and polyclonal T-like cytotoxic cells. These problems must be resolved before the LAK effector cell is described definitively by serological analyses.

Characterizing the phenotype of the precursor has been even more difficult. In the mouse some would argue that the precursors are sensitive to treatment with anti-Thy1+C (40,43,65,67). Others have observed that the effectors arise from precursors that are not affected by this treatment (15,63,69). The murine LAK precursor has also been described as asialo $GM_1^+$ in some studies (63,68, 69) and asialo $GM_1^-$ in others (65), depending upon when the LAK effector cells are enumerated. Most precursors for murine LAK cells are asialo $GM_1^+$ if cytotoxicity is measured early after culture initiation and asialo $GM_1^-$ if measured after long-term culture (63,65).

Distinctions between LAK and NK precursors have been shown utilizing an adoptive transfer system in which donor bone marrow (syngeneic) was fractionated on Percoll discontinuous gradients. In this system LAK precursors were demonstrated in all bone marrow fractions. One fraction, however (>65% Percoll) was devoid of NK precursors (70). Therefore, at the level of the bone marrow, there was a distinction between NK and LAK precursor cells.

In humans, the precursors were seen as distinct from both mature T cells and classic NK. They have been described as OKM1⁻, OKT3⁻, LEU1⁻, LEU7⁻, OKT9⁻, OKT10⁻, Tac⁻, and OKT11⁻ (55,59,67). One study demonstrated that NK-depleted peripheral blood cells were able to provide precursors for in vitro LAK activity (71). A number of investigators performed extensive serological studies which have undoubtedly shown that the human LAK "precursor" is derived from a phenotypically heterogeneous population of cells (61,72) with some suggesting that NK cells provide the majority of activity (61).

## VI. COMPARISON OF LAK CELLS WITH OTHER CYTOTOXIC LYMPHOCYTES

Activation of classic CTL requires two signals, antigen and a proliferative signal (IL-2), while LAK cells require only IL-2. CTL lyse specific targets and are restricted by the MHC, while LAK cells are neither restricted nor specific. After culture, CTL activity is optimal within 5-6 days. Both LAK and CTL effectors can be detected around 2-3 days. Both CTLp and LAKp are sensitive to treatments which inhibit cell division whereas as effectors both are shown to be resistant to these same treatments (40). In a study by Grimm and Wilson (42) LAK and memory CTL were distinguished by at least two characteristics. LAKp were not OKT3⁺, whereas memory CTL were and the generation of LAK activity required proliferation whereas memory CTL did not. Though this novel effector population shares many characteristics with classic CTL, it lacks the same functional restrictions. The placement of the LAK cell within the CTL lineage cannot be accomplished using traditional characteristics.

Natural killer effector cells exhibit spontaneous cytolytic activity against a limited range of susceptible targets and their response requires no previous antigenic stimulation. Murine NK reactivity was observed to be labile in culture and was usually not seen by 48 hr (26). Many investigators suggest that NK cells are not a single cell type but rather are a heterogeneous population of cells sharing the capability of selective cytotoxicity (46,73). Morphologically, these cells are described as large granular lymphocytes (LGL) which bear Fc receptors (54).

Interferons have been shown to be regulators of NK activity (54). It was suggested that IL-2 can stimulate the development of NK precursors which lack certain NK markers. In this study IL-2 was seen to act directly on LGL isolated from PBL and IL-2 induced a rapid increase in the proportion of OKM1+ cells (54). It was suggested that IL-2 may have promoted the differentiation of immature NK to mature NK. Others have shown augmentation of NK activity by IL-2 (26,46,74). Exposure of PBL to rIL-2 has been shown to increase cytolytic activity of PBL in a short-term CRA (4 hr exposure to IL-2) (75). Exposure of PBL to

rIL-2 directly activated NK via a process requiring protein but not DNA synthesis. Four phenotypically distinct NK populations were observed: LEU11+LEU7−,
LEU11+LEU7+, LEU11−LEU7+, and LEU11−LEU7−. The most potent cytotoxic cells were LEU11+ and all NK stimulated by rIL-2 were confined to this
subset of lymphocytes (75).

It is clear that NK activity is augmented by both IFN and IL-2 (46,54). NK
cells show a narrower range of susceptible targets, while effectors activated by
IL-2 lyse all NK-sensitive and -insensitive targets. Cells driven by IL-2 to display
cytotoxic activity do not seem to belong conclusively in either the NK or CTL
class of cytotoxic cells. Some investigators align LAK with NK, some with CTL
and others suggest that the LAK population provides a link between conventional
cytotoxic populations. Precursors for LAK can be found in the LEU11+ lymphocyte cell fractions (41). In fact, the highest nonspecific cytotoxic activity induced
by IL-2 was shown to arise from the LEU7−,11+ fraction of LGL. Lanier et al.
(75) had reported that the most potent IL-2-driven NK-like effectors were LEU11+
as well. Other studies (76) suggest that NK, CTL, and LAK may share a common
precursor pool in bone marrow and represent different stages of differentiation
of cytotoxic effector cells. Nieminen and Saksela (76) used a new monoclonal
antibody NK9+, which recognizes practically all peripheral blood LGL. They
showed that the precursor for both nonspecific and antigen-specific cytotoxic
cells may at least be phenotypically related. These cytotoxic cells appeared to be
harbored in the NK9+ pool of bone marrow. These results differ from that of the
mouse in which a fraction of bone marrow was shown to lack NK precursors but
contain LAK cytotoxic precursors (70).

The generation of LAK, NK, and CTL was also studied after bone marrow
transplantation (BMT) and irradiation (77,78). It was reported that lethally irradiated mice could generate LAK in response to IL-2 as early as 7 days after
bone marrow transplant. CTL were not active until 4 weeks after transplant (77).
In addition, LAK and CTL precursors could be distinguished by their relative sen-
sitivities to gamma irradiation. CTL precursors were more sensitive to gamma
irradiation than were LAK precursors and LAK activity could be demonstrated
sooner after sublethal irradiation than that of CTL (65).

Brooks and Henney (46) explain the interrelationship of NK and CTL derived
from IL-2-supplemented cultures in the following way. In short-term cultures,
the predominant system involves IL-2 potentiating NK activity through IFN production. During longer incubation periods, IL-2 and IFN together induce cells
from the CTL lineage to express NK-like activity. In long-term cultures young
cells may acquire the CTL-like phenotype or more mature CTL may be triggered
to express IL-2 receptors by recent exposure to antigen, serum proteins, traces
of lectins, or other lymphokines. Once triggered, these CTL can acquire NK-like
activity through interaction with IL-2 alone. In an early study it was reported
that IFN was not produced in IL-2-stimulated spleen cell cultures and the use
of an anti-gamma IFN antibody did not abrogate the generation of murine LAK

cells (40). This indicated that IFN-$\gamma$ was probably not necessary for the generation of murine effectors. Nishimura and Hashimoto (48) investigated the relationship between the induction of LAK and the production of gamma IFN. They detected IFN-$\gamma$ in the cultures and suggested that the production of this lymphokine was related to the development of LAK. They also observed that IFN was produced in the culture prior to the observed LAK activity. Nishimura and Hashimoto suggested that IFN may play a role in the early phase of LAKp differentiation. In a report by Itoh et al. (45) data was presented which suggest that IFN-$\gamma$ does play a role in LAK generation. The cytotoxic activity in relation to IFN-$\gamma$ was examined after 3 days in culture. They observed that the addition of IFN-$\gamma$ to rIL-2 cultures or the pretreatment of PBL with IFN-$\gamma$ resulted in an augmented NK response and the generation of activated killer cells. These data suggest that IFN-$\gamma$ can induce LAK, but it is also possible that this "early" nonspecific activity is only due to the survival of NK. The relationship of IFN-$\gamma$ and LAK cell generation remains unclear.

By the addition of N-acetyl-D-galactosamine (NADG) at the initiation of culture, the culture-derived NK-like cells could be distinguished from CTL and LAK (79). NK-like activity was inhibited and CTL and LAK were not affected. This was shown by adding the antisera OKT3 as well as NADG to the culture system. LAK and CTL were inhibited by the OKT3 antibody and when NADG was present the effectors capable of lysing the NK-sensitive target K562 were not generated. This inhibition of the NK-like activity was reversed when conditioned media was added to the culture.

Experiments were designed to test the effect of parental injections of antithymocyte serum (ATS) or antiasialo GM$_1$ on NK, LAK and CTL generation precursors (65). NK cells were not affected by ATS, but were removed after in vivo injection of antiasialo GM$_1$. In these experiments, some cytotoxic activity against the NK-insensitive target P815 was generated after 24 hr. This "early" cytotoxic activity was slightly reduced in the spleen cell cultures from ATS-pretreated mice and fully removed in the spleen cultures from the antiasialo GM$_1$-pretreated mice. These "early" generated cytotoxic effects seemed to be derived from an ATS-resistant, antiasialo, GM$_1$-susceptible, precursor pool. After 7 days in culture, LAK cells were derived from a AST-sensitive, antiasialo, GM$_1$-resistant pool. The LAK cells generated after ATS pretreatment of mice were never completely eliminated by ATS. Classic CTL were derived from an ATS-sensitive, antiasialo, GM$_1$-resistant precursor population. These results suggest IL-2 is capable of stimulating a mixed population of cells, both T cell and non-T cell to become cytotoxic and that LAK cells appear to be closely aligned with classic CTL. It is becoming apparent that CTL can no longer be thought of as an end cell of differentiation (46,47). It was suggested that NK and CTL each represent one of several stages of differentiation. Rather than the LAK effector system being unique, it may be categorized somewhere between classical CTL and NK (46,65).

## VII. IN VIVO STUDIES OF LAK CELLS

The appearance of a novel nonspecific cytotoxic system, capable of lysing a variety of tumor targets, has helped to renew interest and research in the field of immunotherapy. Many investigators have recognized the potential of this nonspecific cytotoxic system activated by IL-2 (for reviews see Refs. 80-83), which provides a means for activating and expanding large numbers of autologous lymphocytes in vitro. By returning them to the donor by infusion these cells may eradicate neoplastic cells and provide the host with a more competent cellular immune response. Animal models are being utilized to test the feasibility of such protocols in clinical trials. In very early studies, investigators utilized primed lymphocytes or lymphocytes from tumor-bearing animals (84,85). They expanded these cells in culture with IL-2 along with the stimulating antigen. When these cells were adoptively transferred into secondary hosts they were effective in killing the tumor in vivo or were able to increase the host's mean survival time (85). The lymphocytes' enhanced cytotoxicity was illustrated in a parallel CRA (84). In Winn neutralization tests, lymphocytes expanded in crude IL-2 delayed or inhibited growth of lymphomas and carcinomas in syngeneic and allogeneic recipients (29). In a study using similar methods, results indicated that rIL-2 could induce killer cells capable of lysing primary tumor explants (86). Mazumder and Rosenberg (87) showed that lymphocytes from tumor-bearing animals, when activated in vitro by IL-2, could inhibit the growth of established melanoma pulmonary metastases. In another adoptive transfer study, Mule et al. (88) added multiple IL-2 injections to the protocol. Here the method was effective in decreasing the number and size of the neoplastic nodules. A subsequent study by Mule et al. (89) outlined the factors necessary for successful in vivo therapy of micrometastases. It was observed that the number of LAK cells infused and the amount of rIL-2 injected was directly related to the success of the treatment in vivo. Another murine model, using hepatic micrometastases, was examined for response to LAK and rIL-2 therapy (90). Effective treatment required rIL-2 alone at high doses or a combination of LAK cell infusion with IL-2 injections. It was also observed that if mice were sublethally irradiated prior to treatment, the effects of rIL-2 alone were removed, but effective therapy could still be obtained if LAK and rIL-2 were used together. In other murine studies, it was observed that some of the precursors of effectors activated by IL-2 were resistant to chemotherapy (91). Since some effectors activated by IL-2 were shown to be spared by certain antineoplastic agents, it may be possible then to combine IL-2 therapy with chemotherapy to achieve greater survival rates and better therapeutic regimes (80).

Through the use of adoptive therapy protocols in animal models, a clear in vivo role for cytotoxic cells activated by IL-2 has been demonstrated (for review see Ref. 83). The latest studies have shown efficacy for LAK cell therapy in combination with IL-2 for murine sarcomas, established pulmonary and hepatic metastases as well as intraperitoneal cancer (92-95). In some systems, the transplanted

tumor cells were eradicated whether or not they were strongly or weakly immunogenic or of different histological types (92). Recently the antitumor effects of
IL-2 and LAK cells on established metastases has been correlated with the cytolytic activity of the LAK effectors (96).

A new approach using tumor-infiltrating lymphocytes as a source of IL-2-
expanded cytotoxic cells (in place of normal lymphocytes) in combination with
IL-2 has been successful (97,98). This approach could be advantageous because
fewer cells may be needed in adoptive transfer experiments. These preliminary
experiments provide a rationale for a similar approach in humans (98).

## VIII. CLINICAL STUDIES

Pilot studies utilizing similar protocols that have been used in the preclinical animal models have begun in clinical settings. Rayner et al. (22) generated, expanded,
and maintained LAK from both normal and tumor-bearing patients. The LAK
were able to lyse a variety of fresh tumor targets derived from single cell suspensions. This study shows that patients have the potential to generate their own
LAK cells which may in turn be used for immunotherapy. Other laboratories
have studied the effects of an in vivo administration of autologous lymphocytes
activated by IL-2 (99). The lymphocytes were injected intralesionally with an
arrest of tumor growth in 8 lesions and a partial regression in 3 lesions. There
was, however, a lack of correlation between enhanced cytotoxicity in vitro and
tumor involution in vivo (99). LAK activity has been demonstrated to occur in
other tissues besides PBL. LAK cells were generated from lamina propria lymphocytes in both normal and malignant intestinal tissues (100). While low NK activity was observed from these same sources, the LAK activity was comparable to
that induced from PBL. Hogan et al. (100) suggest that the LAK effector population may represent the in vivo mechanism for the irradication of abnormal tissue in the intestine.

The latest clinical trials of LAK cells in patients have met with reasonably
good success (81,102-106). Generally the use of LAK and IL-2 has shown therapeutic effects in patients for which no other effective therapy is available (105).
Complete objective regressions (>50% reduction in tumor volume) have been observed in many cases (102). The most recent study has shown encouraging results
with a number of complete and partial remissions (105). Toxicity with IL-2 therapy has included the following problems: malaise, weight gain, minimal renal and
hepatic toxicity, mild anemia, and severe fluid retention (81,101,102,104,105). The
toxicity has been studied in experimental animals in order to elucidate the mechanisms and control for their effects in clinical trials with IL-2 and IL-2/LAK therapy (107,108). Using a system to measure vascular leakage of $[^{125}I]$albumin in
mice, corticosteroids were shown to alleviate the toxicity associated with IL-2,
however the therapeutic effects were negated (107). The vascular leak syndrome
induced by IL-2, which is the cause of the severe fluid retention in patients, seems

to require T cells and therefore may be mediated by a T-cell product or effect (108). A recent study by Damle et al. (109) has shown that both T cells and non-T cells stimulated with IL-2 exhibit enhanced adhesion to normal vascular endothelial cells and cause their lysis. It was suggested that the systemic toxicity of IL-2 is due in part to the destruction of endothelial cells by IL-2-stimulated lymphocytes (109).

## IX.  SUMMARY

Many more questions still have to be addressed. Does this effector population ever occur naturally and if it does, what functional role does it play? Wherever IL-2 may be released in vivo, do physiological concentrations or excess amounts produce this nonspecific cytotoxic potential? Do LAK cells play a role in immune surveillance? Do LAK cells cause or contribute to graft rejection, enhance graft versus host (GVH) disease or exacerbate chronic inflammation? Are LAK cells indeed unique?

## REFERENCES

1. Williams, A.F. The T-lymphocyte antigen receptor-elusive no more. Nature 308: 108, 1984.
2. Butterworth, A.E. Nonspecific cytotoxic effects of antigen-transformed lymphocytes. Kinetics, cell requirements and the role of recruitment. Cell Immunol. 7: 357-369, 1973.
3. Butterworth, A.E., and Franks, D. Nonspecific cytotoxic effects of antigen-transformed lymphocytes III. Relationship to specific cytotoxicity. Cell. Immunol. 16: 74-81, 1975.
4. Alvarez, J.M., de Landazuri, M.O., Bonnard, G.D., and Herberman, R.B. Cytotoxic activities of normal cultured human T cells. J. Immunol. 121: 1270-1275, 1978.
5. Ortaldo, J.R., Bonnard, G.D., Kind, P.D., and Herberman, R.B. Cytotoxicity by cultured human lymphocytes: Characteristics of effector cells and specificity of cytotoxicity. J. Immunol. 122: 1489-1494, 1979.
6. Seeley, J.K., and Golub, S.H. Studies on cytotoxicity generated in human mixed lymphocyte cultures I. Time course and target spectrum of several distinct concomitant cytotoxic activities. J. Immunol. 120: 1415-1422, 1978.
7. Karre, K., and Seeley, J.K. Cytotoxic Thy 1.2-positive blasts with NK-like target selectivity in murine mixed lymphocyte cultures. J. Immunol. 123: 1511-1518, 1979.
8. Seeley, J.K., Masucci, G., Poros, A., Klein, E., and Golub, S.H. Studies on cytotoxicity generated in human mixed lymphocyte cultures II. Anti-K562 effectors are distinct from allospecific CTL and can be generated from NK-depleted T cells. J. Immunol. 123: 1303-1311, 1979.
9. Merluzzi, V.J., Kenney, R.E., Last-Barney, K., O'Reilly, R.J., and Faanes, R.B. Anomalous killer cells: thymus cell dependency, precursor frequency,

and response to immunosuppressive therapy. Clin. Immunol. Immunopathol. 24: 83-92, 1982.

10. Masucci, M.G., Klein, E., and Argov, S. Disappearance of the NK effect after explantation of lymphocytes and generation of similar nonspecific cytotoxicity correlated to the level of blastogenesis in activated cultures. J. Immunol. 124: 2458-2463, 1980.

11. Bartlett, S.P., and Burton, R.C. Studies on natural killer (NK) cells III. The effects of in vitro culture on spontaneous cytotoxicity of murine spleen cells. J. Immunol. 128: 1070-1075, 1982.

12. Hurrell, S.M., and Zarling, J.M. Ly-2+ effectors cytotoxic for syngeneic tumor cells: Generation by allogeneic stimulation and by supernatants from mixed leukocyte cultures. J. Immunol. 131: 1017-1023, 1983.

13. Strassmann, G., Bach, F.H., and Zarling, J.M. Depletion of human NK cells with monoclonal antibodies allows the generation of cytotoxic T lymphocytes without NK-like cells in mixed cultures. J. Immunol. 130: 1556-1560, 1983.

14. Ezaki, T., Skinner, M.A., and Marbrook, J. Spontaneous cytotoxic T cells in murine spleen cell cultures II. Distinguishing between spontaneous cytotoxic T cells and NK cells according to kinetics and target selectivity. Immunology 50: 351-357, 1983.

15. Ezaki, T., Skinner, M.A., and Marbrook, J. Spontaneous cytotoxic T cells in murine spleen cell cultures I. Some characteristics of effector and precursor cells. Immunology 50: 343-349, 1983.

16. Price, G.B., Teh, H.-S., and Miller, R.G. Specific spontaneous cytotoxic activity in human T cell colonies. J. Immunol. 124: 2352-2355, 1980.

17. Shortman, K., Wilson, A., Scollay, R., and Chen, W.-F. Development of large granular lymphocytes with anomalous, nonspecific cytotoxicity in clones derived from Ly-2+ T cells. Proc. Natl. Acad. Sci. USA 80: 2728-2732, 1983.

18. Shortman, K., Wilson, A., and Scollay, R. Loss of specificity in cytolytic T lymphocyte clones obtained by limit dilution culture of Ly-2+ T cells. J. Immunol. 132: 584-593, 1984.

19. Yron, I., Wood Jr, T.A., Spiess, P.J., and Rosenberg, S.A. In vitro growth of murine T cells V. The isolation and growth of lymphoid cells infiltrating syngeneic solid tumors. J. Immunol. 125: 238-245, 1980.

20. Mule, J.J., Forstrom, J.W., George, E., Hellstrom, I., and Hellstrom, K.E. Production of T cell lines with inhibitory or stimulatory activity against syngeneic tumors in vivo. A preliminary report. Int. J. Cancer. 28: 611-614, 1981.

21. Lotze, M.T., Grimm, E.A., Mazumder, A., Strausser, J.L., and Rosenberg, S.A. Lysis of fresh and cultured autologous tumor by human lymphocytes cultured in T-cell growth factor. Cancer Res. 41: 4420-4425, 1981.

22. Rayner, A.A., Grimm, E.A., Lotze, M.T., Wilson, D.J., and Rosenberg, S.A. Lymphokine-activated killer (LAK) cell phenomenon. IV. Lysis of LAK cell clones of resh human tumor cells from autologous and multiple allogeneic tumors. JNCI 75: 67-75, 1985.

23. Mazumder, A., Grimm, E.A., and Rosenberg, S.A. Lysis of fresh human solid tumor cells by autologous lymphocytes activated in vitro by allosensitization. Cancer Immunol. Immunother. 15: 1-10, 1983.

24. Mazumder, A., Grimm, E.A., and Rosenberg, S.A. Characterization of the lysis of fresh human solid tumors by autologous lymphocytes activated in vitro with phytohemagglutinn. J. Immunol. 130: 958-964, 1983.
25. Mazumder, A., Rosenstein, M., and Rosenberg, S.A. Lysis of fresh natural killer resistant tumor cells by lectin activated syngeneic and allogeneic murine splenocytes. Cancer Res. 43: 5729-5734, 1983.
26. Henney, C.S., Kuribayashi, K., Kern, D.E., and Gillis, S. Interleukin-2 augments natural killer cell activity. Nature 291: 335-338, 1981.
27. Domzig, W., Stadler, B.M., and Herberman, R.B. Interleukin 2 dependence of human natural killer (NK) cell activity. J. Immunol. 130: 1970-1973, 1983.
28. Grimm, E.A., Mazumder, A., Zhang, H.Z., and Rosenberg, S.A. Lymphokine-activated killer cell phenomenon. Lysis of natural killer-resistant fresh solid tumor cells by interleukin 2-activated autologous human peripheral blood lymphocytes. J. Exp. Med. 155: 1823-1841, 1982.
29. Kedar, E., Gorelik, E., and Heberman, R.B. Natural cell-mediated cytotoxicity in vitro and inhibition of tumor growth in vivo by murine lymphoid cells cultured with T cell growth factor (TCGF). Cancer Immunol. Immunother. 13: 14-23, 1982.
30. Dorfman, N.A., Winkler, D., and Wunderlich, J.R. Supplement induced cytotoxic cells (SICC) generated from mouse thymus or spleen cells cultured in the presence of interleukin 2 and/or polyinosinic acid. Cell. Immunol. 81: 253-267, 1983.
31. Trinchieri, G., Matsumoto-Kobayashi, M., Clark, S.C., Seehra, J., London, L., and Perussia, B. Response of resting human blood natural killer cells to interleukin 2. J. Exp. Med. 160: 1147-1169, 1984.
32. Gronvik, K.-O., and Andersson, J. The role of T cell growth stimulating factors in T cell triggering. Immunol. Rev. 51: 35-59, 1980.
33. Chang, A.E., Hyatt, C.L., and Rosenberg, S.A. Systemic administration of recombinant human interleukin-2 in mice. J. Biol. Res. Mod. 3: 561-572, 1984.
34. Lotze, M.T., Robb, R.J., Sharrow, S.O., Frana, L.W., and Rosenberg, S.A. Systemic administration of interleukin-2 in humans. J. Biol. Res. Mod. 3: 475-482, 1984.
35. Teh, H.-S., and Teh, S.-J. Direct evidence for a two-signal mechanism of cytotoxic T-lymphocyte activation. Nature 285: 163-165, 1980.
36. Vohr, H.-W., and Hunig, T. Induction of proliferative and cytotoxic responses in resting Lyt-2+ T cells with lectin and recombinant interleukin 2. Eur. J. Immunol. 15: 332-337, 1985.
37. Minato, N., Reid, L., and Bloom, B.R. On the heterogeneity of murine natural killer cells. J. Exp. Med. 154: 750-762, 1981.
38. Kedar, E., Ikejiri, B.L., Timonen, T., Bonnard, G.D., Reid, J., Navarro, N.J., Sredni, B., and Heberman, R.B. Antitumor reactivity in vitro and in vivo of lymphocytes from normal donors and cancer patients propagated in culture with T cell growth factor. Eur. J. Cancer. 19: 757-773, 1983.
39. Grimm, E.A., Robb, R.J., Roth, J.A., Neckers, L.M., Lachman, L.B., Wilson, D.J., and Rosenberg, S.A. Lymphokine activated killer cell phenomenon.

III. Evidence that IL-2 is sufficient for direct activation of peripheral blood lymphocytes into lymphokine activated killer cells. J. Exp. Med. 158: 1356-1361, 1983.

40. Merluzzi, V.J., Savage, D.M., Mertelsmann, R., and Welte, K. Generation of nonspecific murine cytotoxic T cells in vitro by purified human interleukin 2. Cell. Immunol. 84: 74-84, 1984.

41. Itoh, K., Tilden, A.B., Kumagai, K., and Balch, C.M. Leu-11+ lymphocytes with natural killer (NK) activity are precursors of recombinant interleukin 2 (rIL 2)-induced activated killer (AK) cells. J. Immunol. 134: 802-807, 1985.

42. Grimm, E.A., and Wilson, D.J. The human lymphokine-activated killer cell system. V. Purified recombinant IL2 activates cytotoxic lymphocytes which lyse both NK-resistant autologous and allogeneic tumors and TNP-modified autologous PBL. Cell. Immunol. 94: 568-578, 1985.

43. Teh, H.-S., and Yu, M. Activation of nonspecific killer cells by interleukin 2 containing supernatants. J. Immunol. 131:1827-1833, 1983.

44. Rosenstein, M., Yron, I., Kaufmann, Y., and Rosenberg, S.A. Lymphokine-activated killer cells: Lysis of fresh syngeneic natural killer-resistant murine tumor cells by lymphocytes cultured in interleukin 2. Cancer Res. 44: 1946-1953, 1984.

45. Itoh, K., Shiba, K., Shimizu, Y., Suzuki, R., and Kumagai, K. Generation of activated killer (AK) cells by recombinant interleukin 2 (rIL2) in collaboration with interferon-γ (IFN-γ). J. Immunol. 134: 3124-3129, 1985.

46. Brooks, C.G., and Henney, C.S. Interleukin-2 and the regulation of natural killer activity in cultured cell populations. In *Contemporary Topics in Molecular Immunology*. Edited by S. Gillis and F.P. Inman. Plenum Press, New York and London, 1985, pp. 63-89.

47. Burns, G.F., Triglia, T., Werkmeister, J.A., Begley, C.G., and Boyd, A.W. TLiSA1, a human T lineage-specific activation antigen involved in the differentiation of cytotoxic T lymphocytes and anomolous killer cells from their precursors. J. Exp. Med. 161: 1063-1078, 1985.

48. Nishimura, T., and Hashimoto, Y. Induction of nonspecific killer T cells from non-immune mouse spleen cells by culture with interleukin 2. Gann 75: 177-186, 1984.

49. Yang, S.S., Malek, T.R., Hargrove, M.E., and Ting, C.-C. Lymphokine-induced cytotoxicity: Requirement of two lymphokines for the induction of optimal cytotoxic responses. J. Immunol. 134: 3912-3919, 1985.

50. LeFrancois, L., Klein, J.R., Paetkau, V., and Bevan, M.J. Antigen independent activation of memory cytotoxic T cells by interleukin 2. J. Immunol. 132: 1845-1850, 1984.

51. Devos, R., Plaetinck, G., and Fiers, W. Induction of cytolytic cells by pure recombinant human interleukin 2. Eur. J. Immunol. 14: 1057-1060, 1984.

52. Rosenberg, S.A., Mule, J.J., Spiess, P.J., Reichert, C.M., and Schwarz, S.L. Regression of established pulmonary metastases and subcutaneous tumor mediated by the systemic administration of high-dose recombinant interleukin 2. J. Exp. Med. 161: 1169-1188, 1985.

53. Nishimura, T., Uchiyama, Y., Yagi, H., and Hashimoto, Y. Administration of slowly released recombinant interleukin 2. Augmentation of the efficacy

of adoptive immunotherapy with lymphokine activated killer (LAK) cells. J. Immunol. Meth. 91: 21-27, 1986.

54. Miyasaka, N., Darnell, B., Baron, S., and Talal, N. Interleukin 2 enhances natural killing of normal lymphocytes. Cell. Immunol. 84: 154-162, 1984.

55. Rayner, A.A., Grimm, E.A., Lotze, M.T., Chu, E.W., and Rosenberg, S.A. Lymphokine-activated killer (LAK) cells. Analysis of factors relevant to the immunotherapy of human cancer. Cancer 55: 1327-1333, 1985.

56. Forni, G., Giovarelli, M., and Santoni, A. Lymphokine-activated tumor inhibition in vivo I. The local administration of interleukin 2 triggers nonreactive lymphocytes from tumor-bearing mice to inhibit tumor growth. J. Immunol. 134: 1305-1311, 1985.

57. Nishimura, T., Yagi, H., Yagita, H., Uchiyama, Y., and Hashimoto, Y. Lymphokine activated cell associated antigen involved in broad-reactive killer cell mediated cytotoxicity. Cell. Immunol. 94: 122-132, 1985.

58. Henkart, P.A., Yue, C.C., Yang, J., and Rosenberg, S.A. Cytolytic and biochemical properties of cytoplasmic granules of murine lymphokine-activated killer cells. J. Immunol. 137: 2611-2617, 1986.

59. Rosenberg, S.A. Immunotherapy of cancer by systemic administration of lymphoid cells plus interleukin-2. J. Biol. Res. Mod. 3: 501-511, 1984.

60. Tilden, A.B., Itoh, K., and Balch, C.M. Human lymphokine-activated killer (LAK) cells: identification of two types of effector cells. J. Immunol. 138: 1068-1073, 1987.

61. Ortaldo, J.R., Mason, A., and Overton, R. Lymphokine activated killer cells: analysis of progenitors and effectors. J. Exp. Med. 164: 1193-1205, 1986.

62. Phillips, J.H., and Lanier, L.L. Dissection of the lymphokine-activated killer phenomenon. Relative contribution of peripheral blood natural killer cells and lymphocytes to cytolysis. J. Exp. Med. 164: 814-825, 1986.

63. Owen-Schaub, L.B., Abraham, S.R., and Hemstreet III, G.P. Phenotypic characterization of murine lymphokine activated killer cells. Cell. Immunol. 103: 272-286, 1986.

64. Merluzzi, V.J., Smith, M.D., and Last-Barney, K. Similarities and distinctions between murine natural cells and lymphokine activated killer cells. Cell. Immunol. 100: 563-569, 1986.

65. Merluzzi, V.J. Comparison of murine lymphokine-activated killer cells, natural killer cells, and cytotoxic T lymphocytes. Cell. Immunol. 94: 95-104, 1985.

66. Ting, C.-C., Hargrove, M.E., Wunderlich, J., and Loh, N.-N. Differential expression of asialo GM1 on alloreactive cytotoxic T lymphocytes and lymphokine activated killer cells. Cell. Immunol. 104: 115-125, 1987.

67. Grimm, E.A., Ramsey, K.M., Mazumder, A., Wilson, D.J., Djeu, J.Y., and Rosenberg, S.A. Lymphokine-activated killer cell phenomenon II. Precursor phenotype is serologically distinct from peripheral T lymphocytes, memory cytotoxic thymus-derived lymphocytes, and natural killer cells. J. Exp. Med. 157: 884-897, 1983.

68. Ballas, Z.K., Rasmussen, W., and van Otegham, J.K. Lymphokine-activated killer (LAK) cells. I. Delineation of distinct murine LAK precursor populations. J. Immunol. 138: 1647-1652, 1987.

69. Yang, J.C., Mule, J.J., and Rosenberg, S.A. Murine lymphokine-activated killer (LAK) cells: phenotypic characterization of the precursor and effector cells. J. Immunol. 137: 715-722, 1986.
70. Merluzzi, V.J., Trail, P.A., and Last-Barney, K. Differential expression of lymphokine-activated killer cells and natural killer cells in adoptive transfer experiments utilizing fractionated bone marrow. J. Immunol. 137: 2425-2427, 1986.
71. Dixon Gray, J., Shau, H., and Golub, S.H. Functional studies on the precursors of human lymphokine-activated killer cells. Cell. Immunol. 96: 338-350, 1985.
72. Damle, N.K., Doyle, L.V., and Bradley, E.C. Interleukin 2-activated human killer cells are derived from phenotypically heterogeneous precursors. J. Immunol. 137: 2814-2822, 1986.
73. Lattime, E.C., Pecoraro, G.A., and Stutman, O. Natural cytotoxic cells against solid tumors in mice III. A comparison of effector cell antigenic phenotype and target cell recognition structures with those of NK cells. J. Immunol. 126: 2011-2014, 1981.
74. Weigent, D.A., Stanton, G.J., and Johnson, H.M. Interleukin 2 enhances natural killer cell activity through induction of gamma interferon. Infect. Immun. 41: 992-997, 1983.
75. Lanier, L.L., Benike, C.J., Phillips, J.H., and Engleman, E.G. Recombinant interleukin 2 enhanced natural killer cell-mediated cytotoxicity in human lymphocyte subpopulations expressing the Leu 7 and Leu 11 antigens. J. Immunol. 134: 794-801, 1985.
76. Nieminen, P., and Saksela, E. Common precursor pool marker for allospecific (CTL) and nonspecific (NK and Activated) cytotoxic cells in the bone marrow. J. Immunol. 134: 699-703, 1985.
77. Merluzzi, V.J., Savage, D.M., Smith, M.D., Last-Barney, K., Mertelsmann, R., Moore, M.A.S., and Welte, K. Lymphokine-activated killer cells are generated before classical cytotoxic T lymphocytes after bone marrow transplantation in mice. J. Immunol. 135: 1702-1706, 1985.
78. Merluzzi, V.J. Production and response to interleukin 2 in vitro and in vivo after bone marrow transplantation in mice. J. Immunol. 134: 2426-2430, 1985.
79. Werkmeister, J.A., Triglia, T., and Burns, G.F. In vitro generation of human activated killer cells II. N-acetyl-D-galactosamine inhibits a distinct subpopulation of human activated lymphocyte killer cells generated in mixed lymphocyte culture. Cell. Immunol. 92: 338-349, 1985.
80. Merluzzi, V.J., and Last-Barney, K. Potential use of human interleukin 2 as an adjunct for the therapy of neoplasia, immunodeficiency and infectious disease. Int. J. Immunopharmacol. 7: 31-39, 1985.
81. Lotze, M.T., and Rosenberg, S.A. Results of clinical trials with the administration of interleukin 2 and adoptive immunotherapy with activated cells in patients with cancer. Immunobiology 172: 420-437, 1986.
82. Mertelsmann, R., and Welte, K. Human interleukin 2: molecular biology, physiology and clinical possibilities. Immunobiology 172: 400-419, 1986.

83. Cheever, M.A., Thompson, J.A., Peace, D.J., and Greenberg, P.D. Potential uses of interleukin 2 in cancer therapy. Immunobiology 172: 365-382, 1986.

84. Mills, G.B., Carlson, G., and Paetkau, V. Generation of cytotoxic lymphocytes to syngeneic tumors by using co-stimulator (interleukin 2): In vivo activity. J. Immunol. 125: 1904-1909, 1980.

85. Cheever, M.A., Greenberg, P.D., and Fefer, A. Specific adoptive therapy of established leukemia with syngeneic lymphocytes sequentially immunized in vivo and in vitro and nonspecifically expanded by culture with interleukin 2. J. Immunol. 126: 1318-1322, 1981.

86. Merluzzi, V.J., Savage, D.M., Souza, L., Boone, T., Mertelsmann, R., Welte, K., and Last-Barney, K. Lysis of spontaneous murine breast tumors by human interleukin 2-stimulated syngeneic T-lymphocytes. Cancer Res. 45: 203-206, 1985.

87. Mazumder, A., and Rosenberg, S.A. Successful immunotherapy of natural killer-resistant established pulmonary melanoma metastases by the intravenous adoptive transfer of syngeneic lymphocytes activated in vitro by interleukin 2. J. Exp. Med. 159: 495-507, 1984.

88. Mule, J.J., Shu, S., Schwarz, S.L., and Rosenberg, S.A. Adoptive immunotherapy of established pulmonary metastases with LAK cells and recombinant interleukin 2. Science 225: 1487-1489, 1984.

89. Mule, J.J., Shu, S., and Rosenberg, S.A. The anti-tumor efficacy of lymphokine-activated killer cells and recombinant interleukin 2 in vivo. J. Immunol. 135: 646-651, 1985.

90. Lafreniere, R., and Rosenberg, S.A. Successful immunotherapy of murine experimental hepatic metastases with lymphokine-activated killer cells and recombinant interleukin 2. Cancer Res. 45: 3735-3741, 1985.

91. Merluzzi, V.J., and Last-Barney, K. Expansion of murine cytotoxic precursors in vitro and in vivo by purified interleukin 2. J. Biol. Res. Mod. 3: 468-474, 1984.

92. Papa, M.Z., Mule, J.J., and Rosenberg, S.A. Antitumor efficacy of LAK cells and recombinant IL2 in vivo: successful immunotherapy of established pulmonary metastases from weakly immunogenic and nonimmunogenic tumors of three distinct histological types. Cancer Res. 46: 4973-4978, 1986.

93. Shiloni, E., Lafreniere, R., Mule, J.J., Schwarz, S.L., and Rosenberg, S.A. Effect of immunotherapy with allogeneic lymphokine activated killer cells and recombinant interleukin 2 on established pulmonary and hepatic metastases. Cancer Res. 46: 5633-5640, 1986.

94. Ettinghausen, S.E., and Rosenberg, S.A. Immunotherapy of murine sarcomas using lymphokine activated killer cells: optimization of the schedule and route of administration of recombinant interleukin 2. Cancer Res. 46: 2784-2792, 1986.

95. Ottow, R.T., Steller, E.P., Sugarbaker, P.H., Wesley, R.A., and Rosenberg, S.A. Immunotherapy of intraperitoneal cancer with interleukin 2 and lymphokine activated killer cells reduces tumor load and prolongs survival in murine models. Cell. Immunol. 104: 366-376, 1987.

96. Mule, J.J., Yang, J., Shu, S., and Rosenberg, S.A. The anti-tumor efficacy of lymphokine-activated killer cells and recombinant interleukin 2 in vivo:

direct correlation between reduction of established metastases and cytolytic activity of lymphokine-activated killer cells. J. Immunol. 136: 3899-3909, 1986.

97. Nishimura, T., Yagi, H., Uchiyama, Y., and Hashimoto, Y. Generation of lymphokine-activated killer (LAK) cells from tumor-infiltrating lymphocytes. Cell. Immunol. 100: 149-157, 1986.

98. Rosenberg, S.A., Spiess, P., and Lafreniere, R. A new approach to the adoptive immunotherapy of cancer with tumor-infiltrating lymphocytes. Science 233: 1318-1321, 1986.

99. Adler, A., Stein, J.A., Kedar, E., Naor, D., and Weiss, D.W. Intralesional injection of interleukin-2-expanded autologous lymphocytes in melanoma and breast cancer patients: A pilot study. J. Biol. Res. Mod. 3: 491-500, 1984.

100. Hogan, P.G., Hapel, A.J., and Doe, W.F. Lymphokine-activated and natural killer cell activity in human intestinal mucosa. J. Immunol. 135: 1731-1738, 1985.

101. Cheever, M.A., and Greenberg, P.D. In vivo administration of interleukin-2. In *Contemporary Topics in Molecular Immunology*. Edited by S. Gillis and F.P. Inman. Plenum Press, New York and London, 1985, pp. 263-282.

102. Rosenberg, S.A., Lotze, M.T., Muul, L.M. et al. Observations on the systemic administration of autologous lymphokine-activated killer cells and recombinant interleukin-2 to patients with metastatic cancer. N. Engl. J. Med. 313: 1485-1492, 1985.

103. Jacobs, S.K., Wilson, D.J., Kornblith, P.L., and Grimm, E.A. Interleukin-2 or autologous lymphokine-activated killer cell treatment of malignant glioma: Phase I trial. Cancer Res. 46: 2101-2104, 1986.

104. Lotze, M.T., Matory, Y.L., Rayney, A.A., Ettinghausen, S.E., Vetto, J.T., Seipp, C.A., and Rosenberg, S.A. Clinical effects and toxicity of interleukin 2 in patients with cancer. Cancer 58: 2764-2772, 1986.

105. Rosenberg, S.A., Lotze, M.T., Muul, L.M. et al. A progress report on the treatment of 157 patients with advanced cancer using lymphokine-activated killer cells and interleukin-2 or high-dose interleukin-2 alone. N. Engl. J. Med. 316: 889-897, 1987.

106. West, W.H., Tauer, K.W., Yannelli, J.R., Marshall, G.D., Orr, D.W., Thurman, G.B., and Oldham, R.K. Constant-infusion recombinant interleukin-2 in adoptive immunotherapy of advanced cancer. N. Engl. J. Med. 316: 898-905, 1987.

107. Papa, M.Z., Vetto, J.T., Ettinghausen, S.E., Mule, J.J., and Rosenberg, S.A. Effect of corticosteroid on the antitumor activity of lymphokine-activated killer cells and interleukin 2 in mice. Cancer Res. 46: 5618-5623, 1986.

108. Rosenstein, M., Ettinghausen, S.E., and Rosenberg, S.A. Extravasation of intravascular fluid mediated by the systemic administration of recombinant interleukin 2. J. Immunol. 137: 1735-1742, 1986.

109. Damle, N.K., Doyle, L.V., Bender, J.R., and Bradley, E.C. Interleukin-2 activated human lymphocytes exhibit enhanced adhesion to normal vascular endothelial cells and cause their lysis. J. Immunol. 138: 1779-1785, 1987.

# 5

# Interleukins 3 and 4

Atsushi Miyajima, Takashi Yokota, Takeshi Otsuka, Shoichiro Miyatake,
Yutaka Takebe, Hajime Hagiwara, [†] Jolanda Schreurs, Kozo Kaibuchi, Frank Lee
Naoko Arai, Tim Mosmann, and Ken-ichi Arai / DNAX Research Institute of
Molecular and Cellular Biology, Palo Alto, California

## I. INTRODUCTION: T-CELL-DERIVED LYMPHOKINES

Helper T cells when activated by antigens or lectins, initiate a cascade of events
that result in the development of an immune response. One of the earliest activities is the production of several lymphokines (1). Activation of helper T cells by
antigen has two distinct aspects: (i) recognition of the antigen by a T-cell antigen
receptor which generates intracellular signals for induction of a variety of lymphokines, and (ii) a T-cell-effector function mediated by the produced lymphokines
which regulate proliferation and differentiation of hemopoietic and lymphoid
target cells. Cytotoxic T cells also produce a battery of lymphokines following
activation (2).

Lymphokines produced by helper T cells may be classified into several types
based on the target cells on which they act (Fig. 1). Interleukin-2 (IL-2) stimulates
predominantly the proliferation of cells belonging to the T-cell lineage, while B-
cell growth factor I [BCGFI (BSFI)] , BCGFII, and B-cell differentiation factor
(BCDF) are thought to stimulate proliferation and differentiation of cells of the
B lineage. However, several lymphokines stimulate more than one type of target
cells, and a proposal was made to rename BSF-1 as IL-4 because of its versatile
action on many cell types (3-5). IL-3 and granulocyte-macrophage-colony-stimu-
laing factor (GM-CSF) stimulate the proliferation and differentiation of various
hemopoietic progenitor cells (Fig. 2).

Does a single T cell produce all lymphokines or do specific subsets of T cells
produce unique lymphokines? Recently, two types of helper T-cell clones have
been recognized in the mouse system based on the pattern of their lymphokine
production and this is indicative of a heterogeneous helper T-cell population (6).

---

[†] Deceased

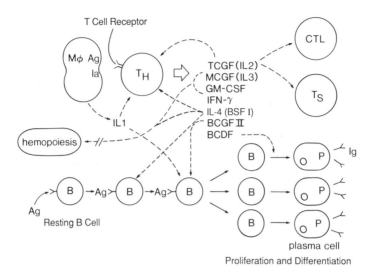

**Figure 1** T-cell lymphokines produced by activated helper T cells. Ag, antigen; B, B cell; CTL, cytotoxic T cell; M, macrophage; P, plasma cell; $T_H$, helper T cell; Ts, suppressor T cell.

Several of these lymphokines such as IL-2 (7-9), IL-3 (10,11), $\gamma$-interferon (IFN-$\gamma$) (12,13), GM-CSF (14-17), and IL-4 (3-5) have now been resolved by purification to homogeneity and/or by molecular cloning of their respective mRNAs and expression of functional polypeptides.

Several aspects of the T-cell lymphokine systems are of basic research interest including: (i) regulation of expression of the T-cell-lymphokine genes, (ii) biological activities of lymphokines, and (iii) the nature of the interaction of lymphokines with their receptors and the subsequent biochemical events. The T-cell antigen receptor-T3 complex plays a central role in transmembrane signaling events to convert antigen-specific signals to nonantigen-specific signals which result in the production of lymphokines. Triggering of the T-cell antigen receptor stimulates the generation of diacylglycerol (DG) and inositol trisphosphate (IP3). This results in the activation of protein kinase C and $Ca^{2+}$ mobilization which have been suggested as early events in T-cell activation (18). However, the mechanisms involved in regulation of coordinate induction of lymphokine genes are largely unknown. The expression of lymphokine genes in normal T cells may be coupled to cell cycle transition from the resting state to early $G_1$ phase. Other proteins, such as the IL-2 receptor, the transferrin receptor and several nuclear oncogene products are also induced during T-cell activation. This process renders T cells "competent" to receive "progression" signals to enter S phase such as that delivered through interaction of IL-2 with the IL-2 receptor (19). The lymphokine-receptor interaction may produce certain intracellular signals which stimulate

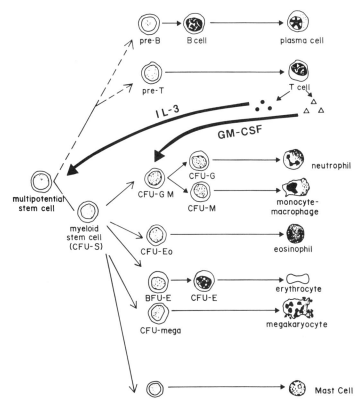

Figure 2   Postulated lineages and relationships of hemopoietic progenitor cells.

proliferation and/or differentiation of target cells. Elucidation of the signal transduction pathways mediated by lymphokines, along with studies of other growth
factors, receptors, and oncogenes, will provide basic knowledge related to control of growth and differentiation of mammalian cells. In this chapter, we summarize molecular biology studies of T-cell-derived lymphokines with an emphasis
on those which affect proliferation and differentiation of hemopoietic cells.

## II.   STRATEGIES FOR ISOLATION OF LYMPHOKINE GENES

### A.   Mammalian cDNA Expression Vector

Supernatants from lectin-activated T-cell clones generally contain multiple lymphokines. Table 1 lists a panel of lymphokines produced by two subsets of mouse
helper T cells (6). One class of T-helper cells produces IL-2, IL-3, GM-CSF, and
INF-γ and the other type of T-helper cells produce IL-3, IL-4, and GM-CSF. One

Table 1   Production of Lymphokines by Mouse Helper T-Cell Clones

| Lymphokines | Cell lines | |
|---|---|---|
| | LB2-1 ($T_H1$) | $C1.L61^{+}2^{-}/9$ ($T_H2$) |
| IL-2 | + | − |
| IL-3 | + | + |
| IL-4 | − | + |
| GM-CSF | + | + |
| IFN-$\gamma$ | + | − |

approach to resolving which proteins are responsible for the various biological activities is to clone and express their genetic coding sequences (cDNAs) separately. In addition to providing materials for biological and biochemical study, this approach provides tools for the study of the corresponding genes and their regulation. Several strategies have been used for the isolation of cDNA clones. One is a chemical approach which utilizes oligonucleotide probes based on protein sequence information. A second is an immunological approach using antibody probes to screen the bacterial lysates (20). The third is a functional approach which relies on the availability of specific biological or enzymatic assays. The protein products, translated following hybrid selection of mRNA, or expressed in cells by cDNA inserts, are assayed for biological activity.

The strategy for isolating lymphokine cDNA clones which mainly relies on the functional approach has proven very useful (8) and has been applied to the cloning of several lymphokine genes. Using a pcD cDNA library prepared with mRNA from Con A-activated mouse and human T-cell lines, we have developed a screening procedure employing transfection of plasmid DNAs into mammalian cells followed by assay of transfected cell supernatants for lymphokine activities of interest. Important aspects of this cloning protocol include (a) the use of a reliable and sensitive bioassay for lymphokine activities, (b) the use of T-cell lines as an enriched source of biologically active lymphokine mRNAs, and (c) the construction of a cDNA library in a pcD mammalian expression vector.

The pcD mammalian expression vector developed by Okayama and Berg (21) which has proven so useful in this strategy contains the SV40 (Simian virus) early promoter, late splicing junction, and origin of replication. This vector permits expression of cDNA inserts in COS7 monkey cells which provide T antigen for replication of the pcD plasmid (Fig. 3). Screening of cDNA libraries can be done by transfection of pools of plasmid DNA into COS7 cells using DEAE-Dextran. Since most lymphokines are secreted proteins composed of a single polypeptide

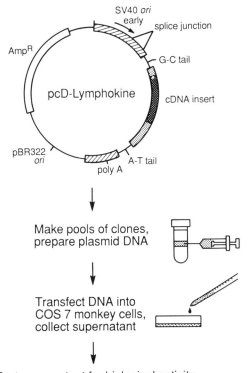

Figure 3   Structure of pcD vector and procedure for screening of cDNA library by direct expression in mammalian cells.

chain, the supernatants from transfected cells can be assayed for biological activity. Positive pools are further divided to identify single cDNA clones which give biological activity after transfection. Successful isolation of several lymphokine genes using this strategy has demonstrated that the identification of full-length cDNA clones for many lymphokines may be achieved entirely on the basis of detection of the functional activity of polypeptides produced in transfected mammalian cells. A set of lymphokine cDNA clones expressible in mammalian cells such as mouse IL-3, mouse and human IL-2, mouse and human IFN-$\gamma$, mouse and human GM-CSF, and mouse and human IL-4 have been isolated from T-cell pcD libraries. Recombinant lymphokines produced in COS7 cells in a pcD vector system are free from other T-cell-specific immunoregulatory products and can be employed for initial characterization of their biological properties. The SV40 early region promoter in the original pcD vector can be replaced by other mammalian promoters and enhancers to accommodate additional features. For example, an expression vector employing the adenovirus major late promoter coupled to a cDNA copy of the adenovirus tripartite leader and the adenovirus VAI and VAII gene region has been described for isolation of a human GM-CSF cDNA clone (17). Recently, a modified pcD vector system was described (4) which relies on the Okayama-Berg principle but employs injection of RNA transcribed by SP6 RNA polymerase in vitro into *Xenopus laevis* oocytes.

### B. Biological Assays

Availability of highly sensitive biological assays is critical for the screening of a cDNA library using the functional approach. The most commonly used assays for hemopoietic growth factors are colony formation assays or cell proliferation assays.

### Colony Formation Assay

The development of semisolid culture systems (22,23) to support the clonal growth of hemopoietic cells made possible the recognition of various hemopoietic precursor cells which are unable to survive or proliferate in vitro without specific stimulation (Fig. 2). This led to the discovery of a group of glycoproteins that stimulate proliferation of hemopoietic cells. These proteins, referred to as colony-stimulating factors (CSF), promote precursor cells to form colonies of progeny cells (24). Several such factors from murine sources have been characterized, each capable of stimulating the development of different types of colonies. Multi-CSF (IL-3) has the ability to stimulate multipotential hemopoietic stem cells to form a variety of colonies including granulocyte, macrophage, erythroid, megakaryocyte, eosinophil, and mast cells. GM-CSF acts on CFU-GM to form colonies of granulocytes, macrophages, or a mixture of these. G-CSF preferentially stimulates the formation of granulocytes and M-CSF the formation of macrophages.

### Proliferation Assay

Various growth factor-dependent cell lines have been established from mouse bone marrow cells or lymphoid cells which respond in vitro to various soluble factors. Many of the cells established from lymphohemopoietic tissues, in the presence of activated T-cell-conditioned medium, share characteristics with mast cells. These cells have been termed persisting (P) cells because of their persistence in cultures after other cell types have disappeared. The unique characteristic of these cells is absolute dependence on growth factors; in other words, removal of the growth factor causes rapid loss of cell viability. These cells, therefore, provide a simple and rapid means to measure the activity of growth factors. A simple colorimetric assay method using 3-(4,5-dimethylthiazol-2-yl)-2,5-diphenyl tetrazolium bromide (MTT) can facilitate this type of assay (25). Using a variety of target cells as listed in Table 2, various growth factor activities in the supernatants of activated T cells can be assayed.

Table 2    Biological Assays Used for cDNA Cloning of Mouse Lymphokines

| Growth factors | Cell lines used for proliferation assays | Colonies formed in bone marrow CSF assays |
| --- | --- | --- |
| IL-2 | HT-2 | |
| IL-3 | MC/9 | GM, G, M, E, Mix, Mt |
| | NFS60 | |
| IL-4 | HT-2 | |
| | MC/9 | |
| | B cells | |
| GM-CSF | NFS60 | GM, G, M |
| G-CSF | NFS60 | G |
| M-CSF | | M |

HT-2 cell is a T-cell line, MC/9 is a mast cell line (30). NFS60 is a myelomonocytic leukemic cell.

Abbreviations: M: macrophage, G: granulocyte, GM: granulocyte-macrophage, E: erythrocyte, Mt: mast cell, Mix: mixture of neutrophil, macrophage, eosinophil, erythrocyte, megakaryocyte, and mast cells.

## III.    BIOLOGICAL PROPERTIES AND cDNA CLONING OF IL-3 AND IL-4

### A.    IL-3

Interleukin-3 was initially defined as a factor which stimulates the production of the enzyme 20$\alpha$-steroid dehydrogenase (20$\alpha$-SDH) by spleen cells from T-cell-deficient (nu/nu) mice (26). As we describe below, recent work from a number of investigators has demonstrated that IL-3 is identical to a factor designated by multiple names including persisting cell-stimulating factor (PSF) (27), mast cell growth factor (MCGF) (28-30), hemopoietic cell growth factor (HCGF), burst-promoting activity (BPA) which stimulates the production of erythroid colonies in the presence of erythropoietin, and multicolony-stimulating activity (multi-CSF) (31) which stimulates multilineage colony formation in vitro from bone marrow cells. IL-3 also stimulates growth of histamine-producing cells (32), induces Thy-1 antigen on spleen and bone marrow cells (26), and inhibits induction of Ia antigens on mast cells by interferon (33).

In addition to the production of these activities by activated T lymphocytes, the myelomonocytic tumor line WEHI-3 was found to produce similar activities (34). This raised the possibility that some or all of the activities could be due to the same molecule. Ihle et al. purified IL-3 to homogeneity from WEHI-3 conditioned medium (35,36) by tracing the 20$\alpha$-SDH activity and the purified protein was shown to stimulate mast cells, P cells, and histamine-producing cells. In addition, homogeneous IL-3 had colony-stimulating factor activity. The purified IL-3 was a 28 kD glycoprotein with a high specific activity ($\sim$ 0.2 ng/ml required for a half-maximal biological response). Clark-Lewis et al. (37) independently purified P-cell-stimulating factor (PSF) from WEHI-3 conditioned medium and the N-terminal amino acid sequence of PSF was determined. The N-terminal amino acid sequence of PSF differed from that of IL-3 in that there were an additional 6 N-terminal amino acid residues, after which the sequence coincided with that of IL-3.

Due to the sensitivity and ease of a proliferation assay employing a cloned mast cell line (MC/9) (30), the MCGF assay was used for isolation of the IL-3 cDNA clone. When mRNA isolated from Con A-stimulated C1.Ly1$^+$2$^-$/9 cells was microinjected into *Xenopus laevis* oocytes, the oocyte incubation medium exhibited MCGF activity. The presence of MCGF activity confirmed that the mRNA isolated from the T cells was biologically active. No MCGF activity could be detected following injection of mRNA from the control uninduced T-cell line, suggesting that production of MCGF mRNA is inducible by Con A. mRNA isolated from the induced T-cell clone was then used to construct a cDNA library using the pcD expression vector. This cDNA library was screened initially by hybrid selection using mRNA from induced C1.Ly1$^+$2$^-$/9 which could be translated by *Xenopus* oocytes into active MCGF. The initial cDNA clone which could selectively hybridize MCGF mRNA was not full length, but was used to isolate additional clones from the cDNA library by hybridization. Several clones which could direct the synthesis of MCGF activity in transfected COS monkey cells were isolated.

The multiple activities of IL-3 were finally confirmed as belonging to a single entity by using recombinant IL-3. The recombinant molecule, expressed in COS cells from the IL-3 cDNA clone, exhibited all the properties described for the purified IL-3 preparations (38). In addition, total chemical synthesis of the IL-3 polypeptide was recently reported (39), and the synthesized IL-3 protein was active in stimulation of growth of mast cell lines, induction of Thy-1 antigen, and the stimulation of multilineage colonies from bone marrow.

Our current picture of the effects of IL-3 in these assays is more complex. Recently, it has become clear that many lymphokines exert a multitude of effects on various cell types, and conversely, many assays detect more than one lymphokine, even using relatively defined proliferative assays with cloned cell lines. The IL-3 assays mentioned above are similarly complex and illustrate this point. The 20$\alpha$-SDH enzyme is induced by IL-3 in spleen cells, but other lymphokines can also induce 20$\alpha$-SDH, and several cell types may be involved (40). Certain mast cell lines respond to IL-4 in addition to IL-3, and these two lymphokines can act synergistically to induce proliferation of these cell lines (3,41,42). HCGF activity is also found associated with another, non-IL-3 lymphokine (43). Several IL-3-dependent cell lines also respond to other lymphokines, such as GM-CSF (44). As a result of these complexities, the unequivocal identification of IL-3 in a crude biological sample is often difficult if biological assays alone are used. For more definitive identification of IL-3, it is desirable to use biochemical tests, preferably in conjunction with biological assays. Such tests might include analysis with either antibodies or nucleic acid probes, or separation by biochemical means before characterizing biological activities.

When the various activities of IL-3 were first discovered, it was not clear initially that the activities were all mediated by the same molecule, and so several names were used to describe the activities. Although IL-3 [originally proposed to describe the 20α-SHD activity (26)] is now used widely, some of the original names are still in use. As discussed above, several of these original names describe activities mediated by other lymphokines in addition to IL-3. For these reasons, in this review we will use the name IL-3 exclusively to describe the molecule whose gene has been cloned (10,11). Based on the same considerations, we will use the name IL-4 instead of BSF-1 (see below).

## B. IL-4

Howard et al. (45), originally described a factor (BCGFI or BSF-1) found in induced mouse EL-4 supernatants that costimulates with anti-IgM antibodies, in short-term cultures of purified B cells, to induce polyclonal B-cell proliferation. A series of findings as described below established that BSF-1 is identical to a factor (produced by a T-cell clone $C1.LyL^+2^-/9$) that has both TCGF and MCGF activities and that this factor is distinct from IL-2 and IL-3.

The mouse T-cell clone $C1.Ly1^+2^-/9$ from which the IL-3 cDNA clone was isolated produces several biological activities, including (i) mast cell proliferation, (ii) T-cell proliferation, (iii) activation of B cells to secrete immunoglobulin, and (iv) formation of hemopoietic colonies of various types (Table 1). While IL-3 cDNA clones express mast cellg rowth factor activity in transfected mammalian cells, even saturating concentrations of IL-3 do not stimulate a cloned mast cell line to the same extent as supernatant derived from original T-cell clone (38). Fractionations of $C1.Ly1^+2^-/9$ cell supernatants demonstrated the existence of a factor distinct from IL-3 that has MCGF activity as well as the ability to enhance the MCGF activity of IL-3. Despite multiple biochemical fractionations, the MCGF activity was found to copurify with a TCGF activity that is distinct from IL-2 (41). These results are consistent with RNA blotting analysis showing that activated $C1.Ly1^+2^-/9$ cells produce TCGF activity but do not produce IL-2 mRNA. Furthermore, the TCGF activity in cell supernatants is not blocked by a monoclonal antibody that completely inhibits the activity of mouse IL-2 (42). These results suggested that the $C1.Ly1^+2^-/9$ cells produced a factor distinct from IL-3 and IL-2, with both MCGF and TCGF activities which were designated as MCGFII/TCGFII. $C1.Ly1^+2^-/9$ cells also produce high levels of three B-cell-stimulating activities. These include costimulation of anti-IgM-activated B cells (46), induction of Ia antigen on resting B cells (46), and enhancement of IgE and IgG1 production in B cells in mixed cultures (47). Recent studies show that anti-IgM costimulation (45,48), Ia induction (49,50), and $IgG_1$ (51) as well as IgE enhancement (52) are all properties of BSF-1. All of these activities in $C1.Ly1^+2^-/9$ supernatants elute following gel filtration with an apparent molecular weight of 20 kD, the same size reported for BSF-1 from EL-4 cells (48). Together, these results suggest that $C1.Ly1^+2^-/9$ cells produce high levels of a factor functionally identical to BSF-1. Several lines of evidence suggested that BSF-1 was identical to the factor having MGCFII/TCGFII activity. When the MCGFII/TCGFII activity was highly purified from $C1.Ly1^+2^-/9$ supernatants, it was found to have Ia-inducing activity on B cells. Another line of evidence demonstrated that BSF-1 purified from EL-4 cells also possesses MCGFII/TCGFII activity and that anti-BSF-1 antibody could block MCGFII/TCGFII activity produced by T cells (42). These observations were all confirmed by following isolation of a novel mouse cDNA distinct from IL-2 and IL-3 that expresses the activity to stimulate B cells, T cells, and mast cells from a $C1.Ly1^+2^-/9$ cDNA library (3). This factor not only stimulates the proliferation of T cell and mast cell lines (3), but also induces Ia expression on resting B cells and enhances $IgG_1$ and IgE production by B cells, two properties of BSF-1. Since the cloned lymphokine exhibited activities on several cell types, the name "IL-4" was proposed (3,4), and we will use this name for the remainder of this chapter.

## IV.  STRUCTURE OF T-CELL-DERIVED LYMPHOKINES WHICH AFFECT GROWTH OF HEMOPOIETIC CELLS

Analysis of several lymphokine cDNA clones derived from activated T cells has revealed that each lymphokine is composed of a single polypeptide encoded by cDNA of about 1 kb in length, containing a hydrophobic signal peptide characteristic of a secretable protein at the $NH_2$-terminal segment. They show no sequence homology with other growth factors (such as EGF, FGF, and PDGF) or oncogenes. In addition, no significant homologies are found among T-cell-derived lymphokines either at the nucleotide sequence or amino acid sequence levels.

### A.  IL-3

The IL-3 cDNA clone which we described (10) was isolated from a mouse T-cell cDNA library on the basis of its ability to direct the synthesis of MCGF activity. The nucleotide sequence of the longest cDNA clone revealed a single long open reading frame of 166 codons. This sequence was identical to that reported for a clone independently isolated from WEHI-3 cells (11). The amino acid sequence of the encoded polypeptide (Figs. 4 and 5) is very hydrophobic at the $NH_2$-terminus, characteristic of a secreted protein. The amino acid sequence beginning with an aspartic acid residue at position 33, is identical to an $NH_2$-terminal

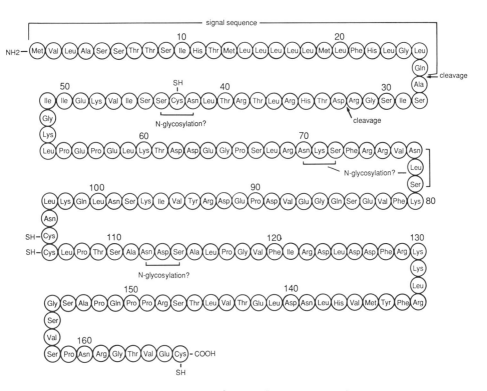

Figure 4   Schematic representation of mouse IL-3 amino acid sequence.

sequence reported for IL-3 purified from WEHI-3 cells (36). Clark-Lewis et al. (37) suggested that the $NH_2$-terminus of IL-3 begins with an alanine residue six amino acids upstream of the aspartic acid residue. Both of these results suggest that the MCGF polypeptide produced by T cells is identical to IL-3 from WEHI-3 cells and that mature IL-3 would consist of 134 or 140 amino acid residues with a calculated molecular weight of about 15 kD. Ihle et al. (35) have shown that mouse IL-3 is glycosylated and has an apparent molecular weight of 28 kD. Judging from the deduced amino acid sequence of the mouse IL-3 clones, there are four potential N-glycosylation sites (Asn-X-Ser) at positions 42-44, 70-72, 77-79, and 112-114. The discrepancy between the reported size of IL-3 and the calculated molecular weight of IL-3 deduced from the cDNA clones may be partly due to glycosylation of the native molecule. Mouse IL-3 expressed in COS7 cells (COS-IL-3) has been used as a convenient source of material to evaluate biological activity (38). Despite the extensive homology between mouse and human cDNAs and proteins for many lymphokines, a human lymphokine homologous to mouse IL-3 has not yet been reported.

```
                 20         40         60         80
Mouse IL-3: MVLASSTTSI HTMLLLLLML FHLGLQASIS GRDTHRLTRT LNCSSIVKEI IGKLPEPELK TDDEGPSLRN KSFRRVNLSK FVESQGEVDP
RAT   IL-3: MVLASSTTSI LCMLLPLLML FHQGLQISDR GSDAHHLLRT LDCRTIALEI LVKLPVSGLN NSDDKANLRN STLRRVNLDE FLKSQEEFDS
                 20         40         60         80

                 20         40         60         80
Mouse IL-2: MYSMQLASCV TLT--LVLLV NSAPTSSSTS SSTAEAQQQQ QQQQQQQHL  EQLLMDLQEL LSRMENYRNL KLPRMLTFKF YLPKQATELK
Human IL-2: MYRMQLLSCI ALSLALVT-- NSAPTSSSTK K-T--QLQ-  --------L  EHLLLDLQMI LNGINNYKNP KLTRMLTFKF YMPKKATELK
                 20         40         60         80

                 20         40         60         80
Mouse GM-CSF: MWLQNLLFLG IVVYSLSAPT RSPITVTRPW KHVEAIKEAL NLLDDMPVTL NEEVEVVSNE -FS--FKKL- --TCVQTRLK IFEQGLRGNF
Human GM-CSF: MWLQSLLLLG TVACSISAPA RSPSPSTQPW EHVNAIQEAR RLLNLSRDTA AEMNETV--E VISEMF-DLQ EPTCLQTRLE LYKQGLRGSL
                 20         40         60         80

                 20         40         60         80
Mouse IL-4: MGLNPQLVVI LLFFLECTRS HIHG--CDKN HLREIIGILN EVTGE-GTPC TEMDVPNVLT ATKNTTESEL VCRASKVLRI FYLKHGK-TP
Human IL-4: MGLTSQLLPP LFFLLACAGN FVHGHKCD-I TLQEIKTLN  SLT-EQKTLC TELTVTDIFA ASKNTTEKET FCRAATVLRQ FYSHHEKDTR
                 20         40         60         80

                 100        120        140        160        166
Mouse IL-3: EDRYVIKSNL QKLNCCLPTS ANDSALPGVF IRDLDDFRKK LRFYMVHLND LETVLTSRPP QPASGSVSPN RGTVEC
RAT   IL-3: QDTTDIKSKL QKLKCCIPAA ASDSVLPGVY NKDLDDFKKK LRFYVIHLKD LQPVSVSRPP QPTSSSDNFR PMTVEC
                 100        120        140        160        166

             100        120        140        160        169
Mouse IL-2: DLQCLEDELG PLRHVLDLTQ SKSFQLEDAE NFISNIRVTV VKLKGSDNTF ECQFDDESAT VVDFLRRWIA FCQSIISTSP Q
Human IL-2: HLQCLEEELK PLEEVLNLAQ SKNFHLRPRD L-ISNINVIV LGLKGSETTF MCEYADETAT IVEFLNRWIT FCQSIISTLT
         80              120        140        160        153

             100        120        140
Mouse GM-CSF: TKLKGALNMT ASYY-QTYCP PTPETDCETQ VTTYADFIDS LKTFLTDIPF ECKKPSQK
Human GM-CSF: TKLKGPLTMM ASHYKQ-HCP PTPETSCATQ IITFESFKEN LKDFLLVIPF DCWEPVQE
             100        120        140

                 100        120        140
Mouse IL-4: CLKKNSSVLM EL-QRLFRAF --RCLDS--- ---SISCTM  ---NESKSTS LKDFLESLKS IMQMDYS
Human IL-4: CLGATAQQFH RHKQ-LIR-F LKR-LDRNLW GLAGLNSCPV KEANQS--T- LENFLERLKT IMREKYSKCS S
                 100        120        140        153
```

**Figure 5** Comparison of mouse and human lymphokine amino acid sequences. Rat IL-3 is compared instead of human IL-3.

## B. GM-CSF

Colony-stimulating factors can be recognized in vitro by their ability to stimulate
the formation of colonies of differentiated cells in semisolid cultures of bone
marrow stem cells. Since many activated T cells produce both GM-CSF and IL-3
(Table 1), and they share many target cells in common in the bone marrow assay,
it is often difficult to demonstrate unequivocally the presence of GM-CSF in
crude mouse T-cell supernatants. The mouse GM-CSF cDNA clone was isolated
from an endotoxin-stimulated mouse cell cDNA library using an oligonucleotide
probe complementary to the putative GM-CSF mRNA based on the partial $NH_2$-
terminal amino acid sequence for mouse GM-CSF (14). Subsequently, a full-length
GM-CSF cDNA clone was isolated from activated T cells (15,53). The mouse
GM-CSF cDNA contains a single open reading frame consisting of 141 codons
(Fig. 5). Analysis of the hydrophobicity of the polypeptide and comparison with
a proposed consensus sequence for the processing of the signal peptides suggest
that processing of the precursor polypeptide would probably occur following
either of the serine residues at positions 15 and 17, or the alanine residue at position 18. The mature protein would consist of 120 amino acid residues corresponding to a protein with a calculated molecular weight of 12 kD while the reported
molecular weight of mouse GM-CSF is 29 kD or 33 kD. This difference could be
explained by posttranslational glycocylation of the molecule. It was suggested
that the hydrophilic region which precedes the putative hydrophobic signal peptide may yield a membrane-bound form of GM-CSF (53). However, S1 mapping
showed that the predominant transcription initiation site of the GM-CSF mRNA
in T-cell clones was 32 base pairs (bp) upstream of the first ATG codon described
above (15). These results suggest that mRNA for a putative membrane-bound
form of GM-CSF may be very rare or absent in T-cell clones.

A human GM-CSF clone (16,17) was identified using an in vitro semisolid
agar colony formation assay with human bone marrow cells. The human GM-CSF
cDNA contains a single open reading frame with 144 codons. The amino acid
sequences of human and mouse GM-CSF are approximately 50% homologous
(Fig. 5) while the nucleotide sequences share approximately 70% homology.
Cleavage of the precursor polypeptide occurs after the Ser residue at position
17 (17,54). There are two potential N-glycosylation sites both in human GM-
CSF (Asn-X-Ser or Asn-X-Thr at positions 44-46 and 54-56) and mouse GM-CSF
(Asn-X-Thr at positions 83-85 and 92-94, respectively). Both human and mouse
GM-CSFs are species-specific (15,16). Human GM-CSF may correspond to CSF-α
which induces colony formation of granulocytes, macrophages, and eosinophils
(55-57).

## C. IL-4

The single open reading frame in the mouse IL-4 cDNA clone encodes a protein
with 140 amino acid residues (Fig. 5). The mature polypeptide would be 120

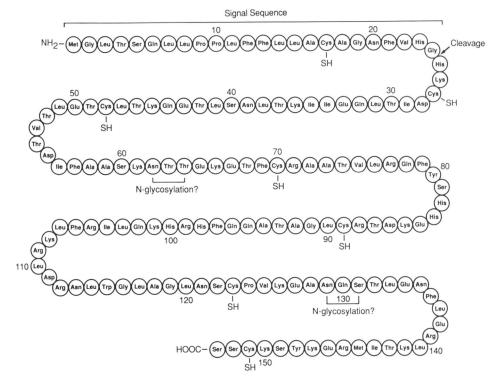

**Figure 6** Schematic representation of human IL-4 amino acid sequence.

amino acid residues long and begin with a histidine residue. This was confirmed by $NH_2$-terminal protein sequencing of mouse IL-4 purified from supernatants of mouse EL-4 cells (58). There are three potential N-glycosylation sequences (Asn-X-Thr and Asn-X-Ser at positions 61-63, 91-93, and 117-119). Despite the biological activities of IL-4 which are similar to activities found for IL-2 and IL-3, there is no significant amino acid sequence homology between IL-4 and either IL-2 or IL-3.

A human IL-4 cDNA clone which is homologous to the mouse IL-4 cDNA and expresses B-cell and T-cell-stimulating activities was isolated (5). This cDNA clone encodes a protein of 153 amino acid residues (Figs. 5 and 6) containing two potential N-glycosylation sequences (Asn-X-Thr or Asn-X-Ser) at positions 62-64 and 129-131, respectively. Analysis of the hydrophobicity of the polypeptide and comparison with the proposed consensus sequence for the processing of signal peptides (59) suggest that cleavage of the precursor polypeptide would occur following the glycine residue at position 24. This was confirmed by the $NH_2$-terminal sequencing of recombinant human IL-4 protein produced in COS7 cells

(60). Amino acid sequences of the mouse and human polypeptides share extensive homology with the exception of about 40 amino acids near the middle portion of the molecule (Fig. 5). Both mouse and human IL-4 contain seven cysteine residues, which are located at similar sites within the IL-4 protein with the exception of cysteine residue at position 107 of mouse IL-4 and that at position 151 in human IL-4 (Figs. 5 and 6). Supernatants of COS7 monkey cells transfected with the human cDNA clone-stimulated proliferation of human helper T-cell clones and anti-IgM-activated human B cells, two of the properties of mouse BSF-1. These results indicate that this human cDNA clone encodes a protein structurally and functionally homologous to mouse IL-4. It is worthwhile to note that prior to these experiments, a human equivalent of mouse BSF-1 had been postulated but never demonstrated.

## V. ORGANIZATION AND EXPRESSION OF LYMPHOKINE GENES

To study the mechanism of coordinate lymphokine induction during T-cell activation and to characterize regions required for regulated expression of lymphokine genes, chromosomal IL-3, GM-CSF, and IL-4 genes were isolated and their structures determined.

### A. Structure of IL-3 Gene

Southern blotting analysis performed with DNA isolated from both spleen and cloned helper T cells showed that there is only one copy of the IL-3 gene in the mouse haploid genome (61). The mouse IL-3 gene contains 5 exons and 4 introns (Fig. 7) (61). Like other lymphokine genes, for which sequences have been determined (mouse and human GM-CSF (15,62), mouse and human IL-2 (63,64) and human IFN-$\gamma$ (65), each intron interrupts the reading frame precisely between codons. The distance between the transcription initiation site determined by S1 mapping and the nucleotide preceding the poly(A) stretch in the IL-3 cDNA clone is 2195 base pairs (bp). A "TATA"-like sequence is found 24 bp upstream from the transcription initiation site. This TATA box is preceded by a GC-rich region about 45 bp long which contains a C block in the sense strand. The sequence GGCCAATCT, which is conserved in the promoter region located ~80 bp upstream of the cap site of many eukaryotic genes (66), is not found upstream of the cap site of the IL-3 gene. In the second intron of the IL-3 gene, there are 9 repeats of a closely related 14 bp sequence, interrupted by two segments of unique sequence. The region encompassing 8 of the repeats can be divided into two 73 bp direct repeats. Within each 73 bp repeat is a sequence homologous to the complementary strand of the enhancer core sequence (67). In addition, the IL-3 14 bp repeats share strong homology with a series of 20 bp repeats in the human genome having enhancer activity in several cell types (68). All of these

118

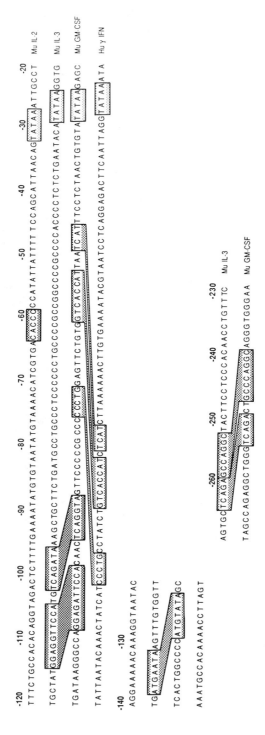

**Figure 7** Schematic representation of mouse IL-3 and GM-CSF genes and the flanking sequences of 4 different lymphokine genes (mouse IL-2, mouse IL-3, mouse GM-CSF, and human IFN-γ).

sequences contain the sequence CCTCCC which is similar to the sequence CCGCCC found in the GC-rich region of the SV40 early promoter.

The rat IL-3 gene has been isolated based on homology with the mouse IL-3 cDNA sequence (69). It consists of five exons interrupted by four introns with similar intron/exon boundaries as with the mouse gene. Extensive nucleotide sequence homology (approximately 90%) is present in the 5' flanking region and the portion of the genes coding for the signal peptide. Several proposed regulatory sequences in the mouse IL-3 gene are consderved in the rat gene and an analogous element to the tandem repeat in the second intron of the mouse gene is present. The predicted amino acid sequence for mature rat IL-3 shows surprisingly low homology (54%) with the mouse counterpart but all four cysteine residues are conserved (Fig. 5).

## B.  Structure of GM-CSF Gene

Southern blotting analysis indicated that there is a single-copy gene encoding GM-CSF in mouse (14) and human (15) haploid genomes, and that both the mouse and human GM-CSF genes (15,62) contain four exons and three introns (Fig. 7). The distance between the transcription initiation site determined by S1 mapping and the nucleotide preceding the poly(A) stretch in the human and mouse cDNA clone is 2376-2378 bp and 2371 bp, respectively. As is the case for several other lymphokine genes, each intron interrupts the reading frame precisely between codons. The consensus sequences for splicing junctions, G/GTAAG, for the donor splice site and AG for the acceptor splice site, were found in all boundaries between introns and exons (70). "TATA"-like sequences are found 20-25 bp upstream from the transcription initiation sites of both genes. In the 5' flanking region of the mouse GM-CSF gene, a stretch of 14 contiguous GT dinucleotides which is known to form a left-handed form of DNA, is found about 1 kb upstream from the cap site. Such a sequence has been reported to have an enhancer activity (71). Both human and mouse GM-CSF genes are organized in a similar manner (15). The sizes of exons 2, 3 and 4 (defined from the beginning of exon 4 to the stop codon TGA) are identical in both species and therefore each exon encodes exactly the same number of amino acid residues in both species. However, exon 1 of the human GM-CSF gene is 9 bp longer than exon 1 of mouse GM-CSF. In addition, the length of each intron is nearly the same in both genes. The mouse GM-CSF gene contains four direct repeats in the second intron, but these repeated sequences are not found in the introns of the human GM-CSF gene. Nucleotide sequences of the mouse and human GM-CSF cDNA clones share ~70% homology and the amino acid sequences share ~50% homology (16). In general, intron sequences show more diversity than exon sequences. However, stretches which show >70% homology are clustered in each intron. The most highly conserved sequences (87% homology) were found in the 5' flanking region extending ~330 bp upstream of putative TATA boxes (Fig. 7). Upstream sequences beyond this point show very little or no homology. The remarkable

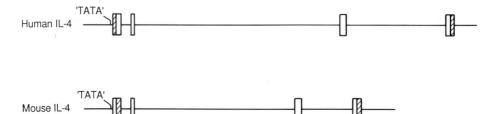

**Figure 8**  Schematic representation of mouse and human IL-4 genes.

conservation of the overall structure as well as the nucleotide sequences of the human and mouse GM-CSF genes indicates that they evolved from a common ancestral gene.

### C.  Structure of IL-4 Gene

The mouse and human IL-4 genes occur as single copies in the haploid genome and no detectable rearrangement has occurred in the mouse helper T-cell clone $Ly1^{+}2^{-}/9$ which expresses IL-4 after Con A stimulation (72,73). Both mouse and human IL-4 genes are composed of four exons and three introns and extend about 6 kb and 8.5 kb in length, respectively (Fig. 8). In view of the relatively small sizes of IL-4 cDNAs, the size of the mouse and human genes is surprisingly longer than that of other lymphokines. The length of exons 1, 2, 3, and 4 of the mouse IL-4 gene are 195 bp, 48 bp, 153 bp, and 191 bp, respectively, and of the human IL-4 gene are 197 bp, 48 bp, 177 bp, and 193 bp, respectively. Introns 2 and 3 of the human IL-4 gene are longer than those of the mouse IL-4 gene. Each intron interrupts the reading frame precisely between codons, begins with the consensus sequence "GT," and ends with consensus sequences "AG." A "TATA"-like sequence, TATATATA, is located 20-30 bp upstream of the transcription initiation sites of both mouse and human genes. The 5' flanking regions of mouse and human IL-4 genes extending 200 bp upstream of putative TATA boxes are highly conserved and share about 85% homology. About 500 bp further upstream sequences of both mouse and human IL-4 genes share about 75% homology (72, 73).

### D.  Comparison of 5' Flanking Regions of Lymphokine Genes

Despite the lack of any convincing homology among the genes for five T-cell-derived lymphokines (IL-2, IL-3, GM-CSF, IL-4, and IFN-γ), some common features can be recognized. All five genes have a relatively short second exon (40-70 bp) while the fourth exon is the longest except for IL-4. The first introns of IL-2, IL-3, and GM-CSF are of nearly the same size (90-100 bp). The 5' flanking region sequences of each lymphokine are more conserved between species than other regions of the gene, suggesting that this region is important for regulated expression in activated T cells.

To find potential consensus sequences which might be involved in regulated expression of lymphokine genes, the 5' flanking region sequences of the lymphokine genes were compared. Some sequence homologies were detected in some of the lymphokine genes (Fig. 7). In the 5' upstream region of mouse IL-3, and mouse GM-CSF, a GC-rich sequence, CCGĆCC, is found about 50 bp and 80 bp from the cap site. A similar sequence, CACCC, is found about 60 bp upstream from the cap site of both mouse and human IL-2 genes. There are some other sequence homologies in the 5' upstream region of mouse IL-3 and human and mouse GM-CSF. One is located about 240-260 bp from the cap site. An additional region of homology between mouse and human GM-CSF and human IFN-$\gamma$ is located 50-70 bp and 80-100 bp upstream of the transcription initiation sites of GM-CSF and IFN-$\gamma$ genes, respectively. These sequence elements may be involved in the coordinate expression of hemopoietic growth factor genes in T cells. Interestingly, both in mouse and human, there is a fairly high degree of homology between IL-4 and IL-2 genes extending more than 200 bp upstream of a "TATA"-like sequence (72,73) composed of numerous patches of homologous sequences. Despite the homologies shared in these regions between mouse IL-4 and IL-2 genes, they are expressed predominantly in different T-cell subsets (6) suggesting other elements may specifically control the expression of IL-4 and IL-2.

## E. Induction of Lymphokine mRNAs and Inhibition by Glucocorticoids

Induction of both human and mouse lymphokine genes at the transcriptional level can be observed in activated T cells after Con A exposure. The induced mRNAs constitute approximately 10% of total T-cell mRNA after 10 hr. As described above, cloned mouse helper T-cell lines can be divided into two distinct subsets on the basis of their pattern of lymphokine production. Both of the subsets (termed $T_H1$ and $T_H2$) (6), produce IL-3 but differ in their production of IL-2 and IFN-$\gamma$. $T_H1$ produces IL-2 and IFN-$\gamma$, whereas $T_H2$ does not produce IL-2 and IFN-$\gamma$. $T_H2$ cells do, however, produce IL-4. The frequency of each induced mRNA is approximately 0.1-1.0% of the total mRNA of the activated T cell. One $T_H1$ clone, MD13-5.1, produces IL-2, IL-3, and IFN-$\gamma$ activities after the addition of Con A. IL-3 levels, measured as MCGF activity, increased rapidly within 2-10 hr after Con A addition, reaching a plateau after 12 hr and continuing at the plateau level up to 24 hr. The kinetics of induction of IL-3 activity in this Con A-activated $T_H1$ clone is similar to that described for a $T_H2$ clone such as the C1.Ly1$^+$2$^-$/9 cells (74) from which a full-length IL-3 cDNA clone was originally isolated. At the mRNA level, IL-3 was strongly induced after Con A addition,

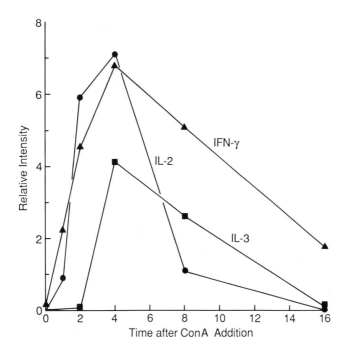

**Figure 9**   Kinetics of accumulation of IL-3, IL-2, IFN-γ mRNAs in Con A-stimulated MD13-5.1 cells. MD13-5.1 cells were stimulated by 6 μg/ml Con A, harvested after 0, 1, 2, 4, 8, or 16 hr and total RNA was isolated. Then 5 μg total RNA were hybridized with [$^{32}$P]endo-labelled probes for IL-3 (■), IL-2 (●), and IFN-γ (▲) and were analyzed using S1 nuclease (150). Autoradiogram showin RNA DNA hybrids separated on a denaturing polyacryleamide gel was analyzed by using densitometric scanning. The intensity of each hybrid in the autoradiogram is shown with arbitrary units.

reaching a maximal level at 4-6 hr. No IL-3 mRNA was detectable prior to activation. Although IL-2 and IFN-γ mRNAs also increased after Con A activation, kinetics of accumulation are different from that of IL-3 mRNA. The rate of accumulation of IL-2 mRNA starts to level off after 8 hr whereas IL-3 and IFN-γ mRNAs were more stable than IL-2 mRNA beyond 8 hr (Fig. 9). These results suggest that the mechanism of lymphokine expression may be different from lymphokine to lymphokine, although they are coordinately induced in this $T_H 1$ clone following Con A treatment. Human helper T-cell clones showed strong induction of GM-CSF, IL-2, and IFN-γ mRNAs after Con A exposure, induced GM-CSF mRNA represented about 0.5-1.0% of the total mRNA. In contrast, HTLV-transformed Mo T cells produced low levels of GM-CSF mRNA constitutively (17).

Glucocorticoids are known to be both immune suppressive and anti-inflammatory. One target of glucocorticoid action in the immune system is the T cell. Dexamethasone has been shown to have an antiproliferative effect on mouse cytotoxic T cells (75) and to inhibit IL-2 production in human peripheral blood lymphocytes (76). Culpepper and Lee (74) have shown that dexamethasone directly inhibits transcription of IL-3 and GM-CSF genes in the T-cell clone $C1.Ly1^+2^-/9$. These findings demonstrate that dexamethasone can inhibit the production of several lymphokines which are produced following mitogen activation. At least part of the immunosuppressive effects of glucocorticoids may result from of specific inhibition of T-cell-derived lymphokines which are necessary for the immune response.

Caput et al. (77) reported that mRNAs encoding for a number of cytokines (IL-1, TNF, fibronectin, interferons, GM-CSF) which may be involved in the inflammatory response have a consensus sequence UUAUUUAU in the 3' untranslated region. Similar AU-rich tracts are also present in the 3' untranslated region of IL-3, IL-4, c-myc, and c-fos mRNAs and are likely to be the target for processing nucleases since the removal of the AU-rich tract increased the stability of mRNAs (78,81). Rapid induction of mRNAs at the transcription level as well as their rapid degradation may be an important feature in regulation of the expression of lymphokine genes in response to the invasion of pathogens.

## F. Constitutive Expression of the IL-3 Gene

Supernatant from the murine meylomonocytic leukemia cell line WEHI-3, which produces IL-3 constitutively, has been commonly used as a source of IL-3. Southern blotting of WEHI-3 genomic DNA revealed that rearrangement had occurred in one allele of the IL-3 chromosomal gene (61). Ymer et al. (79) showed that an intracisternal A particle (IAP) genome analogous to a proviral form of retrovirus was inserted 215 base pairs upstream of the putative IL-3 TATA box in WEHI-3 chromosome.

The inserted IAP genome is positioned with its 5' long terminal response (LTR) close to the promoter region of the IL-3 gene which may result in the constitutive production of IL-3. Activation of a gene due to insertional mutation by an IAP has also been reported for the cellular oncogene c-mos (80). A similar observation was made after inserting the SV40 early region promoter into the chromosomal IL-3 gene at an *EcoR1* site, about 700 bp upstream of the TATA box. The bovine papilloma virus (BPV) plasmid carrying this modified IL-3 gene directed the synthesis of IL-3 in mouse fibroblasts at 10-fold higher levels than a control plasmid carrying the original IL-3 gene (81). These observations suggest that constitutive expression of the IL-3 gene in WEHI-3 is due to the insertion of the IAP sequence into one allele of the IL-3 gene. The enhancer element in the LTR may elevate transcription from the IL-3 promoter or the insertion of the IAP genome may inactivate a negative regulatory element upstream of the IL-3 promoter.

Constitutive expression of the IL-3 gene was also observed in stable transformants of L cells established by cotransfection of IL-3 genomic DNA with pSV2neo which specifies G418 resistance. Eleven of twelve G418-resistant transformants produced relatively high levels of IL-3 activity (61). Southern blotting analysis suggested that multiple copies of the IL-3 gene were integrated into the mouse chromosome. By contrast, very little IL-3 activity was detected in the supernatant of L cells 48 hr after transfection with IL-3 genomic DNA. The result of the transient expression experiment indicated that the IL-3 promoter works inefficiently in L cells. The elevated expression of IL-3 in L cell-stable transformants might be due to the high copy number of the IL-3 gene, expression of IL-3 under the control of SV40 promoter in the pSV2neo plasmid juxtaposed to the IL-3 gene, by a cellular transcription enhancer in the chromosome that activated the integrated IL-3 gene, or by a combination of these possibilities.

The IL-3 promoter works in vitro at levels similar to the adenovirus major late promoter in crude extracts from either HeLa cells or from the T-cell hybridoma FS6.14.13 (82). Since IL-3 may not be naturally expressed at high levels in cells other than activated T cells, these results may indicate that transcription of IL-3 is not regulated in the L cell stable transformants, and cell extracts. Further study of the regulation of lymphokine genes during T-cell activation requires establishment of improved experimental systems. These include a method for introducing genes into T-cell clones and preparation of T-cell transcription extracts after activation.

Southern blotting analysis of the human GM-CSF gene performed with chromosomal DNA isolated from HeLa cells, which are nonproducers, and Mo cells, which are constitutive producers of GM-CSF, showed the same hybridization pattern indicating that each human haploid genome contains a single copy of the gene. No detectable rearrangements were found in the GM-CSF gene in the Mo cell line (15). Therefore, constitutive production of lymphokines in Mo T cells may depend on a certain activator rather than a gene rearrangement.

## VI. EXPRESSION OF RECOMBINANT LYMPHOKINES IN VARIOUS HOST-VECTOR SYSTEMS

While the transient expression of cloned cDNAs in COS cells provides a convenient and rapid means to obtain small amounts of gene product, biochemical studies of lymphokines and their receptors as well as in vivo experiments require large amounts of pure material. Various host-vector systems including mammalian, bacteria, yeast, and insect have been developed to obtain large quantities of recombinant proteins. In addition to the expression systems which employ live cells, recent progress in the chemistry of peptide synthesis enables the synthesis of relatively large segments of proteins with good yield. In this section we describe various systems that have been used to produce lymphokines with an emphasis on IL-3 and GM-CSF.

## A. Mammalian Cells

Since this is the most natural system for expression of lymphokines, specific engineering of the cloned gene such as removal of the signal peptide is not necessary. However, there are many areas of mammalian expression systems and cell culture which require further improvements; these include amplification of copy number of the gene in a chromosomally integrated form or in the extrachromosomal state, use of a strong promoter-enhancer elements, development of a regulatable promoter, improved stability of mRNA or efficiency of translation, and the selection of optimal host cell types for maximum expression (83). The possibility that the nature of posttranslational modification may be different in different cell types needs to be considered.

### Transient Expression System

If cDNA is cloned in a mammalian expression vector, this plasmid can be used in a transient expression system without further manipulation. Human GM-CSF was purified from the supernatant of COS cells transfected with cDNA which was placed downstream of the adenovirus promoter (17,54). Although the amount of protein obtained was not very high (10 $\mu$g from 1 liter of COS medium), the production level was much better than a natural source (1 $\mu$g per 10 liters of Mo T cell medium). Takebe et al. (81) replaced the SV40 promoter in the pcD vector with strong promoters to express IL-3 or IL-4 cDNAs in COS cells or L cells in transient expression system and obtained sufficient amount of recombinant IL-3 or IL-4 (1 mg/ liter). One advantage of the transient expression system is its speed and the ease with which small amounts of recombinant lymphokines for purification can be obtained.

### Stable Transformants

In order to obtain large amounts of recombinant lymphokines, establishment of stable cell lines which produce high levels of recombinant lymphokines by transfecting with the gene may be the method of choice since it is time consuming to accumulate a large volume of COS supernatant in a transient expression system. For example, mouse L cell lines expressing MCGF activity were established by cotransfection with the IL-3 cDNA in the pcD vector and pSVneo. The expression level in these cells was comparable to that of the transient expression system using COS cells and IL-3 was purified from these L-cell-stable transformants (84). The bovine papilloma virus (BPV) vector (85) has been used to express human IFN-$\alpha$5 and IFN-$\gamma$ in mouse cells (86). The advantages of this vector are: (a) the recombinant plasmid is maintained extrachromosomally at high copy number and enables high level expression, and (b) no serum is required to grow the transformed cells which makes purification easy. This system was used to produce IL-3 and GM-CSF (81). IL-3 purified from the mammalian source was active in proliferation and differentiation assays in vitro and seemed to be glycosylated, although the structure of added carbohydrate has not yet been determined.

The Epstein-Barr virus (EBV) vector carrying the replication origin (*oriP*) can replicate as an episome in EBV-transformed human B cells which provide the EBNA1
product to activate *oriP* (87). The expression level of recombinant IL-4 in EBV-
transformed B cells using the EBV vector was lower than that achieved with the
BPV vector in fibroblasts (88).

### B. Bacteria

*Escherichia coli* is the most commonly used prokaryote host organism for expression of large amounts of recombinant proteins although it lacks a glycosylation
system. Since *E. coli* does not normally cleave the mammalian secretion precursor, several modifications to the cDNA are usually required for expression in *E.
coli*. Elements to achieve a high level of expression are shown in Figure 10. The
signal sequence in the original lymphokine cDNA must be removed and the mature lymphokine coding sequence has to be fused immediately downstream of

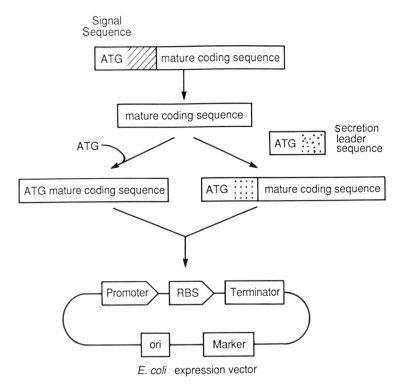

Figure 10  Schematic representation of *E. coli* expression systems. ori; replication origin, marker; selection marker, RBS; ribosome binding site.

the ATG codon or the sequence for secretion in *E. coli.* High level expression of mouse GM-CSF was achieved by inserting the mature protein coding sequence of GM-CSF with an ATG codon downstream of the pL promoter of lambda phage and the ribosome binding site from the *nerl* gene of bacteriophage Mu (89). Since mouse GM-CSF expressed in *E. coli* accumulated in refractile bodies, guanidine-HCl extraction and renaturation steps were necessary to obtain active mouse GM-CSF. The purified mouse GM-CSF was shown to stimulate the growth of granulocyte and macrophage colonies of mouse bone marrow cells. Lee et al. (90) expressed mouse IL-3 using a general cDNA expression vector Tac-RBS that contains the Tac promoter and ribosome binding site (RBS) and showed that accumulated IL-3 is labile in bacteria, being degraded within 30 min if protein synthesis is inhibited by chloramphenicol. The lability of expressed IL-3 was reduced if a *lon⁻ E. coli* host strain is used. Kindler et al. (91) expressed IL-3 in *E. coli* using the pL promoter and the ribosome binding site from T4 gene 32, which constitutes 15% of total *E. coli* protein under derepressed conditions. IL-3, purified and renatured after extraction with guanidine-HC1 was active in vitro in the proliferation and differentiation of various hemopoietic progenitor cells at 1 pM and it was also active in vivo (91). While various cytokines and growth factors have been expressed in *E. coli* in large quantities, proteins highly expressed in *E. coli* tend to accumulate in refractile bodies and have to be renatured after extraction with guanidine-HC1. These problems can sometimes be avoided by using secretion vectors. Kastelein and Van Kimmenade expressed both human and mouse GM-CSFs in the periplasmic space in soluble forms by fusing the signal sequence of *E. coli* lipoprotein (*lpp*) to the mature coding sequence (92).

## C. Yeast

*Saccharomyces cerevisiae* has been used as an alternate host microorganism to produce recombinant proteins because of its ability to secrete and glycosylate proteins. Generally, the secretion sequence of the yeast mating pheromone α-factor precursor has been used to secrete proteins, although in some cases such as IFN-β, yeast cells recognized the mammalian signal sequence and secreted processed proteins into the medium. Miyajima et al. (93) constructed a general secretion vector using the promoter and secretion sequence of the α-factor gene. Mature lymphokine coding sequences were fused to the α-factor secretion sequence. Correctly processed IL-2, IL-3, and GM-CSF were obtained in the culture medium, although the expression level was different in each case with best results obtained with GM-CSF. Figure 11 shows the procedure used to make fusion genes using GM-CSFs (94). Yeast carrying the mouse GM-CSF gene secreted GM-CSF activity into the medium. Although molecular weight heterogeneity was observed, this was due to different degrees of N-linked glycosylation. This was demonstrated by elimination of each of the two potential N-linked glycosylation sites as shown in Figure 11. Although the N-terminus of the secreted mGM-CSF was

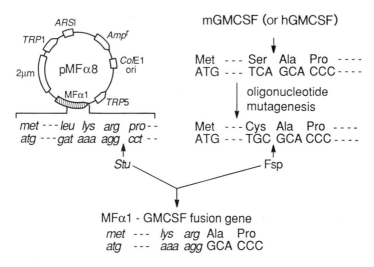

Figure 11  Structure of the yeast secretion vector pMFα8 and construction of MFα1-GM-CSF fusion genes.

4 amino acids shorter than that expected by cleavage at the processing site, it was fully active in proliferation and differentiation assays in vitro and supported colony formation of blast cell as well as granulocyte-macrophage colonies (95). Functional human GM-CSF was produced in the same way as above (94,96). IL-3 expressed using the same vector system stimulated the proliferation and differentiation of various hemopoietic progenitors (Table 3). Since there is a cleavage site within IL-3 recognized by the yeast enzyme which processes the α-factor precursor, the expression level of IL-3 was not high.

Table 3  Summary of Mouse IL-3 Biological Activities (38)

|                                                         | Purified IL-3 | COS-IL-3 | Yeast-IL-3 |
|---------------------------------------------------------|---------------|----------|------------|
| Induction of 20α-SDH                                    | Yes           | Yes      | Not done   |
| Thy 1-inducing activity                                 | Yes           | Yes      | Not done   |
| P-cell-stimulating factor, mast cell growth factor (MCGF) | Yes         | Yes      | Yes        |
| Growth factor of hematopoietic cell lines               | Yes           | Yes      | Yes        |
| Burst-promoting activity (BPA)                          | Yes           | Yes      | Yes        |
| Maintains CFU-S in culture                              | Yes           | Yes      | Not done   |
| Multilineage CSF                                        | Yes           | Yes      | Yes        |

## D. Insect

Because of the high capability of insect cells to produce proteins in vitro and in vivo, *Baculovirus* vector systems have been developed and applied to express IL-2 and interferons. Smith et al. made a recombinant infectious nuclear poly-hedrosis virus carrying IL-2 cDNA, which was placed downstream of the strong promoter of the polyhedrin gene, and used this to infect cultured cells of the moth *Autographa californica*. A few days after infection, the infected cells se-creted functional IL-2 at a level of 20-40 mg/liter of culture (97). Maeda et al. developed a similar vector which can transduce recombinant DNA in silk worm cells and succeeded in high level expression of IFN-α in silk worm larvae (98). IL-3 has been expressed at a high level in the silk worm system using the same vector (99). The IL-3 precursor carrying the signal sequence was correctly proc-essed to yield mature IL-3 and the protein was glycosylated.

## E. Chemical Synthesis

Recent improvements in the chemistry of solid-phase peptide synthesis together with the development of a fully automated peptide synthesizer opened the pos-sibility for synthesis of small proteins such as lymphokines. Using this technology, Clark-Lewis et al. (39) synthesized IL-3 chemically with 41% of the resulting mol-ecules having the correct IL-3 sequence. Refolded synthetic IL-3 was active in inducing proliferation of factor-dependent cells, and in stimulation of colony formation of bone marrow cells. The synthetic IL-3 was 0.5-30% as active as the native IL-3 due to the difficulties with separation of active IL-3 from inactive components. The same authors also synthesized peptide fragments correspond-ing to various regions of IL-3 and showed that the first 7 N-terminal amino acids are not essential for activity which is consistent with results from the yeast expres-sion system (93). In the near future this approach may play a major role in the study of protein structure-function relationship.

## VII. BIOLOGICAL ACTIVITIES OF RECOMBINANT LYMPHOKINES

## A. IL-3

As described above, more than 10 biological activities are associated with IL-3, which different investigators have referred to by different names (26-33). Rennick et al. confirmed most of the activities found with natural IL-3 in vitro using re-combinant-produced materials (38). Recombinant IL-3 expressed in COS7 cells and in yeast induces 20α-SDH, induces Thy-1 expression, and supports the growth of IL-3-dependent cell lines. Furthermore, it is in fact a multi-CSF and has burst-promoting activity and maintains CFU-S in culture (Table 3) (38). Mouse bone marrow cells incubated with recombinant IL-3 gave rise to colonies of various types. The majority of colonies composed of granulocyte, macrophage, or granulocyte/

macrophage mixtures, while some colonies of mixed composition were composed of multiple cell types including eosinophils, mast cells, and megakaryocytes in various combinations. These results established that COS-IL-3 and yeast-IL-3 stimulate the growth and differentiation of a wide spectrum of hemopoietic cell types including multipotential stem cells and various committed progenitor cells. Large-scale production of recombinant lymphokines made it possible to investigate the effect of these molecules in vivo. Purified recombinant IL-3 from *E. coli* was infused into normal and irradiated mice and hemopoietic progenitor cell numbers in spleen and bone marrow were evaluated using in vitro colony assays. The results are summarized as follows (91): (a) Doses of IL-3 infused at the rate of 2.5-5 ng/g of body weight per hour were sufficient to increase the numbers of hemopoietic progenitors in normal mice at least twofold within 3 days. (b) In mice with progenitor cell levels depressed by sublethal irradiation, 7-day treatment with IL-3 resulted in a tenfold increase to near normal levels. (c) The erythroid and myeloid lineages appeared to be enhanced to the same extent. (d) Enhancement of hemopoiesis occurred primarily in the spleen, but hemopoietic foci were also evident in the liver; in contrast, total cell and progenitor cell numbers were decreased in the bone marrow.

## B.  GM-CSF

COS-GM-CSF or yeast GM-CSF stimulates predominantly the formation of granulocyte and macrophage colonies in bone marrow assays (16). Both human and mouse recombinant GM-CSFs produced by COS-7 cells are species-specific (Table 4). Mouse GM-CSF does not stimulate colony formation using human cord blood cells. Human GM-CSF is not active in the mouse system, although it induces colony formation of granulocytes, macrophages, and eosinophils in semisolid human bone marrow cultures. This suggests that activity of the cloned human GM-CSF is similar to what has been described for CSF-α (55-57). Recent work has shown

Table 4  Species Specificity of Mouse and Human COS-GM-CSF by Colony Formation Assay

| cDNA clone transfected | Human | | Mouse |
|---|---|---|---|
| | Bone marrow | Cord blood | Bone marrow |
| | Colonies per $10^5$ cells | | |
| Mock transfection | $<5$ | $<5$ | $<5$ |
| Mouse GM-CSF | N.D. | 0 | 230 |
| Human GM-CSF | 56 | 186 | 0 |

*Source*: From Ref. 16.

that human CSF-$\beta$, which is active in the mouse system, corresponds to human G-CSF (100-102). Human (100) and mouse (103) G-CSF cDNAs contain a single open reading frame consisting of 207 codons and mature human (100,102) and mouse (103) G-CSF consist of 177 and 178 amino acid residues, respectively. No evidence is available thus far for the production of G-CSF by activated T cells.

By using purified yeast-produced mouse GM-CSF, blast cell colonies were formed in cultures of spleen cells from 5-fluorouracil-treated mice. Serial replating of washed blast cell colonies in cultures with GM-CSF formed various types of colonies including multilineage colonies, providing evidence for the direct effects of GM-CSF on proliferation of multipotential blast cells (95). Using an assay based upon the delayed addition of erythropoietin that minimizes or eliminates BPA-independent erythroid colony formation, purified recombinant human GM-CSF from COS cells, yeast, and *E. coli* had significant burst-promoting activity on circulating human erythroid progenitors (104,105). The in vivo effect of recombinant human GM-CSF was also investigated (106). Continuous infusion of GM-CSF in healthy monkeys rapidly elicits a dramatic leukocytosis and a substantial reticulocytosis. A similar effect has been observed in one pancytopenic, immunodeficient rhesus macaque (106).

For in vivo experiments using recombinant lymphokines, there are several problems to be solved such as rapid clearance of the injected materials. The half-life of recombinant IL-3 derived from *E. coli* has been estimated to be 3-4 min (107). Although no direct evidence is available, one reason for rapid clearance may be the difference in glycosylation, because *E. coli*-produced proteins are not glycosylated. Other experiments indicated that 10% of injected human GM-CSF derived from CHO cells remained in the circulation 2 hr after intravenous injection into the macaque. Even with recombinant lymphokine derived from mammalian cells, continuous infusion is necessary to maintain certain levels of concentration in the blood. In the experiments mentioned above, continuous infusion pumps were used.

## C. IL-4

As described above, T-cell clone Cl.Ly1$^+$2$^-$/9 cells produce a TCGF activity and a second MCGF activity distinct from IL-2 and IL-3, respectively. These activities are mediated by IL-4. The dose-response curves of COS-mouse IL-4 tested for TCGF activity on HT-2 cells reached the same maximal level as seen with the supernatant from Cl.Ly1$^+$2$^-$/9 cells. However, COS-IL-4 did not achieve the same level of stimulation obtained with recombinant IL-2 even at saturating levels (Fig. 12A). Human IL-2 stimulates proliferation of mouse T cells at high levels similar to human T cells while mouse IL-2 stimulates human T cells at lower efficiency. In contrast, the TCGF activity of mouse and human IL-4 appear to be species-specific (108). When COS-IL-4 was tested on MC/9 mast cells, the maximal stimulation was approximately the same as with COS-IL-3 (Fig. 12B). Combinations

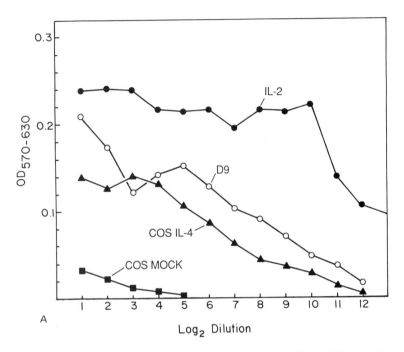

Figure 12   TCGF and MCGF activities of COS-IL-4: (A) TCGF activity was determined with HT-2 T-cell line by using a colorimetric assay (25). D9 and IL-2 denote Cl.Ly $1^+2^-/9$ cell supernatant and COS-IL-2, respectively. (B) MCGF activity was determined by using MC/9 mast cells and a colorimetric assay. IL-3 and D9 denote COS-IL-3 and supernatant of Cl.Ly $1^+2^-/9$ cell, respectively.

of COS-IL-3 and COS-IL-4 reconstituted the full MCGF activity observed with that of supernatant from Cl.Ly$1^+2^-/9$ cells. Several activities of recombinant mouse and human IL-4s on T cells, B cells, and hemopoietic cells are listed in Table 5. More activities may be found as larger quantites of pure recombinant IL-4 become available.

## VIII.   INTERACTIONS WITH RECEPTORS AND MECHANISM OF ACTION

### A.   Cell Cycle Control: Lymphokines as Hemopoietic Growth Factors

Progression of the cell cycle in mammalian cells from $G_0/G_1$ to S phase is controlled by the interaction of growth factors with specific membrane receptors. Studies of growth control of fibroblasts have revealed at least two distinct types of growth factors, "competence factors" and "progression factors," which act at different stages of the $G_1$ phase. Exposure of quiescent fibroblasts to competence

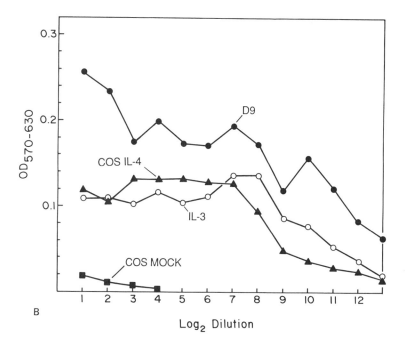

Figure 12B

Table 5   Multiple Activities of Recombinant IL-4

|                        | Mouse | Human |
|------------------------|-------|-------|
| T cell                 |       |       |
|   TCGF       | +     | +     |
| B cell                 |       |       |
|   BCGF       | +     | +     |
|   Ia inducing | +    | +     |
|   IgG$_1$ inducing | + | +   |
|   IgE enhancing | +  | +     |
|   FcεR expression | + | +    |
| Hemopoietic cell       |       |       |
|   MCGF       | +     | ?     |
|   Effect on macrophage | + | ? |
|   Colony formation | ? | ?   |
| Thymocyte stimulating  | +     | +     |

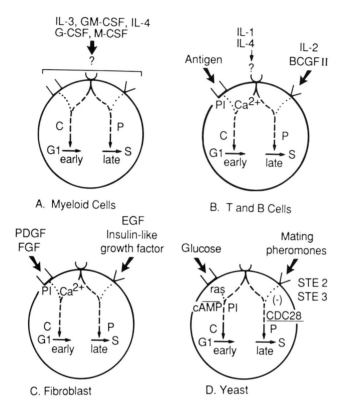

**Figure 13** Schematic representation of the cell cycle progression from $G_0/G_1$ to S phase in eukaryotic cells. C, competence pathway; P, progression pathway; PI, phosphoinositide turnover; $Ca^{2+}$, calcium mobilization. Mating pheromones α and a block the progression of the cell cycle in late $G_1$ phase in *S. cerevisiae*. *STE2* and *STE3* encode receptors for the α and a factor, respectively.

factors such as platelet derived growth factor (PDGF) or fibroblast growth factor (FGF) renders the cell competent to enter S phase upon further stimulation by a progression factor such as insulin or somatomedin (Fig. 13C). Activation of the competence pathway involves stimulation of phosphoinositide turnover, $CA^{2+}$ mobilization, activation of protein kinase C, and expression of nuclear oncogenes such as c-myc, c-fos, and p53. Insulin activates the progression pathways in competent cells by interacting with a receptor having a large cytoplasmic domain with tyrosine kinase activity (109,110).

Two distinct stages have also been recognized in the $G_1$ phase of the yeast *Saccharomyces cerevisiae* (Fig. 13D). The growth of yeast is arrested by nutritional limitation at an early $G_1$ phase and the cell enters into a resting $G_0$ stage. The progression from the early $G_1$ phase is controlled by the cAMP cascade (111).

Glucose stimulates cAMP formation and phosphoinositide turnover as well as $Ca^{2+}$ mobilization in a manner similar to that of growth factors in mammalian cells. *Ras* proteins are involved in regulation of this glucose-induced cAMP formation and phosphoinositide turnover in yeast (112). The late $G_1$ phase is controlled by the *CDC28* gene product (113) and mating pheromone's arrest of the cell cycle at this stage may occur through interaction with their putative receptors (the *STE2* and *STE3* products) (114). In light of these findings, it is tempting to speculate that proliferation of eukaryotic cells is regulated by two distinct signals which act at early and late $G_1$ phase, although the target substrates of both pathways remain to be determined. If this is the case, each lymphokine might be classified as either a competence or a progression factor, or a combination of these based on the signals generated by interaction with specific receptors. Therefore, it is particularly important to characterize the lymphokine receptors and their intracellular signals.

Antigenic stimuli delivered through interaction with a T-cell receptor (18) or a membrane-bound IgM receptor on B cells activates phosphoinositide turnover and renders the cells competent in a manner similar to the effect of PDGF or FGF on fibroblast (Fig. 13B). IL-1 and IL-4 may be costimulators for T-cell and B-cell activation at the early $G_1$ phase. In contrast to fibroblasts, hemopoietic cells are unable to rest in $G_0$ stage in vitro and die in the absence of growth factors (Fig. 13A). Of particular interest is the existence of myeloid cell lines whose survival and proliferation can be sustained by multiple growth factors such as IL-3, GM-CSF, and G-CSF. IL-4 also stimulates proliferation of numerous myeloid cell lines. These cell lines may serve as useful models to understand the nature of intracellular signaling through interaction of lymphokines with their receptors.

## B. Lymphokine Receptors

Genes for several growth factor receptors have already been cloned and their nucleotide sequence has been determined. The receptors for PDGF, epidermal growth factor (EGF), and insulin are transmembrane proteins having a large cytoplasmic domain with tyrosine kinase activity and a phosphorylation site (Fig. 14). Recently the M-CSF receptor was identified as a protein encoded by the cellular oncogene c-fms and nucleotide sequence analysis revealed that the overall structure of the M-CSF receptor is very similar to that of the PDGF receptor (115). Interestingly, membrane fractions of cells transformed with the viral oncogene v-fms had higher phospholipase C activity than similar fractions of normal cells (116) suggesting that the M-CSF receptor may interact with phospholipase C in a manner similar to that of the PDGF receptor.

Unlike receptors carrying a tyrosine kinase domain, the IL-2 receptor, a 55 kD glycoprotein having only a 13 amino acids in its cytoplasmic domain (117, 118), is unlikely to generate intracellular signals such as protein phosphorylation

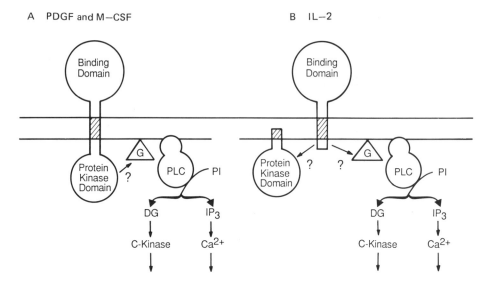

Figure 14 Schematic representation of lymphokine receptors. (A) PDGF and M-CSF receptors. (B) IL-2 receptor.

by itself. Recent studies suggest that a membrane-bound protein may interact with a low affinity IL-2 receptor to convert it into a high affinity form (119). This protein may be an effector molecule or a transducer protein connecting the IL-2 receptor to the effector molecule (Fig. 14). Palaszynski and Ihle (120) developed an assay for the IL-3 receptor on factor-dependent cell lines and showed that binding of [125]I-labeled IL-3 to these cells was specific, saturable, reversible, and time and temperature dependent. Cell lines 32D-cl23 had 4000-5000 specific binding sites with a kD of $5.4 \times 10^{-11}$. Other groups (121) identified the IL-3 receptor on the factor-dependent cell FDC-P2 as a protein of molecular weight 72 kD using crosslinking of [125]I-labeled IL-3. They estimated the number of binding sites to be about 400/cell with a Ka of $8.7 \times 10^9$ $M^{-1}$. Additional studies with an iodinated photoreactivatable cross-linking reagent indicated that the IL-3 receptor is a single polypeptide chain of 67 kD and an isoelectric point of 6.2 (122). Walker and Burgess (123) measured specific binding of radiolabeled GM-CSF to bone marrow cells, peritoneal neutrophils, and myelomonocytic cells and recognized two classes of binding sites: one with high affinity (Kd = 20 pM) and the other with low affinity (Kd = 0.8-1.2 nM). Cross-linking studies indicated that the GM-CSF receptor was a single polypeptide with an apparent molecular weight of 51 kD and the number of high affinity receptors may be 700-1000/cell assuming that 5-10% of bone marrow cells had high affinity receptors. In contrast, myelomonocytic cells had only high affinity GM-CSF receptors, 1000-5000 sites/cell with a Ka of $10^8$-$10^9$ $M^{-1}$, and a molecular weight of 130 kD (124), a value substantially different from that reported by Walker and Burgess. Although there are many discrepancies between the reports, the number of IL-3 or GM-CSF receptors seems in general to be substantially lower than that of IL-2 or EGF receptors. A cellular oncogene c-fes/fps, a 98-kD phosphoprotein with tyrosine kinase activity, was considered as a candidate for the GM-CSF receptor since it is expressed specifically in granulocytes and macrophages (125). Membrane fractions of v-fes/fps-transformed cells had higher phosphoinositide turnover than that of normal cells. However, the exact relationship between c-fes/fps and the GM-CSF receptor remains to be determined. Growth factor receptors thus far characterized seem to have single transmembrane segment in contrast to rhodopsin (126) or the β-adrenergic receptor (127) which have multiple transmembrane segments. At present, it is not clear whether IL-3 and GM-CSF receptors are of the EGF receptor type with a large cytoplasmic domain, or of the IL-2 receptor type having no obvious cytoplasmic domain; or are different from both. Molecular cloning and expression of the receptor genes may clarify these issues.

Expression of growth factor receptors is a critical step in the regulation of cell growth. Alteration of a receptor gene such as those for M-CSF or EGF can lead to oncogenesis due to continued stimulation of cell growth. Walker et al. (128) proposed that there are interactions between CSF receptors which result in a hierarchy in receptor down regulation. They observed that IL-3 suppressed the binding of the other three CSFs (GM-CSF, G-CSF, and M-CSF) to their receptors and GM-CSF suppressed the binding of G-CSF and M-CSF to their receptors. The physiological significance of these results is presently unknown. Although it cannot stimulate colony formation by peritoneal exudate macrophages and blood monocytes, IL-3 enhances the proliferative capacity of both cell types in response to suboptimal concentrations of M-CSF by increasing the number of available M-CSF receptor sites (129). It is noteworthy that some myeloid cells have low affinity IL-2 receptors (130) and certain IL-3-dependent cells switch factor dependency from IL-3 to IL-2 (131,132). Presumably, this change may be accompanied by the appearance of a functional high affinity receptor.

## C.  Autocrine and Nonautocrine Mechanisms for Autonomous Growth of Factor-Dependent Cells

Several mechanisms can be considered which will lead to the autonomous growth of factor-dependent cells (Fig. 15). Factor-dependent cells can become factor independent by expressing the factor required for growth (autocrine growth) (Fig. 15A). For example, some of the factor-independent variants isolated from PSF (IL-3)-dependent cells secreted PSF (IL-3) activity into the medium (133). Factor-dependent FDC-P1 cells transfected with cloned GM-CSF cDNA constitutively produce GM-CSF and grow independently of exogenous GM-CSF and, further, induce tumors in syngeneic mice (134). These results suggest the possibility of an autocrine growth mechanism mediated by lymphokines and their receptors.

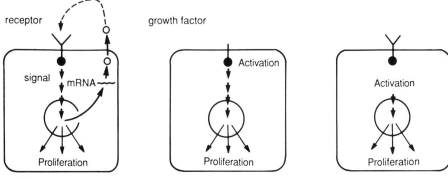

**Figure 15** Abrogation of factor-dependent growth.

Abrogation of factor dependence by a nonautocrine mechanism was also demonstrated using neoplastic transformation of mast cells by Abelson murine leukemia virus (Ab-MuLV) (135). Ab-MuLV has an oncogenic sequence (v-abl) carrying tyrosine kinase activity and causes a variety of tumors including nonthymic lymphoma and hemopoietic tumors. Ab-MuLV infection of normal mast cells eliminated IL-3 dependence for growth without causing expression of IL-3. A similar result was obtained using a factor-dependent myeloid cell line (136). These phenomena were specific to Ab-MuLV and neither Harvey, BALB, or Moloney murine sarcoma viruses (MSV) were able to relieve IL-3 dependence, although Harvey MSV could immortalize the cells while maintaining IL-3 dependence for growth. In contrast, Chung et al. (137) observed GM-CSF production by Ab-MuLV-induced mast cell lines. The possibility exists that v-abl protein abrogates the IL-3 requirement by interacting with the IL-3 receptor (Fig. 15B) or by activating an IL-3-dependent signal transduction cascade downstream (Fig. 15C). Likewise, v-myc expression in IL-2-dependent cells and IL-3-dependent cells obviated the IL-2 or IL-3 requirement for growth (138). This is consistent with the observation that removal of IL-3 from IL-3-dependent cells results in dramatic decrease of c-myc and c-fos mRNA levels and that addition of IL-3 results in rapid recovery of mRNA levels (139). These results suggest that c-myc expression plays a role in the signal transduction events initiated by interaction of IL-3 with its receptor.

Induction of c-myc usually requires activation of protein kinase C and mobilization of $Ca^{2+}$ which are caused by breakdown of phosphoinositides. PDGF or FGF activates phospholipase C which cleaves phosphoinositides to generate diacylglycerol (DG) and inositol trisphosphate ($IP_3$) through interaction with the receptor (140). DG serves as a second messenger to activate protein kinase C and $IP_3$ mobilizes $Ca^{2+}$ from intracellular storage. The observation that IL-3 stimulates the translocation of protein kinase C from the cytoplasmic to the membrane fraction in FDC-P1 cells (141) suggests that protein kinase C is involved in the IL-3-dependent signal transduction cascade. However, activation of phospholipase C by IL-3 needs to be demonstrated to support this view. If this turns out to be true, the function of IL-3 may be analogous to that of PDGF and FGF in fibroblasts. It is conceivable that the IL-3 system is linked to a certain type of GTP binding protein (142) which has been postulated for activation of phospholipase C in the "competence pathway." Depletion of growth factor leads fibroblast cells to enter the $G_0$ state while depletion of IL-3 from factor-dependent hemopoietic cells causes rapid loss of viability. Therefore, IL-3 must have some role in maintaining viability of hemopoietic cells. Whetton and Dexter (143) observed that intracellular adenosine triphosphate (ATP) levels of FDC-P2 cells decreased quickly in the absence of IL-3 and cell viability was maintained up to 48 hr by the addition of an ATP-regenerating system. Furthermore, high concentrations of extracellular glucose or its metabolites prevented cell death and IL-3 stimulated lactate production and hexose uptake (144). These results suggest that IL-3 maintains cell viability by stimulating glucose transport, thereby maintaining cellular metabolic activity.

## IX. ROLE OF T-CELL-DERIVED LYMPHOKINES IN "INDUCIBLE" HEMOPOIESIS IN AN INFLAMMATORY RESPONSE

T cells produce two of the four known CSFs (i.e., IL-3, GM-CSF, G-CSF, and M-CSF) which are known to control proliferation and differentiation of granulocytes and macrophages. What is the role of T-cell-derived CSFs and IL-4 in regulation of hemopoiesis? Hemopoietic cells are produced and destroyed continuously under precise control mechanisms in the bone marrow which we refer to as "constitutive" hemopoiesis. Evidence indicates that all hemopoietic cells are ultimately derived from self-renewing multipotential stem cells (145). During this normal, "constitutive" hemopoiesis, stem cells are usually in the resting $G_0$ state but can be mobilized into a proliferative state when required. The factors which direct stem cells to self-renew or to differentiate are not known. There are two different views about the process of stem cell differentiation. One model assumes that the differentiation of stem cells is a sequential and ordered process characterized by the successive restriction of differentiation potential (in the order macrophage, eosinophil, granulocyte-macrophage, granulocyte, megakaryocyte, erythroid) (146). The other model predicts that stem cells differentiate in a progressive and stochastic manner (147,148). Several lines of evidence indicate that bone marrow stromal cells have a major role in regulation of this "constitutive" hemopoiesis (149). Stromal cells may influence the growth and differentiation of multipotential stem cells and

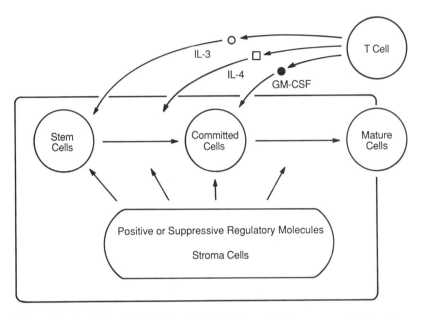

**Figure 16** Possible effect of T-cell-derived lymphokines on constitutive hemopoiesis in the stromal environment of the bone marrow.

committed progenitor cells either in a positive or in a restrictive manner. This may be achieved by the production of soluble mediators or by complex cellular interactions which maintain the microenvironment for stem cells. Do CSFs produced by T cells play a role in regulating the "constitutive" hemopoiesis in the bone marrow? CSFs produced by T cells in response to various immunological stimuli, such as invasion of foreign substances into the body, may affect hemopoiesis in the bone marrow; however, they may not play a major role in "constitutive" hemopoiesis which proceeds in the marrow microenvironment in the absence of immunological stress (Fig. 16). Rather it is tempting to speculate that the T-cell-generated lymphokine cascade may have evolved as an "emergency device" whose major function is to promote rapid expansion and maturation of committed progenitor cells at or near the sites of an acute inflammation reaction. We suggest that this type of hemopoiesis controlled by T cells be called "inducible" or "SOS" hemopoiesis to distinguish it from the normal "constitutive" hemopoiesis which occurs in the bone marrow. The in vivo IL-3 experiments (91) showed that IL-3 induced the enhanced hemopoiesis in spleen and liver, but not in the bone marrow. This observation might be an additional evidence for the role of IL-3 in "inducible" but not "constitutive" hemopoiesis.

GM-CSF and IL-3 produced by activated T cells may trigger rapid proliferation and differentiation of various committed progenitor cells. IL-4 produced by

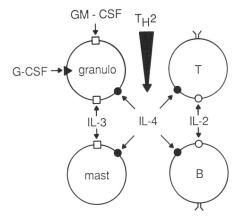

Figure 17  Coordination of cellular interactions by IL-4.

a certain type of activated T cells (5,8) may coordinate the function of mast cells, myeloid cells, T cells, and B cells by virtue of its multiple biological activities (Fig. 17). A general picture is emerging of the functional link between hemopoietic cells, T cells, and B cells in an immune response mediated by multiple lymphokines produced by activated T cells. Although the exact role of T-cell-induced CSFs in normal, constitutive hemopoiesis remains to be determined, abnormal production of CSFs by T cells may contribute to the etiology of some hemopoietic disorders. Hemopoietic diseases may also be related to abnormal production of CSFs by stromal cells (paracrine mechanism) or hemopoietic progenitor cells (autocrine mechanism), or to abnormal expression of CSF receptors in hemopoietic progenitor cells. Studies on the regulation of expression of hemopoietic growth factor genes should shed light on the role of these factors in both normal and abnormal hemopoiesis.

## X.  CONCLUDING REMARKS

Rapid progress has been made in characterizing the molecular nature of T-cell-derived lymphokines. Many lymphokine genes have now been cloned from activated T cells by using mammalian cDNA expression vectors and their products have been expressed in mammalian, bacterial, yeast, and insect cells. Among them are IL-3, GM-CSF, and IL-4 which affect hemopoiesis. Use of these recombinant lymphokines has provided the opportunity to evaluate biological activities in vitro and in vivo and the mechanism of lymphokine action in promoting proliferation and differentiation of hemopoietic cells and lymphoid cells. Characterization of the structure of lymphokine genes will provide information about their regulated expression during T-cell activation. IL-3 and GM-CSF produced by activated T cells in response to immunological stimuli can trigger rapid expansion and maturation of various hemopoietic cells while IL-4, by virtue of its diverse biological activities, may have a role in coordinating the function of hemopoietic cells, T cells and B cells in an inflammatory response. Elucidation of the mechanisms by which T cells regulate the interaction of various hemopoietic stem cells, mast cells, macrophages, T cells and B cells through the production of lymphokines may contribute to understanding the etiology of various hematological disorders.

## ACKNOWLEDGMENT

The authors would like to thank colleagues of DNAX Research Institute in the Department of Molecular Biology (Dov Zipori, Robert Kastelein, Gerard Zurawski, Craig Smith, Martha Bond, Kunihiro Matsumoto, Naoki Nakayama, Hisao Masai, Ron Conaway, and Joan Conaway), in the Department of Immunology (Donna Rennick, Robert Coffman, Albert Zlotnik, John Abrams, Marilyn Kehry, and Maureen Howard), and at the UNICET Immunology Laboratory (Jacques Banchereau and Jan De Vries) for their collaboration on T-cell-derived lymphokines and on the control of cell growth, as well as for sharing information with us. We thank Hiroto Okayama for the pcD expression vector and Susumu Maeda for the silkworm expression vector.

## NOTES ADDED IN PROOF

After this review was completed, the human IL-3 gene was isolated and the second chain of the IL-2 receptor was identified. Young et al. isolated Gibbon IL-3 cDNA based on the activity to support growth of human circulating blast cells of chronic myelogenous leukemia patients. It has 43% homology at the nucleotide level and only 29% homology at amino acid level with mouse IL-3. Human IL-3 cDNA isolated from activated T cells is almost identical to gibbon IL-3 and encodes a protein of 152 amino acid residues with multi-CSF activity and stimulates basophil growth. However, it is not clear at present whether human IL-3 stimulates the growth of mast cells. The high affinity IL-2 receptor (Kd = 10 pM) is composed of both 55 kD and 75 kD molecules. The second chain of the IL-2 receptor (75 kD) binds IL-2 at higher affinity (Kd = 1 nM) than the 55 kD IL-2 receptor (Kd = 10 nM) and transmits an IL-2 signal.

## REFERENCES

1. Nabel, G., Greenberger, J.S., Sakakeeny, M.A., and Cantor, H. Proc. Natl. Acad. Sci. USA 78: 115, 1981.
2. Prystowsky, M., Ely, J., Beller, D., Eisenberg, L., Goldman, J., Goldman, M., Goldwasser, E., Ihle, J., Quintans, J., Remold, H., Vogel, S., and Fitch, F.J. Immunol. 129: 2337, 1982.

3. Lee, F., Yokota, T., Otsuka, T., Meyerson, P., Villaret, D., Coffman, R., Mosmann, T., Rennick, D., Roehm, N., Smith, C., Zlotnik, A., and Arai, K. Proc. Natl. Acad. Sci. USA 83: 2061, 1986.

4. Noma, Y., Sideras, P., Naito, T., Bergstedt-Lindquist, S., Azuma, C., Severinson, E., Tanabe, T., Kinashi, T., Matsuda, F., Yaoita, Y., and Honjo, T. Nature 319: 640, 1986.

5. Yokota, T., Otsuka, T., Mosmann, T., Banchereau, J., DeFrance, T., Blanchard, D., De Vries, J., Lee, F., and Arai, K. Proc. Natl. Acad. Sci. USA 83: 5894, 1986.

6. Mosmann, T.R., Cherwinski, H., Bond, M.W., Giedlin, M.A., and Coffman, R.L. J. Immunol. 136: 2348, 1986.

7. Taniguchi, T., Matsui, H., Fujita, T., Takaoka, C., Kashima, N., Yoshimoto, R., and Hamuro, J. Nature 302: 305, 1983.

8. Yokota, T., Arai, N., Lee, F., Rennick, D., Mosmann, T., and Arai, K. Proc. Natl. Acad. Sci. USA 82: 68, 1985.

9. Kashima, N., Nishi-Takaoka, C., Fujita, T., Taki, S., Yamada, G., Hamuro, J., and Taniguchi, T. Nature 313: 402, 1985.

10. Yokota, T., Lee, F., Rennick, D., Hall, C., Arai, N., Mosmann, T., Nabel, G., Cantor, H., and Arai, K. Proc. Natl. Acad. Sci. USA 81: 1070, 1984.

11. Fung, M.C., Hapel, A.J., Ymer, S., Cohen, D.R., Johnson, R.A., Campbell, H.D., and Young, I.G. Nature 307: 233, 1984.

12. Gray, P.W., Leung, D.W., Pennica, D., Yelverton, E., Najarian, R., Simonsen, C.D., Derynck, R., Sherwood, P.J., Wallace, D.M., Berger, S.L., Levinson, A.D., and Goeddel, D.V. Nature (London) 295: 503, 1982.

13. Gray, P.W., and Goeddell, D.V. Proc. Natl. Acad. Sci. USA 80: 5842, 1983.

14. Gough, N.M., Gough, J., Metcalf, D., Kelso, A., Grail, D., Nicola, N.A., Burgess, A.W., and Dunn, A.R. Nature 39: 763, 1984.

15. Miyatake, S., Otsuka, T., Yokota, T., Lee, F., and Arai, K. EMBO J. 4: 2561, 1985.

16. Lee, F., Yokota, T., Otsuka, T., Gemmell, L., Larson, N., Luh, J., Arai, K., and Rennick, D. Proc. Natl. Acad. Sci. USA 82: 4360, 1985.

17. Wong, G.G., Witek, J.S., Temple, P.A., Wilkens, K.M., Leary, A.G., Luxenberg, D.P., Jones, S.S., Brown, E.L., Kay, R.M., Orr, E.C., Shoemaker, C., Golde, D.W., Kaufmann, R.J., Hewick, R.M., Wang, E.A., and Clark, S.C. Science 248: 810, 1985.

18. Weiss, A., Imboden, J., Hardy, K., Manger, B., Terhorst, C., and Stobo, J. Ann. Rev. Immunol. 4: 593, 1986.

19. Smith, K. Ann. Rev. Immunol. 2: 319, 1984.

20. Young, R.A., and Davis, R.W. Proc. Natl. Acad. Sci. USA 80: 1194, 1983.

21. Okayama, H., and Berg, P. Mol. Cell. Biol. 3: 280, 1983.

22. Bradley, T.R., and Metcalf, D. Aust. J. Exp. Biol. Med. Sci. 44: 287, 1966.

23. Ichikawa, Y., Pluznik, D.H., and Sachs, L. Proc. Natl. Acad. Sci. USA 56: 488, 1966.

24. Metcalf, D. *The Hemopoietic Colony Stimulating Factors.* Elsevier, Amsterdam, 1984.

25. Mosmann. T. J. Immunol. Methods 65: 55 (1983).

26. Ihle, J.N., Pepersack, L., and Rebar, L. J. Immunol. 126: 2184, 1981.

27. Schrader, J.W., Lewis, S.J., Clark-Lewis, I., and Culvenor, J.G. Proc. Natl. Acad. Sci. USA 78: 323, 1981.
28. Yung, Y.P., Eger, R., Tertian, G., and Moore, M.A.S. J. Immunol. 127: 794, 1981.
29. Raxzin, E., Cordon-Cardo, C., and Good, R.A. Proc. Natl. Acad. Sci. USA 78: 2559, 1981.
30. Nabel, G., Galli, S.J., Dvorak, A.M., Dvorak, H.R., and Cantor, H. Nature 291: 332, 1981.
31. Bazill, G.W., Haynes, M., Garland, J., and Dexter, D.M. Biochem. J. 210: 747, 1983.
32. Dy, M., Label, B., Kamoun, P., and Hamburger, J. J. Exp. Med. 153: 293, 1981.
33. Wong, G.H.W., Clark-Lewis, I., Hamilton, J.A., and Schrader, J.W. J. Immunol. 133: 2043, 1984.
34. Lee, J.C., Hapel, A.J., and Ihle, J.N. J. Immunol. 128: 2393, 1982.
35. Ihle, J.N., Keller, J., Henderson, L., Frederick, K., and Palaszynski, E. J. Immunol. 129: 2431, 1982.
36. Ihle, J.N., Keller, J., Oroszlan, S., Henderson, L.E., Copeland, T.D., Fitch, F., Prystowsky, M.B., Goldwasser, E., Schrader, J.W., Palaszynski, E., Dy, M., and Lebel, B. J. Immunol. 131: 282, 1983.
37. Clark-Lewis, I., Kent, S.B.H., and Schrader, J.W. J. Biol. Chem. 259: 7488, 1984.
38. Rennick, D.M., Lee, F.D., Yokota, T., Arai, K., Cantor, H., and Nabel, G.J. J. Immunol. 134: 910, 1985.
39. Clark-Lewis, I., Aebersold, R., Ziltener, H., Schrader, J.W., Hood, L.E., and Kent, S.B.H. Science 231: 134, 1986.
40. Hapel, A.J., Osborne, J.M., Fung, M.C., Young, I.G., Allan, W., and Hume, D.A. J. Immunol. 134: 2492, 1985.
41. Smith, C.A., and Rennick, D.M. Proc. Natl. Acad. Sci. USA 83: 1857, 1986.
42. Mosmann, T.R., Bond, M.W., Coffman, R.L., Ohara, J., and Paul, W.E. Proc. Natl. Acad. Sci. USA 83: 5654, 1986.
43. Dy, M., Lebel, B., and Schneider, E. J. Immunol. 136: 208, 1986.
44. Hapel, A.J., Warren, H.S., and Hume, D.A. Blood 64: 786 (1984).
45. Howard, M., Farrar, J., Hilfiker, M., Johnson, B., Takatsu, K., Hamaoka, K., and Paul, W.E. J. Exp. Med. 155: 914, 1982.
46. Roehm, N.W., Leibson, J.H., Marrack, P., Cambier, J.C., Kappler, J.W., Rennick, D.M., and Zlotnik, A. In Cellular and Molecular Biology of Lymphokines. Edited by C. Sorg and A. Schimpl. Academic Press, Orlando, Florida, 1985, pp. 195-204.
47. Coffman, R.L., and Carty, J. J. Immunol. 136: 949, 1986.
48. Ohara, J., Lahet, S., Inman, J., and Paul, W.E. J. Immunol. 135: 2518, 1985.
49. Noelle, R., Krammer, P.H., Ohara, J., Uhr, J.W., and Vitetta, E.S. Proc. Natl. Acad. Sci. USA 81: 6149, 1984.
50. Reohm, N.W., Leibson, H.J., Zlotnik, A., Kappler, J.W., Marrack, P., and Cambier, J.C. J. Exp. Med. 160: 679, 1984.
51. Vitetta, E.S., Ohara, J., Myers, C., Layton, J., Krammer, P.H., and Paul, W.E. J. Exp. Med. 162: 1726, 1985.

52. Coffman, R.L., Ohara, J., Bond, M.W., Carty, J., Zlotnik, A., and Paul, W.E. J. Immunol. 136: 4538, 1986.
53. Gough, N.M., Metcalf, D., Gough, J., Grail, D., and Dunn, A.R. EMBO J. 4: 645, 1985.
54. Gasson, J.C., Weisbert, R.H., Kaufman, S.E., Clark, S.C., Hewick, R.M., Wong, G.G., and Golde, D.W. Science 226: 1339, 1984.
55. Nicola, N.A., Metcalf, D., Johnson, G.R., and Burgess, A.W. Blood 54: 614, 1979.
56. Das, S.K., Stanley, E.R., Guilbert, L.J., and Forman, L.W. Blood 58: 630, 1981.
57. Lusis, A.J., Quan, D.H., and Golde, D.W. Blood 57: 13, 1981.
58. Grabstein, K., Eisenman, J., Mochizuki, D., Shanbeck, K., Conlon, P., Hopp, T., March, C., and Gillis, S. J. Exp. Med. 163: 1405, 1986.
59. Perlman, D., and Halvoson, H.O. J. Mol. Biol. 167: 391, 1983.
60. Le, H.V., Ramanathan, L., Labon, J.E., et al. (submitted).
61. Miyatake, S., Yokota, T., Lee, F., and Arai, K. Proc. Natl. Acad. Sci. USA 82: 316, 1985.
62. Stanley, E., Metcalf, D., Sobieszczuk, P., Gough, N.M., and Dunn, A.R. EMBO J. 4: 2569, 1985.
63. Fujita, T., Takaoka, C., Matsui, H., and Taniguchi, T. Proc. Natl. Acad. Sci. USA 80: 7437, 1983.
64. Fuse, A., Fujita, T., Yasumitsu, H., Kashima, N., Hasegawa, K., and Taniguchi, T. Nucleic Acids Res. 8: 127, 1980.
65. Gray, P.W., and Goeddel, D.V. Nature 289: 859, 1982.
66. Benoist, C., O'Hare, K., Breathnach, R., and Cambon, P. Nucleic Acids Res. 8: 127, 1980.
67. Weiher, H., Konig, M., and Gruss, P. Science 219: 626, 1983.
68. Rosenthal, N., Kress, M., Gruss, P., and Khoury, G. Science 222: 749, 1983.
69. Cohen, D.R., Hapel, A.J., and Young, I.G. Nucleic Acids Res. 14: 3641, 1986.
70. Breathnach, R., Benoist, C., O'Hare, K., Gannon, F., and Chambon, P. Proc. Natl. Acad. Sci. USA 75: 4853, 1978.
71. Hamada, H., Seidman, M., Howard, B.H., and Gorman, C.M. Mol. Cell. Biol. 4: 2622, 1984.
72. Otsuka, T., Villaret, D., Yokota, T., Takebe, Y., Lee, F., Arai, N., and Arai, K. Nucleic Acids Res. 15: 333, 1987.
73. Arai, N., Nomura, D., Villaret, D., et al. (submitted).
74. Culpepper, J.A., and Lee, F. J. Immunol. 135: 3191, 1985.
75. Gillis, S., Crabtree, G.R., and Smith, K.A. J. Immunol. 123: 1624, 1979.
76. Arya, S.K., Wong-Staal, F., and Gallo, R.C. J. Immunol. 133: 273, 1984.
77. Caput, D., Beutler, B., Hartog, K., Thayer, R., Brown-Schimer, S., and Cerami, A. Proc. Natl. Acad. Sci. USA 83: 1670, 1986.
78. Shaw, G., and Kamen, R. Cell 46: 659, 1986.
79. Ymer, S., Tucker, W.Q.J., Sanderson, C.J., Hapel, A.J., Campbell, H.D., and Young, I.G. Nature 317: 355, 1985.
80. Horowitz, M., Luria, S., Rechavi, G., and Givol, D. EMBO J. 3: 2937, 1984.
81. Takebe, Y., Yokota, K., Hoy, P., and Arai, N. Unpublished results.

82. Otsuka, T., Miyatake, S., Yokota, T., Conaway, J., Conaway, R., Arai, N., Lee, F., and Arai, K. In *Lymphokines*, Vol. 13. Edited by D.R. Webb and D. Goeddel. Academic Press, New York, 1987, pp. 261-273.

83. Arathoon, W.R., and Birch, J.R. Science 232: 1390, 1986.

84. Takebe, Y., Schreurs, J., and Arai, N. Unpublished results.

85. Low, M.F., Lowy, D.R., Dvoretzky, I., and Howley, P.M. Proc. Natl. Acad. Sci. USA 78: 2727, 1981.

86. Fukunaga, R., Sokawa, Y., and Nagata, S. Proc. Natl. Acad. Sci. USA 81: 5086, 1984.

87. Yates, J.L., Warren, N., and Sugden, B. Nature 313: 812, 1985.

88. Takebe, Y., Hayakawa, H., Yokota, K., and Arai, N. Unpublished results.

89. DeLamarter, J.E., Mermod, J.J., Liang, C.M., Eliason, J.F., and Thatcher, D.R. EMBO J. 4: 2575, 1985.

90. Lee, F., Abrams, J., Arai, K., Arai, N., Miyajima, A., Miyatake, S., Mosmann, T., Rennick, D., Schreurs, J., Smith, C., Takebe, Y., Yokota, T., Zurawski, G., and Zurawski, S. *Lymphokines.* Edited by J. Schrader. Academic Press, New York (in press).

91. Kindler, V., Thorens, B., DeKossodo, S., Allet, B., Eliason, J.F., Thatcher, D. Farber, N., and Vassalli, P. Proc. Natl. Acad. Sci. USA 83: 1001, 1986.

92. Kastelein, R., and Van Kimmenade, A. Unpublished results.

93. Miyajima, A., Bond, M.W., Otsu, K., Arai, K., and Arai, N. Gene 137: 155, 1985.

94. Miyajima, A., Otsu, K., Schreurs, J., Bond, M.W., Abrams, J., and Arai, K. EMBO J. 5: 1193, 1986.

95. Koike, K., Ogawa, M., Ihle, J.N., Miyake, T., Shimizu, T., Miyajima, A., Yokota, T., and Arai, K. J. Physiol. Chem. 131: 458, 1987.

96. Cantrell, A.M., Anderson, D., Cerretti, D.P., Price, V., McKereghan, K., Tushinski, R.J., Mochizuki, D.Y., Larsen, A., Grabstein, K., Gillis, S., and Cosman, D. Proc. Natl. Acad. Sci. USA 82: 6750, 1985.

97. Smith, G.E., Ericson, B.L., Moschera, J., Lahm, H.W., Chizzonite, R., and Summers, M.D. Proc. Natl. Acad. Sci. USA 82: 8404, 1985.

98. Maeda, S., Kawai, T., Obinata, M., Fujiwara, H., Horiuchi, T., Saeki, Y., Sato, Y., and Furusawa, M. Nature 315: 592, 1985.

99. Miyajima A., Schreurs, J., Otsu, K., Kondo, A., Arai, K., and Maeda, S. Gene 58: 273, 1987.

100. Nagata, S., Tsuchiya, M., Asano, S., Kaziro, Y., Yamazaki, T., Yamamoto, O., Hirata, Y., Kubota, N., Oheda, M., Nomura, H., and Ono, M. Nature 319: 415, 1986.

101. Nagata, S., Tsuchiya, M., Asano, S., Yamamoto, O., Hirata, Y., Kubota, N., Oheda, M., Nomura, H., and Yamazaki, T. EMBO J. 5: 575, 1986.

102. Souza, L., Boone, T., Gabrilove, J., Lai, P.H., Zsebo, K.M., Murdock, D., Chazin, V.R., Bruszewski, J., Lu, H., Chen, K.K., Barendt, J., Platzer, E., Moore, M.A.S., Mertelsmann, R., and Welte, K. Science 232: 61, 1986.

103. Tsuchiya, M., Asano, S., Kaziro, Y., and Nagata, S. Proc. Natl. Acad. Sci. USA 83: 7633, 1986.

104. Sieff, C.A., Emerson, S.G., Donahue, R.E., Nathan, D.G., Wang, E.A., Wong, G.G., and Clark, S.C. Science 230: 1171, 1985.

105. Donahue, R., Emerson, S.G., Wang, E.A., Wong, G.G., Clark, S.C., and Nathan, D.G. Blood 66: 1479, 1985.
106. Donahue, R.E., Wang, E.A., Stone, D.K., Kamen, R., Wong, G.G., Schgal, P.K., Nathan, D., and Clark, S.C. Nature 321: 872, 1986.
107. Schrader, J.W., Clark-Lewis, I., Crapper, R.M., Wong, G.H.W., and Schrader, S. *Contemporary Topics in Molecular Immunology: The Interleukins.* Edited by S. Gills and F.P. Inman. Plenum, New York, 1985, pp. 10, 121.
108. Mosmann, T.R., Yokota, T., Kastelein, R., Zurawski, S.M., Arai, N., and Takebe, Y. J. Immunol. 138: 1813, 1987.
109. Ebina, Y., Ellis, L., Jarnagin, K., Edery, M., Graf, L., Clauser, E., Ou, J.H., Masiarz, E., Kan, Y.W., Goldfine, I.D., Roth, R.A., and Rutter, W.J. Cell 40: 747, 1985.
110. Ullich, A., Bell, J.R., Chen, E.Y., Herrera, R., Petruzzelli, L.M., Dull, J.J., Gray, A., Coussens, L., Lia, Y.C., Tsubokawa, M., Mason, A., Seeburg, P.H., Grunfeld, C., Rosen, O.M., and Ramachandran, J. Nature 313: 756, 1985.
111. Ishikawa, T., Uno, I., Matsumoto, K. Bioassays 4: 52, 1986.
112. Kaibuchi, K., Miyajima, A., Arai, K., Matsumoto, K. Proc. Natl. Acad. Sci. USA 83: 8172, 1986.
113. Pringle, J.R., and Hartwell, L.H. In *Molecular Biology of the Yeast Saccharomyces.* Edited by J.N. Strathern, E.W. Jones, and J.R. Broach. Cold Spring Harbor, New York, 1981.
114. Nakayama, N., Miyajima, A., and Arai, K. EMBO J. 4: 2643, 1985.
115. Sherr, C.J., Rettenmier, C.W., Sacca, R., Ronssel, M.F., Look, A.T., and Stanley, E.R. Cell 41: 665, 1985.
116. Jackowski, S., Rettenmier, C.W., Sherr, C.J., and Rock, C.O. J. Biol. Chem. 261: 4978, 1986.
117. Leonard, W.J., Depper, J.M., Crabtree, G.R., Rudikoff, S., Pumphrey, J., Robb, R.J., Kronke, M., Svetlik, P.B., Peffer, N.J., Waldmann, T.A., and Greene, W.C. Nature 311: 626, 1984.
118. Nikaido, T., shimizu, A., Ishida, N., Sabe, H., Teshigawara, K., Maeda, M., Uchiyama, T., Yodoi, J., and Honjo, T. Nature 311: 631, 1984.
119. Shimizu, A., Kondo, S., Sabe, H., Ishida, N., and Honjo, T. Immunol. Rev. 92: 103, 1986.
120. Palaszynski, E.W., and Ihle, J.N. J. Immunol. 132: 1872, 1984.
121. Park, L.S., Friend, D., Gillis, S., and Urdal, D.L. J. Biol. Chem. 261: 205, 1986.
122. Sorensen, P., Farber, N.M., and Krystal, G. J. Biol. Chem. 261: 9094, 1986.
123. Walker, F., and Burgess, A.W. EMBO J. 4: 933, 1985.
124. Park, L.S., Friend, D., Gillis, S., and Urdal, D.L. J. Biol. Chem. 261: 4177, 1986.
125. Samarut, J., Mathey-Prevot, B., and Hanafusa, H. Mol. Cell. Biol. 5: 1067, 1985.
126. Nathans, J., and Hogness, D.S. Cell 34: 807, 1983.
127. Dixon, R.A.F., Kobilka, B.K., Strader, D.J., Benovic, J.L., Dohlman, H.G., Frielle, T., Bolanowski, M.A., Bennett, C.D., Rands, E., Diehl, R.E., Mum-

ford, R.A., Slater, E.E., Sigal, I.S., Caron, M.G., Lefkowitz, R.J., and Strader, C.D. Nature 321: 75, 1986.
128. Walker, F., Nicola, N.A., Metcalf, D., and Burgess, A.W. Cell 43: 269, 1985.
129. Chen, C.D-M., and Clark, C.R. J. Immunol. 137: 563, 1986.
130. Koyasu, S., Yodoi, J., Nikaido, T., Tagaya, Y., Taniguchi, Y., Honjo, T., and Yahara, I. J. Immunol. 136: 984, 1986.
131. Warren, H.S., Hargreaves, J., and Hepel, A.J. Lymphokine Res. 4: 195, 1985.
132. Le Gros, G.S., Gillis, S., and Watson, J.D. J. Immunol. 135: 4009, 1985.
133. Schrader, J.W., and Crapper, R.M. Proc. Natl. Acad. Sci. USA 80: 6892, 1983.
134. Lang, R.A., Metcalf, D., Gough, N.M., Dunn, A.R., Gonda, T.J. Cell 43: 531, 1985.
135. Pierce, J.H., DiFionne, P.P., Aaronson, S.A., Potter, M., Pumphrye, J., Scott, A., and Ihle, J.N. Cell 41: 685, 1985.
136. Cook, W.D., Metcalf, D., Nicola, N.A., Burgess, A.W., and Walker, F. Cell 41: 677, 1985.
137. Chung, S.W., Wong, P.M.C., Shen-Ong, G., Ruscetti, S., Ishizaka, T., and Eaves, C.J. Blood 68: 1074, 1986.
138. Rapp, U.R., Cleveland, J.L., Brightman, K., Scott, A., and Ihle, J.N. Nature 317: 434, 1985.
139. Conscience, J.F., Verrier, B., and Martin, G. EMBO J. 5: 317, 1986.
140. Kaibuchi, K., Tsuda, T., Kikuchi, A., Tanimoto, T., Yamashita, T., and Takai, Y. J. Biol. Chem. 261: 1187, 1986.
141. Farrar, W.L., Thomas, T.P., and Anderson, W.B. Nature 315: 235, 1985.
142. Gillman, A. Cell 36: 577, 1984.
143. Whetton, A.D., and Dexter, T.M. Nature 303: 629, 1983.
144. Whetton, A.D., Bazill, G.W., and Dexter, T.M. EMBO J. 3: 409, 1984.
145. Dexter, T.M., Heyworth, C., and Whetton, A.D. BioEssays 2: 154, 1985.
146. Nicola, N.A., and Johnson, G.R. Blood 60: 1019, 1982.
147. Suda, T., Suda, J., and Ogawa, M. Proc. Natl. Acad. Sci. USA 80: 6689, 1983.
148. Ogawa, M., Porter, P.N., and Nakahata, T. Blood 61: 823, 1983.
149. Zipori, D. In Experimental Hematology Today—1985. Edited by S.J. Baum, D.H. Pluznik, and L.A. Rosenszajn. Springer-Verlag, New York, 1986, pp. 55-63.
150. Berk, A.J., and Sharp, P.A. Proc. Natl. Acad. Sci. USA 75: 1274, 1978.

# 6

# B-Cell Growth and Differentiation Factors

David Greenblatt / George Washington University, Washington, D.C.

Maureen Howard / DNAX Research Institute of Molecular and Cellular Biology, Palo Alto, California

B-cell function is regulated by a family of soluble glycoproteins collectively referred to as B-cell stimulatory factors (BSF). The precise number of BSF is currently unclear, and elucidation of this number is impeded by the pluripotency of some [e.g., interleukin-4 (1)] if not all BSF, by synergistic and inhibitory interactions between BSF [e.g., gamma interferon (2) or BCGF II (3,4)], by the promiscuity of various BSF bioassays [e.g., BCGF II (3)], and by the fact that few BSF have yet been cloned and/or purified to homogeneity. Bearing these difficulties in mind, this chapter will attempt to consolidate a large volume of information concerning BSF, and produce an integral picture of factor-mediated B-cell growth factors which are distinct from IL-4; such factors may or may not (1) interleukin-4 (IL-4), an extensively characterized lymphokine with multiple biological activities including induction of B-cell growth and differentiation; (2) B-cell growth factors which are distinct from IL-4, such factors may or may not additionally induce immunoglobulin synthesis; and (3) B-cell differentiation factors, which cause differentiation of B cells without induction of DNA synthesis. Consideration will be given to both the human and murine counterparts of these various types of BSF.

## I. INTERLEUKIN-4 (IL-4)

### A. Murine IL-4

Murine interleukin-4 (IL-4) is a T-cell-derived glycoprotein first identified by Howard et al. as a B-cell growth factor for highly purified small B lymphocytes activated with soluble affinity-purified IgM antibodies (5,6). At low cell density

149

($5 \times 10^4$ B cell/well), supernatant from phorbol myristate acetate- (PMA) stimulated $EL_4$ thymoma cells was found to induce polyclonal proliferation of B cells
stimulated with suboptimal amounts of anti-IgM antibodies. Biochemical characterization of the costimulating moiety in the $EL_4$ supernatant revealed a new
factor not previously identified (5,6). The factor was initially designated BCGF
(5); subsequently renamed BCGF 1 (7), then BSF-1 (8), and most recently has
received the designation interleukin-4 (9). While IL-4 is the only lymphokine
known to date to be capable of inducing polyclonal proliferation of highly purified small dense murine B cells costimulated with anti-immunoglobulin, several
other lymphokines are capable of modulating the effect of IL-4 in this assay.
Specifically, IL-1 (10) and a separate T-cell-derived B-cell growth factor (see Section II; Ref. 11) are both capable of augmenting the polyclonal proliferation obtained when B cells are stimulated with anti-immunoglobulin and a saturating
amount of IL-4, gamma interferon ($\gamma$-IFN) abrogates this same response (2). IL-4
is found in numerous T-cell sources, including supernatant from alloreactive T-
cell clones, (12) induced or constitutive supernatants from T-cell hybridomas
(13,14), and supernatants from some though not all antigen-induced long-term
normal T-cell lines (15,16). Howard, Farrar, and colleagues initially reported
that murine IL-4 had an approximate molecular weight of 16.5-18.5 kD by gel
filtration analysis and a somewhat smaller size of 12-15 kD by sodium dodecyl-
sulfate polyacrylamide gel electrophoresis (SDS-PAGE) (5,6). Utilizing isoelectric
focusing (IEF) they demonstrated two major peaks of activity migrating with pIs
of 6.4-6.6 and 7.4-7.6 (6). A single peak of activity migrating with a pI of 9.3
was obtained following neuraminadase treatment. More recently, Ohara et al.
estimated a molecular weight of 18-21.7 kD for IL-4 which was purified from
PMA-stimulated $EL_4$ cells by a combination of reverse phase and gel filtration
high pressure liquid chromatography (HPLC) (17). Radioiodination of this material followed by SDS-PAGE revealed several bands between 14 and 30 kD with
a prominent band at 20 kD. A single peak of activity migrating at a pI of 6.3
was determined using IEF. These biochemical properties were confirmed by
Grabstein et al., who recently purified murine IL-4 to homogeneity and showed
a single band of 18.4 kD on SDS-polyacrylamide gels (18). Protein sequence analysis of this material elucidated the first 20 amino acid residues, His-Ile-His-Gly-Cys-
Asp-Lys-Asn-His-Leu-Arg-Glu-Ile-Ile-Gly-Ile-Leu-Asp-Glu-Val.

Initial kinetic studies analyzing the role of IL-4 in the anti-IgM B-cell costimulator assay demonstrated a need for its presence early in the course of this response. A delay of even 4 hours in the addition of IL-4-containing supernatant
resulted in a diminution of thymidine incorporation measured 30-42 hours after
culture initiation; delays greater than 12 hours completely abrogated the costimulatory response (19). Such studies suggested that IL-4 acted early in $G_1$ phase,
but could not exclude the possibility of a direct action on resting B cells. Indeed,
evidence supporting a direct action of IL-4 on $G_0$ B cells was subsequently provided by two sets of observations. Rhoem et al. demonstrated that IL-4-containing

supernatant derived from the T-cell hybridoma FS6-14.3 could induce in a concentration-dependent fashion an 8-10-fold increase in class II (Ia) major histocompatibility complex (MHC) antigen expression on resting B cells (20). The IL-4 costimulator activity and the class II antigen-inducing activity coeluted under conditions of gel filtration chromatography. Neither recombinant interleukin-2 (IL-2) nor recombinant $\gamma$-IFN had detectable B-cell class II antigen-inducing activity at concentrations as high as 1000 units/ml. The increase of class II antigen expression occurred on nearly all B cells and a small percentage of cells demonstrated an increase in cellular RNA indicative of entry into $G_1$. In a concurrent and independent investigation, Noelle et al. showed that IL-4 purified from PMA-stimulated $EL_4$ cells by HPLC caused an increased expression of class II MHC antigens on resting B cells (21). In contrast, IL-4 caused only a minimal increase in surface immunoglobulin and class I MHC antigen expression. Further evidence that IL-4 acted directly on resting B cells was provided by Rabin and colleagues (22). Using highly enriched small dense B cells and HPLC-purified IL-4 derived from PMA-stimulated $EL_4$ cells, they were able to show that IL-4 prepared resting B cells to enter S phase more rapidly than control cultures when subsequently stimulated with anti-IgM antibodies. A 24-hr preculture in the presence of IL-4 alone caused an increase in cell volume and accelerated subsequent entry into S phase by approximately 12 hours. Similarly, Oliver et al., using IL-4 and anti-IgD antibody coupled to Sepharose beads in a sequential culture protocol, demonstrated that IL-4 rendered $G_0$ B cells susceptible to anti-IgD-mediated entry into $G_2/S$ phase of the cell cycle (23). Confirmation that both of these effects on small dense $G_0$ cells were mediated by IL-4 was provided by experiments involving a monoclonal antibody specific for IL-4, designated 11B11, which blocked IL-4 costimulatory activity (24). This antibody also blocked the induction of class II MHC antigens and the preparation of resting B cells for more rapid entry into cell cycle by IL-4-containing supernatants (22,25).

The above data indicate roles for IL-4 in both B-cell activation and proliferation. IL-4 has also been implicated as a differentiation factor for B cells. Isakson et al. initially showed that the addition of supernatants from concanavalin A (con A) induced alloreactive T-cell lines, PK 7.1.1a and 7.1.2, or a T-cell hybridoma, FS 7-6.18, to lipopolysaccharide-stimulated splenic B cells resulted in a marked increase in $IgG_1$ secretion, a decrease in $IgG_{2b}$ and $IgG_3$ secretion, and little to no effect on IgM secretion (26). Removal of surface IgG-positive B cells from the splenic B-cell preparations did not reduce the IgG plaque forming cell (PFC) response, leading to the proposal that the activity represented an isotype switching factor, subsequently designated BCDF-gamma (BCDF-$\gamma$). Recently, Isakson has demonstrated that BCDF-$\gamma$ induces the same isotype distribution when added to anti-IgM activated B cells (27). To investigate the molecular mechanism of BCDF-$\gamma$-induced isotype regulation, Jones et al. isolated cytoplasmic RNA from B cells cultured with either lipopolysaccharide (LPS) alone, or LPS plus BCDF-$\gamma$-containing supernatant, PK 7.1 (28). Northern blot analysis revealed that cultures receiving PK 7.1 supernatant had an increase of $IgG_1$ mRNA with a concomitant decrease in $IgG_{2b}$ and $IgG_3$ mRNA levels, supporting the notion of an isotype "switch." Pure et al. confirmed these findings and demonstrated that BCDF-$\gamma$ had an apparent molecular weight of less than 20 kD when analyzed by gel filtration chromatography (12). More extensive biochemical characterization of BCDF-$\gamma$ was provided by Sideras et al. (29). Using supernatant from a con A-stimulated T-cell line designated 2.19, they found that BCDF-$\gamma$ had a molecular size of 20 kD by gel filtration, and showed some heterogeneity by IEF, with major peaks of activity at pI 7.2-7.4 and 6.2-6.4. The close resemblance of these biochemical properties to those of IL-4 prompted speculation that the two molecules may be identical. This suspicion was subsequently confirmed by Vitetta and colleagues, who showed that highly purified IL-4 mediated BCDF-$\gamma$-like activities, and that monoclonal anti-IlL-4 antibody blocked them (30).

A related activity of IL-4 was recently identified by Coffman and Carty, who showed that supernatant obtained from the T-cell clone, D9.1, contained an activity that enhanced the IgE production of LPS-stimulated T-cell-depleted murine spleen cells (31). This factor not only stimulated Balb/c mice, but also the IgE low and nonresponder strains, SJA/9 and SJL/J. Supernatants containing this activity also caused a 10-fold increase in $IgG_1$ and IgA, as well as a 10-fold decrease in $IgG_3$ levels in the same cultures. Further studies attempting to purify this IgE enhancing activity were unable to separate it from IL-4 activity (32). Similarly, highly purified IL-4 derived from $EL_4$ thymoma cells enhanced IgE production by LPS blasts to the same extent as D9.1 supernatant, and monoclonal anti-IL-4 antibody inhibited these activities. Interestingly, IL-4 did not appear to be responsible for IgA regulation in these cultures (32).

In addition to its roles in polyclonal B-cell responses, studies from our laboratory have recently shown that IL-4 also plays a critical role in antigen-specific B-cell proliferative responses (33,34). Antigens can be subdivided into three categories based on their immunogenicity in certain immunodeficient mouse strains: (1) type 1 thymus-independent (TI-1) antigens induce antibody formation in both congenitally athymic (nude) mice and in mice bearing the X-linked immunodeficiency gene, xid; (2) type 2 thymus-independent (TI-2) antigens induce antibody formation in nude mice but not xid-bearing mice; and (3) thymus-dependent (TD) antigens induce antibody formation in xid-bearing mice but not nude mice. To test the role of IL-4 in antigen-specific B-cell proliferation, we cultured affinity-purified TNP-binding resting B cells with prototype antigens from each of these categories. As is summarized schematically in Figure 1, our data indicated that: (i) the TI-1 antigens TNP-lipopolysaccharide (LPS) and TNP-*Brucella abortus* induced proliferation of hapten-specific B cells in the absence of exogenous B-cell stimulatory factors; (ii) TNP-Ficoll, a TI-2 antigen, absolutely required IL-4 to induce antigen-specific proliferation; and (iii) TD antigens such as TNP-ovalbumin (OVA) absolutely required the presence of carrier-specific helper T cells for induction of antigen-specific B-cell proliferation (33). When such helper T cells did

1. T.I. - 1 antigens (e.g.,TNP - LPS)

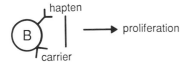

2. T.I. - 2 antigens (e.g.,TNP - Ficoll)

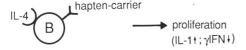

3. T.D. antigens (e.g.,TNP - OVA)

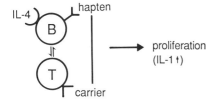

Figure 1   Role of IL-4 in antigen-specific B-cell proliferation.

not themselves produce IL-4, exogenous IL-4 was absolutely required as well (34). Confirmation that IL-4 was required for antigen-specific proliferation induced by TI-2 and TD antigens was provided by experiments showing the blocking of these responses with the anti-IL-4 monoclonal antibody, 11B11 (34). As in the case of IL-4-dependent polyclonal B-cell proliferation induced by anti-immunoglobulin (10), the IL-4-dependent proliferation of T1-2 or TD antigen-induced B cells was augmented by IL-1 (33,34). Interestingly, the effects of $\gamma$-IFN on these B-cell proliferative responses differed. Recombinant $\gamma$-IFN profoundly suppressed both anti-immunoglobulin-induced IL-4-dependent polyclonal B-cell proliferation (2) and T1-2 antigen-induced IL-4-dependent specific B-cell proliferation (33). However, $\gamma$-IFN had no effect on TD-induced IL-4-dependent B-cell proliferation (35). The reason for this difference in sensitivity to $\gamma$-IFN is currently unclear.

In an exciting new development in this field, recent evidence has indicated that IL-4 acts on a variety of cell types other than B cells. Mosmann and colleagues discovered that BSF-1 enhanced IL-2-dependent T-cell proliferation, and IL-3-dependent mast cell proliferation (36); it was also capable of inducing short-term T-cell proliferation in the absence of IL-2 (37). Rennick and colleagues demonstrated that IL-4 enhanced GM-CSF- and G-CSF-dependent proliferation of granulocytes and macrophages, and decreased M-CSF-dependent proliferation of

Table 1   Biological Properties of IL-4

| | |
|---|---|
| Murine | Stimulates proliferation of anti-immunoglobulin or antigen-activated B cells |
| | Increases class II MHC antigen expression on resting B cells |
| | Prepares B cells for entry into S phase |
| | Enhances $IgG_1$ and IgE secretion of activated B cells |
| | Enhances IL-2-dependent T-cell proliferation |
| | Enhances IL-3-dependent mast cell proliferation |
| | Induces short-term T-cell proliferation |
| | Enhances GM-CSF and G-CSF proliferation of granulocytes and macrophages |
| | Induces Fc epsilon receptor on normal B cells |
| | Enhances antigen presentation by B cells and some macrophages |
| Human | Stimulates proliferation of anti-immunoglobulin activated B cells |
| | Enhances IL-2-dependent T-cell proliferation |
| | Enhances the yield of BM-CSF-induced granulocyte-macrophage colonies |
| | Induces Fc epsilon receptor on normal B cells and EBV-transformed B-cell lines |

macrophages (38). In addition, Zlotnik et al. found that IL-4 increased antigen-presenting cell function of a subset of macrophages (39). The effects of murine IL-4 on T cells and IL-3-dependent cell lines have recently been confirmed by Grabstein et al. (18), and by Fernandez-Botran and colleagues (40). These data collectively illustrate that IL-4 may best be regarded as a competence enhancing factor which acts on all hemopoietic cell types. Whether or not IL-4 also acts on cells outside the hemopoietic lineage is currently unclear.

Confirmation that all of the aforementioned activities (summarized in Table 1) were indeed attributable to a single lymphokine has been provided by the recent isolation and characterization of DNA clones which encoded for a single protein with multiple activities (1,41). Lee et al. (1) utilized a cDNA library constructed from mRNA of the murine helper T-cell clone Cl.Ly1+2−/9. The plasmid DNA was pooled, transfected into COS monkey cells, and the resultant supernatants screened for T-cell growth, mast cell growth, B-cell class II antigen induction, and $IgG_1$ and IgE enhancement activities. Isolation and analysis of a cDNA-clone which was positive in all assays revealed a 585 base pair insert excluding the poly A tail with a single long open reading frame consisting of 140 codons. The deduced protein was 120 amino acids long and had a molecular weight of approximately 14,000. The existence of three posttranslational glycosylation sites suggested that the discrepancy between this deduced molecular weight and the molecular weight of biochemically purified IL-4 (i.e., 18 kD, Ref. 18) reflected carbohydrate content of the mature potein. Indeed, the predicted initiation site and deduced polypeptide sequence of the first 20 amino acid residues proposed by Lee et al. (1) was subsequently confirmed when IL-4 was purified to homogeneity and partially sequenced (18). Interestingly, there was no significant nucleotide sequence homology between the cDNA for IL-4 and either IL-2 or IL-3 cDNA sequences. In a concurrent but independent study, Noma et al. (41) constructed two cDNA libraries from mRNA of the murine T-cell line 2.19; one for total poly(A)$^+$ RNA and the other for selected mRNA obtained from sucrose gradient fractionation. The second library was enriched for mRNA known to contain IgG$_1$ activity. Linearized DNA from each library was used to prepare capped RNA and this RNA was injected into *Xenopus* oocytes. The resultant supernatants were screened for IgG$_1$-inducing activity on LPS-stimulated B cells. Analysis of a positive clone revealed an open reading frame of 140 codons with a sequence which was identical to that described by Lee et al. (1). The deduced polypeptide had a molecular weight of approximately 14,000 and contained three N-glycosylation sites as described above. These investigators demonstrated that the recombinant material had not only IgG$_1$-inducing activity, but also anti-IgM costimulatory activity and Ia-inducing activity.

## B.  Human IL-4

Identification of a human homologue of murine IL-4 has eluded investigators until very recently. Several laboratories have identified a factor(s) in supernatant of phytohemagglutinin- (PHA) stimulated human peripheral blood lymphocytes which caused polyclonal proliferation of anti-immunoglobulin-stimulated purified human B cells (42-44). However, this factor(s) failed to display the other biological activities now associated with murine IL-4 (see Table 1). Indeed, positive identification of human IL-4 has been achieved only recently subsequent to the cloning of mouse IL-4. Using the murine IL-4-specific probe to cross-hybridize with cDNA libraries generated from human T-cell line mRNAs, it was possible to isolate a human homologue for this lymphokine (45). This human IL-4 was clearly distinct from previously described BCGF(s). It showed 70% DNA sequence homology with murine IL-4, and little to no significant homology with other human lymphokines (45). The biological properties ascribed to it to date include costimulation of anti-Ig activated human B cells (45), augmentation of IL-2-dependent human T-cell proliferation (45), and an increase in the number of granulocyte-macrophage colonies obtained from bone marrow-colony-stimulating factor-stimulated human bone marrow cells (46). Studies using the recombinant IL-4 have also led to the identification of a new activity of IL-4, namely its ability to induce Fc epsilon receptors on purified normal B cells and Epstein-Barr virus- (EBV) transformed B-cell lines (47). This finding has recently been reproduced on mouse B cells using recombinant murine IL-4 (48). In contrast to some other lymphokines such as IL-1 and IL-2, IL-4 shows tight species specificity, that is, mouse and human IL-4 show no cross-reactivity on human and mouse cells, respectively (49).

## II.  B-CELL GROWTH FACTORS DISTINCT FROM IL-4

### A.  Murine BCGF II

The existence of a second T-cell-derived factor active on murine B cells and distinct from IL-4 was initially suggested by Swain and Dutton (50). They identified a growth-promoting activity in culture supernatant derived from the alloreactive T-cell line C.C3 11.75, more commonly designated DL, which caused increased in vitro uridine incorporation by in vivo passaged $BCL_1$ lymphoma cells, by dextran sulfate- (DXS) stimulated B cells, and by B cells receiving no other exogenous stimuli (7,50). IL-4 had no activity in these assays, and DL supernatant had no activity in the B-cell anti-IgM costimulator assay described above (7). Such studies clearly demonstrated the existence of two distinct factors leading to their designations, BCGF I (i.e., IL-4) and BCGF II (7). BCGF II could be absorbed by untreated or glutaraldehyde-fixed $BCL_1$ cells, whereas a separate differentiation factor, DL-TRF present in the DL supernatant was unaffected. Biochemical characterization of BCGF II derived from PMA stimulated $EL_4$ cells revealed an approximate molecular weight of 55 kD by gel filtration analysis and a mean pI of 5.5 by IEF (51).

Recently several groups have shown that BCGF II is not only a growth-inducing factor, but that it also plays a role in polyclonal and antigen-specific B-cell differentiation. Swain showed that partially purified BCGF II caused enhanced IgM secretion by $BCL_1$ lymphoma cells while recombinant IL-2, recombinant $\gamma$-IFN, and purified IL-4 had no such activity (3). The differentiation activity copurified with the proliferative activity in a variety of chromatographic separations. Similarly, Pike et al. using antigen-specific B cells in a single cell assay showed that conditioned media derived from con A-stimulated $EL_4$ thymoma cells contained a proliferation and differentiation activity (52). When the con A-induced supernatant was subjected to gel filtration chromatography in the presence of 6 molar guanidine hydrochloride, both activities coeluted over a range corresponding to 25-60 kD.

The discovery that BCGF II caused both growth and differentiation of activated B cells prompted speculation that this factor might be identical to a number of B-cell stimulatory activities identified using other B-cell assays (see Table 2). In particular, Takatsu and Hamaoka had identified a B-cell differentiation factor (initially designated B151-TRF, but recently renamed B151-TRF1) in constitutive supernatants from the murine T-cell hybridoma B151K12 sometime before the initial identification of a second B-cell growth factor (53,54). Their assay for

Table 2 Properties and Designations of Murine BCGF II

| Designation | Biological properties | Biochemical[a] properties | References |
|---|---|---|---|
| BCGF-II | Proliferation and Ig secretion of $BCL_1$ cells, $DXSO_4$-stimulated B cells, and unstimulated B cells | 55 kD pI 5.5 | 3,7,50,51 |
| BGDF | Proliferation and Ig secretion of antigen-activated B cells | 25-60 kD | 52 |
| B151-TRF1 | Ig secretion of antigen-activated B cells; proliferation and Ig secretion of $BCL_1$ cells; proliferation of $DXSO_4$ activated B cells | 50-60 kD 18 kD (SDS-PAGE) pI 5.0 | 53,54,55 |
| BCGF-II | Proliferation of anti-Ig-activated B cell blasts and $DXSO_4$-activated B cells | 40-50 kD | 59 |
| EDF | Eosinophil development from bone marrow precursors proliferation of $BCL_1$, in vivo-activated B cells, and anti-Ig B cell blasts | 45 kD 45 kD (SDS-PAGE) pI 5.5 | 60,62 |
| B-BCGF II | Proliferation of in vivo-activated B cells and $DXSO_4$-activated small B cells; proliferation and Ig; secretion of $BCL_1$ | 20 kD pI 4.5 | 63 |

[a]Molecular weight determined by gel filtration unless otherwise indicated.

B151-TRF1 measured IgG anti-DNP-specific PFC responses of B cells derived from DNP-KLH-primed Balb/c mice cocultured with supernatants containing B151-TRF1 and TNP-OVA. Extensive purification of B151-TRF1 revealed it to be a glycoprotein containing N-acetylgalactosamine residues with an apparent molecular weight of 50-60 kD on gel permeation chromatography, 18 kD on SDS-PAGE under reducing conditions, and had a pI of 5.0 by IEF (55-58). The purified material was shown to be distinct from IL-1, IL-2, IL-4, and $\gamma$-IFN. Speculation that the biochemically similar B151-TRF1 and BCGF II factors were identical was confirmed when highly purified B151-TRF1 was found capable of inducing proliferation and immunoglobulin secretion by $BCL_1$ lymphoma cells, and proliferation of DXS-activated normal B cells (56,58). The B-cell-specific monoclonal antibody, 9T1, which preferentially blocked B151-TRF1-dependent PFC responses also blocked BCGF II-induced proliferation of $BCL_1$ cells (56,58). Furthermore, both differentiation and proliferative activities of B151-TRF1 could be antagonized by the addition of appropriate amounts of N-acetylgalactosamine to the assay systems (55,58).

While BCGF II was initially distinguished from IL-4 by its inability to induce proliferation of anti-immunoglobulin-activated B cells, two groups have identified conditions under which a BCGF II-like factor could cause proliferation of B cells stimulated with anti-immunoglobulin. Müller et al. showed that B cells stimulated for 48 hours with high doses of anti-IgM proliferated and differentiated in response to a factor in PMA-induced $EL_4$ supernatant (59). Biochemical analysis employing gel filtration and reverse phase HPLC revealed that the proliferation- and differentiation-inducing activities copurified. The active component had an apparent molecular weight of 40-50 kD, and was capable of inducing proliferation of DXS-stimulated B cells. Similarly, Nakanishi et al. showed that B cells activated with low dose anti-IgM and saturating IL-4 proliferated in response to the BCGF II contained in B151K12 T-cell hybridoma supernatant (4); the same source that Hamaoka and Takatsu used to identify B151-TRF1 (53).

Recently, a novel activity of BCGF II has been proposed by Sanderson et al. (60). Using supernatants derived from alloreactive T-cell clones and hybrids, these investigators have identified an eosinophil differentiation factor (EDF) (61) which appeared to additionally display BCGF II activity (60). EDF was assayed by incubating bone marrow cells derived from *Mesocestoides corti*-infected mice with test supernatants, and measuring eosinophil development at 5 days by a colorimetric assay for eosinophil peroxidase. BCGF II activity was determined by the short-term $BCL_1$ proliferation assay described earlier. Gel filtration chromatography revealed an apparent molecular weight of 45-46 kD for both activities. Attempts to separate the activities by IEF and/or lentil lectin, phenyl-Sepharose, DEAE-Sepharose, and reverse phase chromatography were unsuccessful. Extending these studies, O'Garra and colleagues examined the effects of partially purified EDF prepared from the T-cell hybrid, NIMP-TH1, on normal resting, endogenously activated, and exogenously activated murine B cells (62).

Importantly, NIMP-TH1 T cells did not produce IL-1, IL-2, IL-3, $\gamma$-IFN, or IL-4, immediately distinguishing EDF from these lymphokines (58). EDF had no effect on Percoll-purified small, dense B cells as measured by thymidine incorporation or increased expression of class II MHC molecules. However, EDF could induce thymidine incorporation as well as immunoglobulin secretion by Percoll-purified large, low density B cells. Similarly, small B cells which had been incubated with $10 \mu g/ml$ $F(ab')_2$ anti-mouse immunoglobulin for 40 hours responded to EDF with enhanced thymidine incorporation. EDF was fractionated by SDS-PAGE in an attempt to separate the B-cell growth-promoting activity from the B-cell differentiation activity. Both activities comigrated in the same fractions corresponding to a molecular weight of 44 kD. EDF was reported to have a pI of 5.5.

A recent study indicates that BCGF II may be produced by B cells in addition to the T-cell sources described previously. Nakajima et al. showed that the murine B lymphoma cell line, WEHI 231, constitutively produced a factor which induces proliferation and IgM secretion in both $BCL_1$ tumor cells and splenic B cells (63). Separation of splenic B cells by a discontinuous Percoll gradient revealed that the WEHI 231-derived factor acted directly on endogenously activated large low density B cells. High density small B cells only responded to this factor when cultured concurrently with DXS. Biochemical analysis employing ion exchange, gel filtration, and phenyl-Sepharose chromatography failed to separate the growth-promoting activity from the differentiation component. The apparent molecular weight of this factor was estimated to be 20 kD by gel filtration chromatography and possessed an isoelectric point between 4.1 and 4.5. The finding that B cells produce BCGF II raises the interesting possibility that this lymphokine may act as an autocrine growth factor in some situations, and second, that it may represent the B-cell analogue of IL-2. Further experimentation will be required to confirm these proposals.

The above data suggest BCGF II is a lymphokine capable of multiple biological activities (summarized in Table 2). In addition to these direct activities, BCGF II appears to synergize with other B-cell stimulatory factors to generate maximal B-cell differentiation. Swain has shown that suboptimal doses of BCGF II synergize with B-cell differentiation factor (BCDF), a lymphokine which induces immunoglobulin secretion but not proliferation of activated B cells (see Section III), to cause optimal IgM secretion by $BCL_1$ cells (3). Higher doses of BCGF II alone led to a nearly equivalent response, however this may have reflected contamination of the partially purified BCGF II preparation with BCDF (discussed in more detail in the following section). Further investigations using normal splenic B cells revealed that BCGF II augmented their BCDF-induced polyclonal PFC responses (3). Interestingly, these experiments also indicated that IL-2 was equally capable of augmenting BCDF-induced polyclonal PFC responses. In contrast, experiments examining antigen-specific responses revealed that IL-2, BCGF II, and BCDF were all required for optimal plaque formation (3). Synergisms between BCGF II and other B-cell stimulatory factors have also been reported by others. Nakanishi et al. showed that the combination of BCGF II, IL-4, and BCDF was required to obtain optimal IgM secretion by anti-IgM-stimulated B cells (4).

For simplicity, we suggest that the above unrelated studies collectively describe a single T-cell-derived protein (summarized in Table 2). It is of course possible that there is more than one BCGF II-like factor under analysis. Indeed biological data presented in the next section suggests this may well be the case. Further clarification of this issue will await isolation of BCGF II, either by protein purification or recombinant DNA technology. Progress in this direction was reported by Honjo and colleagues at the VIth International Congress of Immunology in Toronto in July 1986. At that time they reported the isolation of a cDNA encoding a product which induced proliferation and IgM secretion of $BCL_1$ cells, and which stimulated dinitrophenyl-specific PFC from DNP-primed B cells, specifically, the B151TRF1 activity described above (refer to Table 2). Further characterization is required to verify that the recombinant product reported by Honjo is identical to any or all of the BCGF II-like factors described above.

## B.  Two Murine BCGF II-Like Factors

In a recent effort to extend the characterization of murine BCGF II, this laboratory has identified the existence of two discrete BCGF II-like molecules (11,64). The prototype sources of these two factors are antigen-stimulated supernatant from a murine T-cell clone, D10.G4.1 designated D10, and a partially purified low molecular weight (l.m.w.) human BCGF obtained from PHA-stimulated peripheral blood lymphocytes. For our present purpose, these two factors are designated BCGF IIA and BCGF IIB, respectively. Importantly, murine sources of BCGF IIB have been identified, eliminating concern that the distinction between BCGF IIA and BCGF IIB might simply reflect species differences. As summarized in Table 3, BCGF IIA and BCGF IIB could both be classified as BCGF II-like molecules by the following criteria: (i) they induced large in vivo-activated B cells to proliferate and secrete immunoglobulin; (ii) they caused DXS-activated B cells to proliferate. However, the two activities could be distinguished by differential responsiveness in other BCGF II assays: BCGF IIA induced $BCL_1$ proliferation and immunoglobulin secretion, whereas, BCGF IIB caused proliferation of unstimulated B cells and augmented proliferation of B cells stimulated with anti-

Table 3    Two Murine BCGF-Like Factors

| Assay | BCGF IIA | BCGF IIB | BCGF IIA + BCGF IIB |
|---|---|---|---|
| $BCL_1$ proliferation | + | − | inhibition |
| $BCL_1$ secretion | + | − | synergy |
| $BCL_1$ PFC | + | − | no change |
| Small B-cell proliferation | − | + | no change |
| Small B-cell secretion | + | + | no change |
| Small B-cell PFC | + | + | no change |
| Small (B+αIg+IL-4) proliferation | − | + | no change |
| Small (B+αIg+IL-4) PFC | − | + | no change |
| Small (B+DXS) proliferation | + | + | no change |
| Large B proliferation | + | + | additive |
| Large B secretion | + | + | synergy |
| Large B PFC | + | + | synergy |

IgM and saturating doses of IL-4. The two BCGF II-like activities were further distinguished by a range of synergistic and inhibitory effects observed when both factor sources were added simultaneously to cultures. As summarized in Table 3, BCGF IIB inhibited BCGF IIA-induced $BCL_1$ proliferation; BCGF IIB synergized with BCGF IIA to produce optimal immunoglobulin secretion by $BCL_1$ cells and in vivo-activated large B cells; BCGF IIB augmented BCGF IIA-induced proliferation of in vivo-activated large B cells. Importantly the various bioactivities summarized in Table 3 were not attributable to IL-1, IL-2, $\gamma$-IFN, or IL-4. The l.m.w. human BCGF preparation used as a prototype BCGF IIB source lacked all of these murine activities except IL-1, and control experiments showed recombinant IL-1 could not substitute for l.m.w. human BCGF in these assays. Similarly, the prototype source of BCGF IIA used throughout our experiments (i.e., D10 supernatant) additionally contained IL-1 and IL-4, however, purified preparations of these lymphokines could not substitute for D10 supernatant.

The two BCGF II-like molecules summarized in Table 3 are remarkably similar to two B-cell stimulatory factors recently distinguished by Ono and colleagues (54). As these investigators generally measured immunoglobulin synthesis, they regarded their BSF as differentiation factors, and have designated them B151-TRF1 and B151-TRF2. B151-TRF1 caused proliferation and immunoglobulin secretion of $BCL_1$ cells and antigen-stimulated B cells (54,56,58) and thus would appear to resemble our BCGF IIA (Table 2). In contrast, B151-TRF2 did not stimulate $BCL_1$ proliferation or immunoglobulin secretion, but did stimulate immunoglobulin secretion by small dense unstimulated B cells (54). By these criteria, B151-TRF2 closely resembles BCGF IIB (Table 3). As B151-TRF1 causes growth and differentiation of activated B cells, it is regarded in this review as a BCGF II-like molecule, and has thus been discussed in the BCGF II section above. As B151-TRF2 has only been observed in immunoglobulin secretion assays in Hamaoka's laboratory, it is regarded by these investigators as a B-cell differentiation factor. It is therefore discussed in more detail in the BCDF section below. The proposed identity of B151-TRF2 and the BCGF IIB described in Table 3 focuses attention on an important complication in this field, namely that factors are frequently designated as growth (BCGF) or differentiation (BCDF) based on the assays used for their detection. The existence of two distinct factors, both of which are capable of causing growth and/or differentiation in some but not all assays (Table 3) means that a BCDF in one laboratory may correspond to a BCGF (e.g., BCGF II) in another. The fact that the biochemical properties generally attributed to BCGF II (details above; see Table 2) and BCDF (details below; see Table 5) are often very similar exacerbates this problem. As mentioned above, such complications make it impossible to definitively enumerate the total number of B-cell stimulatory factors at this point in time. The data presented in this section, however, provide compelling support for the notion that there are at least two discrete factors capable of causing growth and differentiation of murine B cells in some but not all B-cell stimulatory factor bioassays.

## C.  Low Molecular Weight Human BCGF (∼ 20 kD BCGF)

The first human BCGF identified was a low molecular weight molecule initially believed to be the human homologue of murine IL-4. Doubt was cast on this assumption when it became clear that l.m.w. human BCGF did not exhibit many of the new bioactivities recently ascribed to murine IL-4, such as induction of class II MHC antigens on B cells (65) and induction of T-cell proliferation (66). Indeed a clear distinction between l.m.w. human BCGF and human IL-4 has now been provided following the cloning of human IL-4 (45; discussed above). The following summarizes what is currently known of low molecular weight human BCGF.

At least four separate laboratories have investigated l.m.w. human BCGF derived from T cells (42-44,67-71). The experimental systems used in these laboratories vary, and it is not yet clear whether the same factor is being investigated by each of the groups. Nevertheless, some uniform conclusions regarding the nature of l.m.w. human BCGF(s) have emerged. Low molecular weight human BCGF is currently used to designate either a material that costimulates with anti-immunoglobulin or other polyclonal B-cell activators to cause DNA synthesis by normal or leukemic human B cells (43,44,68,69,72), or alternatively a material that maintains the proliferation of activated purified human B lymphocytes in suspension culture (42,67,71,73). Obviously, these two functions may well be mediated by different moieties. Low molecular weight human BCGF defined by both assays could be found in supernatants of lectin-activated normal T lymphocytes (43,44, 67,71) and also in T-cell hybridoma supernatants (68,70,74). Low molecular weight human BCGF could be distinguished from human IL-2 by its relatively delayed appearance after lectin stimulation of human T cells and by cellular absorption studies with either normal human T cell blasts or long-term IL-2-dependent T-cell lines (43,68,69,71). Such cells removed IL-2 but did not diminish l.m.w. BCGF activity in culture supernatants. The existence of T hybridomas that secreted l.m.w. human BCGF and not IL-2 (68,70,74), and of conditioned media that lacked one or the other activity (75), verified this distinction. Low molecular weight human BCGF derived from 72-hour lectin-stimulated peripheral blood lymphocytes has an approximate molecular weight of 17-20 kD (43, 68,69, 70,77) or 12-13 kD (42,76) by gel filtration analysis, and an isoelectric point of 6.5-6.9 (42,43,77), and could be distinguished from IL-1, γ-IFN, and BCDF on the basis of biochemical properties, or sources containing restricted activities (72, 74,76-78). Direct binding of l.m.w. human BCGF to B-cell blasts has been demonstrated by its absorption on human leukemic B cells activated with anti-immunoglobulin or anti-idiotypic antibodies (43,68,77).

In an attempt to extend the characterization of l.m.w. human BCGF and to correlate this factor with murine B-cell stimulatory factors, we have recently tested this lymphokine in a range of well-defined mouse B-cell stimulatory factor bioassays. A commercially available preparation of partially purified l.m.w.

human BCGF induced proliferation of unstimulated murine B cells, DXS-activated murine B cells, and murine B cells activated with anti-IgM and saturating IL-4 (11). In contrast, it lacked murine IL-4 activity, and was unable to induce $BCL_1$ proliferation and IgM secretion (11). These studies indicated that l.m.w. human BCGF possessed some but not all of the biological properties ascribed to murine BCGF II (see Sect. II.B.).

Recently, Sharma and colleagues have succeeded in isolating and characterizing a DNA clone which appears to encode a l.m.w. human BCGF (78). In their report, poly(A)+ RNA was isolated from PHA-stimulated T cells, fractionated on agarose-methyl mercury hydroxide gel, and microinjected into *Xenopus laevis* oocytes. Secreted products were screened for l.m.w. human BCGF activity using long-term BCGF-responsive B-cell lines developed in their laboratory (73). Such lines have been shown to be extremely sensitive to limiting quantities of l.m.w. human BCGF when compared to the conventional anti-IgM costimulatory assay. Fractions exhibiting the greatest l.m.w. BCGF activity were used to construct a cDNA library in the bacterial expression vector, pUC9. Analysis of a positive cDNA-clone revealed a 700 base pair insert with a single open reading frame of 372 nucleotides. The deduced protein was 124 amino acids long and had an estimated molecular weight of 12,000. This predicted molecular weight did not take into account a single potential posttranslation glycosylation site. No significant homology to human IL-1, IL-2, or GM-CSF (granulocyte/macrophage-colony-stimulating factor) was found. Interestingly, the carboxy terminal end of the protein contained 32 amino acids derived from a nucleotide sequence showing an 87% homology to the Alu repeat family. Total cellular RNA from unstimulated and PHA-stimulated peripheral blood lymphocytes was examined by Northern blot analysis using an Alu-free fragment of the cDNA. Specific hybridization with a 15-16 S RNA band was seen using unstimulated cells; upon stimulation a new 11-12 S RNA band in addition to the 15-16 S RNA band was seen. The recombinant BCGF enhanced thymidine incorporation by BCGF-responsive long-term B-cell lines as well as anti-IgM-stimulated normal peripheral blood B cells.

In addition to T-cell-derived l.m.w. human BCGF, it has recently become clear that a factor with very similar biological and biochemical properties could be obtained from *Staphylococcus aureus* Cowan 1- (SAC) stimulated human B cells and human B-cell lines (79,80). As in the case of murine BCGF II (details above), the production of l.m.w. human BCGF by B cells raises the interesting possibility that it may in some situations behave as an autocrine growth factor, and furthermore, that it may represent the B-cell analogue of IL-2.

## D. High Molecular Weight Human BCGF (~ 60 kD BCGF)

Several laboratories have identified a high molecular weight (h.m.w.) human BCGF which is distinct from IL-1, IL-2, IL-4, γ-IFN, BCDF, and l.m.w. human BCGF. High molecular weight BCGF is produced by alloreactive T-cell clones, human

T-cell leukemia virus- (HTLV) transformed T-cell lines, and normal T cells stimulated with the combination of PHA and PMA (43,81). Supernatants from these
sources caused growth of anti-immunoglobulin-activated human B cells, anti-
idiotype-activated B-CLL leukemic cells, DXS-activated murine B cells, unstimulated murine B cells, and murine $BCL_1$ cells (43,81). In addition, they induced
$BCL_1$ IgM secretion (81). Biochemical analysis of the active component in these
supernatants has revealed a glycoprotein of 50-60 kD by gel filtration (43,81)
with a pI of 5-6 (81). High molecular weight human BCGF has been found to
synergize with the low molecular weight human BCGF described above to produce optimal proliferation of anti-immunoglobulin-activated human B cells or
anti-idiotype-stimulated B-CLL cells (43). Such a high molecular weight human
BCGF which maintained proliferation of long-term B-cell lines has been extensively purified from the cytoplasm of human peripheral blood mononuclear cells
by Sahasrabuddhe et al. (82,83). However, unlike the secreted high molecular
weight BCGF studied in other laboratories, this cytoplasmic BCGF failed to induce proliferation of anti-immunoglobulin or DXS-activated human B cells. The
discrepancy in biological properties of these two factors may have simply reflected
a difference in the target B cells used in each laboratory, or a difference between
intracellular and exported high molecular weight human BCGF.

     As in the case of low molecular weight human BCGF, high molecular weight
human BCGF has also been obtained from B-cell as well as T-cell sources. Ambrus
and Fauci (84) recently showed that PHA-stimulated supernatants from the human B lymphoma Namalva contained a high molecular weight human BCGF similar if not identical to that produced by PHA-stimulated T-ALL cells (85), which
caused proliferation of tonsillar B cells stimulated with SAC or anti-IgM, or in
vivo-activated density gradient purified tonsillar B cells. The active molecule from
both B- and T-cell sources had a molecular weight of 60 kD by gel filtration and
SDS-PAGE, and a pI of 6.7-7.8. Highly purified radiolabelled high molecular
weight human BCGF specifically bound to SAC activated human B cells, but not
resting B cells, resting T cells, or PHA-activated T cells.

### E.  Correlations Between Human and Mouse BCGFs

The preceding sections have provided evidence suggesting the existence of two
murine BCGF II-like molecules (BCGF IIA/B151-TRF1 and BCGF IIB/B151-
TRF2) and two human BCGF molecules (low and high molecular weight human
BCGFs). All four molecules are distinct from IL-4 (see Sect. I). Comparison of
these human and mouse factors suggest possible correlations between them (see
Table 4). Low molecular weight human BCGF and murine BCGF IIB/B151-TRF2
both cause proliferation of B cells stimulated with anti-IgM and IL-4, fail to induce $BCL_1$ proliferation and immunoglobulin secretion, and have a molecular
weight of 20-30 kD. Similarly, high molecular weight human BCGF and murine
BCGF IIA/B151-TRF1 both induce $BCL_1$ proliferation and immunoglobulin

Table 4   Correlations Between Human and Mouse B-Cell Growth Factors

| Property | Human l.m.w. BCGF | Murine BCGF IIB/B151-TRF2 | Human h.m.w. BCGF | Murine BCGF IIA/B151-TRF1 |
|---|---|---|---|---|
| B+ anti-IgM + IL-4 proliferation | + | + | | − |
| BCL$_1$ proliferation and immunoglobulin secretion | − | − | + | + |
| Molecular weight by gel filtration (kD) | 20 | 30 | 50-60 | 50-60 |

secretion, and have a molecular weight of 50-60 kD. Further experimentation is required to confirm the identity of these murine and human B-cell stimulatory factors, however, the data currently available make this possibility a serious consideration.

## III.  B-CELL DIFFERENTIATION FACTOR (BCDF)

B-cell differentiation factor (BCDF) induces activated B cells to secrete IgM and/ or IgG. It may be distinguished operationally from the BCGF II-like activities described above in terms of its inability to induce B-cell proliferation, in contrast to the BCGF II-like activities which generally induce both proliferation and immunoglobulin secretion. However, as will be outlined in detail below the biochemical properties of BCDF somewhat resemble those of BCGF II (e.g., compare Tables 2 and 5). Thus the distinction between BCDF and BCGF II might become obscured in some studies due to the use of partially purified factor preparations enriched for one of these lymphokines but contaminated with small amounts of the other. This confusion is obviously exacerbated in cases where B-cell function is measured by immunoglobulin secretion, an assay which detects both BCDF and many, if not all, BCGF II-like activities. Thus, it is conceivable that some of the above studies on BCGF II may in fact reflect the behavior of BCGF II contaminated with BCDF, and vice versa. Despite this complication in deciphering the current literature, sufficient data exist to justify classification of two major classes of B-cell stimulatory factors: BCGF II-like factors which induce proliferation and immunoglobulin secretion by B cells, and BCDF which induces immunoglobulin secretion but not proliferation of B cells. The following describes what we currently know of the latter molecule(s).

The most compelling data in support of a discrete BCDF has been provided by the laboratories of Kishimoto and Onoue using supernatants derived from human sources. Their studies indicated the existence of a factor(s) present in culture supernatants from mitogen-stimulated T cells (86-88), a human T-cell hybrid (74), and a HTLV-transformed T-cell line (89) which induced IgG (86) or IgM (90) secretion by EBV-transformed human B-cell lines. BCDF detected in such assays did not affect proliferation of the Epstein-Barr virus (EBV)-transformed cells, nor did the blocking of cell proliferation with hydroxyurea inhibit BCDF-mediated induction of immunoglobulin synthesis (86,88,89). The mechanism of action of BCDF included an increase in biosynthesis of secretory type heavy chains of immunoglobulin as well as their mRNA (91). Separate studies have indicated that BCDF also induced IgM and IgG secretion in SAC-activated normal human B cells (74,92-94). Following extensive biochemical characterization in several laboratories (87,88, 94), this lymphokine has recently been purified to homogeneity by Hirano et al. (89). Together these studies showed that BCDF has a molecular weight of 30-35 kD by gel filtration analysis, 20 kD by SDS-PAGE, and an isoelectric point of 5.0-5.1. A partial amino acid sequence of the purified BCDF has been obtained, and antibodies raised to synthetic peptides constructed from the sequence were found to absorb biological activity (95). Isolation of a cDNA encoding human BCDF was reported by Kishimoto at the VIth International Congress of Immunology in Toronto in July 1986.

Table 5   B-Cell Differentiation Factors

| General name | Other names | Biological properties | Biochemical[a] properties |
|---|---|---|---|
| Human BCDF | BSF-2 | Induces Ig secretion by EBV-transformed B-cell lines or SAC-activated normal B cell | 30-35 kD 20 kD (SDS-PAGE) pI 5.0 |
| | | Does not induce or require proliferation | |
| Murine BCDF | BCDF EL-TRF DL-TRF | Induces Ig secretion by murine B lymphomas or activated normal B cells | 30-50 kD 32 kD (SDS-PAGE) |
| | | Does not induce or require proliferation | pI 4.5 |
| | BMF-T B151-TRF2 | Induces Ig secretion by "resting" small dense B cells | 30-55 kD 16 kD (SDS-PAGE) pI 5-6 (BMF-T) pI 4.5 (B151-TRF2) |

[a]Molecular weight determined by gel filtration unless otherwise indicated.

A murine BCDF resembling human BCDF in terms of biological and biochemical properties has been identified in several laboratories (Table 5). This murine homologue induced IgM secretion by murine B lymphoma cells (26,96), normal murine B cells activated with anti-immunoglobulin, IL-4 and BCGF II (4,97), and murine B cells activated with antigen, BCGF-II, and IL-2 (50). Murine BCDF was found in induced or constitutive supernatants from murine T-cell lines, clones, and hybridomas. Its range of designations include BCDF (26), EL-TRF (4), and DL-TRF (50). It is a late-acting factor, as evidenced by the fact that it could be added in the final 16 hours of a 4 day assay measuring immunoglobulin secretion by B cells stimulated with anti-immunoglobulin, IL-4, and BCGF-II without significant diminution of the response (4). Murine BCDF appeared to have no effect on the proliferation of transformed or activated normal B cells (4,96). Biochemical characterization of this factor has revealed a molecular weight of 30-35 kD by gel filtration analysis (96,97), 32 kD by SDS-PAGE (97), and an isoelectric point of 4.5 (4).

Recently, two laboratories have independently identified a murine BCDF-like molecule capable of inducing Percoll-purified small B cells to secrete immunoglobulin without concomitant proliferation. This activity has been designated BMF-T (98,99) and B151-TRF2 (54) by the two laboratories, respectively. It is not yet clear whether this activity corresponds to the murine and human BCDFs described in the preceding paragraphs. However, the fact that BMF-T/B151-TRF2 causes immunoglobulin secretion with little or no proliferation and has similar biochemical properties to those of murine BCDF makes this proposed identity a serious consideration. Furthermore, BMF-T at least was capable of inducing IgM secretion by murine B lymphomas in a manner similar to murine BCDF (98,99). BMF-T and B151-TRF2 were found in supernatants from a T-cell clone and a T-cell hybridoma, respectively. Biochemical analysis of BMF-T revealed a molecular weight of 50-55 kD by gel filtration analysis, 12-16 kD by SDS-PAGE, and an isoelectric point of 5-6 (99). B151-TRF2 had slightly different biochemical properties, with a broad range of activity peaking at 30 kD on gel filtration, and an isoelectric point of 4-5 (54). Both factors acted on neonatal B cells and mice of most MHC haplotypes, including athymic (nude) mice, LPS-unresponsive C3H/ HeJ mice, and BCGF II- (i.e., B151-TRF1) unresponsive DBA/2Ha mice. No consensus has yet been reached by the two laboratories as to whether or not the factor is capable of acting on CBA/N B cells. Even though the sources of BMF-T and B151-TRF2 also contained BCGF II, the latter has been distinguished biochemically in both cases (54,98,99). In addition, B151-TRF2 has no activity on $BCL_1$ lymphoma cells (54) an assay routinely used for detection of BCGF II (Sect. II.A.). The fact that BMF-T/B151-TRF2 acts on normal resting B cells to drive them into terminal differentiation prompts speculation that this factor may be responsible for clonal abortion of immature autoreactive B cells and/or polyclonal activation of B cells in autoimmune disease. Indeed, proliferating T cells in enlarged nodes and spleens of MRL/1pr autoimmune mice spontaneously secreted in vitro abnormally high levels of a factor (L-BCDF) which induced terminal differentiation of B cells into immunoglobulin-secreting cells (100). Furthermore, Dobashi et al. have recently provided evidence that B151-TRF2 induced striking autoantibody production both in vivo and in vitro (101). Both reports suggest a role for MMF-T/B151-TRF2 in the development of autoimmune diseases.

Several other laboratories have described factors which act on small dense resting B cells. However, in contrast to B151-TRF2 and BMF-T, these factors induce both proliferation and immunoglobulin secretion of the small B-cell population. Such factors have received a variety of designations, including B-cell replication and maturation factor (i.e., BRMF;102) B-cell activation factor (i.e., BCAF; 103,104), and BCGF IIB (11); Table 3). To correlate these B-cell stimulatory factors with the others described throughout this chapter the following possibilities must be considered: (i) that such factors represent a separate set of BCGF II-like factors, distinguishable from other BCGF II-like factors (Sect. II) by their ability to act on resting B cells; (ii) that such factors in fact reflect the activity of B151-TRF2/BMF-T which causes immunoglobulin secretion, contaminated with BCGF-II which causes proliferation; (iii) that such factors are identical to B151-TRF2/BMF-T, and that the growth-promoting activity of the latter has gone unrecognized in Hamaoka's and Sidman's laboratories. While continued experimentation will undoubtedly shed light on these various possibilities, resolution of the issue will probably await isolation of each of the activities by biochemical purification or recombinant DNA technology.

## IV. CONCLUSION

The previous paragraphs review our developing knowledge of the biochemistry and mode of action of a group of lymphokines which regulate B-cell function. The current data suggest the existence of three distinct types of murine B-cell stimulatory factors: (i) IL-4, which activates resting B cells to move out of the $G_0$ phase and to increase class II MHC antigens, (ii) BCGF II, which induces activated B cells to proliferate and secrete immunoglobulin, and (iii) BCDF which induces activated B cells to cease proliferation and commence high rate immunoglobulin synthesis and/or secretion. The BCGF II subgroup appears to contain two distinct members, designated as BCGF IIA and BCGF IIB in this review (Table 3), and probably corresponding to the B151-TRF1 and B151-TRF2 factors recently described by Hamaoka and colleagues (54). Both molecules cause proliferation and immunoglobulin secretion of in vivo-activated large B cells, but can be distinguished in other BCGF II bioassays, for example, only BCGF IIA/B151-TRF1 induces $BCL_1$ proliferation and immunoglobulin secretion, and only BCGF IIB/B151-TRF2 induces proliferation and immunoglobulin secretion of small B cells stimulated with anti-IgM and IL-4 (Table 3). In addition, BCGF IIB/B151-TRF2 has the intriguing property of directly stimulating small dense resting

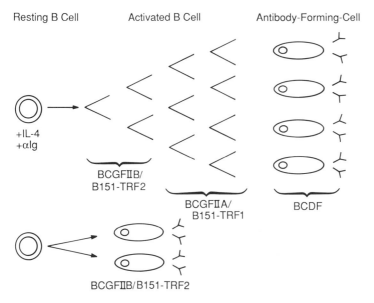

**Figure 2**   Model of factor-mediated murine B-cell development.

B cells to terminal differentiation. An analogous situation exists in the human system consisting of human IL-4, low and high molecular weight human BCGF which correspond to murine BCGF IIB and BCGF IIA, respectively, and human BCDF.

In Figure 2, we attempt to integrate these data into a model of factor-mediated murine B-cell development. For simplicity, we have proposed a linear model suggesting that the factors all work on the same B-cell population in a sequential fashion, with product-precursor relationships existing between each factor-responsive stage. Such a linear model is purely speculative, and the current data are equally consistent with the notion of distinct factors stimulating distinct B-cell subsets. The model depicted in Figure 2 shows IL-4 as the initial factor operating in lymphokine-mediated B-cell development, accommodating several reports that this lymphokine acts directly on small dense resting B cells. We then propose that BCGF IIB/B151-TRF2 is the next factor in this linear sequence, as this factor augments proliferation of B cells stimulated with anti-immunoglobulin and IL-4 (Table 3). BCGF IIA/B151-TRF1 lacks this property, but is, however, capable of stimulating large in vivo-activated B cells to proliferate and secrete immunoglobulin (Tables 2, 3). Thus BCGF IIA/B151-TRF1 may act later in this linear scheme on B cells activated by anti-immunoglobulin, IL-4, and BCGF IIB/B151-TRF2. Such a proposal is readily amenable to experimental analysis. The final factor in this linear model is BCDF, a lymphokine which acts on fully differentiated cells, causing terminal immunoglobulin secretion. BCDF is distinguished from BCGF IIA/B151-TRF1 by the observation that only the latter induces proliferation. It is possible however that this distinction reflects differences in the assays rather than differences in the factors, that is, that this is in fact a single lymphokine which causes growth and immunoglobulin secretion by some target cells, and immunoglobulin secretion without growth by others. BCGF IIB/B151-TRF2 has the additional property of activating small dense B cells to terminal immunoglobulin secretion (Fig. 2).

Several other lymphokines are known to modulate B-cell function, specifically IL-1 (10), IL-2 (97,105), and γ-IFN (105-107). The effects of these factors on B-cell development have been reviewed extensively elsewhere (19,58,108), and therefore were not considered here.

It is anticipated that enormous progress will be made in the next few years on the purification and cloning of all of the B-cell stimulatory factors depicted in Figure 2. Such accomplishments will pave the way for the quantitation and characterization of the receptors for these factors, and to investigation of how receptor expression is modulated in the immune response. It will also permit careful cell cycle analysis to reveal the proportion of cells responding to each lymphokine, and whether or not B-cell development proceeds as depicted in the linear model outlined in Figure 2. The accumulation of such information will hopefully lead to a new physiologically based pharmacology for the manipulation of antibody responses in human disease and in responses to vaccines.

## REFERENCES

1. Lee, F., Yokota, T., Otsuka, T., Meyerson, P., Villaret, D., Coffman, R., Mosmann, T., Rennick, D., Roehm, N., Smith, C., Zlotnik, A., and Arai, K. Isolation and characterization of a mouse interleukin cDNA clone that expresses B-cell stimulatory factor 1 activities and T-cell and mast-cell stimulating activities. Proc. Natl. Acad. Sci. (USA) 83: 2061, 1986.
2. Mond, J.J., Finkelman, F.D., Sarma, C., Ohara, J., and Serrate, S. Recombinant interferon-γ inhibits the B cell proliferative response stimulated by soluble but not by sepharose-bound anti-immunoglobulin antibody. J. Immunol. 135: 2513, 1985.
3. Swain, S.L. Role of BCGF II in the differentiation to antibody secretion of normal and tumor B cells. J. Immunol. 134: 3934, 1985.
4. Nakanishi, K., Howard, M., Muraguchi, A., Farrar, J., Takatsu, K., Hamoaka, T., and Paul, W.E. Soluble factors involved in B cell differentiation: identification of two distinct T cell-replacing factors (TRF). J. Immunol. 130: 2219, 1983.
5. Howard, M., Farrar, J., Hilfikar, M., Johnson, B., Takatsu, K., Hamaoka, T., and Paul, W.E. Identification of a T cell-derived B cell growth factor distinct from interleukin 2. J. Exp. Med. 155: 914, 1982.

6. Farrar, J.J., Howard, M., Fuller-Farrar, J., and Paul, W.E. Biochemical and physiochemical characterization of mouse B cell growth factor: a lymphokine distinct from interleukin 2. J. Immunol. 131: 1838, 1983.
7. Swain, S.L., Howard, M., Kappler, J., Marrack, P., Watson, J., Booth, R., Wetzel, G.D., and Dutton, R.W. Evidence for two distinct classes of murine B cell growth factors with activities in different functional assays. J. Exp. Med. 158: 822, 1982.
8. Paul, W.E. Proposed nomenclature for B cell stimulating factors. Immunol. Today 4: 332, 1983.
9. Proposed VIth International Congress of Immunology. Toronto, Canada, July, 1986.
10. Howard, M., Mizel, S.B., Lachman, L., Ansel, J., Johnson, B., and Paul, W.E. Role of interleukin 1 in anti-immunoglobulin induced B cell proliferation. J. Exp. Med. 157: 1529, 1983.
11. Ennist, D.L., Greenblatt, D., Coffman, R., Sharma, S., Maizel, A., and Howard, M. Activity of a partially purified human BCGF on murine assays for B-cell stimulating factors. I. BCGF II-like activity of human BCGF. Cell. Immunol. 110: 77, 1987.
12. Pure, E., Isakson, P.C., Kappler, J.W., Marrack, P., Krammer, P.H., and Vitetta, E.S. T cell-derived B cell growth and differentiation factors: dichotomy between the responsiveness of B cells from adult and neonatal mice. J. Exp. Med. 157: 600, 1983.
13. Leanderson, T., Lundgren, E., Ruuth, E., Borg, H., Persson, H., and Coutinho, A. B-cell growth factor: distinction from T-cell growth factor and B-cell maturation factor. Proc. Natl. Acad. Sci. (USA) 79: 7455, 1982.
14. Leanhardt, W., Corbel, C., Wall, R., and Melchers, F. T cell hybridomas which produce B lymphocyte replication factors only. Nature 300: 355, 1982.
15. Howard, M., Matis, L., Malek, T., Shevach, E., Kell, W., Cohen, D., Nakanishi, K., and Paul, W.E. Interleukin 2 induces antigen-reactive T cell lines to secrete BCGF-I. J. Exp. Med. 158: 2024, 1983.
16. Mosmann, T.R., Cherwinski, H., Bond, M.W., Giedlin, M.A., and Coffman, R.L. Two types of murine helper T cell clones: I. definition according to profiles of lymphokine activities and secreted proteins. J. Immunol. 136: 2348, 1986.
17. Ohara, J., Lahet, S., Inman, J., and Paul, W.E. Partial purification of murine B cell stimulatory factor (BSF)-1. J. Immunol. 135: 2518, 1985.
18. Grabstein, K., Eisenman, J., Mochizuki, D., Shanebeck, K., Conlon, P., Hopp, T., March, C., and Gillis, S. Purification to homogeneity of B cell stimulating factor: a molecule that stimulates proliferation of multiple lymphokine-dependent cell lines. J. Exp. Med. 163: 1405, 1986.
19. Howard, M., and Paul, W.E. Regulation of B cell growth and differentiation by soluble factors. Ann. Rev. Immunol. 1: 307, 1983.
20. Roehm, N.W., Leibson, H.J., Zlotnik, A., Kappler, J., Marrack, P., and Cambier, J.C. Interleukin-induced increase in Ia expression by normal mouse B cells. J. Exp. Med. 160: 679, 1984.
21. Noelle, R., Krammer, P.H., Ohara, J., Uhr, J.W., and Vitetta, E.S. Increased expression of Ia antigens on resting B cells: an additional role for B-cell growth factor. Proc. Natl. Acad. Sci. (USA) 81: 6149, 1984.

22. Rabin, E.M., Ohara, J., and Paul, W.E. B-cell stimulatory factor 1 activates resting B cells. Proc. Natl. Acad. Sci. (USA) 82: 2935, 1985.

23. Oliver, K., Noelle, R.J., Uhr, J.W., Krammer, P.H., and Vitetta, E.S. B-cell growth factor (B-cell growth factor I or B-cell stimulating factor, provisional 1) is a differentiation factor for resting B cells and may not induce cell growth. Proc. Natl. Acad. Sci. (USA) 82: 2465, 1985.

24. Ohara, J., and Paul, W.E. Production of a monoclonal antibody to and molecular characterization of B-cell stimulatory factor 1. Nature 315: 333, 1985.

25. Rabin, E.M., Mond, J.J., Ohara, J., and Paul, W.E. B cell stimulatory factor 1 (BSF-1) prepares resting B cells to enter S phase in response to anti-IgM and lipopolysaccharride. J. Exp. Med. 164: 517, 1986.

26. Isakson, P.C., Pure, E., Vitetta, E.S., and Krammer, P.H. T cell-derived B cell differentiation factor(s): effect on the isotype switch of murine B cells. J. Exp. Med. 155: 734, 1982.

27. Isakson, P.C., Antiimmunoglobulin-treated B cells respond to a B cell differentiation factor for IgG$_1$. J. Exp. Med. 164: 303, 1986.

28. Jones, S., Jung-Wu, C., Isakson, P., Layton, J., Pure, E., Ward, C., Krammer, P.H., Tucker, P., and Vitetta, E.S. Effect of T cell-derived lymphokines containing B cell differentiation factor(s) for IgG (BCDFγ) on γ-specific mRNA in murine B cells. J. Immunol. 131: 3049, 1983.

29. Sideras, P., Bergstedt-Lindquist, S., MacDonald, H.R., and Severinson, E. Secretion of IgG$_1$ induction factor by T cell clones and hybridomas. Eur. J. Immunol. 15: 586, 1985.

30. Vitetta, E.S., Ohara, J., Myers, C.D., Layton, J.E., Krammer, P.H., and Paul, W.E. Serological, biochemical and functional identity of B cell-stimulatory factor 1 and B cell differentiation factor for IgG$_1$. J. Exp. Med. 162: 1726, 1985.

31. Coffman, R.L., and Carty, J. A T cell activity that enhances polyclonal IgE production and its inhibition by interferon. J. Immunol. 136: 949, 1986.

32. Coffman, R.L., Ohara, J., Bond, M.W., Carty, J., Zlotnik, A., and Paul, W.E. B cell stimulatory factor-1 enhances the IgE response of lipopolysaccharide-activated B cells. J. Immunol. 136: 4538, 1986.

33. Stein, P., Dubois, P., Greenblatt, D., and Howard, M. Induction of antigen-specific proliferation in affinity-purified small B lymphocytes: requirement for BSF-1 by type 2 but not type 1 thymus-independent antigens. J. Immunol. 136: 2080, 1986.

34. Dubois, P., Stein, P., Ennist, D., Greenblatt, D., and Howard, M. Requirement for BSF-1 in the induction of antigen-specific B cell proliferation by a thymus dependent antigen and carrier-reactive T cell line. J. Immunol. 139: 1927, 1987.

35. Dubois, P., Stein, P., and Howard, M. (manuscript in preparation).

36. Mosmann, T.R., Bond, M.W., Coffman, R.L., Ohara, J., and Paul, W.E. T cell and mast cell lines respond to B cell stimulatory factor-1. Proc. Natl. Acad. Sci. (USA) 83: 5654, 1986.

37. Mosmann, T., Cherwinski, H., Cher, D., Bond, M., and Coffman, R. Two types of mouse helper T cell clone differ in function and produce distinct

sets of lymphokines. Presented at the VIth International Congress of Immunology, Toronto, Canada. July 1986.

38. Rennick, D. personal communication.

39. Zlotnik, A., Fischer, M., Roehm, N., and Zipori, D. Evidence for effects of interleukin 4 (B cell stimulatory factor 1) on macrophages: enhancement of antigen presenting ability of bone marrow-derived macrophages. J. Immunol. 138: 4275, 1987.

40. Fernandez-Botran, R., Krammer, P.H., Diamantstein, T., Uhr, J.W., and Vitetta, E.S. B cell-stimulatory factor 1 (BSF-1) promotes growth of helper T cell lines. J. Exp. Med. 164: 580, 1986.

41. Noma, Y., Sideras, P., Naito, T., Bergstedt-Lindquist, S., Azuma, C., Severinson, E., Tanabe, T., Kinashi, T., Matsuda, F., Yaoita, Y., and Honjo, T. Cloning of cDNA encoding the murine $IgG_1$ induction factor by a novel strategy using SP6 promoter. Nature 319: 640, 1986.

42. Maizel, A., Sahasrabudde, C., Mehta, S., Morgan, J., Lachman, L., and Ford, R. Biochemical separation of a human B cell mitogenic factor. Proc. Natl. Acad. Sci. (USA) 79: 5998, 1982.

43. Yoshizaki, K., Nakagawa, T., Fakunaga, K., Kaieda, T., Maruyama, S., Kishimoto, S., Yamamura, Y., and Kishimoto, T. Characterization of human B cell growth (BCGF) from cloned T cells or mitogen-stimulated T cells. J. Immunol. 130: 1241, 1983.

44. Maraguchi, A., and Fauci, A.S. Proliferative responses of normal human B lymphocytes development of an assay system for human B cell growth factor (BCGF). J. Immunol. 129: 1104, 1982.

45. Yokota, T., Otsuka, T., Mosmann, T., Banchereau, J., DeFrance, T., Blanchard, D., De Vries, J.E., Lee, F., and Arai, K. Isolation and characterization of a human interleukin cDNA clone, homologous to mouse B-cell stimulating factor 1, that expresses B cell and T cell stimulating activities. Proc. Natl. Acad. Sci. (USA) 83: 5894, 1986.

46. Banchereau, J. personal communication.

47. Banchereau, J., Defrance, T., Spits, H., Rousset, F., Blanchard, D., Yssel, H., Bonnefoy, J.Y., Aubry, J.P., Mosmann, T., Takebe, Y., Arai, N., Lee, F., Otsuka, T., Yukota, T., Arai, K., and de Vries, J.E. The multiple biological activities of a novel recombinant human lymphokine homologous to mouse BSF-1. Presented at the VIth International Congress of Immunology, Toronto, Canada. July 1986.

48. Kehry, M. personal communication.

49. Mosmann, T.R., Yokota, T., Kastelein, R., Zurawaski, S., Arai, N., and Takebe, Y. Species specificity of T cell stimulatory activities of IL-2 and BSF-1 (IL-4): comparison of normal and recombinant mouse and human IL-2 and BSF-1 (IL-4). J. Immunol. 138: 1813, 1987.

50. Swain, S.L., and Dutton, R.W. Production of a B cell growth-promoting activity, (DL) BCGF from a cloned T cell line and its assay on the $BCL_1$ B cell tumor. J. Exp. Med. 156: 1821, 1982.

51. Dutton, R.W., Wetzel, G.D., and Swain, S.L. Partial purification and characterization of a BCGF II from $EL_4$ culture supernatants. J. Immunol. 132: 2451, 1984.

52. Pike, B.L., Vaux, D.L., Clark-Lewis, I., Schrader, J.W., and Nossal, G.J.V. Proliferation and differentiation of single hapten-specific B lymphocytes is promoted by T-cell factor(s) distinct from T-cell growth factor. Proc. Natl. Acad. Sci. (USA) 79: 6350, 1982.
53. Takatsu, K., Tanaka, K., Tominaga, A., Kumahara, Y., and Hamaoka, T. Antigen-induced T cell-replacing factor (TRF): III establishment of a T cell hybrid clone continuously producing TRF and functional analysis of released TRF. J. Immunol. 125: 2646, 1980.
54. Ono, S., Hayashi, S., Takahama, Y., Dobashi, K., Katoh, Y., Nakanichi, K., Paul, W.E., and Hamaoka, T. Identification of two distinct factors, B151-TRF1 and B151-TRF2, inducing differentiation of activated B cells and small resting B cells into antibody-producing cells. J. Immunol. 137: 187, 1986.
55. Takatsu, K., Harada, N., Yoshinobu, H., Yousuke, T., Yamada, G., Doabshi, K., and Hamaoka, T. Purification and physiochemical characterization of murine T cell replacing factor (TRF). J. Immunol. 134: 382, 1985.
56. Harada, N., Kikuchi, Y., Tominaga, A., Takaki, S., and Takatsu, K. BCGF II activity on activated B cells of a purified murine T cell-replacing factor (TRF) from a T cell hybridoma (B151K12). J. Immunol. 134: 3944, 1985.
57. Hara, Y., Takahama, Y., Murakami, S., Yamada, G., Ono, S., Takatsu, K., and Hamaoka, T. B cell growth and differentiation activity of a purified T cell-replacing factor (TRF) molecule from B151-T cell hybridoma. Lymphokine Res. 4: 243, 1985.
58. Hamaoka, T., and Ono, S. Regulation of B-cell differentiation: interactions of factors involved and corresponding receptors. Ann. Rev. Immunol. 4: 167, 1986.
59. Müller, W., Kuhn, R., Goldman, W., Tesch, H., Smith, F.I., Radbruch, A., and Rajewsky, K. Signal requirements for growth and differentiation of activated murine B lymphocytes. J. Immunol. 135: 1213, 1985.
60. Sanderson, C.J., O'Gara, A., Warren, D.J., and Klaus, G.G.B. Eosinophil differentiation factor also has B cell-growth factor activity: proposed name interleukin 4. Proc. Natl. Acad. Sci. (USA) 83: 437, 1986.
61. Sanderson, C.J., Warren, D.J., and Strath, M. Identification of a lymphokine that stimulates eosinophil differentiation in vitro: its relationship to interleukin 3, and functional properties of eosinophils produced in cultures. J. Exp. Med. 162: 60, 1985.
62. O'Garra, A., Warren, D.J., Holman, M., Popham, A.M., Sanderson, C.J., Klaus, G.G.B. Interleukin-4 (B cell growth factor-II/eosinophil differentiation factor) is a mitogen and differentiation factor for preactivated murine B lymphocytes. Proc. Natl. Acad. Sci. (USA) 83: 5228, 1986.
63. Nakajima, K., Hirano, T., Takatsuki, F., Sakaguchi, N., Yoshida, N., and Kishimoto, T. Physiochemical and functional properties of murine B cell-derived B cell growth factor II (WEHI-231-BCGF-II). J. Immunol. 135: 1207, 1985.
64. Ennist, D.L., Elkins, K., Cheng, S., and Howard, M. Synergy between two distinct BCGF II-like factors in promoting B cell differentiation. J. Immunol. 139: 1525, 1987.

65. Kehrl, J.H., Muraguchi, A., and Fauci, A.S. The modulation of membrane Ia on human B lymphocytes. Cell. Immunol. 92: 391, 1985.
66. Banchereau, J. personal communication.
67. Sredni, B., Sieckmann, D., Kumagai, S., House, S., Green, I., and Paul, W.E. Long term culture and cloning of nontransformed human B lymphocytes. J. Exp. Med. 154: 1500, 1981.
68. Kishimoto, T., Yoshizaki, K., Okada, M., Miki, Y., Nakagawa, T., Yoshimur, N., Kishi, H., and Yamamura, Y. Activation of human monoclonal B cells with anti-Ig and T cell derived helper factor(s) and biochemical analysis of the transmembrane signaling in B cells. Proc. UCLA Symp. Molecular Cell. Biol. 24: 375, 1982.
69. Muraguchi, A., Kasahara, T., Oppenheim, J.J., and Fauci, A.S. B cell growth factor and T cell growth factor produced by mitogen-stimulated normal human peripheral blood lymphocytes are distinct molecules. J. Immunol. 129: 2486, 1982.
70. Butler, J.L., Muraguchi, A., Lane, H.C., and Fauci, A.S. Development of a human T-T cell hybridoma secreting B cell growth factor. J. Exp. Med. 157: 60, 1983.
71. Ford, R.J., Mehta, S.R., Franzini, D., Montagna, R., Lachman, L.B., and Maizel, A.L. Soluble factor activation of human B lymphocytes. Nature 294: 261, 1981.
72. Muraguchi, A., Butler, J.L., Kehrl, J.H., and Fauci, A.S. Differential sensitivity of human B cell subsets to activation signals delivered by anti-$\mu$ antibody and proliferative signals delivered by a monclonal B cell growth factor. J. Exp. Med. 157: 530, 1983.
73. Maizel, A.L., Morgan, J.W., Mehta, S.R., Louttab, N.M., Bator, J.M., and Schasrabuddhe, C.G. Long-term growth of human B cells and their use in a microassay for B-cell growth factor. Proc. Natl. Acad. Sci. (USA) 80: 5047, 1983.
74. Okada, M., Sakaguchi, N., Yoshimura, N., Hara, H., Shimizu, K., Yoshida, N., Yoshizaki, K., Kishimoto, S., Yamamura, Y., and Kishimoto, T. B cell growth factors and B cell differentiation factor from human T hybridomas: two distinct kinds of B cell growth factor and their synergism in B cell proliferation. J. Exp. Med. 157: 583, 1983.
75. Rosenberg, Y.J., and Chiller, J.M. Ability of antigen-specific helper cells to effect a class-restricted increase in total Ig-secreting cells in spleen after immunization with the antigen. J. Exp. Med. 150: 517, 1979.
76. Mehta, S.R., Conrad, D., Sandler, R., Morgan, J., Montagna, R., and Maizel, A.L. Purification of human B cell growth factor. J. Immunol. 135: 3298, 1985.
77. Butler, J.L., Ambrus, Jr, J.L., and Fauci, A.S. Characterization of monoclonal B cell growth factor (BCGF) produced by a human T-T hybridoma. J. Immunol. 133: 251, 1984.
78. Sharma, S., Mehta, S., Morgan, J., and Maizel, A. Molecular cloning and expression of a human B cell growth factor gene in Escherichia coli. Science 235: 1489, 1987.

79. Jurgensen, C.H., Ambrus, Jr, J.L., and Fauci, A.S. Production of B cell growth factor by normal human B cells. J. Immunol. 136: 4542, 1986.

80. Muraguchi, A., Nishimoto, H., Kawamura, N., Hori, A., and Kishimoto, T. B cell-derived BCGF functions as autocrine growth factor(s) in normal and transformed B lymphocytes. J. Immunol. 137: 179, 1986.

81. Shimizu, K., Hirano, T., Ishibashi, K., Nakano, N., Taga, T., Sugamura, K., Yamamura, Y., and Kishimoto, T. Immortalization of BCDF (BCGF II) and BCDF-producing T cells by human T cell leukemia virus (HTLV) and characterization of human BGDF (BCGF II). J. Immunol. 134: 1728, 1985.

82. Sahasrabuddhe, C.G., Morgan, J., Sharma, S., Mehta, S., Martin, B., Wright, D., and Maizel, A. Evidence for an intracellular precursor for human B-cell growth factor. Proc. Natl. Acad. Sci. (USA) 81: 7902, 1984.

83. Sahasrabuddhe, C.G., Martin, B., and Maizel, A.L. Purification and partial characterization of human intracellular B cell growth factor. Lymphokine Res. 5: 127, 1986.

84. Ambrus, Jr., J.L., and Fauci, A.S. Human B lymphoma cell line producing B cell growth factor. J. Clin. Invest. 75: 732, 1985.

85. Ambrus, Jr., J.L., Jurgensen, C.H., Brown, E.J., and Fauci, A.S. Purification to homogeneity of a high molecular weight human B cell growth factor; demonstration of specific binding to activated B cells; and development of a monoclonal antibody to the factor. J. Exp. Med. 162: 1319, 1985.

86. Muraguchi, A., Kishimoto, T., Miki, Y., Kuritani, T., Kaieda, T., Yoshizaki, K., and Yamamura, Y. T cell replacing factor-induced IgG secretion in a human B blastoid cell line and demonstration of acceptors for TRF. J. Immunol. 127: 412, 1981.

87. Yoshizaki, K., Nakagawa, T., Kaieda, T., Muraguchi, A., Yamamura, Y., and Kishimoto, T. Induction of proliferation and Igs-production in human B leukemic cells by anti-immunoglobulins and T cell factors. J. Immunol. 128: 1296, 1982.

88. Teranishi, T., Hirano, T., Arima, N., and Onoue, K. Human helper T cell factor(s) (ThF). II. Induction of IgG production in B lymphoblastoid cell lines and identification of T cell replacing like factor(s). J. Immunol. 128: 1903, 1982.

89. Hirano, T., Taga, T., Nakano, N., Yasukawa, K., Kashiwamura, S., Shimizu, K., Nakajima, K., Pyun, K., and Kishimoto, T. Purification to homogeneity and characterization of human B cell differentiation factor (BCDF or BSF p-2). Proc. Natl. Acad. Sci. (USA) 82: 5490, 1985.

90. Saiki, O., and Ralph, P. Clonal differences in response to T cell replacing factor for IgM secretion and TRF receptors in a human B lymphoblast cell line. Eur. J. Immunol. 13: 31, 1983.

91. Kikutani, H., Taga, T., Akira, S., Kishi, H., Miki, Y., Saiki, O., Yamamura, Y., and Kishimoto, T. Effect of B cell differentiation factor (BCDF) on biosynthesis and secretion of immunoglobulin molecules in human B cell lines. J. Immunol. 134: 990, 1985.

92. Hirano, T., Teranishi, T., Lin, B., and Onoue, K. Human helper T cell factor(s). IV. Demonstration of a human late-acting B cell differentiation factor

acting on *Staphylococcus aureus* Cowan I-stimulated B cells. J. Immunol. 133: 798, 1984.

93. Teranishi, T., Hirano, T., Lin, B., and Onoue, K. Demonstration of interleukin 2 in the differentiation of *Staphylococcus aureus* Cowan I-stimulated B cells. J. Immunol. 133: 3062, 1984.

94. Butler, J., Falkoff, R., and Fauci, A. Development of a human T cell hybridoma secreting separate B cell growth and differentiation factors. Proc. Natl. Acad. Sci. (USA) 81: 2475, 1984.

95. Kishimoto, T. personal communication.

96. Pure, E., Isakson, P., Takatsu, K., Hamaoka, T., Swain, S., Dutton, R., Dennert, G., Uhr, J., and Vitetta, E. Induction of B cell differentiation by T cell factors. I. Stimulation of IgM secretion by products of a T cell hybridoma and a T cell line. J. Immunol. 127: 1953, 1981.

97. Nakanishi, K., Malek, T., Smith, K., Hamaoka, T., and Paul, W.E. Both interleukin 2 and a second T cell-derived factor in EL-4 supernatant have activity as differentiation factors in IgM synthesis. J. Exp. Med. 160: 1605, 1984.

98. Sidman, C., Paige, C., and Schreier, M. B cell maturation factor (BMF:; A lymphokine or family of lymphokines promoting the maturation of B lymphocytes. J. Immunol. 132: 209, 1984.

99. Sidman, C., and Marshall, J. B cell maturation factor: Effects on various cell populations. J. Immunol. 132: 845, 1984.

100. Prud'homme, G., Park, C., Fieser, T., Kofler, R., Dixon, F., and Theofilopoulos, A. Identification of a B cell differentiation factor spontaneously produced by proliferating T cells in murine-lupus strains of the 1pr/1pr genotype. J. Exp. Med. 157: 730, 1983.

101. Dobashi, K., Ono, S., Murakami, S., Takahama, Y., Katoh, Y., and Hamaoka, T. Polyclonal B cell activation by a B cell differentiation factor, B151-TRF2. III. B151-TRF2 is a B cell differentiation factor closely associated with autoimmune disease. J. Immunol. 138: 780, 1987.

102. Melchers, F., Andersson, J., Lernhardt, W., and Schreier, M. H-2-unrestricted polyclonal maturation without replication of small B cells induced by antigen-activated T cell help factors. Eur. J. Immunol. 10: 679, 1980.

103. Leclercq, L., Bismuth, G., and Theze, J. Antigen-specific helper T-cell clone supernatant is sufficient to induce both polyclonal proliferation and differentiation of small resting B lymphocytes. Proc. Natl. Acad. Sci. (USA) 81: 6491, 1984.

104. Bowen, D.L., Ambrus, J.L., and Fauci, A.S. Identification and characterization of a B cell activation factor (BCAF) produced by a human T cell line. J. Immunol. 136: 2158, 1986.

105. Yoshizaki, K., and Kishimoto, K. Effect of IL2 and -IFN on proliferation and differentiation of human B cells. J. Immunol. 134: 959, 1985.

106. Sidman, C.L., Marshall, J.D., Shultz, L.D., Gray, P.W., and Johnson, H.M. γ-Interferon is one of several direct B cell-maturing lymphokines. Nature 309: 801, 1984.

107. Leibson, H.J., Gefter, M., Zlotnik, A., Marrack, P., and Kappler, J.W. Role of γ interferon in antibody-producing responses. Nature 309: 799, 1984.

108. Kishomoto, T. Factors affecting B-cell growth and differentiation. Ann. Rev. Immunol. 3: 133, 1985.

# Part III

**Lymphokines and Cytokines as Modulators
for Biological Responses
and Their Application in Therapy**

# 7

# Human Lymphotoxin, Macrophage Toxin, and Tumor Necrosis Factor

Bruce J. Averbook,* Thomas R. Ulich, S. Orr, Robert S. Yamamoto, I. Masunaka, and Gale A. Granger / University of California at Irvine, Irvine, California

## I. BACKGROUND: TUMOR NECROSIS FACTOR, LYMPHOTOXINS, AND MACROPHAGE CYTOTOXINS

Human macrophages and lymphocytes produce a family of proteins that are growth inhibitory and lytic for cells in vivo and in vitro. Cytolytic lymphocytes can produce two different types of cell lytic effector molecules in vitro; cytoplasmic granule-associated proteins that cause rapid (5-10 min), nonspecific cell lysis (1) and secreted proteins that cause protracted (12-24 hr), selective lysis of tumor but not normal cells (2). These latter effector molecules were originally termed lymphotoxins (LT). Subsequent in vitro studies revealed macrophages can also be induced to release cell lytic materials, those that were macromolecular and protein were termed macrophage toxins (MT) (3). The participation of LT and MT in cell-mediated tissue destruction has been debated for over a decade and there is evidence both for and against such a role. It is not our purpose here to reopen that debate; however, it is clear that these molecules are released when a cytolytic effector cell contacts its target, and they can induce important effects separate from target cell lysis. We will consider some of the newly understood roles for these mediators. In the mid-1970s, factors with antitumor activity were identified in the serum of sensitized animals challenged with antigen or endotoxin and were termed tumor necrosis factors (TNF) (4-6). It is now clear that MT, LT, and TNF are interrelated.

The terminology of these effector molecules is confusing, for LT and MT both have TNF activity and certain forms of LT and MT are referred to as TNF (7,8). Historically, most investigators consider TNF as macrophage derived; this material has also been termed TNF-alpha (7,9). In keeping with tradition we will

---

*Present affiliation: University of California at Irvine Medical Center, Orange, California

181

employ LT when molecules are from lymphocytes and MT-TNF when they are
derived from macrophages.

## II. SOURCES, CHARACTERISTICS, AND RELATIONSHIPS
## OF LT AND TNF

Each class of human lymphocyte can produce common and distinct LT forms.
Alpha-LT, which we will term LT-1, is produced by many different types of lymphocytes and lymphoid cell lines, when induced in vitro with the proper activating agents (2). Because it causes TNF effects in vivo, the LT-1 protein has also
been referred to as TNF-beta (8,9). We have found two additional LT forms,
termed LT-2 and LT-3, that can be produced in vitro by specific and nonspecific
cytolytic T cells when they are stimulated with lectins, phorbol esters, or contact
with target cells (10,11). Biochemical and immunologic studies indicate that LT-2
is similar to MT-TNF. Thus, specific and nonspecific cytolytic T lymphocytes
and activated macrophages have the capacity to release MT-TNF. In contrast,
the LT-3 form appears to be released only by cytolytic T lymphocytes. The LT-3
form is very interesting for it is lytically active on many more types of target cells
in vitro than either the LT-1 or LT-2. While LT-3 is distinct from LT-1 and LT-2,
both functionally and physically, it is also related, for LT-3 shares immunologic
reactivity with both TNF and LT-2 proteins. Exhaustive studies indicate that
cytolytic T cells produce LT-1 when induced with IL-2 but switch to the production of LT-2 and LT-3 when stimulated with lectins or when they contact
target cells in vitro. Thus these cells can produce different LT forms in response
to different membrane signals. Natural killer (NK) lymphocytes produce LT-1
and NK-cytotoxic factor, here designated as LT-4. This latter material is the
least understood member of this family of lymphocyte effector molecules (12,
13). However, we have found LT-4 shares immunologic reactivity with LT-2
and LT-3 and thus they appear to be related (10). One of the interesting aspects
of LT, MT, and TNF is that these molecules have inhibitory effects on continuous cells but have no effect or stimulate the growth of primary cells in vitro.
Finally, each of the LT forms affects a different constellation of target cells in
vitro. Thus, cytolytic effector cells possess a panel of distinct but related effector molecules that they may employ against target cells. The data shown in Table
1 summarize the current relationships between type of lymphocyte and class of
LT produced in vitro.

Recent studies have characterized the LT-1 protein. The human LT-1 molecule is isolated from lymphoblastoid cell lines and exists in several different but
related molecular forms: (a) a nonglycosylated 25,000 molecular weight (m.w.)
peptide that assembles into a molecule of 50-70,000 m.w., this molecule is available from a "recombinant" source (7,8), (b) a glycosylated 27,000 m.w. peptide
that can assemble into a 90-100,000 m.w. form (this is a "native" LT form) (14),
and (c) a "native" form in which the 27,000 m.w. peptide is associated with an

Table 1    Release of Lymphotoxins by Human Lymphocyte Subsets In Vitro

| | LT form released | | | |
|---|---|---|---|---|
| Lymphocyte subset | LT-1[a] | LT-2[b] | LT-3 | LT-4[c] |
| Specific cytotoxic T cells | + | + | + | ? |
| Nonspecific cytotoxic T cells | + | + | + | ? |
| Natural killer cells | + | − | − | + |
| B lymphocytes | + | − | − | − |

[a]Also termed alpha lymphotoxin or TNF-beta.

[b]May be similar, if not identical, to MT and TNF-alpha.

[c]Also termed NK cytotoxic factor.

unrelated 76,000 m.w. peptide (14). The 25-27,000 m.w. peptide in each of these LT forms is similar, however, the large peptide in the later form is distinct. The MT-TNF molecule is an assemblage of a common, nonglycosylated 17,000 m.w. peptide to give a molecule of 55-65,000 m.w. (9,15). The MT-TNF peptide shares 28% amino acid homology with the 25,000 m.w. recombinant LT peptide. These two effector molecules are distinct but related.

Interesting and important studies have been conducted with purified LT-1 from native and recombinant sources. The in vitro functional capacities of the recombinant and native LT-1 molecule are beginning to be clarified. Each form has growth inhibitory and lytic effects on certain continuous cell lines; however, these molecules have other functions as well. Both LT-1 forms have the ability to synergize with all classes of interferon (IFN) and very low levels of a variety of metabolic inhibitors, to induce increased cell lysis (16). Our studies reveal that this is most evident when cells are pretreated with very low levels of IFN followed by nonlytic levels of LT; thus very low levels become cytolytic. Recombinant LT-1 and MT-TNF can activate leukocytes in vitro (17), stimulate bone resorption by osteoclasts (18), and stimulate fibroblast proliferation (9). MT-TNF can alter lipid metabolism, apparently by inhibition of lipoprotein lipase activity, and can cause cachexia in animals (19,20).

## III.  PHARMACOKINETICS AND BIODISTRIBUTION OF HUMAN LT-1 IN MICE

We have examined the pharmacokinetics and distribution of radioiodinated native LT-1 in the tissues of normal and Meth-A-bearing Balb/C mice (21,22). In vitro testing of blood samples, from LT-injected tumor and normal Balb/C mice, indicates this material has a functional 2-3 hr half life in circulation. The LT-1 molecule itself, after loss of lytic activity in circulation, however, persists in the blood vascular system for longer periods of time with a half life on the order of 16-20 hours. We found that these animals can tolerate 200,000 units in a single injection or 50,000 units given every other day for 5 injections without showing any overt detrimental effects. A unit of LT activity is equivalent to 100 pg of protein and will destroy 7500 L929 cells in vitro within 16 hr. Parenterally injected, lytically active, radioiodinated LT is distributed evenly throughout the tissues of both normal and tumor-bearing animals. Labelled material is removed from circulation and tissues and apparently excreted by the kidney. These studies also revealed that when the molecule was administered parenterally it did not localize in tumor tissues above that noted for other body organs such as the spleen or liver.

The pharmacokinetics of TNF has been examined by Beutler who showed that TNF was cleared from circulation with a half life of about 6 minutes. Beutler found that TNF distributed broadly to liver, skin, kidney, lung, and gastrointestinal tract (23). Tumor necrosis factor levels in brain and adipose tissue were found to be low. This latter point is of interest since TNF appears to affect lipid metabolism, and yet, has a low affinity for adipose tissue.

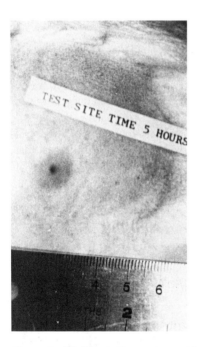

Figure 1   Visible, inflammatory skin reaction in a New Zealand White (NZW) Rabbit 5 hours after intradermal injection with 4200 units of LT (10 μl). The skin reaction at this time exhibits erythema, edema, and hyperthermia.

## IV. INFLAMMATORY CAPABILITIES OF LT AND TNF IN VIVO

The native and recombinant forms of human LT-1 are powerful inducers of inflammation in vivo (24). The native form can induce inflammation when given intradermally in the skin of mice, rabbits, and guinea pigs. The mouse inflammatory skin reaction is only evident by histological examination of tissue. The recombinant form of LT has been tested in rabbits. Single injections of 1000 units or more of these molecules induce erythema and edema that begins about 5 hr after injection (Fig. 1), peaks at 24-36 hr, and then subsides by 72 hr. The degree of visible skin reactivity is dose dependent. Doses less than 1000 units show less erythema, edema, and do not persist as long. Histologic examination of rabbit skin reactions to the native molecule indicate the response is characterized by polymorphonuclear neutrophils (PMN) and edema which is consistent with acute inflammation. Leukocytic infiltration can be seen as early as 3 hours after treatment. Figure 2B demonstrates PMN infiltration into rabbit dermal tissue 6 hours after LT injection (4500 units) into the site biopsied as compared to its control in Figure 2A. Of note is that repeated daily injections of LT for 3 days into the same rabbit skin site result in a greater degree of inflammation and edema with up to 1 cm of palpable induration 24 hours after the third injection. Histologic examination of a chronically injected site (injected with 4500 units every 24 hr for 3 days) revealed acute inflammation with microabscesses composed of PMNs and their debris (Fig. 2C). In contrast, recombinant human TNF at the same or greater levels (up to 60,000 units) does not induce these inflammatory changes. Thus LT but not TNF induces visible signs of inflammation. Histologic studies of TNF-treated rabbit skin are in progress to observe for occult inflammatory reactions.

## V. ANTITUMOR EFFECTS OF LT IN VIVO: REGRESSION, NECROSIS, IMMUNITY, AND HISTOLOGY

Native and recombinant LT-1 have antitumor effects in Meth-A-bearing Balb/C mice in vivo (8,21,22). Initial studies with native LT-1 demonstrated that 1000 to 5000 units suppressed completely the appearance of nonvascularized Meth-A tumors when the two were coinjected into the same intradermal sites. However, the same levels of LT had no effect on the appearance of these tumors when injected at a subcutaneous site 1-2 cm from the site of tumor cell injection. In addition, high levels were without effect on nonvascularized Meth-A tumors when administered intraperitoneally. Thus the molecule can exert a local, suppressive effect on small nonvascularized clusters of tumor cells. We then made direct comparisons of the ability of this molecule to destroy Meth-A cells in vitro and suppress the appearance of tumors when coinjected with these cells in vivo. We found the molecule is up to 300 times more effective in vivo than in vitro. This material also causes a dose-dependent growth inhibition or necrosis of vascularized, 10-14 day subcutaneous Meth-A tumors growing in Balb/C mice. Figure 3

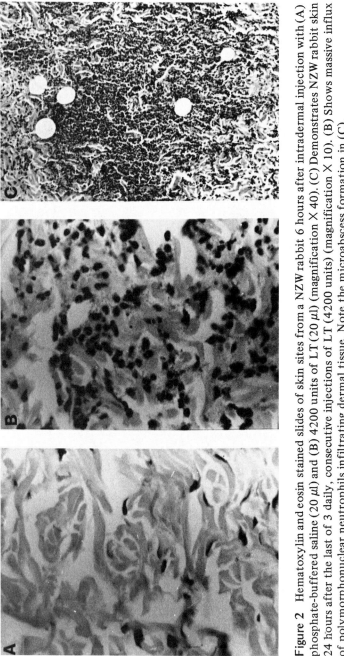

**Figure 2**  Hematoxylin and eosin stained slides of skin sites from a NZW rabbit 6 hours after intradermal injection with (A) phosphate-buffered saline (20 μl) and (B) 4200 units of LT (20 μl) (magnification × 40). (C) Demonstrates NZW rabbit skin 24 hours after the last of 3 daily, consecutive injections of LT (4200 units) (magnification × 10). (B) Shows massive influx of polymorphonuclear neutrophils infiltrating dermal tissue. Note the microabscess formation in (C).

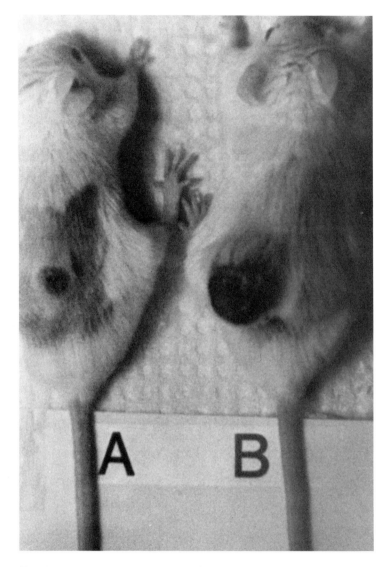

Figure 3 (A) Growth inhibition of a one-month-old Meth-A sarcoma in a Balb/C mouse from low dose LT administration. (B) Control Balb/C mouse with a one-month-old Meth-A tumor.

demonstrates growth inhibition in an LT-treated mouse alongside its control. Low levels, administered via intraperitoneal, intravenous, or intratumor routes, induce growth inhibition and high levels administered via the same routes induce tumor necrosis. This material is effective when administered parenterally; however, the most effective route is direct injection into the tumor. Necrosis is visible grossly 8-12 hr after injection, and when high levels of LT are given, continues to increase for 2-3 days. Figure 4 shows a tumor undergoing necrosis 24 hours after LT treatment. If necrosis is complete tumors do not reappear. However, if necrosis is only partial, the tumor will regrow and kill the animal. In a similar fashion, tumors that are only growth inhibited for 10-12 days will restart and grow progressively to kill the animal in 30-35 days. Animals that exhibited complete necrosis of their tumors have remained completely free of tumor for the one year period of these studies. In addition, these animals have developed immunity to the tumor since they showed greater resistance to rechallenge with fresh Meth-A tumor cells over controls who had tumors removed surgically. Indeed, no mouse who had tumors destroyed with LT regrew tumor after repeated rechallenge. Resistance is specific for these Balb/C mice, who are fully susceptible to challenge with NS-1 myeloma tumor cells.

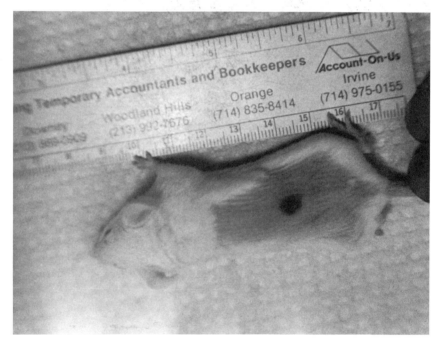

**Figure 4**  Complete necrosis of an 8-day-old Meth-A sarcoma in a Balb/C mouse 24 hours after a high dose administration of LT.

## VI. HISTOLOGIC STUDIES OF LT- AND TNF-TREATED METH-A TUMORS IN BALB/C MICE

Histologic studies of LT-treated subcutaneous tumors indicate that necrosis becomes evident at different sites in LT-injected, Meth-A tumors; (a) at the base, (b) at the center, and (c) in areas around tumor blood vessels (23). The overlying epithelium is usually ulcerated or dead with an underlying layer of hemorrhage. This hemorrhage gives the gross appearance of a spreading black scab in necrosing tumors. Infiltration of host polymorphonuclear neutrophils (PMN) is apparent by 3 hr, increases to 24 hr, and then declines, followed by the gradual infiltration of a few mononuclear cells. Figure 5 demonstrates the neutrophilic

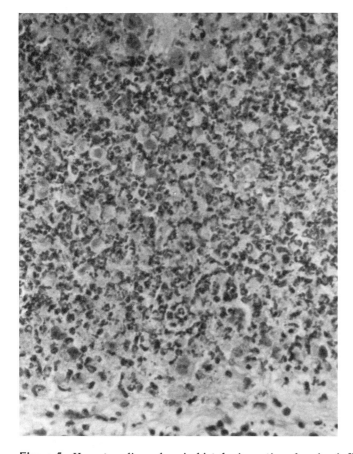

Figure 5 Hematoxylin and eosin histologic section showing infiltration of polymorphonuclear neutrophils in a Balb/C mouse Meth-A sarcoma 24 hours after direct intratumor injection of LT (magnification X 25).

infiltration in tumor at 24 hours. Host cells invade the tumor in large numbers from the vascular bed below the tumor mass and around scattered blood vessels within the tumor. Necrosis in the base of the tumor is associated with cellular infiltration however, necrosis at the center of the tumor is frequently free of host inflammatory cells and is typical of coagulation necrosis. In addition, there are focal areas of liquifaction necrosis associated with leukocytic debris. Untreated tumors or tumors treated with control preparations also show a variable degree of central ischemic, coagulation necrosis.

The mechanism of in vivo tumor cell destruction by TNF and LT may, in part, be mediated by an alteration in the vasculature. This is suspected since the surface of necrotizing tumors after treatment are seen to be hemorrhagic. The literature, however, has not previously had any good histologic descriptions of TNF- or LT-treated tumors. We have seen PMN infiltration, superficial hemorrhage, and ischemic type necrosis in LT-treated tumors, but no obvious vessel thrombi in specimens.

Of interest is that histologic study of TNF-treated Meth-A tumors undergoing necrosis does not demonstrate any significant PMN infiltration. This may reflect a diminished capacity of TNF to activate PMNs when compared with LT, however, this is purely speculative at this time. In LT-treated tumors on immunosuppressed mice who previously received 600 rads of total body irradiation, necrosis progressed without PMN infiltration. Long-term survival and followup of irradiated mice after LT treatment of their tumors is not yet conclusive. It is apparent that PMNs are not required to induce necrosis, but their role in achieving complete eradication of tumor tissue and promoting long-term survival cannot be discounted at this time.

## VII.  VASCULAR AND INFLAMMATORY EFFECTS OF LT AND TNF: INTERACTION WITH NEUTROPHILS AND COAGULATION

The following section will focus on new discoveries of LT actions: its effects on coagulation, vascular endothelium, neutrophils, and its possible relation to sepsis and endotoxic shock. Recent, in vitro findings have demonstrated a variety of previously unknown functions of LT and TNF. These findings may aid in the understanding of cytokine-induced tumor cytolysis and in the roles these biological response modifiers may play in both normal and pathological functions. TNF has been shown to induce procoagulant activity on contact with vascular endothelium (25,26). This not only raises the possibility of a "new" modulator of the clotting mechanism, but lends credence to the concept of LT-TNF vascular interaction having a role in the destruction of vascularized tumors. From day to day use of LT in our experiments, we have seen that LT activity is consumed from serum if a blood sample being assayed is allowed to clot. The role of TNF in septic shock has been considered along with the possibility of monitoring its presence in patients to aid in clinical management. Indeed, passive immunization against TNF has been shown to protect mice from the lethal effects of endotoxemia (27). There is the possibility that TNF may be, in part, responsible for disseminated intravascular coagulation.

TNF has been shown to induce receptor proliferation for itself and IL-1 on cultured endothelium in vitro. In addition, in vitro studies reveal that TNF causes overt morphologic alterations in cultured bovine endothelium to become elongated, to overlap, to rearrange actin filaments, and to lose stainable fibronectin matrices (28). These morphologic changes may be responsible for local edema and possible migration of effector cells across vascular beds in vivo. It has also been speculated, that TNF or LT may be partially responsible for atherosclerotic changes in vessels since it interacts with endothelium and also alters lipid metabolism. Lastly, LT and TNF have been shown to activate PMNs in vitro, however, this effect appears to be much greater for LT than it is for TNF (17,29). TNF will induce neutrophils to adhere to endothelium (30). Adherence occurs either when PMNs are preincubated with TNF prior to exposure to endothelium and when endothelium is pretreated with TNF prior to exposure to untreated PMNs. The mechanism of adherence appears, at least in part, to be mediated by receptors. Of note, however, is that coincubation with protein synthesis inhibitors and RNA synthesis inhibitors cannot prevent TNF-treated PMN adherence to untreated endothelium. In contrast, treatment of vascular endothelium with these inhibitors concomitantly with TNF completely blocks neutrophil adherence.

## VIII.  MECHANISMS OF LT ACTION

Our studies indicate lymphotoxins may exert their antitumor effects via several different mechanisms. LT and MT-TNF can cause direct lysis of transformed cells in vitro without apparent effects on normal cells (9-11). Thus, these molecules may be capable of direct lysis of tumor cells in vivo. This is supported by our finding that LT blocks the appearance of Meth-A tumors when coinjected into the same site with tumor cells. Because of its short half life this molecule must induce this suppressive effect by acting directly and locally on the tumor cells themselves. However, the finding that the molecule is 300 times more effective in vivo than in vitro may indicate that some form of host antitumor mechanism may be participating in this effect. It has been suggested that MT-TNF may act by destroying the vascular supply of tumors. Since LT-1 and MT-TNF are similar, they may both have direct antitumor effects by action on the vascular bed of the tumor(s). These mechanisms may explain the necrosis that occurs in the areas of tumor that are not infiltrated with host inflammatory cells. Our present studies indicate LT-1 can also have several indirect antitumor effects. It is clear that this molecule induces infiltration of host inflammatory cells into tumor tissues. If this LT-1 form can also activate the inflammatory cells in these sites, as has been reported for TNF and recombinant LT-1 in vitro, these cells could participate in nonspecific destruction of tumor tissue. Finally, LT-1 treatment of Meth-A-bearing animals somehow enhances a specific antitumor response that could also participate in destruction of tumor tissues.

## IX.  THE LT/TNF RECEPTOR

There has been considerable interest in isolating a receptor for both LT and TNF for the obvious reasons of understanding how these effector molecules cause their effects on cells and tissues. Correlation of receptor density to cell lysis has been suggested (31,32) but does not appear at this time to be panning out. The average number of receptors seen on all cells examined, both normal and transformed lines, have only a range of 2000-5000 receptors present on them. Also, the lytic activity of these effectors has not shown significant direct correlation to cell lysis and thus there may be other mechanisms operating in cytotoxicity not related to the receptor density or affinity (33,34). The TNF molecule has been shown to become internalized and degraded upon binding to both resistant and sensitive cell lines (33). Initial studies suggest that the receptor for LT and TNF are the same and can be up-regulated by gamma-interferon (35). It has been shown previously that $\gamma$-interferon synergizes with LT to inhibit cell growth of certain tumor lines in vitro (36). Full clarification of the significance of the LT/TNF receptor and its relation to cell lysis and other functions will require further elucidation.

## X.  CONCLUSION

Interaction of an effector lymphocyte with a target cell can result in the release of LT and MT-TNF forms. Irrespective of their role(s) in contact-mediated cell lysis these molecules are going to be involved in a variety of reactions that can occur subsequent to lysis of a single target cell. It is already apparent these molecules can promote the destruction of certain cells and tissues both in vivo and in vitro. Moreover, they have roles in inflammation and cellular activation that were not previously suspected and the list of their functional capacities may not yet be fully elucidated. The understanding of these proteins and their roles in cell-mediated immunity has been made possible by the availability of purified and recombinant forms for study. Clearly, much new information will be forthcoming over the next few years about these interesting mediators.

## REFERENCES

1. Henkart, P., Millard, P., Reynolds, C., and Henkart, M. Cytolytic activity of purified cytoplasmic granules from cytotoxic rat large granular lymphocyte tumors. J. Exp. Med. 106: 75, 1985.
2. Devlin, J.J., Klostergaard, J., Orr, S.L., Yamamoto, R.S., Masunaka, I.K., Plunkett, J.M., and Granger, G.A. Lymphotoxins: After fifteen years of research. In *Lymphokines*, Vol. 9. Edited by E. Pick. Academic Press, New York, 1984, p. 313.

3. Kramer, J., and Granger, G. The *in vitro* induction and release of a cell toxin by immune C57B1/6 mouse peritoneal macrophages. Cell. Immunol. 3: 88, 1972.
4. Ruff, M., and Gifford, G. Tumor necrosis factors. In *Lymphokines*, Vol. 2. Edited by E. Pick. 1981, p. 235.
5. Carswell, E., Old, L., Kassel, R., Green, S., Fieore, N., and Williamson, B. An endotoxin-induced serum factor that induces necrosis of tumors. PNAS 72: 3666, 1975.
6. Old, L.J. Tumor necrosis factor. Science 230: 630, 1985.
7. Aggarwal, B., Kohr, W., Hass, P., Moffat, B., Spencer, S., Henzel, W., Bringman, T., Nedwin, G., Goeddel, D., and Harkins, R. Human tumor necrosis factor: Production, purification, and characterization. J. Biol. Chem. 260: 2345, 1985.
8. Grey, P., Aggarwal, B., Benton, C., Bringman, T., Henzel, W., Jarrett, J., Lung, D., Moffat, B., Ng, P., Sevedersky, L., Palladino, M., and Nedwin, G. Cloning and expression of cDNA for human lymphotoxin, a lymphokine with anti-tumor activity. Nature 312: 721, 1984.
9. Sugarman, B., Aggarwal, B., Hess, P., Figari, I., Palladino, M., and Sheppard, M. Recombinant human tumor necrosis factor-alpha: Effects on proliferation of normal and transformed cells *in vitro*. Science 230: 943, 1985.
10. Yamamoto, R.S., Ware, C.F., and Granger, G.A. The human LT system: XI. Identification of LT and TNF-like LT forms from stimulated natural killers, specific and nonspecific cytotoxic human T cells *in vitro*. J. Immunol. 137: 1878, 1986.
11. Kobayashi, M., Plunkett, J.M., Masunaka, I.K., Yamamoto, R.S., and Granger, G.A. The human LT system: XII. Purification and functional studies of LT and TNF-like forms from a continuous human T cell line that resembles LT forms from human cytolytic T cells. J. Immunol. 137: 1885, 1986.
12. Wright, S., and Bonivida, B. Selective lysis of NK sensitive target cells by a soluble mediator released from mouse spleen cells and human peripheral blood lymphocytes. J. Immunol. 126: 1516, 1981.
13. Granger, G., Weitzen, M., Devlin, J., Innins, E., and Yamamoto, R. Lymphotoxins: An NK-like system. In *The Biologic Response Modifiers*. Edited by N. Hill and A. Kahn. Academic Press, New York, 1982, p. 495.
14. Granger, G., Kobayashi, M., Orr, S., Masunaka, I., Plunkett, M., and Yamamoto, R. Human lymphotoxins: A multicomponent family of proteins with selectivity for transformed cells *in vitro* and *in vivo*. In *Recent Advances in Chemotherapy*. Edited by J. Ishigami. University of Tokyo Press, Tokyo, 1985, p. 86.
15. Wang, A., Creasey, A., Ladner, M., Lin, L., Strickler, J., Van Aresdell, J., Yamamoto, R., and Mark, D. Molecular cloning of the cDNA for human tumor necrosis factor. Science 228: 149, 1985.
16. Aggarwal, B., Moffatt, B., Lee, S., and Harkins, R. In *Thymic Hormones and Lymphokines*. Edited by A. Goldstein. Plenum, New York, 1984.
17. Shalaby, M.R., Aggarwal, B.B., Rinderknecht, E., Svedersky, L.P., Finkle, B.S., and Palladino, Jr., M.A. Activation of human polymorphonuclear neutrophil functions by interferon-gamma and tumor necrosis factor. J. Immunol. 135(3): 2069, 1985.

18. Bertolini, D.R., Newdin, G.E., Bringman, T.S., Smith, D.D., and Mundy, G.R. Stimulation of bone resorption and inhibition of bone formation *in vitro* by human tumour necrosis factors. Nature 319: 816, 1986.

19. Buetler, B., and Cerami, A. Cachectin and tumour necrosis factor as two sides of the same biological coin. Nature 320: 584, 1986.

20. Beutler, B., Mahoney, J., Le-Trang, N., Pekala, P., Cerami, A. Purification of cachectin, a lipoprotein lipase-suppressing hormone secreted by endotoxin-induced RAW 264.7 cells. J. Exp. Med. 161(5): 984, 1985.

21. Jeffes, E.W.B., Averbook, B.J., Ulich, T.R., and Granger, G.A. Human alpha lymphotoxin (LT): Studies examining the mechanism(s) of LT-induced inflammation and tumor destruction *in vivo*. Lymphokine Res. 6(2): 141, 1987.

22. Averbook, B.J., Yamamoto, R.S., Ulich, T.R., Jeffes, E.W.B., Masunaka, I., and Granger, G.A. Purified native and recombinant human alpha lymphotoxin [tumor necrosis factor (TNF)-beta] induces inflammatory reactions in normal skin. J. Clin. Immunol. 7(4): 333, 1987.

23. Beutler, B.A., Milsark, I.W., and Cerami, A. Cachecton/tumor necrosis factor: Production, distribution, and metabolic fate *in vivo*. J. Immunol. 136 (6): 3972, 1985.

24. Averbook, B., Yamamoto, R., Masunaka, I., Orr, S., and Granger, G. Human alpha lymphotoxin: Pharmacokinetics and effects on Meth-A tumors in Balb/c mice. Fed. Proc. 45(3): 271 (Abstr. 682), 1986.

25. Bevilacqua, M.P., Pober, J.S., Majeau, G.R., Fiers, W., Cotran, R.S., and Gimbrone, M.A. Recombinant tumor necrosis factor induces procoagulant activity in cultured human vascular endothelium: characterization and comparison with the actions of interleukin 1. Proc. Natl. Acad. Sci. (USA) 83: 4533, 1986.

26. Nawroth, P., Bank, I., Cassimeris, J., Chess, L., Stern, D. Endothelium is a target tissue for tumor necrosis factor. Fed. Proc. 45(4): 942 (Abstr. 4579), 1986.

27. Beutler, B., Milsark, I.W., and Cerami, A.C. Passive immunization against cachectin/tumor necrosis factor protects mice from lethal effect of endotoxin. Science 299 (1716): 869, 1985.

28. Stolpen, A.H., Guinan, E.C., Fiers, W., and Pober, J.S. Recombinant tumor necrosis factor and immune interferon act singly and in combination to reorganize human vascular endothelial cell monolayers. Am. J. Pathol. 123 (1): 16, 1986.

29. Klebanoff, S.J., Vadas, M.A., Harlan, J.M., Sparks, L.H., Gamble, J.R., Agosti, J.M., and Waltersdorph, A.M. Stimulation of neutrophils by tumor necrosis factor. J. Immunol. 136 (11): 4220, 1986.

30. Gamble, J.R., Harlan, J.M., Klebanoff, S.J., and Vadas, M.A. Stimulation of the adherence of neutrophils to umbilical vein endothelium by human recombinant tumor necrosis factor. Proc. Natl. Acad. Sci. (USA) 82: 8667, 1985.

31. Hass, P.E., Hotchkiss, A., Mohler, M., and Aggarwal, B.B. Characterization of specific high affinity receptors for human tumor necrosis factor on mouse fibroblasts. J. Biol. Chem. 260 (22): 12214, 1985.

32. Baglioni, C., McCandless, S., Tavernier, J., and Fiers, W. Binding of human tumor necrosis factor to high affinity receptors on HeLa and lymphoblastoid cells sensitive to growth inhibition. J. Biol. Chem. 260 (22): 13395, 1985.
33. Tsujimoto, M., Yip, Y.K., and Vilcek, J. Tumor necrosis factor: specific binding and internalization in sensitive and resistant cells. Proc. Natl. Acad. Sci. (USA) 82: 7626, 1985.
34. Kull Jr., F.C., Jacobs, S., and Cuatrecasas, P. Cellular receptor for 125I-labeled tumor necrosis factor: specific binding, affinity labeling, and relationship to sensitivity. Proc. Natl. Acad. Sci. (USA) 82: 5756, 1985.
35. Aggarwal, B.B., Eessalu, T.E., and Hass, P.E. Characterization of receptors for human tumour necrosis factor and their regulation by gamma-interferon. Nature 318 (19): 665, 1985.
36. Lee, S.H., Aggarwal, B.B., Rinderknecht, E., Assisi, F., and Chiu, H. The synergistic anti-proliferative effect of gamma-interferon and human lymphotoxin. J. Immunol. 133 (3): 1083, 1984.

# 8

# Interferons: Biology, Clinical Trials, and Effects on Hematologic Neoplasms

René I. Jahiel / New York University Medical Center, New York, New York

Mathilde Krim / St. Luke's-Roosevelt Hospital Center, New York, New York

## I. INTRODUCTION

Only in the past three or four years have the results of a large number of clinical trials yielded a realistic assessment of interferons as antitumor agents in humans. These results show that a clinical response to interferons can be achieved in most cases of hairy cell leukemia, chronic myeloid leukemia (in the stable phase), and juvenile laryngeal papillomatosis, and in a smaller but significant number of cases of low-grade non-Hodgkin's lymphoma, cutaneous T-cell lymphoma, Kaposi's sarcoma, multiple myeloma, renal cell carcinoma, metastatic malignant melanoma, certain urinary bladder tumors, and certain endocrine neoplasms, they showed minimal if any effect against another group of malignancies such as metastatic carcinomas of the lung, stomach, colon, and exocrine pancreas (1-4a). In addition to the clinical studies, there have been many basic biological or preclinical investigations which have shed some light on the antitumor actions of interferons.

It is not yet possible to assess the eventual role of the interferons in cancer therapy. There are three reasons for this state of affairs. First, the recently acquired knowledge of the molecular biology of the interferons, their biological effects on cells, and their interactions with other cytokines has not been fully sorted out and utilized in cancer studies. Second, most interferon clinical trials have been done in rather restricted conditions, i.e., Phase I or II studies of advanced cancer patients, short duration of interferon therapy, and no combined therapy with other antitumor agents or biological response modifiers (BRM). Phase III trials on less advanced cases, or studies with longer duration of interferon therapy or combination therapy including interferons, are, for the most part, just getting under way, and they have been reported in only a few instances.

Third, the response to interferons is very characteristic of the tumor involved, and even, within a given tumor type, of the tumor subtype or the individual patient.

This review focuses on two areas that are critical for further research—the biology of the interferons (exclusive of their immunology, which has been extensively reviewed) and comparative studies of the effects of alpha interferons on human hematologic neoplasms.

## II. BIOLOGY OF THE INTERFERONS

### A. Historical Overview

The history of the biology of the interferons may be divided into five overlapping approaches, each of which contributed a different aspect to the concept of interferons.

### The Antiviral Effect

The history of the interferons can be traced back to 1957, when Isaacs and Lindemann found that cells infected with viruses produced a protein which made other, uninfected cells temporarily resistant to subsequent viral infection. They named this protein, which appeared to be the mediator of viral interference, interferon (5). Alick Isaacs went on to develop the concept of interferon as the mediator of a general antiviral defense mechanism which develops within hours of the infection, in contrast with antibodies or sensitized cells which become detectable days after initial infection. While antibodies react directly with the microorganism, interferon does not neutralize the virus or prevent its entry into the cell, but it induces some modification of the cell that makes it resistant to some phase(s) of intracellular viral development. While antibodies are effective against the specific microorganism in any host, interferons are most effective in the host species in which they are induced, and they are effective against a wide variety of challenge viruses.

During the next 15 years, interferon research was conducted mainly within the domain of virology. The kinetics of interferon production and antiviral action were described in several systems. It was shown that the induction of interferon is followed by a period of refractoriness to the inducing agent. Several kinds of interferons were recognized, and they were classified according to interferon-producing cell, inducing agent, and physical/chemical properties of the interferon. They were called leukocytic (alpha) and fibroblastic (beta) interferons which were grouped together as type I interferon and immune (gamma) or type II interferon. Viruses, certain microbial products, and certain synthetic compounds, especially double-stranded RNA (dsRNA) were used to induce type I interferons. Mitogenic agents or specific antigens were used to induce type II interferon in lymphocytes or sensitized lymphocytes, respectively. Natural beta and gamma interferons are glycosylated, but human alpha interferon is not. Work done during that period firmly established that RNA and protein synthesis were needed to produce the antiviral state in interferon-treated cells, and, therefore, some mediating agent of the antiviral action had to be produced or activated under the influence of interferon. This early work has been reviewed in Refs. 6 to 8.

## Multiple Biological Effects

Although some other than antiviral effects of interferons had been noted in the early 1960s, it was only about 1970 and in the next few years that mounting evidence was provided by Gresser and others that the interferons have multiple biological effects. These studies, which were initially performed in murine systems with impure preparations of alpha/beta interferons and were sometimes preceded by work with interferon inducers, showed that administration of interferon preparations protects against certain tumors, inhibits cell multiplication, interferes with the pre-erythrocytic development of a malaria parasite, modulates in a dose-dependent manner antibody response, enhances the cytotoxicity of sensitized lymphocytes and of natural killer cells, increases the expression of major histocompatibility antigens on the cell surface, and, in certain doses delays allograft rejection and modulates the differentiation of several cell types (reviewed in Refs. 9-12). During the 1960s and early 1970s, the majority of interferon workers were reluctant to interpret these phenomena as effects of interferons, because of the presence of impurities in the preparations. However, when pure preparations became available, late in the 1970s, and the findings were, in general, confirmed with such preparations, the concept of interferons as inducible biological agents with pleiotropic effects on cells became generally accepted.

## Molecular Biology of Interferons

In the few years from 1976 through 1982, the concept of the interferons evolved from agents identifiable only through their effects on cells or organisms, to a family of small proteins of known amino acid sequence, available to experimenters in pure form, and whose mechanisms of production and action became increasingly more accessible at the molecular level. The landmarks of this breakthrough period are: The synthesis of interferons in cell-free systems with interferon mRNAs in 1975; the discovery, in 1976-1977, of two dsRNA-dependent, interferon-inducible or -activated enzyme systems: a protein kinase which inhibits peptide chain initiation and an endonuclease, ribonuclease L, which is activated by $2'5'$-oligoadenylates (thereafter abbreviated as 2-5A) whose production from adenosine triphosphate (ATP) is catalyzed by the interferon-inducible enzyme 2-5A synthetase; high yield purification of interferons, reaching homogeneity in 1979-1980; preparation of monoclonal antibodies to interferons in 1980-1981; cloning of interferon DNA and expression in bacterial cells of recombinant human interferon beta in 1979-1980, alpha in 1980, and gamma in 1982; and the demonstration of high affinity cell membrane receptors specific for types I and II interferons in 1980-1981. During the same period, the amino acid and nucleotide sequences of the interferons and their cDNAs, respectively, were determined, and, in the following years, several mRNAs and polypeptides induced by interferons were discovered, ushering the analysis of interferon action at the molecular level (reviewed in Refs. 13-17).

Physiological Interferon Production

In 1981, Bocci put forward the concept of physiological interferon response, contrasting it with the acute interferon response following the administration of interferon inducers. It is based on the following premises: (a) trace amounts of exogenous and endogenous inducers act as physiological stimuli in various sites; (b) occasionally, a few stimulated cells switch on the production of interferon; (c) most of the interferon released is consumed locally; (d) the effects of the released interferon are exerted mainly in the vicinity of the producing cells; and (e) since only a few cells produce interferon, the state of generalized refractoriness which follows the acute response does not develop (18,19).

Reports of the "spontaneous" production of interferons are compatible with this concept. Reports published prior to 1980 are reviewed by Bocci (18). Since then, interferons (along in some instances with interferon inhibitors) have been demonstrated in several cells or body fluids associated with gestational (20-24), lymphatic (25), or hematopoietic (26-28) tissues, which had not been pretreated with inducers.

Experimental studies in mice with specific anti-interferon sera have given additional evidence for physiological production of interferon. Treatment with anti-interferon serum abolished the ability of normal mouse lymphoid cells (29) or peritoneal macrophages (30) to confer the antiviral state to other cells, and decreased the 2-5A synthetase level of peritoneal macrophages (31) or mouse embryo fibroblasts (32). Furthermore, treatment with anti-interferon antibodies reduced the S-phase-associated endogenous production of interferon and increased level of 2-5A synthetase in mouse embryo fibroblasts (32). The proliferative response of human melanoma cells in culture to serum was enhanced by the addition of antibodies to human fibroblast interferon (33).

Because of such findings, the concept of interferons as proteins that are present in small amounts and active under physiological conditions is now becoming widely accepted.

A System of Interacting Cytokines

The concept of interferons as cytokines which interact with other cytokines had been advanced in the 1970s, but it was not until well into the 1980s that the extent and complexity of these interactions was fully appreciated. Early in the 1980s, cytokines such as interleukins 1, 2, and 3 (IL-1, 2, 3), tumor necrosis factor (TNF) alpha (cachectin) and beta (lymphotoxin), B-cell-stimulating factors (BSF-1, BSF-2), platelet-derived growth factor (PDGF), and various colony-stimulating factors (CSF) became available as pure, well characterized products.

Many cytokines, once thought to have a single function on a few cell targets, were found to have multiple effects on many cell types.

Interactions between interferons and other cytokines have been demonstrated in many systems. Such interactions include production by cells of one cytokine when stimulated by another; priming by one cytokine of the effect of another on the cell; down regulation by one cytokine of receptors to another cytokine, inhibition of action of one cytokine by another; and, additive or synergistic effects of two cytokines. An example of such networks which involves interferon is shown by Kohase et al. (34). Thus, the last aspect of the concept of interferon involves positive and negative feedback processes taking place among interferons and other cytokines. Positive feedback might result in the amplification of a response under physiological conditions, or leverage in therapeutic intervention. Negative feedback might provide a mechanism for homeostasis at the cellular level as well as limitation of action in therapeutic intervention.

## B. Definition and Classification of the Interferons

It is evident from this brief historical survey that the conceptualization of the interferons has evolved considerably since their discovery in 1957. A contemporary description might be: The interferons are a group of small proteins, with various degrees of amino acid sequence homology, the products of several genes which are usually expressed only to a small extent under physiological conditions and to a much larger extent under the influence of several exogenous or endogenous inducers; the interferons bind to high-affinity receptors on the cell surface and their interaction with the cell results in the modulation of a relatively large number of the cell's mRNA and protein molecular species (including, among others, 2-5A synthetase) and of the proliferation, differentiation or functional activity of the cell; in general, they decrease the cell's ability to support the growth of various viruses; such modulation is controlled in part by the type of interferon, the genetic constitution and physiological state of the cell, the actions of other BRMs and, in the instance of the antiviral effect, certain viruses. Interferons vary in species specificity from strict specificity to significant cross-species reactivity. The interferons are part of a broader class of BRMs which regulate in part one another's production.

Current definitions of the interferons are compatible with this description (e.g., Refs. 15, 35). In contrast with earlier definitions of interferons (6-8) which tended to include very specific criteria, current definitions tend to be more general, except when it is necessary to demonstrate that the substance in question is indeed an interferon (e.g., Ref. 35).

Classification

Table 1 shows the current approach to the classification of the interferons. Types I and II interferons are defined according to their specific receptors on the cell

Table 1  Classification and Nomenclature of Human Interferons

| Receptors | Type I | | | Type II |
|---|---|---|---|---|
| Antigenicity | Alpha[a] | Beta | | Gamma |
| Molecular species | 15 species | Beta-1 | Beta-2[b] | |
| Location of gene on chromosome number: | 9 | 9 | 7 | 12 |
| Number of amino acid residues: | 166 | 166 | 212 | 146 |
| Highly related gene nucleotide sequences: | beta-1 | alpha | no | no |

[a]Nomenclature of alpha interferons used in clinical trials:
   Cloned recombinant interferons:

rIFN-alfa-2a = rIFN-alpha-A = Roferon-A (Hoffman-La Roche)
rIFN-alfa-2b = rIFB-alpha-2 = Intron-A (Schering)
rIFN-alfa-2c (Boehringer)

Natural alpha interferons:

IFN-alfa-N1 = IFN-alpha-Ly = Lymphoblastoid IFN (Wellferon)
IFN-alpha-Le = Leukocyte interferon (several preparations, e.g., Finnish Red Cross)

[b]Whether beta-2 is indeed an interferon is still disputed by some investigators (see text).

surface (36). Interferons are classified as alpha, beta, or gamma, on the basis of their neutralization by specific antisera (37). Finer classification of interferons is based on nucleotide hybridization and amino acid sequence studies. The human alpha interferon genes consist of at least 15 nonallelic functional molecular species, along with allelic variants and nonfunctional pseudogenes. They are all located on chromosome 9 and they show considerable nucleotide homology. The mature interferon alpha proteins usually have 166 amino acid residues (38). The human beta interferons consist of at least two molecular species (38). The interferon beta-1 gene shows considerable nucleotide sequence homology with the interferon alpha genes, and, like them, it is located on chromosome 9. The mature interferon beta-1 protein has 166 amino acid residues (38).

    Interferon beta-2 (39,40) shows considerable differences with interferons alpha and beta-1. The beta-2 gene is larger and the mature beta-2 protein has 212 amino acid residues. The interferon beta-2 gene is on chromosome 7 (41). Its nucleotide sequence has been determined (42,43). While no cross-hybridization was demonstrable between beta-2 cDNA and beta-1 mRNA or vice versa, the interferon beta-2 protein has a 92-amino acid-long sequence which shares 39 amino acid residues in conserved locations with a comparable segment of the beta-1 protein (43). Part of the same region is highly conserved between interferon beta-1 and all the interferons alpha that have been sequenced (38). The amino acid sequence of interferon beta-2 is identical to that of the B-cell differentiation factor BSF-2 (44). Other workers have isolated a glycoprotein with the same molecular weight as interferon beta-2 (26 kD) following induction with poly(I)•Poly (C) or with IL-1-beta which has B-cell differentiation-inducing activity, but does not produce the antiviral effect (45). It is not clear if this protein has the same amino acid sequence as the one described as beta-2. If the two proteins are found to have the same amino acid sequence, the discrepancy between the results of the different investigators concerning its antiviral effect would have to be resolved before these proteins can be definitely classified.

Only one interferon gamma gene has been found in human tissues. The mature human interferon gamma protein has 146 amino acids. Its gene is on chromosome 12. Although there is no detectable homology between the interferons gamma and alpha or beta genes, several parts of the interferon gamma protein share a significant number of amino acid residues in conserved locations with alpha or beta interferons (38,46). It is now agreed that interferon gamma is a macrophage-activating factor (MAF) (47,48).

Table 1 shows naturally occurring interferons which have been expressed in bacteria following recombination and cDNA cloning. Their molecules differ in some respects from their naturally occurring counterparts, for instance in the lack of glycosylation of certain interferons whose natural counterparts are glycosylated (interferons beta and gamma).

There are several other naturally occurring interferons besides those listed in Table 1. Some are being discovered by more refined analysis and cDNA cloning of mRNA species in induced cells, for instance additional types of human beta interferons, such as interferon-beta-3 (49). Studies with novel cosmid libraries have revealed interferon-alpha species in families with interferon polymorphism (50) which are probably allelic variants (51).

Some interferons found in normal body fluids or tissues that have been discussed earlier, or those found in some pathological states (52) have distinctive features (e.g., acid-labile alpha interferons). Interferons induced in hamster embryonic tissues appear to differ from those induced in adult tissues of the same species (53).

Modified Interferons

*Genetically Modified Interferons.* Site-specific mutagenesis has been used to produce interferons with substituted amino acid(s) at one or more site(s) of the interferon molecule (54-57). Recombinant genetic engineering techniques have been used to produce interferons missing some part of the original molecule (58), or cDNA upstream of interferon-coding genes that have inserted oligonucleotides (59) or missing sequences (60). Hybrid interferons where one part of the molecule is coded by one gene and another part by another gene have been constructed with the help of restriction enzyme treatment of the respective nucleic acids (61-65). Recently, in vivo recombination systems have been used to obtain many hybrids with different recombination sites (66). Genetic modification of interferons changes in some instances the secondary or tertiary structure of the interferon protein (57,65). In another example of the versatility of genetic engineering methods, a recombinant "consensus" interferon alpha gene was constructed to code for the most frequent amino acid residues known to occur in the various molecular species of human interferon alpha (67).

*Phenotypically Modified Interferons.* Interferons have been modified by controlled proteolysis (e.g., Refs. 67,69) or by treatment with monoclonal antibodies against specific epitopes on the interferon molecule (e.g., Ref. 70).

*Comments on the Definition and Classification of the Interferons.* As the definition of interferon has evolved from a narrow focus on a special type of antiviral effect to a broader one, based on multiple structural and functional parameters, certain boundary problems in the use of terminology have arisen. The well characterized cloned interferons may be grouped into two categories. The first category would include alpha and beta-1 interferons, which have significant, though variable, nucleotide sequence gene homology, and a strong antiviral effect relative to their other biological effects. The second category would include gamma and beta-2 interferons, having very little nucleotide sequence homology with alpha and beta-1 interferons. However, the proteins have a significant number of amino acid residues conserved in common with alpha and beta-1 interferon in specific locations in certain parts of the molecule. These interferons have weaker antiviral activity relative to their other biological effects than alpha or beta interferons and they have unique sets of biological effects in addition to those they have in common with alphas and beta-1 interferons. So far, it has not appeared necessary to place any of these molecules outside the boundary of the interferon family—except insofar that there is a 26 kD protein/interferon-beta-2 controversy (35,45). However, if greater dissociation were to be found between antiviral effect and other functions of interferons, such as antiproliferative effects, either in natural or modified interferons, the question of defining the boundaries of the interferon family might become more pressing.

There are similar problems with respect to classification. Interferon classification is hierarchical, starting with receptor-specific sites on the interferon molecule (classes I and II), and continuing with the antibody-neutralizable sites (interferons alpha, beta, and gamma), and, finally, nucleotide or amino acid sequence homology (which tends to be closest among molecular species of the same antigenic type). Recently, several investigators discovered a new class I interferon gene coding for a 172-amino acid-long protein with about 60% and 26% homology with interferon-alpha and -beta-1, respectively. This interferon was coinducible with alpha interferons in human peripheral blood lymphocytes or lymphoid cell lines (71-73). In tests done with monoclonal antibodies, this interferon, variously called omega-1 or alpha-11-I, shows no immunological cross-reactivity with recombinant alpha, beta, or gamma interferons, although it does react with polyclonal antibodies prepared against natural human leukocytic or lymphoblastic interferons (74).

Eventually, the questions of definition and classification will have to be examined at the functional-molecular level. That is, after defining the role of different parts of the interferon molecule regarding the interferon's functions and interactions with cells, and the range of variation in the molecular composition of these parts, a more rational basis for definition and classification would be available. It is likely that this enterprise would have to consider the three-dimensional structure of the interferon molecule (75) and the functions of critical sites rather than only the one-dimensional amino acid sequence.

*Phylogeny of the Interferons.* Interferons have been found in all vertebrate species that have been investigated (38). A protein(s) with several functional and physicochemical similarities with interferon has been found in plants (76,77). Computations, making use of assumptions on the constancy of mutation rates, suggest that divergence of interferon alpha genes began at least 75 millennia ago, possibly antedating the mammalian convergence, and that divergence of interferon beta from alpha took place much earlier (38). Several parts of the interferon genes have been highly conserved evolutionarily (78), as well as some sequences 5' distal to interferon alpha and beta genes (79, pp. 59-60). The ubiquity of interferons, as well as the long evolutionary conservation of areas of their genomes and of 5' distal parts significant for initiation of their transcription, suggests that interferons must have fundamental biological functions.

## C.  Production of Interferons

Knowledge of the production of interferon is relevant to the use of interferons as antineoplastic agents in several respects. First, interferon inducers are still under consideration as potential antineoplastic agents. Indeed, as discussed later, certain BRMs used against cancer, such as tumor necrosis factor (TNF) might act in part through induction of interferon. Second, the possibility of combining interferon and interferon inducers for a therapeutic effect might be considered. Third, elucidating the circumstances of the physiological production of interferons may provide clues to their biological functions.

### Production of Interferons; Effect of Inducers

*Diversity of Inducers and Producing Cells.* Inducers of interferons include polyanions (viral or synthetic dsRNA, polyphosphates, polysulfates, and polycarboxylates), amines, antibiotics, bacterial endotoxin, complete viruses, bacteria, mycoplasma, chlamydiae, rickettsiae, and protozoa; inducers of interferon gamma include mitogens, specific antigens, mixed lymphocyte cultures, and antilymphocytic antibody (10,80,81). More recently, there have been reports of the induction of interferons by growth factors, such as platelet-derived growth factor (PDGF) (82), IL-1 (83), colony-stimulating factor (CSF) (84,85), TNF (86), and IL-2 (87-89), as well as leukotrienes (90,91) and calcium ionophores (92). A wide variety of cell types can be induced to produce interferons, including but not limited to fibroblasts, epithelial cells, monocytes/macrophages, various lymphocytes (93), and tumor cells. The kind of interferon produced depends in part on the cell and on the inducer. The same cell population may produce two kinds of interferons with the same inducer (94,95).

*Characteristics of the Induction of Interferons.* The induction of interferons has been studied much more extensively with synthetic dsRNA, especially polyinosinic-polycytidylic acid [poly(I).poly(C)] than with other inducers. Unless otherwise stated, the following description is based on research with these much studied inducers. Induction of interferons has the following kinetic and quantitative characteristics: (a) There is a lag of from 1 to 8 hours before interferon can be detected; the lag period depends upon the cell and the inducer. However, with some, though not all, mitogenic agents or growth factors, the lag period may be as long as 24 to 48 hours. (b) Maximum rate of interferon production is reached within 2 to 12 hours in different cell systems. (c) Interferon synthesis is switched off within several hours after induction, even in the continued presence of the inducer. (d) Induction of interferon is followed by a period of refractoriness to repeated interferon induction (hyporesponsiveness) which lasts several hours to several days. Hyporesponsiveness is less pronounced or, in a few cell systems, may not occur. (e) Treatment of interferon-producing cells with inhibitors of RNA or protein synthesis results in enhanced production of interferon (superinduction). (f) Treatment of cells with interferon a few hours before exposing them to interferon inducers shortens the lag period and increases the amount of interferon that is produced (priming) (10).

*Molecular Biology of Interferon Induction.* Studies conducted with dsRNAs, especially poly(I).poly(C), have yielded the following findings.

1. Dose-response curves are compatible with the Poisson distribution model for interferon induction by one particle of dsRNA (96).
2. Microinjected poly(I).poly(C) induces interferon production in HeLa cells. This is compatible with the hypothesis that interferon induction by poly(I).poly(C) is mediated by an intracellular target (97).
3. Human interferon beta-1 genes with several 5' distal deletion mutants were introduced in mouse cells and induced with poly(I).poly(C), providing a powerful tool to analyze the regulation of interferon production (98-102). In one system, two negative control elements were found, one of which repressed constitutive expression of the gene, while the other repressed an enhancer element responsible for the induced expression of the gene (100,101). Re-

pressor molecules attached to the two negative control elements were released within two hours after exposure to the inducer (101). Another group of workers have identified a nuclear protein which binds specifically to the interferon beta-1 upstream regulatory region (103).

4. Within 4 hours of treatment of human fibroblasts with poly(I).poly(C), some 23 new mRNAs are synthesized. This synthesis is not triggered by the interferon produced in response to poly(I).poly(C), because it occurs in the presence of cycloheximide, when interferon synthesis is markedly inhibited, and the newly synthesized polypeptides corresponding to these mRNAs are different from those found in interferon-treated cells (104).

5. In the same system, the production of interferon mRNA (but not that of other mRNAs) begins to decrease 3 hours after treatment with poly(I).poly(C) until, by 8 hours, no interferon mRNA is detectable in the cytoplasm of the treated cells. However, when induction is allowed to continue in the presence of cycloheximide, interferon mRNA continues to accumulate. This is compatible with the explanation that the termination of interferon production in this system is due to specific degradation of interferon mRNA by a regulatory protein coinduced with interferon (105,106). These observations may provide an explanation for the phenomena of induced hyporesponsiveness and superinduction.

6. In addition to its effect on transcription, dsRNA has a posttranscriptional effect in human fibroblasts, stabilizing interferon beta-1 mRNA (98).

7. Other observations are relevant to priming. When HeLa cells, which are poorly inducible by poly(I).poly(C), were fused with highly inducible mouse cells, the heterokaryons became highly inducible by poly(I).poly(C) for the production of human beta-1 interferon (102). This suggests that certain cells have a factor necessary for interferon induction which is missing in other cells. Whether this factor is induced by interferon in these cells remains to be determined. Priming by interferon was associated with an increased level of novel mRNAs in poly(I).poly(C) induced cells (105).

These studies have been conducted mainly in one system namely, induction of interferon beta-1 with poly(I).poly(C) in human fibroblasts. While they cannot be generalized to other systems, such as Newcastle disease virus systems (106), they do provide a model for interferon induction at the molecular level. It is of considerable interest that this model, with its repressive transcriptional control of constitutive as well as induced interferon production and its posttranscriptional control of the duration of interferon production, allows for strong control and limited duration of the interferon response.

Constitutive Production of Interferons

Constitutive interferon production has been engineered in bacteria or eukaryotic cells by the insertion of recombinant interferon cDNA with its promoter elements and without repressive sequences (e.g., Refs. 78, 100,101). Natural production of interferon in in vitro cell systems has been observed in the absence of added inducers. Whether it is due to constitutive production or induced production triggered by endogenous inducers has not been established yet. For instance, several cell lines produce interferon during logarithmic growth but not during the lag phase, irrespective of initial cell population density (107). This is compatible with constitutive production interrupted by a repressor during the lag phase, or with production triggered by an endogenous inducer whose concentration builds up during the lag phase. The cyclic elevation in level of interferon and interferon-induced proteins during the cell cycle in synchronized mouse fibroblasts (32) is open to similar interpretations. Posttranscriptional events might also play a role in such cyclic variation.

## Physiological Production of Interferons

Physiological production of interferons might represent a constitutive production or an induced production in response to endogenous inducers or common exogenous inducers. For instance, 1% and 3.5% of adult and newborn blood mononuclear cells, respectively, contain gamma interferon (26). This might mean that a small fraction of the cells produce gamma interferon continuously, or that most cells produce interferon cyclically during a small part of the cell cycle, or a small fraction of the cells has been induced exogenously or endogenously to produce interferon. However, the cells may also contain interferon because they have internalized circulating interferon rather than produced it.

Recently, the use of RNA blot hybridization with interferon nucleic acid probes of high specific activity has provided a sensitive method to detect and measure the amount of specific interferon mRNA molecular species in organs or tissues of normal individuals. Interferon-alpha-1 and -2 mRNAs have been detected with this method in human liver, kidney, spleen, and peripheral blood leukocytes, but no interferon beta-1, alpha-4,5,6,7,8, or 14, or gamma mRNAs were found (except for one case with interferon gamma mRNA in the spleen) (108). Again, such interferon mRNA may have been produced constitutively or inductively by the cells which contained it, or internalized by these cells. A method for detecting interferon mRNA in individual cells by in situ hybridization with specific interferon DNA probes has been used to demonstrate interferon mRNA in uninduced cells (109). This method might well become an important tool to identify cells containing interferon mRNA in normal organs and tissues.

## D.  Biological Activities of Interferons

### Initial Interactions with Cells

The initial interaction of interferons with cells involves their binding to the cell membrane at the site of high affinity receptors (110), as well as other sites with much lower affinity (nonspecific binding). The type I interferon receptor is coded in humans by the IFRC locus on chromosome 21 (reviewed in Ref. 111). The type II interferon receptor is coded by chromosome 6. However, following binding of interferon gamma to the type II receptor, a second event is needed, which requires chromosome 21, before interferon gamma can exert one of its biological actions, the induction of the class I major histocompatibility antigen HLA (112). Kinetic studies of the binding of interferon-alpha-2 to its membrane receptors on Daudi cells showed a biphasic process, where the second, slower step, was associated with a much higher affinity. It was suggested that the first step might involve binding of interferon to the receptor, and the second might involve transfer of interferon to an activation complex on the cell membrane (113).

Tracer and electron microscopic studies show that following binding, interferons are internalized and their receptors are down-regulated (114-117). Internalization takes place by receptor-mediated endocytosis (117,118). In L929 fibroblasts, internalization of beta interferon is followed by binding of this interferon or its fragments to nuclear membrane receptors (118) and transport into the nucleus within 3 minutes after contact with the cell surface (119).

Two models have been proposed for the transmission of the interferon signal. According to the first model, exogenous interferon reacts with cell surface receptors to elicit the release of "second messenger(s)" which carry the signal into the cell. Evidence for this model includes (a) the prevention of the antiviral effect when specific anti-interferon antibody is added to the cell population in which interferon is produced, (b) induction of the antiviral state by interferon bound to particles that do not enter the cell, (c) the inability to induce the antiviral effect when interferon is microinjected into the cell (120), and (d) elicitation of the antiviral state or induction of 2-5A synthetase by interferon in the presence of agents that inhibit its internalization (114). The putative messenger for alpha or beta interferon is unknown. It does not appear to be cAMP or cGMP (121) nor $Ca^{2+}$ (122). The signal transduction system that involves the breakdown of phosphatidylinositol 4,5 biphosphate into diacylglycerol and inositol triphosphate which act as second messengers to activate protein kinase C and mobilize intracellular calcium has recently been implicated in the mediation of several effects of interferon gamma on macrophages (122a).

According to the second model, internalized interferon or its fragments would themselves carry the signal into the nucleus. The evidence for the transport of interferon or its immunologically specific fragments into the cell nucleus (119) is compatible with this model. A recently described system provides some support for this model. A mouse cell line was transformed by a truncated human gamma interferon DNA lacking the sequence for the signal peptide which is needed for secretion of interferon, so that interferon accumulates intracellularly. These cells exhibit resistance to viral infection and other characteristics of interferon-treated cells (122b).

In summary, there is support for both models. There may be different mechanisms for the transmission of the interferon signal in different cell systems or with different interferons. It is also conceivable that the mode of interferon signal transmission differs for different biological actions of interferon. Thus, one possible explanation for the conflicting results might be that interferons (or their degradation fragments) might have several points of impact on the cell: at the cell membrane, and additionally, at the nuclear membrane or at other intracellular sites. Different messengers or mediators might be involved at the different sites.

### E.  Biological Effects of Interferons: Molecular Level

The activity of several enzyme systems and the amounts of several cell proteins are changed after treatment with interferons (reviewed in Refs. 123 and 124). These effects are dependent upon the cell as well as the interferon species. For instance, in one system, interferon gamma induced 24 proteins, only 12 of which were induced by interferons alpha or beta (125). On the other hand, interferon alpha or beta, but not gamma, induced the Mx protein (126) or Ind-1 and Ind-2 proteins (122).

Several mechanisms may be involved in the molecular effects of interferons, for example, activation or inhibition of enzymes, induction or suppression of transcription, increased or decreased turnover of mRNA, enhancement or inhibition of translation, increased or decreased turnover of proteins. Such effects may require (or be inhibited by) other factors provided by the cell. Interferon may exert its effects directly through a messenger, or indirectly by inducing proteins which would mediate the effects. There is evidence supporting most of these mechanisms in various biological systems. In this section, we shall discuss only a few mechanisms which have been recently elucidated or which are of critical relevance to neoplasms.

### Stimulation of Transcription of Specific Genes by Interferons

In the early 1980s, several investigators had shown that interferon-treated cells had several new or increased mRNA species and proteins. By 1983-1984, cDNA clones had been isolated which were complementary to mRNAs unique to or increased in interferon-treated cells (122,127,128). Furthermore, unique mRNAs were detected within 4- minutes of exposure of cells to interferons (129). This set the stage for study of the mechanisms of induction of new mRNAs by interferon. Three main tools were used. Specific cDNA probes were used to detect and quantify the induced mRNA. The transcription rate of nascent-labeled mRNA in isolated nuclei was measured by annealing the labeled mRNA with specific cDNA. Protein synthesis inhibitors, such as cycloheximide, were used to ascertain whether synthesis of new protein was a factor in the induction of the new mRNAs, and also to find if proteins were synthesized which might affect the intracellular level of the specific interferon-induced mRNAs.

With this battery of techniques, several groups of investigators, working with different interferon-induced mRNA species found that (a) the rate of transcription of the new mRNA rose within 5 to 10 minutes after exposure to interferon and reached a maximum by 30 to 60 minutes (122,130,131); (b) in some instances such as with Ind-1, Ind-2 (122) or protein 1-8 (130), the rate of transcription decreased after some 6-12 hours and the cell became "desensitized" (i.e., it failed to respond to a second treatment with interferon) for as long as 48-72 hours. In other instances, such as 2-A, an mRNA with marked homology to that of an HLA antigen, transcription continued at a high rate for over 24 hours, (c) studies with cycloheximide showed that interferon stimulated the synthesis of a protein(s) which, after a few hours, inhibited transcription of the specific interferon-induced mRNAs but not that of other mRNAs, such as actin (132).

The discovery that a given interferon molecular species induces the transcription of several genes raised the possibility that a common nucleotide sequence responsive to interferon might be involved. Searches undertaken with interferon alpha for such element yielded highly related nucleotide sequences upstream of the 5' end of human HLA and metallothionein genes (133). Sequences partly homologous to this sequence were found in the promoter regions of a number of mouse class I histocompatibility genes (134-137) and the mouse cDNA clone 202 (138,139). However, an unrelated interferon alpha-responsive nucleotide sequence upstream of the gene of the 15 kD protein induced that gene (140-141) and another unrelated sequence in the promoter region of a major histocompatibility complex (MHC) class II gene was responsible for activation of that gene by interferon gamma (141a). Thus, with only a few of the interferon-activated genes examined so far, there appear to be at least three interferon-sensitive nucleotide enhancer sequences.

At least two of these sequences have the characteristics of an inducible enhancer since they are capable of conferring interferon-induced enhancement of the promoter irrespective of orientation (137,139,141). Gene activation by the interferon-sensitive sequences may be enhanced (137) or it may require (135) additional genetic elements. The demonstration of several interferon-responsive gene-activator sequences as well as the requirement of additional elements in some instances could provide a framework for the modulation of the set of interferon-induced proteins in different cells or in response to different interferon molecular species.

The biological functions of some of the proteins induced by interferons are known. The 2-5A synthetase and DsRNA-dependent protein kinase have functions related to the antiviral effect. The histocompatibility antigens type I induced by alpha, beta, and gamma interferons (133-137) and type II, induced by interferon gamma only (141a) have functions in cell recognition and immunological responses. The metallothioneins (133) play a role in heavy metal binding, free-radical scavenging, and resistance to radiation damage. Ubiquitin, which is partly homologous with the interferon-induced 15 kD protein (142) is one of the most highly conserved eukaryotypic proteins. It readily adducts to other proteins and it has been suggested that it may function inside the nucleus in regulating chromatin structure and outside the nucleus in modulating the function of various membrane-bound or soluble cytoplasmic proteins (reviewed in Ref. 142). Other interferon-induced proteins are enzymes for reactions involved in the metabolism of amino acids (143,144). A very large additional set of metabolic effects of interferons or of interferon inducers which have not yet been elucidated at the molecular genetic level have been reviewed (124).

Many of the mRNAs and corresponding proteins induced by interferons are present, at lower concentrations, in untreated cells. Others are not detectable in untreated cells but this does not rule out their being produced below detectable levels. It is possible that endogenous interferon might induce these proteins in untreated cells. Studies of 2-5A synthetase reported above would be compatible with this possibility. However, proteins such as metallothionein have several other known inducers besides interferon.

The relationships between the interferon-induced mRNAs or proteins and neoplastic diseases is not known. Inspection of the functions of these proteins readily brings to mind hypothetical ways in which deficiency of endogenous interferon may promote neoplastic changes or in which administration of interferons may enhance defenses against neoplastic processes, but there is little relevant experimental evidence.

Selective Inhibition of Protein Synthesis by Interferons

Interferons may inhibit the synthesis of specific proteins via specific inhibition of RNA transcription, increased RNA turnover, or inhibition of translation. In some instances, some molecular forms of enzymes are induced while other forms of the same enzymes are suppressed (144). The 2-5A synthetase induced by interferons contributes to inhibition of protein synthesis by providing the 2-5 oligonucleotides necessary for the activation of ribonuclease L.

An important inhibitory role of interferons is mediated by the induction or activation of proteins which inhibit with some specificity, after a given time interval, the induction of specific mRNAs by interferons (132). This provides a mechanism for regulation of the duration and extent of induction of new mRNAs and their proteins.

*Inhibition of Oncogenes.* Interferon alpha or beta inhibits c-*myc* RNA and protein (145-149) and *ras* oncogene products (150). The effects of interferons on oncogenes may be complex. Interferons may enhance the expression of some oncogenes while suppressing that of others in the same cell population (151).

Because the activation of cellular oncogenes may be a factor in the development of human neoplasms (152), the ability of interferons to selectively suppress certain oncogenes might be an important factor in their antineoplastic actions.

Effects on Growth Factors and Lymphokines

Growth factors may play a role in the activation of cellular oncogenes and other molecules in various physiological or pathological conditions (153,154). Therefore, the interaction of interferons with growth factors might be relevant to normal growth and differentiation as well as neoplastic diseases. Platelet-derived growth factor (PDGF) is one of the serum constituents which confer on resting $3T_3$ cells the ability to reenter the cell cycle and undergo DNA synthesis. For this reason it is sometimes called a "competence factor." PDGF directly activates the expression of several genes, including the oncogenes c-*fos* and c-*myc* and the gene of the first enzyme in polyamine biosynthesis, ornithine decarboxylase (ODC) and of beta-actin. Induction of c-*fos* by PDGF is maximal at 10-20 minutes and decreases thereafter. Mouse interferon alpha/beta inhibited the PDGF-activated expression of c-*fos*, ODC, and beta-actin in the absence of protein synthesis and that of c-*myc* through a process that required protein synthesis (155). The action of PDGF is self-limited under physiological or benign pathological conditions, as one would expect. In this connection, it is recalled that PDGF and dsRNA stimulate expression of the same genes in 3T3 cells, including dsRNA-induced interferons (82). More recent work has shown that PDGF-treatment of cells increases the expression of at least two growth inhibitors, transforming growth factor-beta and interferon-beta-2 (Heldin, cited in Ref. 154). Thus, interferon alpha and beta appear to participate in the feedback inhibition of oncogene activation by PDGF.

The effects of interferons on the expression of lymphokines often depend upon the type of cell treated with interferon, the type of interferon used, and other factors. For instance, interferon alpha augments the lipopolysaccharide (LPS) -induced production of interleukin-1 (IL-1) and prevents prostaglandin E2 (PGE-2) suppression of LPS-induced IL-1 production in mouse peritoneal cells, while, in the same system, interferon gamma markedly inhibits LPS-stimulated IL-1 production (156). However, in other macrophage/monocyte systems, interferon gamma stimulated IL-1 production (reviewed in Ref. 152). Future work should elucidate the relation of the stage of differentiation or activation of the monocytes and of their microenvironment to the stimulation of lymphokine production by interferons.

In one of the few investigations at the molecular genetic level, interferon gamma enhanced the transcription of tumor necrosis factor alpha (TNFα), IL-1, and urokinase-type plasminogen activator genes which were shown to be under the control of short-lived repressors in mouse peritoneal macrophages (157).

Effects on Receptors

Treatment of Marbin-Darby bovine kidney cells with human alpha-2 interferon resulted in a dose-dependent decrease in number and ligand affinity of epidermal growth factor (EGF) receptors as well as inhibition of cell multiplication. Human beta or gamma interferons had no such effects (158). PDGF, which is an interferon inducer, causes a transient reduction in EGF receptor number and affinity (reviewed in Ref. 158).

Human interferon alpha-2 induced rearrangement of T-cell antigen receptor alpha-chain genes, and maturation to cytotoxicity in T lymphocyte precursor clones (159).

The effects of interferon on receptors may depend upon the host cell as well as the interferon species. Treatment of HeLa or HT-29 cells with interferon gamma increased the binding of tumor necrosis factor (TNF), but alpha or beta interferons had this effect only on HeLa cells (160). Interferon gamma, but not alpha or beta interferons, increased the number of TNF receptors in ME-180, another human cell line (161).

Interferon gamma induced interleukin-2 receptor (IL-2R) mRNA as well as IL-2R in human monocytes and the monocytic cell line U937 (162), but not in T lymphocytes (reviewed in Ref. 162).

### Effects of Interferons on Cell Surface Antigens

It has long been demonstrated that alpha, beta, and gamma interferons increase the expression of class I major histocompatibility (MHC) antigens and that interferon gamma increases the expression of class II MHC antigens, as well as that of surface antigens that might be specific for given tumor cell types (163). More recent reports have shown that interferons increase the expression of tumor-associated antigens, especially in human melanoma (e.g., Ref. 164) or human colon carcinoma cells (165).

These properties of interferon provide rationales for several tumor therapy approaches. In the first place, interferon treatment would be expected to increase reactivity of tumor cells with specific or nonspecific killing cells. Second, interferon treatment might enhance the effectiveness of specific monoclonal antibodies to specific tumor antigens in reacting with their target cells in diagnostic studies or in clinical trials. These approaches are currently under investigation in several laboratories.

### Other Effects of Interferons on Cell Membrane or Cytoskeleton

Treatment of human fibroblasts for three days with large amounts of interferon (640 U/ml) was followed by increased mean cell surface and volume, increased size and number of microfilament bundles, reduced motility of cells, and other changes in the cell membrane. However, it is not clear to what extent these changes represent direct effects of interferon on the cell organelles or are mediated by inhibition of cell multiplication (166).

### F.  Biological Effects of Interferons: Cellular Level

### Effects on Cell Proliferation

The interferons have several inhibitory effects on the cell cycle (reviewed in Refs. 123,167). They fall into two groups (123, p. 349): inhibition of the $G_0/G_1$ transition and prolongation or even inhibition of various phases of the cell cycle.

Both effects have considerable significance for oncologists. The former effect is of particular interest since one of the characteristics of many neoplasms is a decreased $G_0$ cell pool or increased $G_0/G_1$ transition. The 3T3-PDGF system has been used extensively to study the interactions among PDGF, c-*fos*, c-*myc*, polyamine metabolism, and interferons in relation to the $G_0/G_1$ transition (v.s.). It would be of interest to extend such studies to a number of human neoplastic cell types.

Also in the 3T3-PDGF system, interferon-beta has inhibitory effects on DNA synthesis which occur late in $G_1$ and appear to be mediated by an effect of interferon on microtubules since they can be prevented by colchicine (168). Earlier, it was shown that colchicine and other antitubule agents inhibit the antigrowth effect of interferon (169). These findings might be of particular interest to experimental oncologists using interferons along with antitumor agents that are active on microtubules, such as vinblastine.

Interferon alpha selectively inhibited histone synthesis in human Daudi cells and mouse ANN-1 cells. In the same systems, up to 50% of newly labeled DNA turns over rapidly in the presence of interferon. This is consistent with the hypothesis that growth inhibition induced by interferon may be related to increased sensitivity of DNA to nucleases in nuclei partly deficient in histones (170). The delayed maturation of chromatin observed in these experiments was compared to the effect of antitumor agents such as hydroxyurea or cytosine arabinoside in inhibiting DNA replication fork movement (170). Thus, it might be of interest to study combined experimental chemotherapy with interferon and hydroxyurea or cytosine arabinoside in the light of these effects on disruption of DNA replication.

While most of the reports on the effects of interferons on cell proliferation have pointed to an inhibition, some reports, especially with interferon gamma, have provided examples of stimulation of cell proliferation. The cell type and the other BRMs that may be present in the system may considerably affect the results. For instance, a synergestic effect of recombinant IL-2 and interferon gamma on the proliferation of human monoclonal lymphocytes from a chronic B-cell lymphocytic leukemia patient has been reported (171). The enhancement of B-cell proliferation demonstrated in this report is particularly significant to oncologists, since it involved a human neoplastic cell.

Effects on Cell Differentiation

The effects of interferons on cell differentiation have been reviewed (123,172, 173). Interferons promoted cell differentiation in some systems and inhibited it in others. The transformation of fibroblasts into adipocytes (inhibited by interferon) and that of myoblasts into muscle cells (inhibited by interferon in embryonic chick myoblasts and stimulated by it in adult human myoblasts) provides instances of the effects of interferons on the differentiation of normal cells. Studies on the differentiation of a human promyelocytic leukemia, HL-60, into granulocytes (enhanced by interferon in the presence of retinoic acid) or macrophages (enhanced by interferon in the presence of conditioned medium of cells treated with phorbol ester or 2-mercaptoethanol), or of Friend leukemia cells into hemoglobin-producing cells after treatment with DMSO (enhanced or inhibited by interferon in small and large doses, respectively) are instances of the effects of interferons on the differentiation of malignant cells (reviewed in more detail in Ref. 173).

The question of the promotion of differentiation of malignant cells by interferons is of considerable importance in neoplastic diseases, because such differentiation might be accompanied by decreased proliferative activity or loss of other malignant characteristics in some instances. Further work is needed regarding the effects of interferons on the differentiation of various human neoplastic cells, at various doses of interferons and in the presence of various factors which might interact with interferon with regard to cell differentiation. This is a vast area of work which has only barely begun.

### Effects on Cell Transformation

The effect of prolonged cultivation of transformed cells in interferon-containing medium on phenotypic markers of malignancy has been the subject of only a few studies since the demonstration in 1970 of phenotypic reversion of murine sarcoma virus (MSV)-transformed mouse fibroblasts after prolonged interferon treatment (174). MSV arose by recombination of Moloney murine leukemia virus with murine *mos* sequences. The transformed cell line is productively infected with the virus. After some 600 cell generations in presence of 50 U/ml of mouse alpha/beta interferon, the transformed line displayed the orderly growth, flat morphology, lack of colony formation in agar, and failure to produce tumors in nude mice which are considered as markers of nonmalignancy. Unexpectedly, the nonmalignant revertant DNA contained an increased number of v-*mos* sites and twice as many copies of the oncogene as in the malignant transformed line's DNA. However, the nonmalignant revertants produced helper MSV but no detectable *mos*-containing virions, suggesting that a posttranscriptional block in the v-*mos* gene had occurred (175). The revertant remained stable during further cultivation in the absence of interferon. Study of the interferon system of the transformed and revertant cells showed that the nonmalignant revertant was producing interferon constitutively at a much higher level than comparison mouse cell lines (176). Therefore, it is possible that the block of the v-*mos* gene was related to the constitutional production of interferon.

In the second system, a human *ras* oncogene transformed a 3T3 cell line into a line with the usual markers of malignancy. The transformed line was cultivated for at least one to two months and cloned in the presence of 200 U/ml of mouse interferon alpha/beta, to yield cultures which were phenotypically alike. These revertant clones retained the transforming c-Ha-*ras* DNA activated by a retroviral long terminal repeat, but they showed a reduced level of *ras* mRNA and protein. They remained stable after interferon treatment was discontinued (177). The persistent revertants cultivated without interferon showed a high level of *ras* protein and were resistant to transformation by RNA tumor viruses bearing the oncogenes v-Ki-*ras*, v-Ha-*ras*, v-*abl*, or v-*fes*, but they were transformed by v-*mos*. Furthermore, they were readily transformed by 5-azacytidine, which alters gene expression by inhibiting DNA methylation (178).

These studies have considerable interest in view of the possibility that they raise that prolonged interferon treatment may revert the malignant phenotype of tumors. In this respect, it may be desirable to use prolonged interferon treatment in clinical trials. They also show that the interaction of interferons with transformed cells that might result in reversion is complex. It is not merely a matter of inhibiting an oncogene. Rather, the interactions of oncogenes with other cellular factors which lead to the expression of the transformed state need to be studied. Finally, as pointed out, (178) they introduce a note of caution, since demethylating drugs such as those used for retransformation in the second system are used in cancer chemotherapy.

## Cell Killing

Very little work has been done to determine if, and in what conditions, interferons might be capable of killing cells directly. Liver necrosis was caused by interferon alpha/beta in vivo in newborn mice (179). Low concentrations (10 to 100 U/ml) of interferon gamma killed murine epidermoid carcinoma cells in monolayer cultures but not in sparsely populated cell cultures (180). Massive necrosis was observed in cells or organotypic cultures of a human epidermoid carcinoma cell line after 2 to 6 days of continuous exposure to 200 U/ml of interferon gamma (181). It is not clear from the descriptions provided whether cell population killing in those instances was of a nearly all-or-none nature (as might occur in a cell-to-cell propagated disturbance in the high cell density systems involved) or whether there were graded lesions.

## Effects of Interferons on Specialized Cells

There is a large literature on the effects of interferons on function or growth of various cell types. We shall mention here only the work which is most pertinent to neoplasms of the bone marrow and lymphoid tissues.

*Effects of Interferons on Hematopoietic Progenitor Cells.* The myelosuppressive effect of interferons is relevant to neoplastic studies both absolutely (with regard to toxicity of administered interferon) and relatively (with regard to relative responses of neoplastic and non-neoplastic cells). Granulocytic progenitor cells from normal and leukemic donors were inhibited to a comparable degree by interferon-alpha or -beta (182).

*Effects of Interferons on Osteoclasts.* Osteoclasts participate in the resorption of bone in the osteolytic lesions associated with several cancers. Therefore, the recently published evidence that interferon gamma inhibits formation of osteoclast-like cells (183) and bone resorption (reviewed in Ref. 184) opens a new approach to control of neoplastic osteolytic lesions. Further work needs to be done to determine if this effect is shared by alpha or beta interferons and how it is affected by other cytokines.

*Effects of Interferons on Endothelial Cells.* Endothelial cells play a role in the vascularization of tumors, the transport of metabolites to tumor cells, the adhesion and emigration of monocyte and other leukocytes, and the presentation of antigens. Studies undertaken recently show that interferons participate in a network of interactions involving endothelial cells—for instance the enhancement by interferon gamma of the production of IL-1 by lipopolysaccharide-stimulated endothelial cells (184).

*Effects of Interferons on Monocytes/Macrophages.* In contrast to endothelial cells, there have been extensive studies with macrophages, including studies of the effects of interferons on the differentiation of monocytes into macrophages and on modification of macrophage functions (185). Among effects of interest to cancer researchers are the stimulation of phagocytosis, priming of macrophages for nonspecific tumoricidal action, enhancement of macrophage oxidative metabolism, enhancement of intracellular cytocidal action of macrophages, and the expression of Ia (human) or DR (mouse) antigens and thereby of antigen presentation. Some of these effects are unique to interferon gamma, while others such as phagocytosis and tumoricidal effects are shared with interferon-beta but appear to involve different mechanisms (reviewed in Ref. 185).

*Effects on Cytotoxic Effector Cells.* The effects of interferons on cytotoxic immune T cells as well as natural killer (NK) cells have been extensively reviewed (e.g., Ref. 186).

*Modulation of Antibody Response.* Enhancement or suppression of antibody response by interferons dependent upon dose of interferon, antigen, the cell populations involved, and interactions with other cytokines has been extensively reviewed (e.g., Ref. 187).

*Effects on Cell-Mediated Immunity.* The effects of interferon on cell-mediated immunity which are of considerable significance for neoplastic diseases have been extensively reviewed (e.g., Ref. 188).

## III.  CLINICAL STUDIES

Therapeutic studies with interferons in humans were started as early as the 1960s (189), but they were not followed up. The main impetus for human trial was provided by the demonstration of a protective effect of interferons against murine tumors by Gresser in 1969. The preparation of human leukocytic interferons in large quantities by Cantell and co-workers was another requirement for the initiation of significant clinical studies that was accomplished early in the 1970s. This was followed by the First Scandinavian clinical trials (190) with osteosarcomas in the mid-1970s and by small-scale trials with other neoplasms in Scandinavian and other countries. Encouraging results with these studies led to the larger scale American Cancer Society clinical trials with natural leukocytic interferon and British trials with lymphoblastic interferon (Wellferon) in the early 1980s.

In the meantime, cloned alpha, beta, and gamma interferons had become available and large-scale production of recombinant interferon alpha, especially what is now known as alpha-2, was undertaken by pharmaceutical companies such as Hoffman-LaRoche and Schering in the early 1980s. Thus in the first half of the 1980s, large-scale clinical trials were conducted with recombinant as well as natural alpha interferons with a wide variety of neoplasms. As usual in such trials, the initial (Phase 1) trials aimed at defining the pharmacodynamics and toxicity of the preparations, with secondary observation of short-term clinical outcomes. These were followed by Phase II trials of to define the most appropriate therapeutic regimens and to initially assess short-term and longer term clinical response, in order to select the most appropriate regimens and tumor types for controlled long-term comparisons with other antitumor agents in Phase III trials.

By mid-1987, Phase I and II trials had been done with several alpha interferons, and selected Phase III studies were undertaken. Less extensive Phase I and a few Phase II studies had been conducted with interferon-gamma. Very few studies were done with interferon beta, most of these were done in Europe or Japan. Several Phase I studies had been undertaken and reports were beginning to appear in 1987 of Phase I studies of interferon alpha or gamma in combination with other interferons or with chemotherapeutic agents and of chemically modified interferons. Studies with alpha interferons were given a further impetus when the FDA granted approval of Roferon and Intron (two interferon-alpha preparations) for the treatment of hairy cell leukemia.

Since, at the present time, most of the studies reported have been done with alpha interferons, this review will be limited to studies with alpha interferons unless stated otherwise.


The material in the following sections is presented according to neoplasm. The reason is that each neoplasm has specific biological features, clinical course, and response to chemotherapy and other treatments which must be considered in assessing the current and potential roles of interferon in its treatment.

Notwithstanding the uniqueness of each neoplasm, there are some general concepts and approaches that cut across the whole field of neoplastic diseases.

*The first*, which has already been discussed, is the division of clinical trials into four phases. At present, only alfa interferons have had extensive Phase II clinical trials.

*The second general concept* concerns the parameters of effectiveness of therapy. These parameters fall under four rubrics: response, duration of response including disease-free interval, survival time, and quality of life. Responses are generally classified as complete response (CR), partial response (PR), minimal response (MR), mixed response (MXR), stable disease (SD), and progressive disease (PD), on the basis of measurements of a stated, quantifiable parameter, such as the product of two diameters of a tumor mass, the number or percentage of neoplastic cells in a tissue section or a blood smear, the amount in the blood, or other body fluid, of a substance secreted specifically by the tumor cells, and so on. CR means that no tumor can be detected with the parameters that are used; PR means a 50% or greater reduction in the measure of the stated parameter; CRs and PRs are usually scored only if they last for a given minimum duration such as four weeks; CR and PR are combined in some reports as "objective response." MR means a 25-50% reduction in the measure of the stated parameter. MXR means that some tumors are regressing and other progressing in the same individual. SD means that the measure of the parameter varies within ± 25% of its initial measure during a stated period of time, usually at least four weeks. The significance of SD depends upon the evolution of the tumor prior to the therapy under test: if the tumor was rapidly progressing, SD might be therapeutically significant; on the other hand, if the tumor growth was relatively slow to start with, SD would be equivalent to no change. PD means that the measure of the parameter has increased by 25% or more during the period of observation. The score no response (NR) is sometimes used; it means that the tumor is evolving at the same rate as before therapy.

The duration of response refers to the disease-free interval following a CR, or to the interval during which a PR, MR, or SD is maintained. Recurrence following cessation of therapy (recurrent disease) is due to the proliferation of remaining tumor cells; this is understandable since CR means only disappearance of detectable tumor cells and there may still be millions of tumor cells in the body, below the level of detectability. Recurrence or progression of a neoplasm during treatment may be due to acquisition of resistance to the therapeutic agent by the tumor cells (refractory disease) or to inactivation of the therapeutic agent in the body of the patient, for instance because of the development of antibodies to that agent. Since there may be $10^{12}$ or more tumor cells at the beginning of therapy, the probability that one or more tumor cells in the body will mutate to become resistant to the therapeutic agent is high, even though the probability of such a mutation per cell is very low. Because of the relatively high number of tumor cells that may remain in the body after CR and the high probability of a mutation to resistance to the chemotherapeutic agent, cytocidal-agent chemotherapy adopts a strategy of maximal tumor cytoreduction in which series of courses of several agents are given at or near the maximal tolerated dose. However, this need not be the best therapeutic strategy with BRMs, since the optimal therapeutic dose might be well below the maximal tolerated dose and eradication of the tumor cell population might not always be the overriding goal.

Survival time addresses the threat of death from not only the tumor but also iatrogenic consequences of antitumor therapy and intercurrent disease. The cumulative proportion surviving through a given interval of time is estimated with the life-table or Kaplan-Meier methods. Quality of life is another significant feature of survival. Quality of life addresses the utility of survival time for the affected person. Its measurement is more complex than that of the other parameters. Disease-specific instruments to assess quality of life or compare it across different therapeutic options have been developed. Because it is still relatively young, interferon literature emphasizes response and duration of response to a greater extent than survival time and quality of life.

*The third general concept* concerns the time required by an agent to achieve its therapeutic effect. In conventional cytocidal cancer therapy, cell killing presumably occurs within a very short time after the administration of the agent. However, with interferons, there is evidence (which will be presented in detail later in this chapter) that it may take, at least in certain instances, weeks or months of ongoing therapy to achieve maximum antitumor effect. This point must be considered in deciding on the duration of the test therapy and on the time when its effect will be scored. With regard to duration of the therapy that is being tested, disease that progresses during therapy presents a dilemma: on the one hand, one would like to give the patient the benefit of a possibly delayed therapeutic effect; on the other hand, one would want to give the patient the benefit of alternative therapies that might prove more effective. In general, this dilemma has been resolved in most studies in favor of the second option, that is, interferon therapy is terminated when disease progression is observed or shortly afterward. With regard to a PR or CR, there are two options: interferon therapy may be continued indefinitely, unless resistance to interferon or untoward effects develop, or, interferon therapy may be stopped to observe the duration of the response after discontinuation of treatment. With regard to SD, investigators usually set a time limit (which may range from one month to four months or longer) before discontinuing interferon therapy.

The results of interferon therapeutic trials are often scored and reported at several time intervals after the onset of therapy. In some instances, the results may be scored after a very brief period of therapy (e.g., 4 or 6 weeks); such data are likely to be found in abstracts or preliminary communications at scientific meetings. When the response is scored after a longer period of time (e.g., 4 or 8 months), the PDs and in some instances the SDs are scored as of the time when these patients' therapy was discontinued. In follow-up studies over long intervals of time, progression of response may occur (e.g., a MR may become a PR), as well as regression of response. In the latter instance, some investigators may present the maximal response, while others report the response at the end of the period of observation. In rare instances, a response may be delayed till after the therapy has been discontinued. For these reasons, studies of the same cohort of patients published at different time intervals may differ in response rates and duration of response.

*Fourth*, patient selection for the trials requires some consideration. The patient population is in general heterogeneous. Within the same general disease category, for example, carcinoma of the breast, there may be several histologically or pathologically distinct entities; conversely, certain pathologically distinct entities may be lumped into one category (e.g., non-Hodgkins' lymphoma). Even within a pathologically homogeneous group, there may be differences in the indolence-aggressiveness dimension among different patients; this may be reflected by the time interval between diagnosis and therapeutic trial in previously untreated patients. The previous treatment history of the patient may also be an important variable. Previously untreated patient populations may in some instances be biased toward more indolent cases. On the other hand, patients who relapsed following previous successful therapy or patients who were refractory to previous therapy, may be at a stage of evolution of the disease when the original tumor cell population may have been replaced by a more aggressive one or when body defense mechanisms which may have played an important adjuvant role in the initial therapy may be significantly weakened. The total tumor load in the body, staging classification of the tumor and localization of the tumor in the body are variables that might also significantly affect the response to therapy. The general functional status of the patient, as reflected by the Karnofsky index or other measure may also affect the response to therapy.

Finally, attrition of patient populations during the therapeutic trial may present some methodological problems. The initial patient population, the "n" of the study, may be reduced by deaths from the tumor, its complications or intercurrent disease; withdrawal of patients from therapy may occur because of therapeutic agent toxicity or for some other patient decision. If these losses have occurred before the end of a minimum duration of therapy, the effect of therapy on these cases cannot be evaluated. Additional cases may be disqualified because they do not meet criteria for inclusion in the study in the first place or because of a failure to carry through the necessary evaluation procedures. This leaves a smaller, "evaluable" patient population, the "$n_{eval}$" of the study. There is some controversy concerning the denominator that should be used, n or $n_{eval}$, in reporting response rates. In an overall therapeutic assessment of an agent and comparison with other agents, n might be more appropriate. However, early in the course of studies with an agent (as in the instance of interferons at present) when one of the main questions is whether the agent has therapeutic efficacy and against what tumors, the use of $n_{eval}$ might provide a more sensitive indicator.

## IV. NEOPLASMS OF MYELOID AND LYMPHOID TISSUES

The neoplasms discussed below are all derived from the lineages of a single cell type, the pluripotent stem cell which gives rise to lymphoid and myeloid stem cells. The lymphoid stem cells give rise to the B- and T-lymphocyte lineages. The myeloid stem cells give rise to granulocytic, monocytic, erythrocytic, and mega-karyocytic lineages. The various stages of differentiation along the different lineages can be identified with batteries of monoclonal antibodies against surface antigens that appear or disappear as cell differentiation progresses (191,192) and by enzyme and other markers.

Cell surface markers provide a rationale for an initial classification of the neoplasms of myeloid and lymphoid tissues. It should be clear, however, that the proliferative cell pool of the neoplasm usually belongs to a stem cell population which is at an earlier stage of differentiation but is already committed to differentiation leading to the characteristic cell type of that particular neoplasm.

Along the lymphocyte B lineage (going from least to most differentiated cell), the cells of non-T acute lymphoblastic leukemias correspond to progenitor B, pre-B or, when they are most differentiated, early B cells; those of chronic lymphocytic leukemia and small-cell lymphocytic lymphoma correspond to intermediate B cells; those of prolymphocytic leukemia and follicular and diffuse small-cleaved and large-cell lymphomas correspond to mature B cells; and, hairy cell leukemia cells have markers of pre-plasma cells, while Waldenstrom's macroglobulinemia and multiple myeloma cells have markers of plasmacytoid and plasma cells, respectively. Similarly, along the T-cell lineage, the cells of T-acute lymphoblastic leukemias range from early thymocyte to early mature thymocyte; those of T-lymphoproliferative disease and some T-chronic lymphocytic leukemias have markers of mature T-suppressor cells, while those of adult T-cell leukemia, cutaneous T-cell lymphomas, peripheral T-cell lymphomas, and some T-cell chronic leukemias have markers of mature T-helper cells. In the myeloblastic series, the cells of acute myeloblastic leukemia have markers of myeloid stem cells or myeloblasts, while those of chronic myelocytic leukemias have markers of mature cells in the chronic phase, giving way to a variety of more immature and, eventually, blast cells as the disease progresses (191,192).

Neoplasms of lymphoid or myeloid tissues also vary with respect to the aggressiveness of the disease. They exhibit a wide range of variability, from very indolent neoplasms such as certain nodular lymphomas (where untreated cases may survive for several decades) to certain acute leukemias (where a fatal outcome may occur in a matter of weeks). Even within a category of neoplasms, there may be much variation in the aggressivity of the disease. Furthermore, many neoplasms of lymphoid and myeloid tissues show sequential replacement of more indolent by more aggressive cell populations, especially, but not only, after courses of chemotherapy.

The proliferative advantage of myeloid or lymphoid neoplastic cells is *not* due to faster progression through the cell cycle. The duration of the S phase or of the entire cell cycle is usually the same as or longer than that of analogous normal cells. However, the neoplastic cell progenitors have a greater probability of $G_0/G_1$ transition than their normal counterparts or a lesser probability of entering $G_0$ following completion of a cell cycle. Pluripotent or partially committed stem cells have a probability of differentiation after the next cell division which may differ in normal and neoplastic cells (193,194). These transitions are controlled by diffusible substances which may be growth promoting or inhibitory or induce differentiation.

The microenvironment of hematopoietic cells offers opportunities for interactions not only among cells in the hematopoietic lineage, but also between these cells and other cells such as fibroblasts, osteoclasts, and fat cells in the bone marrow, reticular cells in the marrow and lymph nodes or epithelial cells in the thymus (195). Interactions between neoplastic and non-neoplastic hematopoietic cells may have an effect on the non-neoplastic cells, such as the inhibition of normal hematopoiesis in response to increased mass of neoplastic cells (196) or the stimulation of osteoclasts by myeloma cells (p. 229), or on neoplastic cells, such as the induction of differentiation-like changes in neoplastic cells by non-neoplastic cells or their products (e.g., Ref. 197). This complex system of interactions has to be taken into account in analyzing the effects of interferons on hematological neoplasms.

The development and evolution of hematological neoplasms is a dynamic process. Three critical points need to be distinguished along the hematopoietic lineage of the neoplastic cell, namely the point where the initial oncogenic event occurs; the point where proliferation of progenitors of the neoplastic cell population takes place; and the point where neoplastic cells accumulate. These events usually have differing locations on the hematological lineage. Furthermore, there often is not a unique population of neoplastic cells. Rather, there is a succession of different populations, usually showing increasing aggressiveness. The possibility of sequential activation of different oncogenes has been discussed earlier. Chromosome studies of neoplastic lymphoid and myeloid cells throw some light on the subject, as many of these neoplasms have characteristic translocations, in some instances involving the sites of known oncogenes. Additional translocations sometimes occur in association with increased aggressiveness of the neoplasm (198-200). The dynamic nature of the neoplasm's evolution must also be taken into account in analyzing the effects of interferons on hematological neoplasms.

Finally, some consideration must be given to factors affecting the life span of the neoplastic cell. Lymphoid and myeloid cells have a characteristic life span, in part related to the probability of clearance of these cells in the spleen and other sites. Changes in the efficiency of clearance by the host, as well as changes in the resistance of the neoplastic cell to clearance, may also play an important role in the evolution of the neoplasm. This is another area of concern in analyzing the effects of interferon therapy.

## A. Hairy Cell Leukemia

Hairy cell leukemia (HCL), a neoplasm initially described as leukemic reticulo-endotheliosis (201), derives its name from the "hairy cells" (HC) which infiltrate the bone marrow, spleen, and, in some instances, the blood of patients with the disease. These cells have a characteristic morphology (202,203) and a specific tartrate-resistant acid phosphatase (TRAP) (204). Their surface shows many long microvilli containing actin-rich filaments, which give the cell its hairy appearance (205,206).

It is now well established that in all but a few cases of HCL,* the HC have several characteristics of B lymphocytes, namely synthesis of IgG (207), B-cell-associated or -restricted surface markers (208,209), and evidence of rearrangement of light as well as heavy chain genes (210). Along the B-cell lineage, HC have more mature markers than other lymphocytic leukemia cells (211) and they have the PCA1 but not the PC1 markers of plasma cells, suggesting that their normal counterparts are preplasma cells (212). Several lines of evidence suggest that HCL is a tumor of already activated B cells: HC respond to phytohemagglutinin-lymphocyte-conditioned medium, PHA-LCM, like activated B cells (212); some monoclonal antibodies prepared against HC are inactive against resting B cells but react with activated B cells (208); HC have the Tac receptor for the T-cell growth factor, IL-2, though in lesser amounts than T cells (213) as do some normal activated B cells (213,214).

Hairy cells can be induced to proliferate in vitro by a B-cell growth factor (BCFG) (215). This finding is especially significant since HC have BCGF-like activity in their cytosol and secrete a high-molecular weight growth factor which is active on autochtonous B cells (216). This is consistent with the hypothesis that HC neoplasms may autostimulate their own growth in a positive feedback (217) that bypasses the negative feedback associated with the control of the size of the non-neoplastic hematopoietic cell population. This does not necessarily mean that HC are the main progenitor cells of the HC cell population in vivo, as the main progenitors might, instead, be more distant cells in the HC lineage (B, pre-B, or even stem cells) which would be committed to HC differentiation as well as responsive to the high molecular weight growth factor secreted by HC cells. Studies of the growth response of various cells along the HC lineage to the HC-secreted high-molecular weight growth factor might help to resolve this point.

No chromosomal markers have been identified in HCL. However, the difficulty in growing HC in vitro has interfered with such studies. Future studies may be facilitated by using BCGF (215). In contrast with T-hairy cell leukemia, no virus has been associated as yet with the predominant B form of HCL.

---

*There are very rare cases of T hairy cell leukemia (see section on T-cell leukemia, p. 236). The discussion in the present section is concerned only with HCL of the B phenotype.

Clinically, HCL is a relatively rare disease, affecting chiefly middle aged men. The U.S. incidence is about 600 cases per year (203). Male to female ratio is 4:1 or greater. It is a slowly progressive disease. Median survival time is 4 to 5 years, and 35% of patients survive 10 years or longer (218-220). The clinical and pathological features have been well described (218,221,222). The disease is characterized by splenomegaly, with infiltration by HC which line pseudosinuses, increased number of splenic macrophages, increased phagocytosis, and the clinical manifestations of hypersplenism; bone marrow changes include infiltration with HC, a marked decrease in the number of normal hematopoietic cells, and an increase in reticulum fibers. The blood shows pancytopenia in at least 50% of cases and at least one cytopenia in most cases. The total white blood count (WBC) may be decreased, or, in the leukemic phase, increased. Other abnormalities include a decrease in the number of circulating T cells, without change in the helper/suppressor ratio (223) and with normal T-cell function (224), a deficiency of NK activity (225) and a deficient interferon-alpha production (226). Severe, recurrent infections with a wide variety of bacteria, fungi or protozoa, and bleeding dominate the later course of the disease and are the main causes of death (203,221,222,227).

At least 10% of patients have a very indolent disease and do not require treatment (228). The majority of patients have splenomegaly. When these patients develop leukopenia, thrombocytopenia, or anemia to a significant extent, splenectomy has, until now, been the primary treatment of choice. It does not affect bone marrow infiltration with HC, but it produces a temporary improvement of the cytopenias. Patients who are refractory to or relapse after splenectomy have been difficult to treat in the past, because single-agent chemotherapy produced only partial responses of short duration, and more aggressive multiagent or other therapy was fraught with complications because severe cytopenia is aggravated by these therapies (203,221,222,227,228). Recently, the chemotherapeutic agent pentostatin (2 -dexycoformycin), an adenosine deaminase inhibitor, has been used with response rates as high as 96%, half of which were complete responses (229-233) and without the severe infections or other cytopenic effects which accompany other aggressive chemotherapy (234).

Interferon Therapy

The report of a therapeutic effect of leukocytic interferon on HCL, by Quesada et al. (235) has been amply confirmed with natural leukocytic (236,237) or lymphoblastic (238) interferons and with recombinant interferons alfa-2a (239-243), alfa-2b (244-250), Boehringer's alfa-2c (251,252), as shown in Table 2. The effective dose of interferon was relatively small, in most instances, 2 $MU/m^2$. 201 (78%) of the 258 evaluable patients had hematological remissions (CR+PR), and 39 also met the stringent CR requirement of total clearance of hairy cells from bone marrow specimens.

Transient myelosuppression was often observed during the first month of therapy (240,247). The first hematological improvement was usually a decrease in the number of circulating hairy cells; this was followed by a sequential increase in the number of platelets, red blood cells (RBC), granulocytes, and lastly, monocytes, in responding patients (240,241,242,247). Monoclonal antibody markers of hairy cells disappeared along with morphologically recognizable hair cells (238,241,243). Bone marrow changes were slower to occur. Bone marrow cellularity usually decreased within the first 3 months, but the percentage of hairy cells and the hairy cell index of the marrow decreased slowly over a period of at least 18 months of therapy (248). Sometimes there was a dissociation between bone marrow and peripheral blood findings, as several instances were reported when patients with minor hematological responses had markedly improved bone marrow biopsy (239,247).

Therapy was associated with marked decrease in incidence and severity of infections (235,242) and, in some instances, with dramatic recoveries from pyogenic (254), atypical mycobacterial (255,256) or mucormycotic (257) infections. Successful therapy was reported with doses as low as $0.2$ MU/m$^2$ although the responses were not as marked as with the higher doses (258-261). Intermittent regimens are also under study (262).

Following discontinuation of interferon therapy, stable remissions of 6-22+ months have been observed (242). The stability of remission following discontinuation of therapy appeared to be related to the duration of interferon therapy as the number of recurrences decreased when the duration of therapy was increased from 7-12 months to 18-29 months (248,253,263,264). The development of resistance to interferon during therapy has not been reported in this disease. Interferon was active in splenectomized as well as nonsplenectomized patients (242). The pros and cons of interferon versus splenectomy as initial therapy have been discussed (265,266).

Investigations of host defenses in HCL as they relate to interferon therapy have been initiated. HCL patients in remission, who have no evidence of residual disease, had a defective interferon system (267). The reportedly depressed natural killing activity of HCL patients' lymphocytes has been reported to be not improved (269) or improved (241,270) following interferon treatment. Enhanced expression of class II HLA antigens was found in hairy cells (271). Several indicators of T-cell function were improved (242). Studies of receptors to interferons or other lymphokines in hairy cells of interferon-treated patients have been initiated (272-274).

In a recent study, the interesting observation was made that cultures of bone marrow (BM) or peripheral blood monocytes (PBMC) of HCL patients showed a type of lymphomyeloid colonies not found in normal individuals. Interferons

Table 2  Response of Hairy Cell Leukemia to Interferons alfa

| Reference | Interferon | Route | Dose MU/m$^2$ | Schedule | Duration (months) | n | n$_{eval}$ | CR | PR | MR | S | PD | % CR + PR n$_{eval}$ |
|---|---|---|---|---|---|---|---|---|---|---|---|---|---|
| 236 | alfa N-Le | im, sc | 2-8 | qd | 6$^+$-10$^+$ | 22 | 22 | 5 | 13 | 4 | — | — | 82 |
| 237 | alfa-N-Le | im, sc | 2 | qd | 6 | 10 | 10 | 1 | 6 | 3 | — | — | 70 |
| 238 | alfa-N1 | im, sc | 2-4 | qd | 6 | 17 | 17 | 2 | 12 | 3 | — | — | 82 |
| 239 | several | sc | 2 | qd, tiw | 4 | 54 | 27 | 2 | 8 | 14 | — | 3 | 37 |
| 242 | alfa-2a | im, sc | 2-8 | qd | 12-18 | 30 | 30 | 9 | 17 | 4 | — | — | 87 |
| 241 | alfa-2a | im, sc | 2-8 | qd | 2-10 | 15 | 14 | 1 | 12 | — | — | 1 | 93 |
| 243 | alfa-2a | im | 2 | qd | 2-8 | 19 | 14 | — | 9 | 3 | — | 2 | 64 |
| 244 | alfa-2b | sc | 2 | tiw | 6-12 | 13 | 13 | 3 | 10 | — | — | — | 100 |
| 245 | alfa-2b | sc | 2 | tiw | 2-13 | 11 | 10 | 2 | 7 | — | — | 1 | 90 |
| 246 | alfa-2b | sc | 2 | tiw | 6 | 10 | 10 | 1 | 8 | 1 | — | — | 90 |
| 247,248 | alfa-2b | sc | 2 | tiw | 6 | 53 | 49 | 10 | 29 | 9 | — | 1 | 80 |
| 250 | alfa-2b | sc | 2 | tiw | 12 | 25 | 24 | — | 23 | 1 | — | — | 96 |
| 251 | alfa-2c | sc | 2-3.3 | qd, tiw | 3-9 | 11 | 11 | 2 | 3 | 5 | — | 1 | 45 |
| 252 | alfa-2c | sc | 2 | qd, tiw | 6 | 9 | 7 | 1 | 5 | — | — | 1 | 86 |
| Total | | | | | | 258 | | 39 | 162 | 47 | 0 | 10 | 78 |
| Percent | | | | | | 100 | | 15 | 63 | 18 | 0 | 4 | |

Abbreviations: interferon, see Table 1; im, intramuscular; sc, subcutaneously; MU, megaunits; qd, daily; tiw, three times a week. Responses (see p. 220).

alpha or beta, but not gamma, inhibited these colonies, but, unexpectedly, they increased the number of monocytes, myeloid, erythroid, or megakaryocytic elements in the colonies. It was hypothesized that HCL patients have an active pluripotent lymphomyeloid primitive stem cell and that interferon alpha or beta modify the growth of these colonies to inhibit their lymphoid differentiation and enhance their myeloid-monocytic differentiation (275).

## B. Multiple Myeloma

Multiple myeloma is a monoclonal tumor of plasma cells. Myeloma cells have retained many immunological surface markers of plasma cells as well as the ability to secrete a unique myeloma protein which may be a complete immunoglobulin or, in some 20% of patients, only lambda or kappa light chains (Bence-Jones proteins). All the cells in a given myeloma case have the same idiotypic marker in the variable region of their immunoglobulin (276). This protein is also present on the surface of B lymphocytes and in the cytoplasm of pre-B cells of the same patient. Thus the oncogenic event that gave rise to the myeloma clone occurred at the level of the pre-B cell or even earlier (277). No chromosomal markers have been reported.

Myeloma has several clinical manifestations, namely: (a) Hyperglobulinemia with the myeloma protein; (b) hypercellular bone marrow, rich in plasma cells and poor in other cellular elements; (c) osteolysis in part due to a factor produced by myeloma cells which stimulates osteoclast proliferation (278), causing pathological fractures, severe bone pain, and hypercalcemia; (d) decreased blood levels of normal globulin; (e) anemia, granulocytopenia, or thrombocytopenia; (f) depressed cell-mediated immunity; (g) increased susceptibility to infections; (h) amyloidosis; and (i) renal failure. At least two of the first three features must be present in order to make a diagnosis of multiple myeloma.

Multiple myeloma is usually an aggressive neoplasm. Prior to the advent of chemotherapy, untreated cases survived, on the average, for 7 months after the time of diagnosis. A very small minority of patients have an indolent course ("smoldering myeloma") without ever receiving chemotherapy (279). Median survival of treated cases is 2 to 3 years (range: $<1$ - $>10$ years) (280). Myeloma cases are staged with the Durie-Salmon criteria which are based in part on clinical and biochemical findings and in part on the calculated myeloma cell mass in the body, which is $<0.6 \times 10^{12}$ cells/$m^2$ and $>1.2 \times 10^{12}$ cells/$m^2$ for stages I and III, respectively (281). Scoring of clinical response is usually based on the Southwest Oncology Group (SWOG) criteria. A complete response (CR) means no detectable serum myeloma protein on two determinations 4 weeks apart or decrease in Bence-Jones protein to less than 0.1 g/24 hr, and return of hematological parameters to normal. Partial (PR) and minor (MR) responses mean a decrease of serum myeloma protein to 50% and 25% of pretreatment level, respectively (282). In myeloma literature, a clinical response usually includes CRs and PRs.

In initial therapy, alkylating agents such as melphalan achieve response rates of 24-41% when used alone, or 32-56% when given together with prednisone. Multiagent chemotherapy has response rates of 33-74%. Median survival time was 18-29 months with melphalan, 19-39 months with melphalan and prednisone, and 25-41 months with multiagent chemotherapy (276).

Response rates of previously treated patients ranged from 0 to 36% of relapsing cases and from 5 to 22% of primary resistant cases. Adding prednisone to combination therapy raised the response rate to 20-50% and 10-42% of relapsing and primary resistant cases, respectively (276).

Interferon Therapy

Table 3 shows the results of several trials with various preparations of alpha interferons (283-294). The response rates were in general lower than those observed with either malphalan/prednisone or multiagent chemotherapy. CRs were rare, of the order of 1-2%. The response rates were rather uniform across studies in relapsing or refractory patients. There was considerable variation across the studies using interferon as initial therapy (13.5 to 75%). Even when the most favorable of the two computations is used, the overall average response rate (28.9%) remains lower than that achieved with the better chemotherapeutic regimens. Randomized clinical trials comparing interferon with chemotherapy as initial treatment have been performed. In both instances, the response rates in the interferon-treated group were lower than those in the chemotherapy group.

The median interval for response ranged from 1 to 3 months, although responses have occurred for as long as 4 to 9 months after beginning interferon treatment. The median duration of response ranged from 2 to 27 months in different series.

Several studies have revealed considerable subjective improvement, especially regarding bone pain, even in patients who did not have a clinical response by the usual criteria.

Thirty previously untreated myeloma patients who received interferon alpha-2 in combination with melphalan/prednisone therapy had a response rate of 75%, with a median response duration of 10+ months (range: 2-15+ months). All responses were partial (295).

In summary, multiple myeloma is an aggressive disease with a relatively poor response to chemotherapy. Although the response rates obtained with interferon are inferior to those obtained with the better chemotherapeutic regimens, interferon may yet play a role in the management of this disease. There are three main avenues that need further exploration. The first question is whether there are clinical forms of myeloma that are more responsive than others to interferon therapy and, if so, how can they be identified? As the number of cases treated with interferon grows it might be possible to ascertain whether cases with less aggressive

**Table 3**  Multiple Myeloma

| Reference | IFN | Dose MU/m$^2$ | Schedule/ route | Months treated | N | CR | PR | MR | No R | % CR + PR |
|-----------|-----|---------------|-----------------|----------------|---|----|----|----|------|-----------|
| Clinical responses in previously untreated patients | | | | | | | | | | |
| 283 | Le | 2 | qd/im | 16-28 | 4 | 2 | 1 | 1 | – | 75 |
| 284 | Le | 2 | qd/im | 4-12 | 4 | – | 1 | – | 3 | 25 |
| 287 | Le | 2-4 | qd/im | NA | 74 | – | 10 | – | 64 | 13.5 |
| 285 | Le | 2-6 | qd/im | 3 | 12 | – | 3 | 2 | 7 | 25 |
| 293 | r-2a | 6-12 | qd/im | 3-12 | 14 | – | 7 | – | 7 | 50 |
| 292 | r-2a | 2-33 | qd/im | 1-11 | 7 | – | 2 | 2 | 3 | 28.5 |
| 294 | r-2c | 6-12 | qd/im | 1-12 | 14 | – | 2 | 4 | 8 | 14.3 |
| Total | | | | | 129 | 2 | 26 | 9 | 92 | 21.7[a] 28.9[b] |
| Clinical response in refractory or relapsing patients | | | | | | | | | | |
| 284 | Le | 2 | qd/im | 5-10 | 5 | – | 1 | – | 4 | 20.0 |
| 285 | Le | 2-6 | qd/im | 3 | 5 | – | 1 | – | 4 | 20.0 |
| 288 | r-2b | 2-6 | tiw/sc | 3-15 | 14 | – | 2 | – | 12 | 14.3 |
| 289 | r-2b | 2-6 | tiw/sc | 3-18 | 38 | 1 | 6 | – | 31 | 18.4 |
| 290 | r-2b | NA | tiw/sc | 3 | 20 | – | 4 | – | 16 | 20.0 |
| 291 | r-2b | NA | tiw/sc | 3 | 20 | – | 2 | 3 | 15 | 10.0 |
| 293 | r-2a | 6-12 | qd/im | 3-12 | 13 | – | 2 | – | 11 | 15.4 |
| 292 | r-2a | 2-33 | qd/im | 1-11 | 39 | – | 8 | 5 | 26 | 20.5 |
| Total | | | | | 154 | 1 | 26 | 8 | 119 | 17.5[a] 17.3[b] |

[a]Overall average of cases.

[b]Average of % CR + PR in different studies.

Abbreviations: as in Table 2.

forms of the disease might show better response to interferon. Are there biological markers associated with favorable response to interferon? The suggestion that IgG myelomas were less responsive than other types (287) has not been confirmed as yet. Studies of the association of various immunological markers with response of myeloma cases to interferon might be worth including in future clinical trials.

The response to interferon in combination with, or alternating with, the more effective chemotherapeutic regimens should be tested in randomized clinical trials, since the first clinical study would indicate that the combination compares well with historical series using chemotherapy alone (295).

Finally, the significance of responses to interferon that fall short of CR or PR but are associated with decreased bone pain, increased resistance to infections, or fewer renal complications must not be underestimated. The decreased bone pain noted in several studies is noteworthy. This observation might stimulate studies to find if interferon has an inhibitory effect on the activation of osteoclasts that occurs in myeloma patients. In clinical trials, more attention might be given to the scoring of stable disease or minor response with regard to these criteria.

## C. Chronic Lymphocytic Leukemia

Chronic lymphocytic leukemia (CLL) is, in the vast majority of cases, due to a monoclonal proliferation of SmIg-positive B lymphocytes, as shown by expression of a single Ig light chain, unique Ig idiotype specificity, a single pattern of glucose-6-phosphate dehydrogenase, immunoglobulin gene rearrangement and, in some instances, clonal chromosomal abnormalities. The cells are usually intermediately differentiated B cells which have not matured to plasma cells, but may give rise to plasma cells following in vitro treatment with phorbol esters (reviewed in Ref. 191, pp. 10-11).

Clinically, it is a disease of older adults (median age 60), which is usually stable, often for several years, before transforming into a more aggressive disease. Its features include peripheral lymphocytosis, lymphadenopathy, infiltration of bone marrow with lymphocytes, anemia, thrombocytopenia, decreased resistance to infection, and autoimmune phenomena (296,297). The findings of lymphocytosis, lymphadenopathy, splenomegaly, anemia, and thrombocytopenia are criteria for stages 0, I, II, III, and IV, respectively (298). Median survival is greater than 4 years for stages 0-II, and less than 2 years for stages III-IV (296, p. 1740). Chemotherapy with alkylating agents gives temporary responses with little change in survival time (296).

Clinical trials of interferon-alpha therapy in advanced cases of CLL have been on the whole disappointing, with low (5 $MU/m^2$) or high (50 $MU/m^2$) doses (299). Review of 57 evaluable patients in six small series revealed no CR and only 8 PR (14%) (300). Furthermore, 5 of 18 patients in one series appear to have had an acceleration of their disease while receiving recombinant alpha interferon (300).

Alpha, beta, or gamma interferons were added in relatively large doses (500 to 5000 U/ml) to B lymphocytes grown in vitro from the blood of CLL patients. Blast-like or plasmacytoid morphological changes were found in the cells of 19/22 patients, and increased thymidine uptake was found in those of 3/29 patients (301). Further work from the same group indicated that addition of interferon-alpha or -beta to mitogen-containing medium increased thymidine uptake by B cells from CLL patients as well as some B cells from the spleen of normal individuals (302).

Thus in vitro as well as in vivo studies provide some hints that interferons might stimulate the growth of some CLL cell subsets, and possibly some lymph spleen B-lymphocyte subsets. Further studies are needed to confirm this finding and further identify the subtype of cells involved and their stage of differentiation.

## D. Non-Hodgkin's Lymphomas

Non-Hodgkin's lymphomas (NHL) originate in lymph nodes or other lymphoid tissues from cells of the lymphocytic series. They form a very heterogeneous group of tumors, by morphological, immunological, or clinical criteria (303-305). According to histological pattern of growth, NHL can be divided into nodular (or follicular) and diffuse groups, resembling the proliferative lymphoid follicles and the medullary cords of lymph nodes, respectively (303, pp. 1629-1630). Another morphological criterion is the size of the cell (small, "lymphocyte-like" or large, "histiocyte-like"). The Rappaport classification is based on these criteria as well as other features of cell differentiation (306). The incidence of various types of NHL according to the Rappaport classification is shown in Table 4. Although several other systems of classification have been proposed, the Rappaport method, or its modification in the "Working Formulation" (303, pp. 1635-1635) are the ones most commonly used by clinicians.

By immunological (monoclonal antibody) criteria, NHL usually show a monoclonal cell population, at least early in the disease (303, p. 1627-1629). The majority of NHL have B-cell markers, while the remainder are composed of T, null, or blast cells (303, p. 1629; 304). Along the B-cell lineage, intermediate B-cell markers are found in Burkitt, diffuse well differentiated lymphocytic (DWDL), and CLL tumors; mature B-cell markers are found in nodular and diffuse poorly differentiated lymphocytic (NPDL and DPDL) tumors; and secretory B-cell markers are found in diffuse histiocytic lymphocytic (DHL) tumors. Along the T-cell lineage, thymocyte markers are found in lymphoblastic lymphomas and mature T-lymphocyte markers are found in some DHL and in Sézary syndrome (304).

Cytogenetic abnormalities involving translocation of the long arm of chromosome 14, usually at band 14q32, with several other chromosomes (#18 in follicular lymphomas, #8 in diffuse undifferentiated lymphomas or various other rearrangements in DHL) are often found. Burkitt's lymphoma shows 8:14, 8:22, or 8:2 translocations, involving the site on chromosome 8 where the c-*myc* oncogene is located (304).

Clinically, the NHL have been aggregated into two broad categories as shown in Table 4, the indolent or low-grade, and the aggressive or high-grade tumors (305). They are staged with the Ann Arbor classification, from most localized (Stage 1) to most disseminated (Stage IV) involvement, further suffixed accord-

Table 4    Prognostic Classification of Non-Hodgkin's Lymphomas

| Histology | % of NHL | Median survival (years)[a] |
|-----------|----------|------------------------|
| Favorable |          |                        |
| Low grade |          |                        |
| DWDL | <5 | >7.5 |
| NWDL | <5 | >7.5 |
| NPDL | 20-30 | 5-7.5 |
| NM | 10-15 | 7.5 |
| Unfavorable |          |                        |
| Intermediate grade |          |                        |
| DPDL | 15-30 | 1.8-3.0 |
| DM | 5-10 | 1.5 |
| NH | <5 | 0.8-3.0 |
| Low grade |          |                        |
| DH | 30 | 0.6-1.1 |
| DU | <5 | 0.6 |

[a]The median survival was that of patients who were treated prior to 1973, i.e., they received primarily single-agent chemotherapy.

Abbreviations (according to Rappaport terminology): DWDL = diffuse well differentiated lymphocytic; NWDL = nodular well-differentiated lymphocytic; NPDL = nodular poorly differentiated lymphocytic; NM = nodular mixed (i.e., lymphocytic and histiocytic); DPDL = diffuse poorly differentiated lymphocytic; DM = diffuse mixed (lymphocytic and histiocytic); NH = nodular histiocytic; DH = diffuse histiocytic; DU = diffuse undifferentiated. Notes: The terms nodular and follicular are used interchangeably. The term histiocytic refers only to the appearance of the cell, not to its origin.

*Source*: Modified from Ref. 306. Authors used data from early studies reported by Jones et al. Cancer 31: 806-823, 1973.

ing to the presence (B) or absence (A) of fever, night sweats, or weight loss. Low-grade NHL seldom present in stage I or II, in contrast with the intermediate or high-grade tumors (306,307). Because the low-grade and high-grade NHL have differing natural history, clinical course, and response to conventional and interferon therapies, they will be discussed separately.

Low-Grade NHL

Low-grade NHL, such as NPDL or DWDL, occur predominantly in older individuals (median age 55-65) with a preponderance of men. Even when they present at stage III or IV, their course is initially indolent and their response to single-agent or combination chemotherapy is excellent, as the complete response rates (CR) range from 65% to 90%. However, this disease, especially the NPDL, has a tendency to convert to a diffuse aggressive form which is much more resistant to therapy. Relapses following successful initial therapy are very common (about 10-15% a year) and the tumor is much more resistant to treatment. Thus few of these patients are cured and most die of the disease after a median survival rate of about 6 years, irrespective of the treatment received (303-308). For this reason, some centers give no initial therapy for this type of tumor, but monitor them for progression at which time therapy is instituted (309). Exceptionally, some of these patients show spontaneous regression (310).

High-Grade NHL

The natural history and response to therapy of high-grade NHL present almost a mirror image to those of the low-grade tumors. High-grade NHL occur predominantly in a younger age group (middle to young adulthood depending upon the type of tumor), they are aggressive and fatal within 1 or 2 years if left untreated or treated only with single-agent therapy. However, a significant number of them, ranging from 25% to over 75%, depending upon the presence of various prognostically significant factors, have a CR following combination chemotherapy (303, 311) and a number of these patients, possibly as high as 30-40% may be cured or at least have very long survival (311,312).

Interferon Therapy

Interferon alfa therapy of low-grade NHL has had only limited success, especially when compared with the more established forms of chemotherapy. The results of several studies are shown in Table 5. The clinical response rates (CR+PR) have been in the range of 35-50% in the majority of studies, but the CR has ranged from 0 to 17% (except for one small initial series) (313-321). Inspection of Table 5 shows that response was somewhat improved when the duration of treatment was longer or the dose higher, but even in the study which satisfied both of these requirements (318), the response rate was only 54% and the CR rate 17%. Even this improved response is considerably inferior to that obtained with combined chemotherapy (303,306). Response duration was short. Although, in general, the interferon study populations probably had more advanced disease than those reported in chemotherapeutic trials, the results obtained to date do not support the use of interferon in lieu of chemotherapy, except possibly when there might be contraindications to chemotherapy.

Patients with high-grade NHL were treated with interferons alfa-2a and -2b, respectively, in doses of 50 MU/m$^2$, in two studies (318,320) with very poor results. The combined study population was 43 subjects, of whom 33 were evaluable. There were no CR and only 4 PR (12%) of short duration. The patients had, in general received prior courses of chemotherapy with initial resistance or relapse. Yet, even when that factor is considered, the results are markedly inferior to those achieved with combined chemotherapy (311,312).

Table 5  Interferon Alpha Therapy of Low-Grade Lymphomas

| Reference | IFN | Route | Dose U/m² | Schedule | Duration (months) | N | CR | PR | MR | No R | %CR+PR |
|-----------|-----|-------|-----------|----------|-------------------|---|----|----|----|------|--------|
| 313 | Le | im | 2-6 | qd | 1 | 6 | 2 | 1 | -- | 3 | 50 |
| 314 | Le | im | 3.3 | bid | 1 | 7 | 1 | 2 | 2 | 2 | 43 |
| 315 | Le | im | 0.3-6 | qd | 1 | 18 | − | 3 | 3 | 12 | 17 |
| 316 | Ly | im | 3.3 | tiw | 2 | 20 | 1 | 4 | − | 15 | 25 |
| 317 | A | im | 2-33 | qd | 3+ | 17 | 2 | 4 | -- | 11 | 35 |
| 318 | A | im | 50 | tiw | 3+ | 24 | 4 | 9 | 2 | 10 | 54 |
| 319 | A | im | 12 | tiw | 2+ | 17 | 1 | 6 | − | 9 | 41 |
| 320 | 2 | sc | 10 | tiw | 3+ | 20 | 1 | 8 | − | 11 | 45 |
| 321 | 2 | sc | 2 | tiw | 3+ | 34 | − | 17 | − | 17 | 50 |
| Total | | | | | | 163 | 12 | 54 | 7 | 91 | 42 |

Abbreviations: im, intramuscular; sc, subcutaneous; qd, daily; bid, twice a day; tiw, 3 times a week; N is N evaluable.

## E.  T-Cell Leukemia

Adult-T cell leukemia is associated with the human T-cell leukemia virus 1 (HTLV-1). It is a relatively rare disease in the United States, but it is endemic in parts of the Far East. The clinical course is variable, but a major problem is the associated immune deficiency. In one series of 6 patients treated with recombinant interferon-beta (24 MU/m² three times a week for 4 weeks or longer by 1-hour intravenous infusion, for a total dose of 216-4824 MU), 2 patients died early, one had no response and three had PRs lasting 1.5 to 12 months, with survival of 2 to 14+ months. Another group of 5 patients was treated with intravenous or intramuscular recombinant interferon gamma, starting with 1 MU and escalating to 8 MU every three days until relapse for a total dose of 34-518 MU. There was one early death, 1 PD, 2 PR, and 1 CR of 2-4 months duration with 1.5-4.5 months survival (322). Thus, beta or gamma interferons, administered in relatively large doses, had very limited effectiveness in these advanced cases, and they appear to be less effective than chemotherapy. Yet they are potential alternatives to chemotherapy when severe immunodeficiency makes it difficult to administer the latter.

## F.  Cutaneous T-Cell Lymphoma

Cutaneous T-cell lymphoma is a tumor of mature T-helper cells (303). These cells migrate extensively and settle in the peripheral blood, skin, and lymph nodes, so that disseminated lesions occur early in the disease, different forms or stages of which are known as mycosis fungoides and Sézary syndrome. The disease, which affects predominantly older men has an indolent course often surpassing 10 years without systemic therapy. In the early stages, local treatment of skin lesions is effective, but in more advanced disease, single or combination chemotherapy must be used. There is clinical response to such therapy in the majority of cases, but complete response occurs in only 20-25% of cases (303), and relapse is universal.

A clinical trial of interferon alfa-2a therapy has been conducted in one center. Treatment consisted of 50 MU/m$^2$ intramuscularly, three times weekly, indefinitely in responders and for 3 months in patients with minor response or stable disease. It was discontinued if disease progressed. The subjects all had advanced lesions and had failed multiple previous courses of therapy (323). There were 20 subjects. There were 2 CR and 7 PR, for a clinical response rate of 45%. The median duration of response was 5.5 months. Three patients had responses of more than 2 years duration. The authors concluded that interferon is the therapy of choice for refractory cutaneous T-cell lymphoma, and they have initiated investigations with lower doses of interferon (300).

### G. Acute Lymphocytic or Lymphoblastic Leukemia (ALL)

ALL is predominantly a disease of children or young adults. The leukemic cells may have T-, B-, or non-T- non-B-markers corresponding to various developmental stages below the intermediate B and the mature T stages. There is good response to combination therapy with 5-year remissions in 50-80% of cases depending upon prognostic group and the disease is apparently curable in some patients (324,325). There have been very few studies with interferon, therefore it is not possible at present to comment on its therapeutic efficacy in this disease.

### H. Acute Nonlymphocytic (Myelogenous) Leukemia (ANLL)

This is an heterogeneous group of diseases of children and young adults with immature myeloid cells at various degrees of initial differentiation along granulocytic, monocytic, megakaryocytic, or erythroid series. Single-agent and combination chemotherapy are followed by CR in about 20-50% and 30-85% of cases, respectively. Initial therapy is usually followed by postremission, maintenance, and intensification courses of therapy to prevent relapses. Eventually, most patients relapse. Optimal salvage therapies may produce short remissions in 25-50% of cases (326).

There have been few trials of interferon therapy. A group of 9 previously untreated patients with contraindications to chemotherapy received relatively short courses of 5-35 MU of IFN alpha-Le. There were 7 PD, 1 SD, and 1 MR (327). A group of 23 patients with refractory or relapsing ANLL IFN were given alpha-Ly for one week in daily doses of 100 MU/m$^2$. Among 18 evaluable patients, 14 had NR, 3 had an MR, and 1 had a PR (328,329). All the responding patients had interferon blood levels $>10^3$ U/ml. Because of the short duration of therapy in both studies, it is difficult to assess the effect of interferon in ANLL, since responses often occur in other neoplasms after weeks or months of interferon therapy. The response of acute leukemia cases to leukocyte interferon which was reported in early case studies (330) warrants that the subject be reexamined.

## I. Chronic Myelogenous Leukemia

Chronic myelogenous (or myelocytic) leukemia (CML) is a biphasic malignant myeloproliferative disorder. In the first, "stable" or "chronic" phase, there is myeloid hyperplasia with near normal hematopoietic cell differentiation, as well as leukocytosis with functional leukocytes. In the second, "acute" or "accelerated" and eventually "blast" phase, maturation of progenitor cells is abnormal, and immature cells accumulate in the bone marrow, blood, and other tissues (331).

Stable CML is a monoclonal disorder of a multipotent stem cell, as shown by the presence of the Philadelphia ($Ph^1$) chromosome and enzyme markers in stem cells as well as their leukemic progeny, but not in bone marrow fibroblasts or other mesenchymal cells (332). The $Ph^1$ chromosome is the result of a balanced translocation, t(9,22)(q34.1:q11.21) (333). The proportion of $Ph^1$-positive cells gradually increases to more than 99% of dividing bone marrow cells. $Ph^1$-negative cells persist in the bone marrow, but their growth and differentiation appear to be suppressed (334,335). The rate of proliferation of $Ph^1$-positive myeloid stem cells is not faster than that of their normal counterparts, but rather, there is an enormous expansion of the pool of committed $Ph^1$-positive progenitors (332). Yet, the growth and differentiation of $Ph^1$-positive cells remain subject to several controls. In vitro, they require colony-stimulating factor (336). In vivo, the granulocyte count of untreated patients typically stabilizes at about $100\text{-}400 \times 10^9$ cells per liter, with spontaneous oscillations. During the chronic phase, the proliferative myeloid cells are present only in the bone marrow, spleen, or liver and they do not invade other tissues (332).

The translocation that gives rise to the $Ph^1$ chromosome involves the rearrangement of two oncogenes. Oncogene c-abl, located in chromosome 9 at band 34, is transferred to $Ph^1$. The human homolog of c-sis, located on chromosome 22 is translocated to the rearranged chromosome 9. The translocation of c-abl results in the formation of a fusion gene which has components from chromosomes 9 and 22. This fusion gene has retained much of the nucleotide chain of c-abl, but it is longer (8 KB instead of 6.7 KB) and its protein product has a tyrosine kinase activity which is not present in the normal c-abl protein (337).

When the disease progresses into the acute phase, there is an expansion of an undifferentiated clone of myeloid (60% of cases), erythroid (10%), lymphoid

(30%), or exceptionally megakaryocytic origin (332). This is usually associated with the appearance of additional chromosome changes, either a second $Ph^1$ chromosome, a trisomy of chromosome 8 or of the long arm of chromosome 17, or some other translocation (338). The disease takes on the characteristics of an acute leukemia, as blast cells appear in the circulation in large numbers and infiltrate various tissues. Altogether, the median survival from the time of diagnosis is 3-4 years. Less than 30% of cases survive 5 years (339). After onset of the acute phase, the disease is fatal within a few weeks or months.

Current therapy of CML during the chronic phase consists of single-agent chemotherapy, bisulfan, or hydroxyurea. This therapy has limited effects because of lack of differential sensitivity of normal and malignant hematopoietic cells to these agents (340). It reduces leukocytosis and associated symptoms, but the bone marrow remains populated with $Ph^1$-positive cells. Median survival time ranges from 35 to 56 months with bisulfan or hydroxyurea to 48-65 months with intensive combination chemotherapy. Encouraging results have been obtained with intensive chemoradiotherapy to attempt to eradicate the $Ph^1$ clone followed by allogeneic or syngeneic marrow transplantation (332,341). Chemotherapy of acute phase CML is unsatisfactory, with low remission rates (except for the lymphoid type where complete response rates as high as 60% may be achieved) and median survival of 2-8 months. Higher rates of complete remission have been achieved with bone marrow transplantation (332,341).

Interferon Therapy

The main interferon clinical trials in CML have been done by Talpaz and coworkers (Table 6). These authors have reported on 51 patients treated with natural leukocytic alpha interferon (342) and 17 patients treated with recombinant interferon alpha A (343). All the cases were in the chronic phase. In both groups complete hematological response occurred in about 70% of patients and a partial hematological response in another 5 to 10%. In the larger series the median time to hematological response was 14 weeks (range 2-55). Bone marrow response (decreased cellularity, increased maturity index) required 6 to 9 months. Partial suppression of $Ph^1$ metaphases and return of normal diploid metaphases in a fraction of the cells occurred after several months of treatment in about 60% of individuals who had a complete hematological response. Not enough time has elapsed to assess the durability of the response. However, in the larger series, the median duration of complete hematological response was 33+ months at the time of publication. A small European study, using recombinant alpha-2 interferon has shown similar response rates (344). Another recent study has shown hematological response of CML patients in the chronic phase to recombinant gamma interferon (345). In the studies of Talpaz et al., the patients who developed the blast phase during interferon therapy had a higher than expected frequency of lymphoid blast pattern, which has a better prognosis (342).

Table 6   Interferon Therapy of CML in the Chronic Phase

| Reference | 362 | 363 |
|---|---|---|
| Interferon | Le | rA |
| Route/schedule | im, qd | im, qd |
| Dose (MU/m$^2$) | 2-6 | 3 |
| Number evaluable | 51 | 17 |
| HR | 36 | 13 |
| PR | 5 | 1 |
| No R | 10 | 3 |
| Ph$^1$ decrease in BM | 20/36HR | 8/13HR |
| Time to HR (weeks | | |
| Median (range) | 14 (2-55) | |

Abbreviations: as in Table 2. HR, hematologic remission.

While these results are at least comparable to those obtained with single-agent chemotherapy, they fall short of the bone marrow improvement seen after bone marrow transplantation. Therefore studies with interferon after, before or during chemotherapy have been performed. Interferon alfa-2b significantly slowed the leukocyte doubling time and lengthened the duration of remission following busulfan therapy in 4 out of 5 patients (346). In another study, 28 patients were treated with multiagent chemotherapy and then maintained on interferon-alpha A. After a median follow up of 24 months, 21 of the patients remained on interferon and projected three year survival is 82%. Temporary complete suppression of the Ph$^1$ chromosome occurred in 11 of these patients (347). Patients treated with interferon who had relapsed or developed a blast phase were successfully treated with chemotherapy (342).

## J.  Comments on Interferons and Hematopoietic Neoplasms

The studies reviewed in the preceding section show that neoplasms of the bone marrow and lymphoid tissues vary in their response to interferon-alfa. Excellent response rates are achieved in hairy cell leukemia and chronic myelogenous leukemia. Responses are also obtained in the majority of patients with cutaneous T-cell lymphomas and "low-grade" NHL. There are much fewer responses in patients with multiple myeloma. Patients with "high-grade" NHL, acute nonlymphocytic leukemia and acute lymphocytic leukemia respond in only rare instances. This response gradient among neoplasms which are initially derived from the same multipotent stem cell offers an opportunity to test some of the hypotheses that might be advanced to explain the relative response rates.

Cell Lineage

The hypothesis that alfa interferons are especially active against tumors in the B-lymphocytic lineage (217) is not supported, since neoplasms with good response rates belong to not only the B lineage (hairy cell leukemia, low grade NHL) but also the T lineage (cutaneous T-cell lymphoma) and myelogenous lineage (chronic myelogenous leukemia), while neoplasms with low or poor response rates include some from the B lineage (multiple myeloma, "high grade" NHL).

Degree of Maturation of the Neoplastic Cells

The hypothesis that interferons may be most active against tumors with the most highly differentiated cell markers relative to the normal hematopoietic lineages is not supported because of the relatively low rate of response of multiple myeloma (a tumor of plasma cell, the most mature form of B lymphocytes) as compared with the higher response rates of hairy cell leukemia or "low-grade" NHL, whose cells have markers corresponding to a lower level of B-cell differentiation than those of multiple myeloma.

Indolent Versus Aggressive Nature of the Tumor

The hypothesis that the effectiveness of interferon and the aggressiveness of the tumor are inversely related is compatible with the results. The most indolent tumors (hairy cell leukemia, chronic myelogenous leukemia in the chronic phase, cutaneous T-cell lymphoma, and "low-grade" NHL) are much more responsive to interferons than the more aggressive tumors (multiple myeloma, "high-grade" NHL, the acute leukemias).

In trying to relate response to interferon to the indolence/aggressiveness feature of the tumor, several possible explanations can be considered. The first, and most trivial one, is that interferon might not have enough time to act in the trials with aggressive tumors. The response time of indolent tumors to interferon varies according to the tumor and the parameter used to assess response, but it is, in general of the order of several weeks and in some instances response does not occur for a few months. Since the research policy is usually to stop experimental therapy when disease progression takes place, in order to try another form of therapy, interferon may not have had enough time to exert its action against aggressive tumors with a propensity to early disease progression.

Another possibility to be considered is that interferons may exert their antitumor effect by decreasing the probability of transition of neoplastic progenitor cells from $G_0$ to $G_1$. If, as might be expected, a much larger fraction of cells undergo that transition in aggressive than in indolent tumors, the same relative decrease in the probability of $G_0$ to $G_1$ transition could be much more effective in moderating the growth of indolent tumors than that of the more aggressive tumors. This hypothesis could be tested by experiments to measure the effect of interferons on the $G_0$-$G_1$ transition of the neoplastic progenitor cells in both types of tumors.

A third possibility is that the control of growth in the indolent tumors is mediated by inhibition of oncogenes or growth factors that are susceptible to interferons while their counterparts in aggressive tumors are not. As data rapidly accumulate on the oncogenes and growth factors which are involved in the tumors in question, it is likely that several systems to test this hypothesis are or will soon become available.

It is possible that indolent and aggressive tumors differ with regard to their interferon receptors or to the down-regulation of these receptors by interferon. As techniques to test this hypothesis are readily available, and, indeed, some data have already been reported, it should be relatively easy to determine if there are quantitative differences in these parameters at the level of the neoplastic progenitor cells of aggressive and indolent tumors.

Finally, it is also possible that the critical difference between indolent and aggressive hematopoietic neoplasms has to do with the host organism's reaction to them. This might be the case if the defenses provided by host macrophages, killer cells, or other host cells were more effectively boosted by interferons in hosts with indolent rather than aggressive tumors. This hypothesis could be tested by studies of the effects of interferons on these defenses in individuals with either type of tumor.

These various hypotheses are not mutually exclusive. Indeed it is more likely that several of the proposed mechanisms might be operative rather than one. However. each calls for a different investigative approach.

### Effect of Interferons on Neoplastic Progression

Several if not most hematopoietic malignancies progress through clinical phases of increasing aggressiveness often associated with cytogenetic changes during their natural history. Such progression is the rule in CML, as it evolves through its chronic, accelerated, and blast phases. The possibility that interferon may prevent or delay progression to the more aggressive phases of the neoplasm is under study, especially in CML. If interferons have such an effect, they should be used preferentially early in the evolution of the tumor, before progression has occurred.

### Indications for Interferon Therapy in Hematopoietic Malignancies and Needs for Further Clinical Research

Currently available data provide some guidance regarding the use of interferon as a therapeutic agent in these malignancies. The relative efficacy of interferon in limiting neoplastic growth has to be taken into account in conjunction with several other factors, each of which would impact on the clinical decision about the selection of a therapeutic modality in a given individual. Among these factors are the relative toxicity of the interferons and other antitumor agents and their effects on the patients' immunological defenses. The relatively low toxicity of the alpha interferons, when they are given in low or moderate doses, and their protective effects against intercurrent infections, some of which may be life-threatening, must be taken into account, along with therapeutic efficacy, in the choice of therapeutic agents.

*Chronic Myelogenous Leukemia.* Interferon alpha is highly effective in controlling the size of the leukemic cell population in chronic myelogenous leukemia, but it is far less effective in decreasing the population of $Ph^1$-positive cells in the bone marrow. The more aggressive chemotherapeutic marrow ablation followed by marrow transplantation appears to be more effective in eradicating $Ph^1$-positive cells. Because of the risks involved in marrow ablation, clinicians might tend to use alpha interferons early in the evolution of the disease and marrow ablation at a later stage. However, there is a need for studies that would guide the selection of the appropriate long-range therapeutic strategy. Experimental animal studies may play a critical role in paving the way for the design of human studies on this question.

*Hairy Cell Leukemia.* There are now two effective drug treatments for hairy cell leukemia: pentostatin and interferon alpha. Pentostatin gives a higher rate of clinical complete responses. There appears to be no cross resistance to the two agents. Clinicians have to decide in what sequence these two drugs are best used and how splenectomy might fit in the long-range therapeutic strategy (348). Controlled clinical trials to answer these questions are in order. The ability of alpha interferons to induce remissions in advanced cases of HCL is noteworthy (348).

*Non-Hodgkin's Lymphomas.* There has been a long-standing controversy in the treatment of the more indolent forms of "low-grade" NHL between chemotherapy and close monitoring without treatment. Now clinicians have a fourfold decision: no initial treatment, interferon alpha, chemotherapy, or combined interferon therapy. In devising clinical studies to compare these therapeutic alternatives, it will be very important to use patient populations that are homogeneous with regard to tumor histology and rate of evolution of the neoplasm. These requirements are not easily met, even in collaborative studies.

*Multiple Myeloma.* According to clinical response criteria, interferon alpha is less effective than the current forms of chemotherapy in the treatment of multiple myeloma, an aggressive neoplasm. The alpha interferons' beneficial effect on bone pain is an important factor in maintaining the quality of life of these patients. For this reason, more extensive trials of interferons in combined therapy of multiple amyeloma are needed.

*Chronic Lymphocytic Leukemia.* The effect of alpha interferons on chronic lymphocytic leukemia serves as a warning that these agents may stimulate the growth of certain neoplastic cells while inhibiting that of others.

These examples show that, according to the data presently available, the alpha interferons are not a "magic bullet" in the treatment of hematological malignancies, but rather an important element in an armamentarium of approaches of increasing effectiveness, and that decisions about sequencing, timing, or combinations of the various approaches, including interferon therapy, will become increasingly critical.

## ACKNOWLEDGMENT

Support by a grant from the Milstein Medical Research Foundation is gratefully acknowledged.

## REFERENCES

1. Sikora, D. (Ed). *Interferons and Cancer.* Plenum Press, New York, 1983.
2. Kirkwood, J.M., and Ernstoff, M.S. Interferons in the treatment of human cancer. J. Clin. Oncol. 2: 336-352, 1984.
3. Krown, S.E. Interferons and interferon inducers in cancer treatment. Sem. Oncol. 13: 207-217, 1986.
4. Goldstein, D., and Laszlo, J. Interferon therapy in cancer: From imaginon to interferon. Cancer Res. 46: 4315-4329, 1986.
4a. Smyth, J.F., Balkwill, F.R., Cavalli, F., Kimchi, A., Mattson, K., Niederle, N.E., and Spiegel, R.J. Interferons in oncology: Current status and future directions. Eur. J. Cancer Clin. Oncol. 23: 887-889, 1987.
5. Isaacs, A., and Lindemann, J. Virus interference. I. The interferon. Proc. R. Soc. London, Series B 147: 258-267, 1957.
6. Isaacs, A. Interferon. Adv. Virus Res. 10: 1-35, 1963.
7. Vilcek, J. *Interferon.* Springer Verlag, Vienna, 1969.
8. Finter, N.B. *Interferons and Interferon Inducers.* Elsevier, New York, 1973.
9. Gresser, I. Commentary. On the varied biologic effects of interferon. Cell. Immunol. 34: 406-415, 1977.
10. Stewart, W.E., II. *The Interferon System.* Springer-Verlag, New York, 1979.
11. Taylor-Papadimitriou, J. Effects of interferons on cell growth and function. In *Interferon 1980,* Vol. 2. Edited by I. Gresser. Academic Press, New York, 1980, pp. 13-46.
12. Vilcek, J., Gresser, I., and Merigan, T.C. (Eds). Regulatory functions of interferons. Ann. NY Acad. Sci. 350: 1-641, 1980.
13. Weissman, C. Cloning of interferon and other mistakes. In *Interferon 1981,* Volume 3. Edited by I. Gresser. Academic Press, New York, 1981, pp. 101-134.
14. Pestka, S. Cloning of the human interferons. Meth. Enzymol. 79: 599-601, 1981.

15. Lengyel, P. Biochemistry of interferons and their actions. Ann. Rev. Biochem. 51: 251-282, 1982.

16. Revel, M. Genetic and functional diversity of interferons in man. In *Interferons 1983*, Volume 5. Edited by I. Gresser. Academic Press, New York, 1983, pp. 205-239.

17. Lengyel, P. On the recent excitement in interferon research. In *Interferons as Cell Growth Inhibitors and Antitumor Factors*. Edited by R.M. Friedman, T. Merigan, and T. Sreevalsan. Alan R. Liss, New York, 1986, pp. xxi-xxxviii.

18. Bocci, V. Production and role of interferon in physiological conditions. Biol. Rev. 56: 49-85, 1981.

19. Bocci, V. The physiological interferon response. Immunol. Today 6(1): 7-9, 1985.

20. Fowler, A.K., Reed, C.D., and Giron, D.J. Identification of an interferon in murine placenta. Nature 286: 266-267, 1980.

21. Lebon, P., Girard, S., Thepot, F., and Chany, C. The presence of alpha-interferon in human amniotic fluid. J. Gen. Virol. 59: 393-396, 1982.

22. Cesario, T., Goldstein, A., Lindsey, M., Dumars, K., and Tilles, J. Antiviral activities of amniotic fluid. Proc. Soc. Exper. Biol. Med. 168: 403-407, 1981.

23. Duc-Goiran, P., Robert-Gallio, B., Lopez, J., and Chany, C. Unusual apparently constitutive interferons and antagonists in human placental blood. Proc. Natl. Acad. Sci. (USA) 82: 5010-5014, 1985.

24. Bocci, V., Paulesu, L., and Ricci, M.G. The physiological interferon response: IV. Production of interferon by the perfused human placenta at term. Proc. Soc. Exper. Biol. Med. 180: 137-143, 1985.

25. Bocci. V., Muscettola, M., Paulesu, L., and Grasso, G. The physiological interferon response. II. Interferon is present in lymph but not in plasma of healthy rabbits. J. Gen. Virol. 65: 101-108, 1984.

26. Martinez-Maza, O., Andersson, U., Andersson, J., Britton, S., and De Ley, M. Spontaneous production of interferon gamma in adult and newborn humans. J. Immunol. 132: 251-256, 1984.

27. Fischer, D.G., and Rubinstein, M. Spontaneous production of interferon gamma and acid-labile interferon alpha by subpopulations of human mononuclear cells. Cell. Immunol. 81: 426-434, 1983.

28. Zoumbis, N.C., Gascon, P., Djeu, Y., and Young, N. Interferon as a mediator of hematopoietic suppression in aplastic anemia in vitro and possibly in vivo. Proc. Natl. Acad. Sci. (USA) 82: 188-192, 1985.

29. Ito, Y., Aoki, H., Kimura, Y., Takano, M., Shimakata, K., and Maeno, K. Natural interferon-producing cells in mice. Infect. Immun. 31: 519-523, 1981.

30. Proietti, E., Gessani, S., Belardelli, F., and Gresser, I. Mouse peritoneal cells confer an antiviral state on mouse cell monolayers: Role of interferon. J. Virol. 57: 456-463, 1986.

31. Gresser, I., Vignaux, F., Belardelli, F., Tovey, M.G., and Maunoury, M-T. Injection of mice with antibody to mouse interferon alpha/beta decreases the level of 2'-5' oligoadenylate synthetase in peritoneal macrophages. J. Virol. 53: 221-227, 1985.

32. Wells, V., and Mallucci, L. Expression of the 2-5A system during the cell cycle. Exper. Cell Res. 159: 27-36, 1985.

33. Creasy, A.A., Eppstein, D.A., Marsh, V.V., Khan, Z., and Merigan, T.C. Growth regulation of melanoma cells by interferon and (2'-5') oligoadenylate synthetase. Molec. Cell. Biol. 3: 780-786, 1983.

34. Kohase, M., May, L.T., Tamm, I., Vilcek, J., and Sehgal, P.B. A cytokine network in human diploid fibroblasts: Interactions of beta-interferons, tumor necrosis factor, platelet-derived growth factor, and interleukin-1. Molec. Cell. Biol. 7: 273-280, 1987.

35. Revel, M., and Zilberstein, A. Interferon beta-2 living up to its name. Nature 325: 581-582, 1987.

36. Rubinstein, M., and Orchansky, P. The interferon receptors. CRC Crit. Rev. Biochem. 21: 249-276, 1986.

37. Committee on Interferon Nomenclature. Interferon nomenclature. Nature 286: 110, 1980.

38. Weissmann, C., and Weber, H. The interferon genes. Progr. Nucl. Acid Res. Molec. Biol. 33: 251-300, 1986.

39. Weissenbach, J., Chernajovsky, Y., Zeevi, M., Shulman, L., Soreq, H., Nir, U., Wallach, D., Perricaudet, M., Tiollais, P., and Revel, M. Two interferons mRNAs in human fibroblasts: In vitro translation and Escherichia coli cloning studies. Proc. Natl. Acad. Sci. (USA) 77: 7152-7156, 1980.

40. Sehgal, P.B., and Sagar, A.D. Heterogeneity of poly(I).poly(C)-induced human fibroblast interferon mRNA species. Nature 288: 95-97, 1980.

41. Sehgal, P.B., Zilberstein, A. Ruggieri, M-R. May, L.T., Ferguson-Smith, A., Slate, D.L., Revel, M., and Ruddle, F.H. Human chromosome 7 carries the beta-2 interferon gene. Proc. Natl. Acad. Sci. (USA) 83: 5219-5222, 1986.

42. Zilberstein, A., Ruggieri, R., Korn, J.H., and Revel, M. Structure and expression of cDNA and genes for human interferon beta-2, a distinct species inducible by growth-stimulatory cytokines. EMBO J. 5: 2529-2538, 1986.

43. May, L.T., Helfgott, D.C., and Sehgal, P.B. Anti-beta interferon antibodies inhibit the increased expression of HLA-B[7] mRNA in tumor necrosis factor-treated human fibroblasts: Structural studies of the beta-2 interferon involved. Proc. Natl. Acad. Sci. (USA) 83: 8957-8961, 1986.

44. Sehgal, P.B., May, L.T., Tamm, I., and Vilcek, J. Human beta-2 interferon and B-cell differentiation factor BSF-2 are identical. Science 235: 731-732, 1987.

45. Poupart, P., Vandenabeele, P., Cayphas, S., Van Snick, J., Haegeman, G., Kruys, V., Fiers, W., and Content, J. B cell growth modulating and differentiating activity of recombinant human 26-kd protein (9BSF-2, HuIFN-beta-2, HPGF). EMBO J. 6: 1219-1224, 1987.

46. Epstein, L.B. The special significance of interferon gamma. In Interferon, Volume 2: Interferons and the Immune System. Edited by J. Vilcek and E. De Maeyer. Elsevier, Amsterdam, 1984, pp. 185-200.

47. Nathan, C.F., Murray, H.W., Wiebe, M.R., and Rubin, B.Y. Identification of interferon gamma as the lymphokine that activates human macrophage oxidative metabolism and antimicrobial activity. J. Exper. Med. 158: 670-689, 1983.

48. Talmadge, K.W., Gallati, H., Sinigaglia, F., Walz, A., and Garotta, G. Identity between human interferon-gamma and "macrophage activating factor" produced by human T lymphocytes. Eur. J. Immunol. 16: 1471-1477, 1986.

49. May, L.T., and Sehgal, P.B. The interferon beta-3 locus on human chromosome 2. J. IFN Res. 6(Suppl. 1): 77 (abstr. II-32), 1986.

50. Von Gabain, A., Lindstrom, E., Cavalli-Sforza, L., and Lundgren, E. Identification of an abnormal restriction pattern of the IFN gamma locus in some individuals. J. of IFN Res. 6(suppl. 1): 67 (abstr. II-12), 1986.

51. Von Gabain, A., Ohlsson, M., Holmgren, E., Josephsson, S., Alkan, S., and Lundgren, E. Differential activities of the IFN-alpha-2 variants differing only in position 23 and 34. J. IFN Res. 6(suppl. 1): 11, 1986.

52. Hooks, J.J., and Detrick-Hooks, B. Interferon in autoimmune diseases and other immunoregulatory disorders. In *Interferons* Volume 2: *Interferons and the Immune System*. Edited by J. Vilcek and E. De Maeyer. Elsevier, Amsterdam, 1984, pp. 165-174.

53. Greene, J.J., and Ts'o P.O. Preferential modulation of embryonic cell proliferation and differentiation by embryonic interferon. Exp. Cell Res. 167: 400-406, 1986.

54. Mark, D.F., Lu, S.D., Creasy, A.A., Yamamoto, R., and Lin, L.S. Site-specific mutagenesis of the human fibroblast interferon gene. Proc. Natl. Acad. Sci. (USA) 81: 5662-5666, 1984.

55. Shafferman, A., Velan, B., Cohen, S., Leitner, M., and Grosfeld, N. Specific residues within an amino-terminal domain of 35 residues of interferon alpha are responsible for recognition of the human interferon alpha receptor and for triggering biological effects. J. Biol. Chem. 226: 6227-6237, 1987.

56. Tymms, M.J., Beilharz, M.W., Nisbet, I.T., Chambers, P.J., McInnes, B., Turton, J.C., Hertzog, P.J., and Linnane, A.W. Amino acid residues affecting antiviral and antiproliferative activity of in IFN-alphas. J. IFN Res. 6(suppl. 1): 13, 1986.

57. Leung, W.C., and Leung, M.F.K. Site specific mutagenesis of human interferon gamma. J. IFN Res. 6(suppl. 1): 76, (abstr. # II-30), 1986.

58. Arakawa, T., Hsu, Y-R., Parker, C.G., and Lai, P.H. Role of polycationic C-terminal portion in the structure and activity of recombinant human interferon-gamma. J. Biol. Chem. 261: 8534-8539, 1986.

59. Zorzopulos, J., Diaz, A., Criscuolo, M., Pesce, A., Denoya, B., Goc, B., Conley, E., and Ruiz Trevisan, A. Enhancing of a recombinant IFN 2 synthesis in *E. coli* by insertion of an 18 bp oligonucleotide into the pre IFN coding region. J. IFN Res. 6(suppl. 1): 88 (abstr. #II-55), 1986.

60. Zinn, K., Di Maio, D., and Manatis, T. Identification of two distinct regulatory regions adjacent to the human beta-interferon gene. Cell 34: 865-879, 1983.

61. Streuli, M., Hall, A., Boll, W., Stewart, W.E. II, Nagata, S., and Weissmann, C. Target specificity of two species of human interferon-alpha produced in *Escherichia coli* and of the hybrid molecules derived from them. Proc. Natl. Acad. Sci. (USA) 78: 2848-2852, 1981.

62. Rehberg, E., Kelder, B., Hoal, E.G., and Pestka, S. Specific molecular activities of recombinant and hybrid leukocyte interferons. J. Biol. Chem. 257: 11497-11502, 1982.

63. Meister, A., Uze, G., Mogensen, K.E., Gresser, I., Tovey, M.G., Grutter, M., and Meyer, F. Biologic activities and receptor binding of two human recombinant interferons and their hybrids. J. Gen. Virol. 67: 1633-1643, 1986.

64. Horisberger, M.A., and Staritzky, K. A recombinant human interferon hybrid with a broad host range. J. IFN Res. 6(suppl. 1): 70 (abstr. #II-18), 1986.

65. Le, H.V., Levine, A.M., Nagabhushan, T.L., Trotta, P.P. Novel pattern of disulfide bond pairing in a recombinant hybrid human alpha interferon. J. IFN Res. 6(suppl. 1): 75 (abstr. #II-28), 1986.

66. Zwarthoff, E.C., Gennissen, A.M.C., Van Heuvel, M., Bosveld, I.J., and Trapman, J. Tailoring of alpha interferons via in vivo recombination of the genes. J. IFN Res. 6(suppl. 1): 9, 1986.

67. Neidhart, J.A., Schmidt, S., Rosenblum, M., Quesada, J.R., Alton, N.K., and Downing, M. Phase I study of recombinant methionyl human consensus interferon (r-metHuIFN-conl). J. IFN Res. 6(suppl. 1): 50 (abstr. # I-23), 1986.

68. Bohm, J., Bar, R., Haase, K., Krehle, K., and Otto, B. Protein-engineering of human IFN gamma. J. IFN Res. 6(suppl. 1): 62 (abstr. # 11-3), 1986.

69. Leinikki, P.O., Calderon, J., and Schreiber, R.D. Loss of receptor binding activity in clostripain treated human IFN. J. IFN Res. 6(suppl. 1): 108 (abstr. # III-34), 1986.

70. Cebrian, M., Yague, E., de Landazuri, M.O., Rodiguez-Moya, M., Fresno, M., Pezzi, N., Llamazares, S., and Sanchez-Madrid, F. Different functional sites on rIFN-alpha 2 and their relation to the receptor binding site. J. Immunol. 138: 484-490, 1987.

71. Capon, D.J., Shepard, H.M., and Goeddel, D.V. Two distinct families of human and bovine interferon-alpha genes are coordinately expressed and encode functional polypeptides. Molec. Cell. Biol. 5: 768-779, 1985.

72. Feinstein, S.Y., Mory, Y., Chernajovsky, Y., Maroteaux, L., Nir, U., and Revel, M. Family of human alpha-interferon-like sequences. Molec. Cell. Biol. 5: 510-517, 1985.

73. Hauptmann, R., and Swetly, P. A novel class of human type I interferons. Nucleic Acids Res. 13: 4739-4749, 1985.

74. Adolf, G.R. Antigenic structure of human interferon omega 1 (interferon alpha11-I): Comparison with other human interferons. J. Gen. Virol. 68: 1669-1676, 1987.

75. Sternberg, M.J.E., and Cohen, F.E. Interferon: A tertiary structure predicted from animo acid sequences. Philos. Trans. R. Soc. London, Series B, 299: 125-127, 1982.

76. Sela, I. Preparation and measurement of an antiviral protein found in tobacco cells after infection with tobacco mosaic virus. Meth. Enzymol. 119: 734-744, 1986.

77. Gera, A., Speigel, S., and Loebenstein, G. Production, preparation and assay of an antiviral substance from plant cells. Meth. Enzymol. 119: 729-734, 1986.

78. Weissmann, C., Nagata, S., Boll, W., et al. Structure and expression of human interferon-alpha genes. Philos. Trans. R. Soc. London, Series B, 199: 7-28, 1982.

79. Collins, J. Interferon genes: Gene structure and elements involved in gene regulation. In *Interferon,* Volume 3: *Mechanisms of Production and Action.* Edited by R.M. Friedman. Elsevier, Amsterdam, 1984, pp. 33-83.

80. Stringfellow, D.A. (Ed.). *Interferon and Interferon Inducers.* Marcel Dekker, New York, 1980.

81. Torrence, P., and De Clercq, E. Interferon inducers: General survey and classification. Meth. Enzymol. 78: 291-299, 1981.

82. Zullo, J.N., Cochran, B.H., Huang, A.S., and Stiles, C.D. Platelet-derived growth factor and double-stranded ribonucleic acids stimulate expression of the same genes in 3T3 cells. Cell 43: 793-800, 1985.

83. Van Damme, J., De Ley, M., Opdenakker, G., Billiau, A., de Somer, P., and Van Beeumen, J. Homogeneous interferon-inducing 22K factor is related to endogenous pyrogen and interleukin 1. Nature 314: 226-268, 1985.

84. Moore, R.N., Larsen, M.S., Horohov, D.W., and Rouse, B.T. Endogenous regulation of macrophage proliferative expansion by colony-stimulating factor-induced interferon. Science 223: 178-181, 1984.

85. Warren, M.K., and Ralph, P. Macrophage growth factor CSF-1 stimulates human monocyte production of interferon, tumor necrosis factor and colony stimulating activity. J. Immunol. 137: 2281-2285, 1986.

86. Kohase, M., Henriksen-De Stefano, D., May, L.T., Vilcek, J., and Sehgal, P.B. Induction of interferon beta-2 by "tumor necrosis factor": a homeostatic mechanism in the control of cell proliferation. Cell 45: 659-666, 1986.

87. Handa, K., Suzuki, R., Matsui, H., Shimizu, Y., and Kamagai, K. Natural killer (NK) cells as responder to interleukin 2 (IL-2). II. IL-2-induced interferon-gamma production. J. Immunol. 130: 988-992, 1983.

88. Vilcek, J., Henriksen-De Stefano, D., Siegel, D., Klion, A., Robb, R.J., and Le, J. Regulation of IFN-gamma induction in human peripheral blood cells by exogenous and endogenously produced interleukin 2. J. Immunol. 135: 1851-1856, 1985.

89. Okamura, H., Wada, M., Nagata, K., Tamura, T., and Shoji, K. Induction of murine gamma interferon production by lipopolysaccharide and interleukin 2 in *Propionibacterium acnes* induced peritoneal exudate cells. Infect. Immun. 55: 335-341, 1987.

90. Johnson, H.M., and Torres, B.A. Leukotrienes: positive signals for regulation of gamma-interferon production. J. Immunol. 132: 413-416, 1984.

91. Rola-Pleszczynsky, M., Bouvrette, L., Gingras, D., and Girard, M. Identification of interferon-gamma as the lymphokine that mediates leukotriene B4-induced immunoregulation. J. Immunol. 139: 513-517, 1987.

92. Dianzani, F., Antonelli, G., and Capobianchi, M.R. Induction of human immune interferon with ionophores. Meth. Enzymol. 119: 69-72, 1986.

93. Kirchner, H., and Marcucci, F. Interferon production by leukocytes. In *Interferon* Volume 2. *Interferons and the Immune System.* Edited by J. Vilcek and De Maeyer. Elsevier, Amsterdam, 1984, pp. 7-34.

94. Havell, E.A., Hayes, T.G., and Vilcek, J. Synthesis of two distinct interferons by human fibroblasts. Virology 89: 330-333, 1978.

95. Le, J., Prensky, W., Henridsen, D., and Vilcek, J. Synthesis of alpha and gamma interferons by a human cutaneous lymphoma with T-cell phenotype. Cell. Immunol. 72: 157-160, 1982.

96. Marcus, P.I. Interferon induction by viruses: One molecule of dsRNA as the threshold for interferon induction. In *Interferon 1983,* Volume 5. Edited by I. Gresser. Academic Press, New York, 1983, pp. 115-180.

97. Silhol, M., Huez, G., and Lebleu, B. An antiviral state induced in HeLa cells by microinjected Poly(rI).Poly(rC). J. Gen. Virol. 67: 1867-1873, 1986.

98. Nir, U., Cohen, B., Chen, L., and Revel, M. A human IFN-beta-1 gene deleted of promoter sequences upstream from the TATA box is controlled post-transcriptionally by dsRNA. Nucl. Acid Res. 12: 6979-6993, 1984.

99. Fujita, T., Ohno, S., Yasumitsu, H., and Taniguchi, T. Delimitation and properties of DNA sequences required for the regulated expression of human interferon-beta gene. Cell 41: 489-496, 1985.

100. Goodburn, S., Burstein, H., and Maniatis, T. The human beta interferon gene is under negative control. Cell 45: 601-610, 1986.

101. Zinn, K., and Maniatis, T. Detection of factors that interact with the human beta-interferon regulatory region by in vivo by DNAase 1 footprinting. Cell 45: 611-618, 1986.

102. Enoch, T., Zinn, K., and Maniatis, T. Activation of the human beta-interferon gene requires an interferon-inducible factor. Molec. Cell Biol. 6: 801-810, 1986.

103. Xanthoudakis, S., and Hiscott, J. Identification of a nuclear DNA binding protein associated with the interferon-beta upstream regulatory region. J. Biol. Chem. 262: 8298-8302, 1987.

104. Raj, N.B.K., and Pitha, P.M. Synthesis of new proteins associated with the induction of interferon in human fibroblast cells. Proc. Natl. Acad. Sci. (USA) 77: 4918-4922, 1980.

105. Raj, N.B.K., and Pitha, P.M. Analysis of interferon mRNA in human fibroblast cells induced to produce interferon. Proc. Natl. Acad. Sci. (USA) 78: 7426-7430, 1981.

106. Raj, N.B.K., and Pitha, P.M. Two levels of regulation of beta-interferon gene expression in human cells. Proc. Natl. Acad. Sci. (USA) 80: 3923-3927, 1983.

107. Pickering, L.A., Kronenberg, L.H., and Stewart, W.E. II. Spontaneous production of human interferon. Proc. Natl. Acad. Sci. (USA) 77: 5938-5942, 1980.

108. Tovey, M.G., Streuli, M., Gresser, I., Gugenheim, J., Blanchard, B., Guymarho, J., Vignaux, F., and Gigou, M. Interferon messenger RNA is produced constitutively in the organs of normal individuals. Proc. Natl. Acad. Sci. (USA) 84: 5038-5042, 1987.

109. Zawatzky, R., De Maeyer-Guignard, J., and De Maeyer, E. The detection of individual cells containing interferon mRNA by in situ hybridization with specific interferon DNA probes. Meth. Enzymol. 119: 474-481, 1986.

110. Aguet, M. High affinity binding of [125]I-labelled mouse interferon to a specific cell surface receptor. Nature 284: 459-461, 1980.

111. Epstein, C.J., McManus, N.H., Epstein, L.B., Branca, A.A., D'Alessandro,

S.B., and Baglioni, C. Direct evidence that the gene product of the human chromosome 21 locus, *IFRC*, is the interferon-alpha receptor. Biochem. Biophys. Res. Commun. 107: 1060-1066, 1982.

112. Jung, V., Rashidbaigi, A., Jones, C., Tischfield, J.A., Shows, T.B., and Pestka, S. Human chromosomes 6 and 21 are required for sensitivity to human interferon gamma. Proc. Natl. Acad. Sci. (USA) 84: 4151-4155, 1987.

113. Mogensen, K.E., and Bandu, M-T. Kinetic evidence for an activation step following binding of human interferon alpha-2 to the membrane receptors of Daudi cells. Eur. J. Biochem. 134: 355-364, 1983.

114. Branca, A.A., Faltynek, C.R., D'Alessandro, S.B., and Baglioni, C. Interaction of interferon with cellular receptors. J. Biol. Chem. 257: 13291-13296, 1982.

115. Anderson, P., Yip, Y.K., and Vilcek, J. Human interferon gamma is internalized and degraded by cultured fibroblasts. J. Biol. Chem. 258: 6497-6502, 1983.

116. Sarkar, F.H., and Gupta, S.L. Interferon receptor interaction. Internalization of interferon alpha-2 and modulation of its receptor on human cells. Eur. J. Biochem. 140: 461-467, 1984.

117. Zoon, K.C., Arnheiter, H., zur Nedden, D., Fitzgerald, D.J.P., and Willingham, M.C. Human interferon alpha enters cells by receptor-mediated endocytosis. Virology 130: 195-203, 1983.

118. Kishnaryov, V.M., MacDonald, H.S., Sedmak, J.J., and Grossberg, S.E. Murine interferon-beta receptor-mediated endocytosis and nuclear membrane binding. Proc. Natl. Acad. Sci. (USA) 82: 3281 3285, 1985.

119. Kushnaryov, V.M., MacDonald, H.S., Debruin, J., Lemense, G.P., Sedmak, J.J., and Grossberg, S.E. Internalization and transport of mouse beta-interferon into the cell nucleus. J. IFN Res. 6: 241-245, 1986.

120. Huez, G., Sihol, M., and Lebleu, B. Microinjected interferon does not promote an antiviral response in HeLa cells. Biochem. Biophys. Res. Commun. 110: 155-160, 1983.

121. Tovey, M.G. Interferons and cyclic nucleotides. In *Interferon 1982*. Volume 4. Edited by I. Gresser. Academic Press, New York, 1982, pp. 23-46.

122. Larner, A.C., Jonak, G., Cheng, Y.S.E., Korant, B., Knight, E., and Darnell, J.E. Transcriptional induction of two genes in human cells by interferon beta. Proc. Natl. Acad. Sci. (USA) 81: 6733-6737, 1984.

122a. Hamilton, T.A., and Adams, D.O. Molecular mechanisms of signal transduction in macrophages. Immunol. Today 8: 151-158, 1987.

122b. Sanceau, J., Sondermeyer, P., Beranger, F., Falcoff, R., and Vaquero, C. Intracellular human γ-interferon triggers an antiviral state in transformed murine L cells. Proc. Natl. Acad. Sci. (USA) 84: 2906-2910, 1987.

123. Clemens, M., and McNurlan, M.A. Regulation of cell proliferation and differentiation by interferons. Biochem. J. 226: 345-360, 1985.

124. Mannering, G.J., and Deloria, L.B. The pharmacology and toxicology of the interferons: an overview. Ann. Rev. Pharmacol. Toxicol. 26: 455-515, 1986.

125. Weil, J., Epstein, C., Epstein, L.B., Sedmak, J.J., Sabra, J.L., and Gross-berg, S.E. A unique set of polypeptides is induced by gamma interferon in addition to those induced in common with alpha and beta interferons. Nature 301: 437-439, 1983.

126. Staheli, P., Horisberger, M.A., and Haller, O. Mx-dependent resistance to influenza virus is induced by mouse interferons alpha and beta but not gamma. Virology 132: 456-461, 1984.

127. Chebath, J., Merlin, G., Metz, R., Benech, P., and Revel, M. Interferon-induced 56,000 Mr protein and its mRNA in human cells: molecular cloning and partial sequence of the cDNA. Nucl. Acids Res. 11: 1213-1226, 1983.

128. Merlin, G., Chebath, J., Benech, P., Metz, R., and Revel, M. Molecular cloning and sequence of partial cDNA for interferon-induced (2'5')oligo(A)synthetase mRNA from human cells. Proc. Natl. Acad. Sci. (USA) 80: 4904-4908, 1983.

129. Colonno, R.J., and Pang, R.H.L. Induction of unique mRNA by human interferons. J. Biol. Chem. 257: 9234-9237, 1982.

130. Friedman, R.L., Manly, S.P., McMahon, M., Kerr, I.M., Stark, G.R. Transcriptional and post-transcriptional regulation of interferon-induced gene expression in human cells. Cell 38: 745-755, 1984.

131. Luster, A.D., Unkeless, J.C., Ravetch, J.V. Gamma-interferon transcriptionally regulates an early-response gene containing homology to platelet proteins. Nature 315: 372-375, 1985.

132. Larner, A.C., Chaudhuri, A., Darnell, J.E. Jr. Transcriptional induction by interferon. New proteins determine the extent and length of the induction. J. Biol Chem. 261: 453-459, 1986.

133. Friedman, R.L., and Stark, G.R. Alpha-interferon induced transcription of HLA and metallothionein genes containing homologous upstream sequences. Nature 314: 637-639, 1985.

134. Samanta, H., Engel, D.A., Kimura, A., Israel, A., Le Bail, O., and Kourilisky, P. Detailed analysis of the mouse H-2K promoter: Enhancer-like sequences and their role in the regulation of class I gene expression. Cell 44: 261-272, 1986.

135. Israel, A., Kimura, A., Fournier, A., Fellous, M., Kourilsky, P. Interferon response sequence potentiates activity of an enhancer in the promoter region of a mouse H-2 gene. Nature 322: 743-746, 1986.

136. Vogel, J., Kress, M., Khoury, G., and Jay, G. A transcriptional enhancer and an interferon-responsive sequence in major histocompatibility complex class I genes. Molec. Cell. Biol. 6: 3550-3554, 1986.

137. Sujita, K., Miyazaki, J-I., Appella, E., and Ozato, K. Interferons increase transcription of a major histocompatibility class I gene via a 5' interferon consensus sequence. Molec. Cell. Biol. 7: 2625-2630, 1987.

138. Samanta, H., Engel, D.A., Chao, H.M., Thakur, A., Garcia-Blanco, M.A., and Lengyel, P. Interferons as gene activators. Cloning of the 5' terminus and the control segment of an interferon activated gene. J. Biol. Chem. 261: 11849-11858, 1986.

139. Gribaudo, G., Toniato, E., Engel, D.A., and Lengyel, P.A. Interferons as

gene activators. Characteristics of an interferon-activable enhancer. J. Biol. Chem. 262: 11878-11883, 1987.

140. Levy, D., Larner, A., Chaudhuri, A., Babiss, L.E., and Darnell, J.E. Jr. Interferon-stimulated transcription: Isolation of an inducible gene and identification of its regulatory region. Proc. Natl. Acad. Sci. (USA) 83: 8929-8933, 1986.

141. Reich, N., Evanms, B., Levy, D., Fahey, D., Knight, E. Jr., and Darnell, J.E. Jr. Interferon-induced transcription of a gene encoding a 15-kDa protein depends on an upstream enhancer element. Proc. Natl. Acad. Sci. (USA) 84: 6394-6398, 1987.

141a. Boss, J.M., and Strominger, J.L. Regulation of a transfected human class II major histocompatibility complex gene in human fibroblasts. Proc. Natl. Acad. Sci. (USA) 83: 9139-9143, 1986.

142. Haas, A.L., Ahrens, P., Bright, P.M., and Ankel, H. Interferon induces a 15-kilodalton protein exhibiting marked homology to ubiquitin. J. Biol. Chem. 262: 11315-11317, 1987.

143. Yasui, H., Takai, K., Yoshida, R., and Hayashi, O. Interferon enhances tryptophane metabolism by inducing pulmonary indoleamine 2,3-dioxygenase: Its possible occurrence in cancer patients. Proc. Natl. Acad. Sci. (USA) 83: 6622-6626, 1986.

144. Adams, D.J., Balkwill, F.R., Griffin, D.B., Hayes, J.D., Lewis, A.S., and Wolf, C.R. Induction and suppression of glutathione transferases by interferon. J. Biol. Chem. 262: 4888-4892, 1987.

145. Jonak, G.J., and Knight, E. Jr. Selective reduction of *c-myc* RNA in Daudi cells by human alpha-interferon. Proc. Natl. Acad. Sci. (USA) 81: 1747-1750, 1984.

146. Einat, M., Resnitzky, D., and Kimchi, A. Close link between reduction of *c-myc* expression by interferon and G0/G1 arrest. Nature 313: 597-600, 1985.

147. Dani, C., Mechti, N., Piechaczyk, Lebleu, B., Jeanteur, P., and Blanchard, J.M. Increased rate of degradation of *c-myc* mRNA in interferon-treated Daudi cells. Proc. Natl. Acad. Sci. (USA) 82: 4896-4899, 1985.

148. Knight, E. Jr., Anton, E.A., Friedland, B., and Jonak, G.J. Regulation of *c-myc* proteins by interferon. In *Interferons as Cell Growth Inhibitors and Antitumor Factors*. Edited by R.M. Friedman, T. Merigan, and T. Sreevalsan. Alan Liss, New York, 1986, pp. 403-411.

149. Kimchi, A., Yarden, A., and Resnitzky, D. Suppression of c-*myc* by growth inhibitors: The role of endogenous interferon, and possible cooperation with tumor necrosis factor. In *Interferons as Cell Growth Inhibitors and Antitumor Factors*. Edited by R.M. Friedman, T. Merigan, and T. Sreevalsan. Alan R. Liss, New York, 1986, pp. 391-402.

150. Samid, D., and Friedman, R.M. Transcriptional regulation of *ras* by interferon. In *Interferons as Cell Growth Inhibitors and Antitumor Factors*. Edited by R.M. Friedman, T. Merigan, and T. Sreevalsan. Alan R. Liss, New York, 1986, pp. 413-422.

151. Canivet, M., Mercier, G., Giron, M-L., Emanoil-Ravier, R., and Peries, J. Differential regulation of V-Ki-*ras*, c-*myc* and IAP gene expression by interferon in a murine cell line transformed by Kirstein mouse sarcoma retro-

virus. In *Interferons as Cell Growth Inhibitors and Antitumor Factors*. Edited by R.M. Friedman, T. Merigan, and T. Sreevalsan. Alan R. Liss, New York, 1986, pp. 319-333.

152. Slamon, D.J. Proto-oncogenes and human cancers. N. Engl. J. Med. 317: 955-957, 1987.

153. Helden, C-H., and Westermark, B. Growth factors: Mechanism of action and relation to oncogenes. Cell 37: 9-20, 1984.

154. Marshall, C.J. Oncogenes and growth control 1987. Meeting Report. Cell 49: 723-725, 1987.

155. Einat, M., Resnitzky, D., and Kimchi, A. Inhibitory effects of interferons on the expression of genes regulated by platelet-derived growth factor. Proc. Natl. Acad. Sci. (USA) 82: 7608-7612, 1985.

156. Brandwein, S.R. Regulation of interleukin 1 production by mouse peritoneal macrophages. Effects of arachidonic acid metabolites, cyclic nucleotides and interferons. J. Immunol. 261: 8624-8632, 1986.

157. Collart, M.A., Belin, D., Vassalli, J-D., de Kossoto, S., and Vassalli, P. Gamma interferon enhances macrophage transcription of the tumor necrosis factor/ cachectin, interleukin 1 and urokinase genes which are controlled by short-lived repressors. J. Exper. Med. 164: 2113-2118, 1986.

158. Zoon, K.C., Karasaki, Y., zur Nedden, D.L., Hu, R., and Arnheiter, H. Modulation of epidermal growth factor receptors by human alpha interferon. Proc. Natl. Acad. Sci. (USA) 83: 8226-8230, 1986.

159. Chen, L-K., Mathieu-Mahul, D., Bach, F.H., Dausset, J., Bensussan, A., and Sasportes, M. Recombinant interferon alpha can induce rearrangement of T-cell antigen receptor alpha-chain genes and maturation to cytotoxicity in T-lymphocyte clones in vitro. Proc. Natl. Acad. Sci. (USA) 83: 4887-4889, 1986.

160. Tsujimoto, M., Feinman, R., and Vilcek, J. Differential effects of type I IFN and IFN-gamma on the binding of tumor necrosis factor to receptors in two human cell lines. J. Immunol. 137: 2272-2276, 1986.

161. Aggarwalt, B.B., and Eessalu, T.E. Induction of receptors for tumor necrosis factor alpha by interferons is not a major mechanism for their synergistic cytotoxic response. J. Biol. Chem. 262: 10000-10007, 1987.

162. Rambaldi, A., Young, D.C., Herrmann, F., Cannistra, S.A.S., and Griffin, J.D. Interferon-gamma induces expression of the interleukin 2 receptor gene in human monocytes. Eur. J. Immunol. 17: 153-156, 1987.

163. Gresser, I. The effect of interferon on the expression of surface antigens. In *Interferon* Volume 2. *Interferons and the Immune System*. Edited by J. Vilcek and E. De Maeyer. Elsevier, Amsterdam, 1984, pp. 113-132.

164. Gaicomini, P., Aguzzi, A., Pestka, S., Fisher, P.B., and Ferrone, S. Modulation by recombinant DNA leucocyte (alpha) and fibroblast (beta) interferons of the expression and shedding of HLA and tumor associated antigens by human melanoma cells. J. Immunol. 133: 1649-1659, 1984.

165. Greiner, J.W., Guadagni, F., Pestka, S., and Schlom, J. Augmentation of antigen expression by recombinant human interferon. In *Interferons as Cell Growth Inhibitors and Antitumor Factors*. Edited by R.M. Friedman, T. Merigan, and T. Sreevalsan. Alan R. Liss, New York, 1986, pp. 17-26.

166. Pfeffer, L.M., Wang, E., Landsberger, F.R., and Tamm, I. Assays to measure plasma membrane and cytoskeletal changes in interferon-treated cells.

Meth. Enzymol. 79: 461-473, 1981.

167. Taylor-Papadimitriou, J. Effects of interferons on cell growth and function. In *Interferon* Volume 1. *General and Applied Aspects*. Edited by A. Billiau. Elsevier, Amsterdam, 1984, pp. 139-166.

168. Taylor-Papadimitriou, J., Higgins, T., Shearer, M., and Rozengurt, E. Inhibition of cell growth by interferon: An analysis using quiescent fibroblasts stimulated by PDGF and other growth factors. In *Interferons as Cell Growth Inhibitors and Antitumor Factors*. Edited by R.M. Friedman, T. Merigan, and T. Sreevalsan. Alan R. Liss, New York, 1986, pp. 481 495.

169. Bourgeade, M.F., and Chany, C. Inhibition of interferon action by cytochalasin B, colchicine, and vinblastine. Proc. Soc. Exper. Biol. Med. 153: 501-505, 1976.

170. Clemens, M.J., and Exley, R. Changes in nuclease sensitivity of newly replicated DNA in human and mouse cells during growth inhibition induced by interferons. In *Interferons as Cell Growth Inhibitors and Antitumor Factors*. Edited by R.M. Friedman, T. Merigan, and T. Sreevalsan. Alan R. Liss, New York, 1986, pp. 455-466.

171. Karray, S., Vazquez, A., Merle-Beral, H., Olive, D., Debre, P., and Galanaud, P. Synergestic effect of recombinant IL-2 and interferon-gamma on the proliferation of human monoclonal lymphocytes. J. Immunol. 138: 3824-3828, 1987.

172. Moritz, T., and Kirchner, H. The effect of interferons on cellular differentiation. Blut 53: 361-370, 1986.

173. Grossberg, S.E., and Taylor, J.L. Interferon effects on cell differentiation. In *Interferon* Volume 3, *Mechanisms of Production and Action*. Edited by R.M. Friedman. Elsevier, Amsterdam, 1984, pp. 299-342.

174. Chany, C., and Vignal, M. Effect of prolonged interferon treatment on mouse embryonic fibroblasts transformed by murine sarcoma virus. J. Gen. Virol. 7: 203-210, 1970.

175. Sergiescu, D., Gerfaux, J., Joret, A-M., and Chany, C. Persistent expression of v-*mos* oncogene in transformed cells that revert to non-malignancy after prolonged treatment with interferon. Proc. Natl. Acad. Sci. (USA) 83: 5764-5768, 1986.

176. Gerfaux, J., Sergiescu, D., Vignal, M., Joret, A.M., and Chany, C. Stable reversion to non malignancy by long term interferon treatment of cells expressing the V-*mos* oncogene. In *Interferons as Cell Growth Inhibitors and Antitumor Factors*. Edited by R.M. Friedman, T.Merigan, and T. Sreevalsan. Alan R. Liss, New York, 1986, pp. 377-389.

177. Samid, D., Chang, E., and Friedman, R.M. Biochemical correlates of phenotypic reversion in interferon-treated mouse cells transformed by a human oncogene. Biochem. Biophys. Res. Commun. 119: 21-28, 1984.

178. Samid, D., Flessate, D.M., and Friedman, R.M. Interferon-induced revertants of *ras*-transformed cells: Resistance to transformation by specific oncogenes and retransformation by 5-azacytidine. Molec. Cell. Biol. 7: 2196-2200, 1987.

179. Gresser, I., Aguet, M., Morel-Maroger, L., Woodrow, D., Puvion-Dutilleul, F., Guillon, J-C., and Maury, C. Electrophoretically pure mouse interferon inhibits growth, induces liver and kidney lesions and kills suckling mice. Am. J. Pathol. 102: 396-408, 1980.

180. Baron, S., Hughes, T.K., Sarzotti-Kelsoe, M., Klimpel, G.R., Fleischmann, W.R. Jr., Weigent, D., Stanton, G.J., Albrecht, C., and Tyring, S. Interferon-mediated cytolysis of tumor cells. In *Interferons as Cell Growth Inhibitors and Antitumor Factors*. Edited by R.M. Friedman, T. Merigan, and T. Sreevalsan. Alan R. Liss, New York, 1986, pp. 447-453.

181. Chang, E.H., Black, R., Zou, Z-Q., Masnyk, T., Ridge, J., Noguchi, P., and Harford, J.B. Gamma-interferon modulates growth of A431 cells and expression of EGF receptors. In *Interferons as Cell Growth Inhibitors and Antitumor Factors*. Edited by R.M. Friedman, T. Merigan, and T. Sreevalsan. Alan R. Liss, New York, 1986, pp. 335-349.

182. Oladipopo-Williams, C.K., Svet-Moldavskaya, I., Vilcek, J., Ohnuma, T., and Holland, J.F. Inhibitory effects of human leukocyte and fibroblast interferons in normal and chronic myelogenous leukemic granulocyte progenitor cells. Oncology 38: 356-360, 1981.

183. Takahashi, N., Mundy, G.R., and Roodman, G.D. Recombinant human interferon gamma inhibits formation of human osteoclast-like cells. J. Immunol. 137: 3544-3549, 1986.

184. Miossec, P., and Ziff, M. Immune interferon enhances the production of interleukin-1 by human endothelial cells stimulated with lipopolysaccharide. J. Immunol. 137: 2848-2852, 1986.

185. Vogel, S.N., and Friedman, R.M. Interferon and macrophages: activation and cell surface changes. In *Interferon 2. Interferons and the Immune System*. Edited by J. Vilck and E. de Maeyer. Elseiver, Amsterdam, 1984, pp. 35-59.

186. Heberman, R.B. Interferon and cytotoxic effector cells. In *Interferon 2. Interferons and the Immune System*. Edited by J. Vilcek and E. de Maeyer. Elsevier, Amsterdam, 1984, pp. 61-84.

187. Sonnenfeld, G. Effects of interferon on antibody formation. In *Interferon 2. Interferons and the Immune System*. Edited by J. Vilcek and E. de Maeyer. Elsevier, Amsterdam, 1984, pp. 85-99.

188. De Maeyer-Guignard, J. Effects of interferon cell-mediated immunity as manifested by delayed hypersensitivity and allograft rejection. In *Interferon. 2. Interferons and the Immune System*. Edited by J. Vilcek and E. de Maeyer. Elsevier, Amsterdam, 1984, pp. 133-145.

189. Falcoff, E., Falcoff, R., Fournier, F., and Chany, C. Production en masse, purification partielle et caractérisation d'un interféron destiné à des essais thérapeutiques humains. Annales de l'Institut Pasteur 111: 562-584, 1966.

190. Strander, H., Kantell, K., Carlstrom, G., and Jakobsson, P.A. Systemic administration of potent interferon to man. J. Natl. Cancer Inst. 51: 733-742, 1973.

191. Foon, K.A., and Todd, R.F., III. Immunologic classification of leukemia and lymphoma. Blood 68: 1-31, 1986.

192. Foon, K.A., Gale, R.P., and Todd, R.F. III. Recent advances in the immunological classification of leukemia. Sem. Hematol. 23: 257-283, 1986.

193. Andreeff, M. Cell kinetics in leukemia. Sem. Hematol. 23: 300-314, 1986.

194. Olsson, I. Is the maturation arrest in myeloid leukemia reversible? Acta Med. Scand. 214: 261-272, 1984.

195. Weiss, L. Cellular regulation in hematopoiesis. In *The Reticuloendothelial*

*System*. Volume 9. *Hypersensitivity*. Edited by S.M. Phillips and M.R. Escobar. Plenum Press, New York, 1987, pp. 1-22.

196. Vincent, P.C. Leukemic cellular proliferation. Ann. NY Acad. Sci. 459: 308-327, 1985.

197. Chiao, J.W., Andreef, M., Freitag, W.B., and Arlin, Z. Induction of in vitro proliferation and maturation of human aneuploid myelogenous leukemic cells. J. Exper. Med. 155: 1357-1369, 1982.

198. Sandberg, A.A. The chromosomes in human leukemia. Sem. Hematol. 23: 201-217, 1986.

199. Showe, L.C., and Croce, C.M. Chromosome translocation in B and T cell neoplasias. Sem. Hematol. 23: 237-244.

200. Sandberg, A.A. Applications of cytogenetics in neoplastic disease. CRC Crit. Rev. Clin. Lab. Sci. 22: 219-274, 1985.

201. Bouroncle, B.A., Wiseman, B.K., and Doan, C.A. Leukemic reticuloendotheliosis. Blood 13: 609-629, 1958.

202. Schreck, R., and Donnelly, W.J. "Hairy" cells in blood lymphoreticular neoplastic disease and "flagellated" cells of normal lymph nodes. Blood 27: 199-211, 1966.

203. Portlock, C.S. Therapeutic approaches to the treatment of hairy cell leukemia. Sem. Oncol. 13(4) suppl. 5: 55-59, 1986.

204. Yam, L.T., Li, C.Y., and Lam, K.W. Tartrate-resistant acid phosphatase isozyme in the reticulum cells of leukemic reticuloendotheliosis. N. Engl. J. Med. 284: 357-360, 1971.

205. Braylan, R.C., Jaffee, E.S., Triche, T.J., Nanba, K., Fowlkes, B.J., Metzger, H., Frank, M.M., Dolan, M.S., Yee, C.L., Green, I., and Berard, C.W. Structural and functional properties of the "hairy" cells of leukemic reticuloendotheliosis. Cancer 41: 210-2, 1978.

206. Caligaris-Cappio, F., Bergui, L., Tesio, L., Corbascio, G., Tousco, F., and Marchisio, P.C. Cytoskeleton organization is aberrantly rearranged in the cells of B chronic lymphocytic leukemia and hairy cell leukemia. Blood 67: 223-239, 1986.

207. Reiber, E.P., Hadass, M.R., Linke, R.P., Saal, J.G., Riethmuller, G., von Heyden, H.W., and Waller, H.D. Hairy cell leukemia: surface markers and functional capabilities of the leukemic cells analyzed in eight patients. Br. J. Haematol. 42: 175-188, 1979.

208. Posnett, D.N., Chiorazzi, N., and Kunkel, H.G. Monoclonal antibodies with specificity for hairy cell leukemia cells. J. Clin. Invest. 70: 254-2??, 1982.

209. Jansen, J., Le Bien, T.W., and Kersey, J.H. The phenotype of the neoplastic cells of hairy cell leukemia studied with monoclonal antibodies. Blood 59: 609-614, 1982.

210. Korsmeyer, S.J., Greene, W.C., Cossman, J., Hsu, S.M., Jensen, J.P., Neckers, L.M., Marshall, S.L., Bakhshl, A., Deppere, J.M., Leonard, W.J., Jaffe, K.E.S., and Waldman, T.A. Rearrangement and expression of IgG genes and expression of tac antigen in hairy cell leukemia. Proc. Natl. Acad. Sci. (USA) 80: 4522-4526, 1983.

211. Jansen, J., Ottolander, G.J., Schuit, H.R.E., Waayer, J.L.M., and Hijmans, W. Hairy cell leukemia: its place among the chronic B cell leukemias. Sem. Oncol. 11: 368-393, 1984.

212. Anderson, K.C., Boyd, A.W., Fisher, D.C., Leslie, D., Schlossman, S.F., and Nadler, L.M. Hairy cell leukemia: a tumor of pre-plasma cells. Blood 65: 620-629, 1985.

213. Korsmeyer, S.J., Greene, W.C., and Waldman, T.A. Cellular origin of hairy cell leukemia: malignant B cells that express receptor for T cell growth factor. Sem. Oncol. 11: 394-400, 1984.

214. Liebson, H.J., Marrack, P., and Keppler, J.W. B cell helper factors: I. Requirement for both interleukin 2 and another 40,000 molecular weight factor. J. Immunol. 129: 1398-1402, 1982.

215. Paganelli, K.A., Evans, S.S., Han, T., and Ozer, H. B cell growth factor induced proliferation of hairy cell lymphocytes and inhibition by type 1 interferon in vitro. Blood 67: 937-943, 1986.

216. Ford, R.J., Lwok, D., Quesada, J., and Sahasrabuddhe, C.G. Production of B cell growth factor(s) by neoplastic B cells from hairy cell leukemia patients. Blood 67: 573-577, 1986.

217. Quesada, J.R., and Gutterman, J.U. Alpha interferons in B cell neoplasms. Br. J. Haematol. 64: 639-646, 1986.

218. Turner, A., and Kjeldsberg, C.R. Hairy cell leukemia: a review. Medicine 57: 477-499, 1978.

219. Sabahoun, G., Bouffette, P., and Flandrin, G. Hairy cell leukemia. Leukemia Res. 2: 187-195, 1978.

220. Golumb, H.M., Catowsky, D., and Golde, D.W. Hairy cell leukemia: a five-year update on 71 patients. Ann. Intern. Med. 99: 485-486, 1983.

221. Cawley, J.C., and Worman, C.P. Hairy cell leukemia (annotation). Br. J. Haematol. 60: 213-218, 1985.

222. Golde, D.W., Jacobs, A.D., Glaspy, J.A., and Champlin, R.E. Hairy cell leukemia: biology and treatment. Sem. Hematol. 23(3) (suppl. 1): 3-9, 1986.

223. Worman, C.P., and Cawley, T.C. Monoclonal antibody-defined T-cell subsets in hairy-cell leukemia. Scand. J. Haemat. 29: 338-344, 1982.

224. Foa, R., Lauria, F., Raspadori, D., Lusso, P., Ferrando, M.L., Fierro, M.T., Giubellino, M.C., and Catovsky, D. Normal helper T-cell function in hairy cell leukemia. Scand. J. Haematol. 31: 322-328, 1983.

225. Fontana, L., De Rossi, G., De Sanctis, G., Ensoli, F., Lopez, M., Annino, L., and Mandelli, F. Decreased NK activity in hairy cell leukemia (HCL): an analysis at the cellular level. Blut 53: 107-113, 1986.

226. Porzsolt, F., Janik, R., Heil, G., Brudler, O., Raghavachar, A., Scholtz, S., Papendick, U., and Heimpel, H. Deficient IFN production in hairy cell leukemia. Blut 52: 185-190, 1986.

227. Glaspy, J.A., Jacobs, A.D., and Golde, D.W. Evolving therapy of hairy cell leukemia. Cancer 59: 652-657, 1987.

228. Golomb, H.M., and Ratain, M.J. Recent advances in the treatment of hairy cell leukemia. N. Engl. J. Med. 316: 870-871, 1987.

229. Spiers, A.S.D., Parekh, S.J., and Bishop, M.B. Hairy cell leukemia: induction of complete remission with pentostatin (2'-deoxycoformycin). J. Clin. Oncol. 2: 1336-1342, 1984.

230. Johnston, J.B., Glazer, R.I., Pugh, L., and Israels, L.G. The treatment of hairy cell leukemia with 2'-deoxycoformycin. Br. J. Haematol. 63: 525-534.

231. Johnston, J.B., Eisenhauer, E., Barr, R., Feldman, L., Maksymiuk, A., Scott, G., Sutton, D., Venner, P., and Walde, D. 2'-deoxycoformycin (DCF) in hairy cell leukemia (HCL); a Canadian phase II trial. Proc. Am. Soc. Clin. Oncol. 5: 159 (#621), 1986.

232. Kraut, E.H., Bouroncle, B.A., and Grever, M.R. Low dose deoxycoformycin in the treatment of hairy cell leukemia. Blood 68: 1119-1122, 1986.

233. Spiers, A.S.D., Moore, D., Cassileth, P.A., Harrington, D.P., Cummings, F.G., Neiman, R.S., Bennett, J.M., and O'Connell, M.J. Remissions in hairy cell leukemia with pentostatin (2'-deoxycoformycin). N. Engl. J. Med. 316: 825-830, 1987.

234. Calvio, F., Castaigne, S., Sigaux, F., Marty, M., Degos, L., Boiron, M., and Flandrin, G. Intensive chemotherapy of hairy cell leukemia in patients with aggressive disease. Blood 65: 115-119, 1985.

235. Quesada, J.R., Reuben, J., Manning, J.T., Hersh, E.M., and Gutterman, J.U. Alpha interferon for the induction of remission in hairy cell leukemia. N. Engl. J. Med. 310: 15-18, 1984.

236. Quesada, J.R., Hersh, E.M., and Gutterman, J.U. Treatment of hairy cell leukemia with alpha interferon. Proc. ASCO 3: 207, 1984.

237. Hagberg, H., Alm, G., Bjorkholm, M., Glimelius, B., Killander, A., Simonsson, B., Sundstrom, C., and Ahre, A. Alpha interferon treatment of patients with hairy cell leukemia. Scand. J. Haematol. 35: 66-70, 1985.

238. Worman, C.P., Catovsky, D., Bevan, P., Cambo, L., Joyner, M., Green, P.J., Williams, H.J.H., Bottomley, J.M., Gordon-Smith, E.C., and Cawley, J.C. Interferon is effective in hairy cell leukemia. Br. J. Haematol. 60: 759-763, 1985.

239. Castaigne, S., Sigaux, F., Cantell, K., Falcoff, E., Boiron, M., Flandrin, G., and Degos, L. Interferon alpha in the treatment of hairy cell leukemia. Cancer 57: 1681-1684, 1986.

240. Flandrin, G., Sigaux, F., Castaigne, S., Billard, C., Aguet, M., Boiron, M., Falcoff, E., and Degos, L. Treatment of hairy cell leukemia with recombinant alpha interferon-I. Quantitative study of bone marrow changes during first month of treatment. Blood 67: 817-821, 1986.

241. Foon, K.A., Maluish, A.E., Abrams, P.G., Wrightington, S., Stevenson, H., Alarif, A., Fer, M.F., Overton, W.R., Poole, M., Schnipper, E.F., Jaffe, E.S., and Herberman, R.B. Recombinant leucocyte alpha interferon therapy for advanced hairy cell leukemia. Therapeutic and immunologic results. Am. J. Med. 80: 351-356, 1986.

242. Quesada, J., Hersh, E.M., Manning, J., Reuben, J., Keating, M., Schnipper, E., Itri, L., and Gutterman, J.U. Treatment of hairy cell leukemia with recombinant alpha interferon. Blood 68: 493-497, 1986.

243. Al-Katib, A., Berman, E., Black, P., and Koziner, B. Hairy cell leukemia: a model for studying the B cell family of diseases. Sem. Oncol. 13(4) (suppl. 5): 48-54, 1986.

244. Thompson, J.A., Brady, J., Kidd, P., and Fefer, A. Recombinant alpha-2 interferon in the treatment of hairy cell leukemia. Cancer Treat. Rep. 69: 791-793, 1985.

245. Ehmann, W.C., and Silber, R. Recombinant alpha-2 interferon for treatment of hairy cell leukemia without prior splenectomy. Am. J. Med. 80: 1111-1114, 1986.

246. Mandelli, F., Annino, L., Cafolla, A., De Rossi, G., Bianco, P., Fontana, L., and Dianzani, F. Hairy cell leukemia: preliminary results with alpha$_2$ (r) interferon. Tumori 72: 153-157, 1986.

247. Ratain, M.J., Golomb, H.M., Vardiman, J.W., Vokes, E.E., Jacobs, R.H., and Daly, K. Treatment of hairy cell leukemia with recombinant alpha 2 interferon. Blood 65: 644-648, 1985.

248. Ratain, M.J., Golomb, H.M., Bardawil, R.G., Vardiman, J.W., Westbrook, C.A., Kaminer, L.S., Lembersky, B.C., Bitter, M.A., and Daly, K. Durability of responses to interferon alfa-2b in advanced hairy cell leukemia. Blood 69: 872-877, 1987.

249. Jacobs, A.D., Champlin, R.E., and Golde, D.W. Recombinant alpha-2 interferon for hairy cell leukemia. Blood 65: 1017-1020, 1985.

250. Glaspy, J.A., Jacobs, A.D., and Golde, D.W. Evolving therapy of hairy cell leukemia. Cancer 59: 652-657, 1987.

251. Bernemen, Z.N., Gastl, G., Cangji, D., Vancamp, B., Jochsman, K., Aulitzky, W., Flament, J., Peetermans, M.E., and Huber, C. Treatment of hairy cell leukemia with recombinant alpha 2 interferon. Eur. J. Cancer Clin. Oncol. 22: 987-991, 1986.

252. Schwarzinger, I., Bettelheim, P., Geissler, K., Herold, C., Jagar, U., Kos, M., Neumann, E., Pabinger, I., and Lechner, K. Recombinant alpha 2 interferon for primary therapy in hairy cell leukemia. Blut 53: 129-130, 1986.

253. Quesada, J.R. Alpha interferons in the treatment of hairy cell leukemia. Immunobiology 172: 250-254, 1986.

254. Aderka, D., Levo, Y., Rahmani, R., Mori, Y., Vaks, B., Horowitz, O., Doerner, T., Shoham, J., Wallach, D., and Revel, M. Rapid improvement in a terminal case of hairy cell leukemia treated with a new human recombinant interferon, IFN-α-C. Isr. J. Med. Sci. 21: 977-981, 1985.

255. Maziarz, R.T., Tepler, I., Kerouac, M., Antin, J., Allowill Churchill, W., Holmes, W., and Rappaport, J. Enhanced reversal of atypical mycobacterial infections in patients with hairy cell leukemia by treatment with alpha interferon. Blood 68: 227a (#785), Sept. 1986.

256. Schnall, S., Barnard, E., Armstrong, D., White, K., and Portlock, C. Treatment of mycobacterium avium intracellularle (MAI) in patients with hairy cell leukemia (HCL): the use of antimycobacterial antibody titer (AMAT). Blood 68: 232a (#807) Sept. 1986.

257. Bennett, C.L., Westbrook, C.A., Gruber, B., and Golomb, H.M. Hairy cell leukemia and mucormycosis. Treatment with alpha 2 interferon. Am. J. Med. 81: 1065-1067, 1986.

258. Gastl, G., Aulitzky, W., Tilg, H., Nachbauer, K., Troppmair, J., Flener, R., and Huber, C. A biological approach to optimize interferon treatment in hairy cell leukemia. Immunobiology 172: 262-268, 1986.

259. Von Wussow, P., Will, W., Diedrich, H., Freund, M., Poliwoda, H., and Deicher, H. Low dosage interferon alpha therapy of hairy cell leukemia. Blut 53: 214-215, 1986.

260. Kloke, O., Niederle, N., Doberauer, C., May, D., Schmidt, C.G. The dosage of alpha interferon in the treatment of hairy cell leukemia. Blut 53: 214, 1986.

261. Smalley, R.V., Tuttle, R.L., Whisnant, J.K., Anderson, S.A., Huang, A.T.,

and Robinson, W.A. Effectiveness of Wellferon at a dose of 0.2 MU/m$^2$ in the treatment of hairy cell leukemia. Blood 68: 223a (# 809), 1986.

262. Clark, R.H., Dimitrov, N.V., Axelson, J.A., Oviatt, D.L., Penner, J.A., Charamehla, I.J., and Walker, W. Intermittent alpha leucocytic inferferon in the treatment of hairy cell leukemia. Blood 68: 220a (# 759), 1986.

263. Dorken, B., Pezzuto, A., Ho, A.D., Hunstein, W., and Pralle, H.L. Stable partial remission after interferon alpha (IFN-α) treatment in patients with hairy cell leukemia (HCL). Blut 53: 215 (# 155), 1986.

264. Aulizky, W., Gastl, G., Tilg, H., v. Luttichau, I., Flener, R., and Huber, C. Recurrence of hairy cell leukemia upon discontinuation of interferon treatment. Blut 53: 215 (# 156), 1986.

265. Porzsolt, E. Primary treatment of hairy cell leukemia: should IFN-therapy replace splenectomy? Blut 52: 265-272, 1986.

266. Porzsolt, E., Digel, W., Heil, G., Bartram, C.R., Raghavachar, A., Kern, W., Seifrid, E., Raghavachar, A., and Heimpel, H. Treatment of hairy cell leukemia with interferon alpha (IFN-α) before and after splenectomy. Blut 53: 213 (# 150), 1986.

267. Quesada, J.R., Lepe-Zuniga, J.L., and Gutterman, J.U. Mid-term observations on the efficacy of alpha interferons in hairy cell leukemia (HCL) and status of the interferon system of patients in remission. J. IFN Res. 6 (suppl. 1): 4, 1986.

268. Kraut, E.H., Neff, J.C., and Grever, M. Immune function in hairy cell leukemia patients in complete remission after 2'-deoxycoformycin (dCF). Blood 68: 225a (# 777), 1986.

269. Gastl, G., Aulizky, W., Leiter, E., Flener, R., and Huber, C. Alpha interferon induces remission in hairy cell leukemia without enhancement of natural killing. Blut 52: 273-281, 1986.

270. Semenzato, G., Pizzolo, G., Agostini, C., Ambrosetti, A., Zambello, R., Trentin, L., Luca, M., Masciarelli, M., Chilosi, M., Vinante, F., Perona, G., and Cetto, G. Alpha interferon activates the natural killer system in patients with hairy cell leukemia. Blood 68: 293-297, 1986.

271. Baldini, L., Cortelezzi, A., Polli, N., Neri, A., Nobili, L., Maiolo, A.T., Lambertenghi-Deliliers, G., Polli, E.E. Human recombinant interferon alpha 2-c enhances the expression of class II HLA antigens on hairy cells. Blood 67: 458-465, 1986.

272. Billard, C., Sigaux, F., Castaigne, S., Valensi, F., Flandrin, C., Degos, L., Falcoff, E., and Aguet, M. Treatment of hairy cell leukemia with recombinant alpha interferon, II. In vivo down-regulation of alpha interferon receptors on tumor cells. Blood 67: 821-827, 1986.

273. Pizzolo, G., Chilosi, M., Ambrosetti, A., Agostini, C., Masciarelli, M., Trentin, L., Zambello, R., Lestani, M., Vinante, F., Dazzi, F., Cetto, G., and Semenzato, G. Soluble interleukin-2 receptors in the sera of patients with hairy cell leukemia: relationship with the effect of alpha interferon therapy on clinical parameters and on natural killer in vitro activity. Blood 68: 228a (# 719), 1986.

274. Reuben, J.M., Ip, S., and Quesada, J.R. Effect of IFN therapy on cellular and plasma IL2R in hairy cell leukemia. Blood 68: 231a (# 801), 1986.

275. Michalevicz, R., and Revel, M. Interferons regulate the *in vitro* differentia-

tion of multilineage lympho-myeloid stem cells in hairy cell leukemia. Proc. Natl. Acad. Sci. (USA) 84: 2307-2311, 1987.

276. Bergsagel, D.E., Rider, W.D. Plasma cell neoplasms. In *Cancer. Principles and Practice of Oncology*. Edited by V.T. DeVita, Jr., S. Hellman, and S.A. Rosenberg. JB Lippincott, Philadelphia, 1985, pp. 1753-1795.

277. Kubagawa, H., Vogler, L.B., Capra, J.D., Conrad, M.E., Lawton, A.R., and Cooper, M.D. Studies on the clonal origin of multiple myeloma. Use of individually specific (idiotype) antibodies to trace the oncogenic event at its earliest point of expression in B-cell differentiation. J. Exper. Med. 150: 792-807, 1979.

278. Mundy, G.R., Raisz, L.G., Cooper, R.A., Schecter, G.P., and Salmon, S.E. Evidence for the secretion of an osteoclast stimulating factor in myeloma. N. Engl. J. Med. 291: 1041-1046, 1974.

279. Kyle, R.A., Greipp, P.R. Smoldering multiple myeloma. N. Engl. J. Med. 302: 1347-1349, 1980.

280. Kyle, R.A. Long term survival in multiple myeloma. N. Engl. J. Med. 308: 314-316, 1983.

281. Durie, B.G.M., and Salmon, S.E. A clinical staging system for multiple myeloma. Correlation of measured myeloma cell mass with presenting clinical features, response to treatment and survival. Cancer 36: 842-854, 1975.

282. Chronic-Leukemia-Myeloma Task Force. Proposed guidelines for protocol studies. II. Plasma cell myeloma. Cancer Chemother. Rep. 1: 17-39, 1968.

283. Mellstedt, H., Bjokholm, M., Johansson, B., Ahre, A., Holm, G., and Strander, H. Interferon therapy in myelomatosis. Lancet 1: 245-247, 1979.

284. Mellstedt, H., Aahre, A., Bjorkholm, M., Johansson, B., Strander, H., Brenning, G., Engstedt, L., Gahrton, G., Holm, G., Lehrner, R., Lonnquist, B., Nordeskjold, B., Killander, A., Stalfeldt, A., Simonsson, B., Ternstedt, B., and Wadman, B. Interferon therapy of patients with myeloma. In *Immunotherapy of Human Cancer*. Edited by W.D. Terry and S.A. Rosenberg. Excerpta Medica, Elsevier, Amsterdam, 1981.

285. Alexanian, R., Gutterman, J., and Levy, H. Interferon treatment for multiple myeloma. Clin. Hematol. 11: 211-220, 1982.

286. Gutterman, J.U., Blumenschein, A.R., Alexanian, R., et al. Interferon-induced tumor regression in human metastatic breast cancer, multiple myeloma and malignant lymphoma. Ann. Intern. Med. 93: 399-406, 1980.

287. Ahre, A., Bjorkholm, M., Mellstedt, H. et al. Human leukocyte interferon and intermittent high-dose melphalan-prednisone administration in the treatment of multiple myeloma: A randomized clinical trial from the myeloma group of Central Sweden. Cancer Treat. Rep. 68: 1331-1338, 1984.

288. Wagstaff, J., Lloynds, P., and Scarffe, J.H. Phase II study of r DNA human alpha-2 interferon in multiple myeloma. Cancer Treat. Rep. 69: 495-498, 1985.

289. Costanzi, J., Cooper, M.R., Scarffe, J.H., Ozer, H., Pollard, R.B., Ferraresi, R.W., and Spiegel, R.J. Use in patients with resistant and relapsing multiple myeloma. A phase II study. In *Interferon alpha-2: Pre-clinical and Clinical Evaluation*. Edited by D.L. Kisner and J.F. Smyth. Martinus Nijhoff, Amsterdam, 1985, pp. 75-85.

290. Cooper, M.R. Interferons in the treatment of multiple myeloma. Sem. Oncol. 13(3) (Suppl. 2): 13-20, 1986.

291. Case, D.C., Sonneborn, H.L., Paul, S.D., et al. Study cited by Cooper M.R. (Ref. 290).

292. Ohno, R., and Kimura, K. Treatment of multiple myeloma with recombinant interferon alfa-2a. Cancer 57: 1685-1689, 1986.

293. Quesada, J.R., Alexanian, R., Hawkins, M., Barlogie, B., Borden, E., Itri, L., and Gutterman, J.U. Treatment of multiple myeloma with recombinant alpha interferon. Blood 67: 275-278, 1986.

294. Ludwig, H., Cortelezzi, A., Scheithauer, W., Van Camp, B.G.K., Kuzmits, R., Fillet, G., Peetermans, M., Polli, E., and Flener, R. Recombinant interferon alfa-2c versus polychemotherapy (VCMP) for treatment of multiple myeloma: a prospective randomized trial. Eur. J. Cancer Clin. Oncol. 22: 1111-1116, 1986.

295. Cooper, M.R., Fefer, A., Thomson, J., et al. Interferon alfa-2b/melphalan/prednisone in previously untreated patients with multiple myeloma: A phase I-II study. Invest. New Drugs, 5 suppl: S41-46, 1987.

296. Canellos, G.P. Chronic leukemias. In Cancer. Principles and Practice of Oncology, Volume 2, second edition. Edited by V.T. De Vita Jr., S. Hellman, and S.A. Rosenberg. JB Lippincott, Philadelphia, 1985, pp. 1739-1742.

297. Gale, R.P., and Foon, K.A. Chronic lymphocytic leukemia: Recent advances in biology and treatment. Ann. Intern. Med. 103: 101-120, 1985.

298. Rai, K.R., Sawitsky, A., Cronkite, E.P., Chanana, A.D., Levy, R.N., and Pasternack, B.S. Clinical staging of chronic lymphocytic leukemia. Blood 46: 219-234, 1975.

299. Foon, K.A., Bottino, G., and Abrams, P.G. Phase II trial of recombinant leukocyte A interferon in patients with advanced chronic lymphocytic leukemia. Am. J. Med. 78: 216-220, 1985.

300. Foon, K.A., and Bunn, P.A. Jr. Alpha-interferon treatment of cutaneous T-cell lymphomas and chronic lymphocytic leukemia. Sem. Oncol. 13 (# 4, suppl. 5): 35-39, 1986.

301. Ostlund, L., Einhorn, S., Robert, K-H., Juliusson, G., and Biberfeld, P. Chronic B-lymphocytic leukemia cells proliferate and differentiate following exposure to interferon in vitro. Blood 67: 152-159, 1986.

302. Robert, K-H., Einhorn, S., Ostlund, L., Juliusson, G., and Biberfeld, P. Interferon induces proliferation in leukemic and normal B-cell subsets. Hematol. Oncol. 4: 113-120, 1986.

303. De Vita, V.T. Jr., Jaffe, E.S., and Hellman, S. Hodgkin's disease and the non-Hodgkin's lymphomas. In Cancer. Principles and Practice of Oncology, 2nd edition, Volume II. Edited by V.T. De Vita Jr., S. Hellman, and S.A. Rosenberg. Lippincott Co., Philadelphia, 1985, pp. 1623-1709.

304. Urba, W.J., and Longo, D.L. Cytologic, immunologic and clinical diversity in non-Hodgkin's lymphoma: therapeutic applications. Sem. Oncol. 12: 250-267, 1985.

305. Jaffe, E.S. Relationship of classification to biologic behavior of non-Hodgkin's lymphomas. Sem. Oncol. 13 (# 4, suppl. 5): 3-9, 1986.

306. Skarin, A.T., and Canellos, G.P. Chemotherapy of advanced non-Hodgkin's lymphoma. Clin. Haematol. 8: 667-683, 1979.

307. Heller, D.G. Non-Hodgkin's lymphomas. Med. Clin. North Am. 68: 741-756, 1984.

308. Qazi, R., Aisenberg, A.C., and Long, J.C. The natural history of nodular lymphoma. Cancer 37: 1923-1927, 1976.

309. Portlock, C.S., and Rosenberg, S.A. No initial therapy for stage III and IV non Hodgkin's lymphomas for favorable histologic types. Ann. Intern. Med. 90: 10-13, 1979.

310. Krikorian, J.G., Portlock, C.S., Cooney, P., and Rosenberg, S.A. Spontaneous regression of non-Hodgkin's lymphoma: a report of nine cases. Cancer 46: 2093-2099, 1980.

311. Honegger, H.P., and Cavalli, F. Current status and perspectives in the treatment of non-Hodgkin's lymphomas. Eur. J. Cancer Clin. Oncol. 20: 305-315, 1984.

312. Skarin, A.T. Diffuse aggressive lymphomas: a curable subset of non-Hodgkin's lymphomas. Sem. Oncol. 13 (# 4, suppl. 5): 10-25, 1986.

313. Gutterman, J.U., Blumenstein, G.R., Alexanian, R., Yap, H., Buzdar, A.U., Cabanillas, F., Hortobaggi, G.N., Hersh, E.M., Rasmussen, S.L., Harmon, M., Kramer, M., and Pestka, S. Leucocyte interferon induced tumor regression in human metastatic breast cancer, multiple myeloma and malignant lymphoma. Ann. Intern. Med. 93: 399-406, 1980.

314. Louie, A.C., Gallagher, J.G., Sikora, K., Levy, R., Rosenberg, S.A., and Merigan, T.C. Follow up observations on the effect of human leucocyte interferon in non-Hodgkin's lymphoma. Blood 58: 712-717, 1981.

315. Horning, S.J., Merigan, T.C., Krown, S.E., Gutterman, J.U., Louie, A., Gallagher, J., McCravey, J., Abramson, J., Cabanillas, F., Oettgen, H., and Rosenberg, S.A. Human interferon alpha in malignant lymphoma and Hodgkin's disease: results of the American Cancer Society Trial. Cancer 56: 1305-1310, 1985.

316. Gams, R., Gordon, D., and Guaspani, A. Phase II trial of human polyclonal lymphoblastoid interferon in the management of malignant lymphomas. Proc. Am. Soc. Clin. Oncol. 3: 65, 1984.

317. Quesada, J.R., Hawkins, M., and Horning, S.J. Collaborative phase I-II study of recombinant-DNA produced leucocyte interferon (clone A) in metastatic breast cancer, malignant lymphoma and multiple myeloma. Am. J. Med. 77: 427-432, 1984.

318. Foon, K.A., Sherwin, S.A., Abrams, P.G., Longo, D.L., Fer, M.F., Stevenson, H.C., Ochs, J.J., Bottino, G.C., Schoenberger, C.S., Zeffren, J., Jaffe, E.S., and Oldham, R.K. Treatment of advanced non-Hodgkin's lymphoma with recombinant leucocyte A interferon. N. Engl. J. Med. 311: 1148-1152, 1984.

319. O'Connell, M.J., Colgan, J.P., Oken, M.M., Ritts, R.E. Jr., Kay, N.E., and Itri, L.M. Clinical trial of recombinant leucocyte A interferon as initial therapy for favorable histology non-Hodgkin's lymphoma and chronic lymphocytic leukemia: an Eastern Cooperative Oncology Group pilot study. J. Clin. Oncol. 4: 128-136, 1986.

320. Leavitt, R.D., Kaplan, S., Bonnem, E., Grimm, M., Ozer, H., Portlock, C., Rathanatharathorn, V., Karanes, C., Vetmann, J., and Rudnick, S. High and low dose treatment for high and low grade non-Hodgkin's lymphoma. In *Interferon alpha-2. Preclinical and Clinical Evaluation*. Edited by D.L. Kirsner and J.F. Smyth. Martinus Nijhoff, Boston, 1985, pp. 57-73.

321. Wagstaff, J., Lloynds, J., and Crowther, D. A phase II study of human r-DNA alpha-2 interferon in patients with low grade non-Hodgkin's lymphoma. Cancer Chemother. Pharmacol. 18: 54-58, 1986.

322. Tamura, K., Makino, S., Araki, Y., Imamura, T., and Seita, M. Recombinant interferon beta and gamma in the treatment of adult T-cell leukemia. Cancer 59: 1059-1062, 1987.

323. Bunn. P.A., Ihde, D.C., and Foon, K.A. The role of recombinant interferon alfa-2 in the therapy of cutaneous T-cell lymphomas. Cancer 57: 1689-1695, 1986.

324. Poplack, D.G., Cassady, J.R., and Pizzo, P.A. Leukemias and lymphomas of childhood. In *Cancer. Principles and Practice of Oncology*. Edited by V.T. De Vita Jr., S. Hellman, and S.A. Rosenberg. Lippincott, Philadelphia, 1985, pp. 1591-1607.

325. Wiernik, P.H. Acute leukemias of adults. In *Cancer. Principles and Practice of Oncology*. Edited by V.T. De Vita Jr., S. Hellman, and S.A. Rosenberg. Lippincott, Philadelphia, 1985, pp. 1711-1737.

326. Gale, R.P., and Foon, K.A. Therapy of acute myelogenous leukemia. Sem. Hematol. 24: 40-54, 1987.

327. Marty, M., Bayssas, M., Gisselbrecht, C., Feuillette-Rhodes, A., Canivet, M., and Boiron, M. A phase I-II trial with human leucocyte interferon in patients with primarily untreated acute granulocytic leukemia. In *The Biology of the Interferon System*. Edited by E. De Maeyer, G. Galass, and H. Schelleekens. Elsevier, Amsterdam, 1981, pp. 431-435.

328. Rohatiner, A.Z.S., Balkwill, F.R., Malpas, J.S., and Lister, T.A. Experience with lymphoblastoid interferon in acute myelogenous leukemia. Cancer Chemother. Pharmacol. 11: 56-62, 1983.

329. Rohatiner, A.Z.S. Growth inhibitory effects of interferon on blast cells from patients with acute myelogenous leukaemia. Br. J. Cancer 49: 805-807, 1984.

330. Hill, N.O., Loeb, E., Pardue, A.S., Dorn, G.L., Khan, A., and Hill, J.M. Response of acute leukemia to leukocyte interferon. J. Clin. Hematol. Oncol. 9: 137-149, 1979.

331. Koeffler, H.P., Golde, D.U. Chronic myelogenous leukemia: new concepts. N. Engl. J. Med. 304: 1201-1209, 1269-1274, 1981.

332. Champlin, R.E., and Golde, D.W. Chronic myelogenous leukemia: recent advances. Blood 65: 1039-1047, 1985.

333. Rowley, J.D., and Testa, S.R. Chromosomal abnormalities in malignant hematologic diseases. Adv. Cancer Res. 36: 103-148, 1982.

334. Dube, I.D., Gupta, C.M., Kalousek, D.K., Eaves, C.J., and Eaves, A.C. Cytogenetic studies of early myeloid progenitor compartment in Ph[1] positive chronic myeloid leukemia. I- Persistence of Ph[1] negative progenitor that are suppressed from differentiating in vivo. Br. J. Haematol. 56: 633-644, 1984.

335. Dube, I.D., Kalousek, D.K., Coulombel, L., Gupta, C.M., Eaves, C.J., and Eaves, A.C. Cytogenetic studies of early myeloid progenitor compartment in Ph[1] positive chronic myeloid leukemia. II- Long term culture reveals the persistence of Ph[1] negative progenitors in treated as well as newly diagnosed patients. Blood 63: 1172-1177, 1984.

336. Metcalf, D., Moore, M.A.S., Sheridan, J.W., and Spitzer, G. Responsiveness

of human granulocytic leukemia cells to colony stimulating factor. Blood 43: 847-859, 1974.

337. Gale, R.P., and Cannani, E. The molecular biology of chronic myelogenous leukemia. Br. J. Haematol. 60: 395-408, 1985.

338. Clarkson, B. The chronic leukemias. In *Cecil's Textbook of Internal Medicine.* Edited by P.B. Beeson and W. McDermott. WB Saunders Co., Philadelphia, 1985, pp. 975-980.

339. Sokal, J.E. Evaluation of survival data for chronic myelocytic leukemia. Am. J. Hematol. 1:493-500, 1976.

340. Goto, N., Nishikuri, M., Arlin, A., Gee, T., Kemper, S., Burchenal, J., Strife, A., Wiesniewski, D., Lambek, C., Little, C., Jhanwar, S., Chaganti, R., and Clarkson, B. Growth characteristics of leukemic and normal hematopoietic cells in $Ph^1$ + chronic myelogenous leukemia and effects of intensive treatment. Blood 59: 793-808, 1982.

341. Griffith, J.D. Management of chronic myelogenous leukemia. Sem. Hematol. 23 (# 3, suppl. 1): 20-26, 1986.

342. Talpaz, M., Kantarjian, H.M., McCredie, K.B., Keating, M.J., Trujillo, J., and Gutterman, J. Clinical investigation of human alpha interferon in chronic myelogenous leukemia. Blood 69: 1280 1288, 1987.

343. Talpaz, M., Kantarjian, H., McCredie, K., Trujillo, M., Keating, M.J., and Gutterman, J.U. Hematologic remission and cytogenetic improvement induced by recombinant human interferon alpha A in chronic myelogenous leukemia. N. Engl. J. Med. 314: 1065-1069, 1986.

344. Geissler, G., Gastl, G., Konwalinka, G., and Huber, C. Antileukemic effect of rIFN-alpha in CML. Comparison in vitro and in vivo. Blut 53: 239-240 (abstr. # 215), 1986.

345. Silver, R.T., Reich, S.D., Coleman, M., Benn, P., Verma, R., Gutfriend, A., and Witman, P. Gamma interferon has activity in treating chronic myeloid leukemia (CML). Blood 68: 232a (abstr. # 808), September 1986.

346. Bergsagel, D.E., Haas, R.H., and Messner, H.A. Interferon alfa-2b in the treatment of chronic granulocytic leukemia. Sem. Oncol. 13 (# 3, suppl. 2): 29-34, 1986.

347. Kantarjian, H., Talpaz, M., Keating, M., Walters, R., Estey, E., Andersson, B., Beran, M., Trujillo, J., McCredie, K., and Freireich, E. Therapy of Philadelphia chromosome (Ph)-positive chronic myelogenous leukemia (CML) with initial intensive chemotherapy (DOAP) followed by maintenance with human leukocyte alpha interferon (IFN-A). Blood 68: 224a (abstr. #776), September 1986.

348. Golomb, H.M., Ratain, M.J., and Vardiman, J.W. Sequential treatment of hairy cell leukemia: a new role for interferon. Important Adv. Oncol. 2: 311-321, 1986.

# 9

# Thymic Factors

Richard S. Schulof, Marcelo B. Sztein, and Allan L. Goldstein / George Washington University Medical Center, Washington, D.C.

## I. INTRODUCTION

It is now well established that the thymus gland is an endocrine organ and that a variety of biologically active polypeptides are secreted from its epithelial framework (1-5). The thymus appears to have the capacity to synthesize many different hormonal-like products which differ in chemical structure. A number of thymic factors (TF) with hormone-like activity have been prepared from thymus tissue and blood and these preparations are in various stages of characterization. The best studied are thymosin fraction 5 (TF5), thymosin $\alpha_1$ (T$\alpha_1$), thymosin $\beta_4$ (T$\beta_4$), thymostimulin (TS), thymulin (FTS-Zn), thymopoietin (TP), thymic humoral factor (THF), and thymic factor X (TFX).

The relatively large numbers of TF that have been described and the lack of a well defined bioassay that detects a unique biological activity for any of them has resulted in a continuing controversy as to whether they are true physiological mediators of the thymic-dependent immune system (1). Nevertheless, an increasing number of TF are being employed therapeutically in patients with a wide variety of diseases including primary immunodeficiency disorders and cancer. In this chapter we will review the increasingly complex nomenclature of the various thymic preparations and biochemical similarities and differences among them. In addition, we will review the recent studies with TF in animal models of human diseases, as well as recent clinical trials in a variety of patients with primary and secondary immunodeficiency diseases.

## II. ENDOCRINE ROLE OF THE THYMUS IN HISTORICAL PERSPECTIVE

### A. Neonatal Thymectomy and Thymic Grafts

The important role of the thymus in the development of immunological responsiveness was not fully appreciated until the early 1960s when it was reported individually from several laboratories (6-8) that animals thymectomized in the perinatal period exhibited severe defects, including a depletion of lymphocytes in the blood, lymph nodes, and spleen. Neonatally thymectomized animals developed a wasting syndrome which was characterized by slowing of growth, recurrent infections, and premature mortality. Immunologically, the animals exhibited defective T-cell immunity including an impaired ability to reject foreign skin grafts and to manifest delayed-type hypersensitivity (DTHS) skin tests.

Following the neonatal thymectomy studies it was demonstrated that thymus glands implanted into neonatally thymectomized animals could prevent wasting, reverse lymph node atrophy, and completely abolish the immunological incompetence that would otherwise develop (8,9). Shortly thereafter it was also observed that the implantation of thymus tissue within cell-impermeable millipore diffusion chambers could partially reverse the effects of neonatal thymectomy including the wasting syndrome (10-12). Further support for an endocrine role of the thymus was provided by the observations that thymic epitheliomas, consisting only of epithelial-stromal cells exhibited immunorestorative effects (13) and that female thymectomized mice were immunologically restored when they became pregnant, presumably by the transplacental passage of an embryonic thymus factor (14).

### B. Replacement Studies with Crude Thymic Extracts

Attempts at preparing extracts of thymus glands in order to isolate putative thymic hormones date back as far as 1896 (4). However, it was not until 1935 that an attempt was made to demonstrate the endocrine function of the thymus as it pertains to the lymphoid system (15). At that time it was reported that the regeneration of the cortical regions of the irradiated thymus occurred only if circulating lymphocytes were allowed to reach the epithelial anlage of the thymus; otherwise the thymus remained epithelial. Such observations were not pursued further until the late 1960s when Drs. A. White, A.L. Goldstein, and colleagues demonstrated that treatment of neonatally thymectomized mice with a crude thymic extract (thymosin) decreased the incidence of wasting disease, improved survival, and restored cell-mediated immunity such as the ability to reject skin grafts (16-18). These observations led, over the ensuing two decades, to the identification of more than 20 different factors with thymic-hormone-like activity isolated from both thymus tissue and blood.

## C.  Thymectomy in Adult Animals

For many years it was thought that the thymus gland functioned primarily in fetal and neonatal life and became relatively unimportant by adulthood. This erroneous conclusion was based on two observations, namely (a) that adult thymectomy in animals had no immediately obvious effect on the physiology of the thymus-deprived animal and (ii) that beginning at puberty the thymus atrophies leaving only a trace of its former self as a stromal-epithelial structure. Re-evaluation of the effects of adult thymectomy in rodents revealed that immunologic competence decreased only gradually after removal of the thymus and became apparent only after a period of 6-9 months, a quarter to a half of the animal's lifespan (19-21).

With the development of more sophisticated immunologic assays, many changes in immunologic competence were demonstrable in animals shortly after adult thymectomy. These included a decrease in proliferative responses of lymphocytes to T-cell mitogens (22) and in mixed leukocyte response (MLR) (23). One major postthymic T-cell subset that remains under the control of the thymus in the adult is the T-suppressor cell. Within 2-4 weeks after adult thymectomy there is a decrease in suppressor T-cell activity, which can be restored by administration of various thymic factors (24-28). This decline is most likely attributed to a turnover of a short-lived postthymic T cell (29,30).

Probably the earliest cellular change which can be detected by one week following thymectomy in adult mice is the disappearance of splenic lymphocytes that form azathioprine-sensitive E-rosettes (31). This latter observation enabled Bach and Dardenne to subsequently develop an in vitro bioassay which was utilized for the detection of circulating levels of thymic hormone-like bioactivity. Thus, there is now ample evidence that in the adult the thymus continues to manifest an important long-term role with regard to the maintenance and regulation of the immune system.

## D.  Thymic Epithelial Cells

The thymus can be viewed as a solid epithelial organ penetrated by blood vessels and infiltrated with thymic lymphocytes (thymocytes) which mature under the influence of its epithelial microenvironment. In man, thymic epithelial cells are concentrated primarily in two separate regions, the subcapsular cortex and the medulla (32-35). In the subcapsular area, thymic epithelial cells form a thin circumferential sheet which encompasses the entire surface of the thymic lobules in the superficial layer of the cortex, whereas in the medullary region they form a meshlike interconnected network of cells extending in various directions throughout the parenchyma.

Ultrastructural and histochemical studies have now demonstrated conclusively that many of the epithelial cells in the thymus have the characteristics of secretory cells (36). Cortical as well as medullary thymic epithelial cells may exhibit membrane-bound electron dense granules also found in a variety of endocrine organs. Epithelial cells containing membrane-bound electron dense granules have now been identified in avia (37-39) and various mammalian thymus glands (40-44) including human thymus glands (45-47). The thymic medulla exclusively contains a population of large epithelial cells which can be distinguished by the presence of numerous rough endoplasmic reticulum as well as by the presence of numerous small, electron dense granules which can be discerned around the golgi and elsewhere in the cytoplasm (48). The morphology of these granules closely resembles the secretory granules of other polypeptide-secreting cells (47). Immunohistochemical studies using specific antisera to a number of well characterized thymic polypeptides have confirmed that it is the thymic epithelial cells which are the major hormone-producing cells of the thymus (49-53). Although most thymic polypeptides are found in both medullary as well as subcapsular cortical epithelial cells, some are produced almost exclusively by epithelial cells localized in the subcapsular region (35).

It is now well established that in most vertebrates the thymus undergoes a gradual age-dependent atrophy or involution in which the thymic parenchymal tissue is infiltrated with adipose cells and fat (54). Maximal thymic size occurs just prior to puberty, and it then begins to gradually decrease in size and weight (54). The loss of hormone-producing epithelial cells begins early in life. In humans, by the second decade the number of hormone-containing medullary thymic epithelial cells has decreased dramatically, whereas the number of hormone-containing cortical epithelial cells appears to decrease more gradually and can still be observed even in the fifth decade of life (35). The age-associated decrease in absolute numbers of hormone-containing thymic epithelial cells correlates with the gradual decrease in thymic-hormone-like bioactivity measured in the blood of both animals (54-56) as well as in humans (57-60).

## III.  COMPARATIVE BIOCHEMISTRY OF THYMIC FACTORS

The thymus appears to be an organ with the capacity to synthesize many products of differing chemical structure. A number of factors with thymic hormone-like activity have been prepared from thymus tissue and blood and these preparations are in various stages of characterization. Among the thymic preparations, thymosin fraction 5 (TF5), thymosin $\alpha_1$, thymulin (facteur thymique serique or FTS-Zn), thymopoietin, thymostimulin (TP-1, or TS), thymic humoral factor (THF), and thymic factor X (TFX) are the best characterized, most thoroughly studied thymic preparations and the ones which have currently been entered in widespread clinical trials. TF5, TP-1, and TFX are partially purified extracts of calf thymus glands and include a number of different biologically active peptides. Several of the active polypeptides identified in TF5, such as thymosin $\alpha_1$ and thymosin $\beta_4$, have been purified to homogeneity and sequenced. Thymulin is a nonapeptide initially isolated from porcine blood, but also found in high concentrations in thymic tissue. Four thymic peptides have been synthesized (thymosin $\alpha_1$, m.w. 3108; thymosin $\beta_4$, m.w. 4982; thymopoietin II, m.w. 5562; and thymulin, m.w. 857) and these peptides appear to be unrelated chemically.

Most of the thymic preparations were first identified as crude thymic extracts with the ability to restore or enhance various parameters of thymic-dependent immunity either in vitro or in vivo using lymphoid cells isolated from various immunodeficient animal models. Purified products were then isolated from the crude extracts and exhibited biological effects similar to the crude preparations. Although many different thymic factors have been described which can induce T-cell differentiation in vitro and/or in vivo in various experimental systems, very few have satisfied all of the requirements for categorization as true thymic hormones. Indeed, detailed thymectomy and thymus reimplantation studies to establish the absolute thymus dependency of circulating bioactivity have only been performed for thymulin (31,61). Although thymosin $\alpha_1$, thymosin $\beta_4$, and thymopoietin are all detectable in serum, strict thymus dependency has not, at this time, been completely established. A summary of the major characteristics of the well defined thymic factors is seen in Table 1.

## A. Thymosin and Its Component Polypeptides

Thymosin was first prepared as a crude extract of mouse or rat thymus glands by Goldstein and White in 1966 and was originally assayed by its "lymphocytopoietic" properties when injected into mice (62-65). Goldstein and colleagues demonstrated that treatment of neonatally thymectomized mice with a crude thymosin preparation decreased the incidence of wasting disease, improved survival and restored cell-mediated immunity such as the ability to reject skin grafts (16-18). During the next decade a number of different in vitro and in vivo murine bioassays were employed, none of them completely satisfactory (1,4,5) with which the final purification procedures for thymosin were developed.

### 1. Thymosin Fraction 5

Thymosin fraction 5 (TF5) is a partially purified mixture of polypeptides prepared from calf thymus glands as starting material (66). The crude thymus extract is purified by a heat step, acetone precipitation, and fractionation with ammonium sulfate. The 25-50% ammonium sulfate precipitate is further subjected to ultrafiltration using an Amicon DC-2 hollow fiber system to yield fraction 5 which is lyophilized. Fraction 5 consists of 10 major and at least 30 minor polypeptides on analytical isoelectric gel focusing (Fig. 1) with molecular weights ranging from 1000-15,000, and is free of lipids, carbohydrates, and endotoxin. TF5 has become a standard preparation in that it has demonstrated a wide range of biological activities in animal systems both in vitro and in vivo (4,5) and it was the first partially purified thymic extract to enter clinical trials in primary immunodeficiency patients in the United States.

**Table 1** Characteristics of Well Defined Thymic Factors

| Agent | Usual source | Chemistry | Molecular weight(s) | Chemically synthesized | Present in Thymic Epithelial Cells — Subcapsular cortical | Medullary | Adapted to Measure Serum Levels — Bioassay | RIA | Decreases in Serum — Post-thymectomy | With age |
|---|---|---|---|---|---|---|---|---|---|---|
| I. Thymosin | Calf thymus | | | | | | | | | |
| Fraction 5 | | Family of heat-stable acidic polypeptides | 1,000-15,000 | | | | | | | |
| Thymosin $\alpha_1$ | | Polypeptide, 28 amino acid residues pI = 4.2 | 3108 | Yes[a] | +[e] | + | No | Yes | No(?) | ±[b] |
| Thymosin $\alpha_7$ | | Polypeptide, pI = 3.5 | 2200 | No | − | −[c] | No | No | | |
| Thymosin $\beta_3$ | | Polypeptide, pI = 5.2 | 5500 | No | +[d] | − | No | No | | |
| Thymosin $\beta_4$ | | Polypeptide, pI = 5.1 | 4982 | Yes | +[d] | − | No | Yes | | |
| II. Thymulin (FTS-Zn) | Pig serum | Nonapeptide, heat labile pI = 7.3 | 847 | Yes | + | ++ | Yes | Yes | Yes | Yes |
| III. Thymopoietin | Calf thymus | | | | | | | | | |
| Thymopoietin II | | Polypeptide, 49 amino acid residues heat stable, pI = 5.2 | 5562 | Yes | +[e] | + | Yes[f] | ±[g] | Yes[f] | Yes[f] |
| TP-5 | | Amino acid residues, 32-36 of thymopoietin | | Yes | | | | | | |
| IV. Thymic humoral factor (THF) | Calf thymus | Polypeptide, 31 amino acid residues, heat labile, pI = 5.7-5.9 | 3200 | No | ? | ? | − | − | − | |

[a] Also synthesized by DNA recombinant techniques.
[b] Decrease demonstrated over the first 10 years of life, but not with further aging.
[c] Primarily found in Hassall's corpuscles.
[d] Also synthesized by macrophages in various tissues.
[e] Also detected in squamous epithelium of skin.
[f] Assay uses thymopoietin as standard but may detect other thymic factors.
[g] RIA developed but not applied to serum.

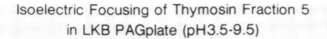

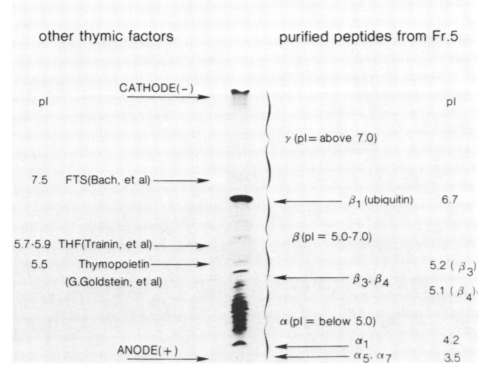

**Figure 1** Isoelectric focusing of thymosin fraction 5 in LKB PAG plate (pH 3.5-9.5). Purified thymosin peptides from the $\alpha$, $\beta$, and $\gamma$ regions are identified. The isoelectric points of other well characterized thymic factors are illustrated for comparison.

## 2. Nomenclature of Thymosin Polypeptides

Analytic isoelectric focusing of TF5 has revealed the presence of a number of components on the preparation. A nomenclature based on the isoelectric focusing pattern of thymosin fraction 5 in the pH range 3.5-9.5 has been described (67) and is illustrated in Figure 1. The separated polypeptides are divided into three regions, the $\alpha$ region consists of polypeptides with isoelectric points below 5.0; the $\beta$ region, 5.0-7.0, and the $\gamma$ region, above 7.0. The subscript numbers, $\alpha_1$, $\alpha_2$, $\beta_1$, $\beta_2$, etc. are used to identify the polypeptides from each region as they are individually isolated.

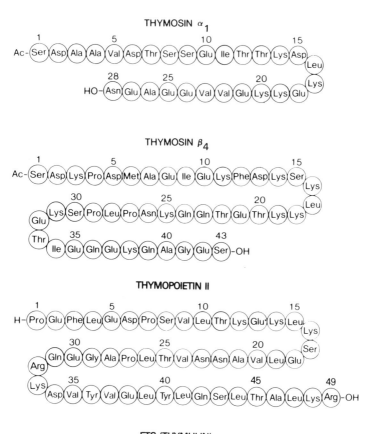

**Figure 2** Sequence analysis of well characterized thymic-peptides: thymosin $\alpha_1$, thymosin $\beta_4$, thymopoietin II, and TFS (thymulin).

Thymosin $\alpha_1$ (T$\alpha_1$). The first thymosin polypeptide isolated from the highly acidic region of bovine fraction 5 has been termed thymosin $\alpha_1$ (T$\alpha_1$) (67-69). Thymosin $\alpha_1$ is a polypeptide consisting of 28 amino acid residues with a molecular weight of 3,108 daltons. T$\alpha_1$ was isolated by ion-exchange chromatography on CM-cellulose and DEAE-cellulose as well as gel filtration on Sephadex G-75. The yield of T$\alpha_1$ from TF5 is only about 0.6%. The complete amino acid sequence (67) of this peptide is shown in Figure 2. The amino terminus of T$\alpha_1$ is blocked by an acetyl group. Human, porcine, and ovine T$\alpha_1$ all appear to have identical amino acid sequences to bovine T$\alpha_1$.

Recent histochemical and immunofluorescence studies have documented the localization of thymosin $\alpha_1$-producing cells primarily to the epithelial cells of the thymus medulla but also to a lesser degree within the ring of subcapsular cortical surface epithelial cells (35,49,50,52,70,72). Using a cell-free wheat germ system to assess the translation of messenger RNA from calf thymus, it was demonstrated that a larger molecular weight radioactive product was immunoprecipitable with antisera against $T\alpha_1$ and the tryptic-isolated peptide products were identical to those expected of tryptic peptides from thymosin $\alpha_1$ (73). Thus, these results suggest that $T\alpha_1$ is indeed synthesized in the thymus. In addition, it has recently been demonstrated that thymus tissue extracted in guanidine-HCl did not express thymosin $\alpha_1$ immunoactivity, whereas tissue extracted in saline did (74). This finding suggested that a precursor molecule was cleaved during the saline extraction procedure to produce thymosin $\alpha_1$. In most recent studies a major immunoreactive form of thymosin $\alpha_1$ has been isolated from rat thymus which appears to represent the prohormone from which thymosin $\alpha_1$ and other fragments are generated during the extraction procedures (75). The purified prohormone consists of 112 amino acid residues with an isoelectric point in the range of 3.55-3.85. Although the complete amino acid sequence of this molecule has not yet been established, the $T\alpha_1$-sequence appears at its $NH_2$ terminus.

It has also recently been demonstrated, using a specific radioimmunoassay (RIA), that $T\alpha_1$ is present in serum and that its serum levels exhibit a circadian rhythm and may be high or low in various disease states (76,77). Thus, $T\alpha_1$ appears to satisfy most criteria for categorization as a true thymic hormone. However, the heterologous rabbit antibody used in the RIA recognizes significant cross-reactivity in fraction 5 equivalent preparations isolated from other bovine tissues. In addition, using the RIA, it has not been possible to establish a strict thymus dependency for circulating levels of $T\alpha_1$ since serum levels are detectable even in elderly subjects and since individuals who have undergone therapeutic thymectomy for myasthenia gravis often do not have a decreased level following surgery (78). It is possible that the background serum levels of $T\alpha_1$ detected in thymectomized or elderly humans may reflect either a nonthymic source of $T\alpha_1$ such as the epithelial layer of the skin (known to produce thymic-hormone-like peptides) (79) or the presence of a biologically inactive $T\alpha_1$-like cross-reacting material. Most recently a variety of monoclonal antibodies specific for $T\alpha_1$ have been prepared (80) and a simple procedure described for removing the material found in human and fetal calf serum which cross reacts with the monoclonal antibodies. It is hoped that such advances will allow for the development of a more specific RIA.

Biologically active $T\alpha_1$ has been chemically synthesized by both solution (81) and solid phase (82) procedures. Most recently the gene for thymosin $\alpha_1$ was synthesized, inserted into a plasmid and biologically active $N^a$-desacetyl thymosin $\alpha_1$ was isolated from *Escherichia coli* by DNA recombinant techniques (83). At the current time, all of the clinical trials using $T\alpha_1$ have employed the chemically synthesized material.

Thymosin $\alpha_5$ ($T\alpha_5$) and $\alpha_7$ ($T\alpha_7$). Both of these partially purified peptides have been isolated from fraction 5 by ion-exchange chromatography on CM-cellulose and DEAE-cellulose and gel filtration on Sephadex G-75 (84). They are highly acidic with isoelectric points around 3.5. The molecular weights of thymosin $\alpha_5$ and thymosin $\alpha_7$ are approximately 3000 and 2200 daltons, respectively. Recently, using heterologous antibodies raised against thymosin $\alpha_7$, this peptide was shown to be present primarily in thymic epithelial cells surrounding Hassall's corpuscles and in a few isolated cells in the medullary epithelium (49, 50,52,72).

Thymosin $\alpha_{11}$ ($T\alpha_{11}$). This peptide was isolated from TF5 by preparative isoelectric focusing and high performance liquid chromatography (85). $T\alpha_{11}$ is homologous to $T\alpha_1$ through its first 28 amino acids and contains seven additional amino acid residues at the carboxy terminus. Preliminary biological studies indicate that $T\alpha_{11}$ is 30 times as active as TF5 and equivalent in biological activity to $T\alpha_1$ with regard to protecting susceptible mice against opportunistic infections.

Polypeptide $\beta_1$. In general, the peptides isolated from the $\beta$ region of thymosin fraction 5 do not appear to be thymus-specific products. The most predominant band on isoelectric focusing of TF5 is polypeptide $\beta_1$ (Fig. 1). It is composed of 74 amino acids and has an isoelectric point of 6.7 and a molecular weight of 4851 (69). This peptide does not possess significant biological activity in any of the in vitro or in vivo bioassays used to monitor the thymosin purification procedures. The sequence of $\beta_1$ (67) was found to be identical to a protein isolated originally from calf thymus glands but also found in many different tissues and termed ubiquitin by G. Goldstein and colleagues (86). Both $\beta_1$ and ubiquitin appear to represent the N terminal 74 amino acids of the nuclear chromosomal protein A24 (87). Thus, it has been postulated that $\beta_1$ (ubiquitin) is a degradation product of A24 (88). Most recently the $\beta_1$ peptide has been shown to be homologous to an ATP-dependent coupling factor ($\alpha$-fetoprotein) involved in proteolysis (89). This observation may account for the ubiquitous distribution of this peptide.

Thymosins $\beta_3$ ($T\beta_3$) and $\beta_4$ ($T\beta_4$). Both of these polypeptides were isolated from TF5 by chromatography on DEAE-cellulose and gel filtration on Sephadex G-75 (90). The isoelectric points and molecular weights of $T\beta_3$ and $T\beta_4$ are 5.2 and 5.1 and approximately 5500 and 4982 daltons, respectively. Thymosin $\beta_4$ was the second thymosin peptide to be sequenced (90) and chemically synthesized (91) (Fig. 2). Thymosin $\beta_3$ and $T\beta_4$ appear to share an identical sequence through most of their amino terminal part and differ in the carboxyl terminal ends. Using immunofluorescent techniques and heterologous antisera to $T\beta_3$ and $T\beta_4$ these peptides were found to localize almost exclusively to the subcapsular thymic epithelial cells covering the thymic cortex and, unlike $T\alpha_1$, they were not present within thymic medullary epithelial cells (35,49,50,52,72).

Recently, a radioimmunoassay for $T\beta_4$ has been developed and it has been identified in both animal and human sera at concentrations much higher than that of $T\alpha_1$ (92). However, $T\beta_4$ does not appear to be a thymus-specific product in that it is also synthesized by both peritoneal as well as splenic macrophages (93). Thus, the peptides of the $\beta$ region appear to have more widespread origins in the body than those of the $\alpha$ region.

Thymosins $\beta_8$, $\beta_9$, and $\beta_{10}$. Recently, three additional thymosin peptides termed thymosin $\beta_8$, thymosin $\beta_9$, and thymosin $\beta_{10}$ have been sequences (94-96). Thymosins $\beta_8$ and $\beta_9$ appear chemically related to $T\beta_4$. However, biological activity similar to thymosin $\beta_4$ has only been described for $T\beta_{10}$.

## B. Thymopoietin

The isolation of thymopoietin (initially termed thymin) by G. Goldstein and colleagues resulted from their interest in myasthenia gravis, a disorder characterized by deficits in neuromuscular transmission and often associated with abnormalities of the thymus gland (97). The original purification procedures were monitored with a bioassay that assessed the ability of the thymic extracts to induce a neuromuscular blockade similar to that seen in myasthenia gravis. Subsequently, the biologically active polypeptides were also found to be capable of inducing the differentiation of bone marrow stem cells into mature T cells in vitro, so that an important physiological role of the preparation was postulated (98-100).

The purification procedure for thymopoietin includes a heat step, two passages on Sephadex G-50 and fractionation on hydroxyapatite and QAE-Sephadex columns (101). Two isopeptides were identified which were related by peptide mapping and immunologic cross reactions. To avoid confusion with the pyrimidine base, thymine, Goldstein changed the nomenclature of his products from thymin to thymopoietins I and II (98,102). These two preparations appeared to be closely related polypeptides which differed by only two amino acid residues. Thymopoietin II has a molecular weight of 5562 daltons and a pI of 5.5. The amino acid sequence of the molecule has been delineated, although a retraction of the original sequence has recently been reported (103) and the corrected sequence is shown in Figure 2. Comparisons of the available data suggest that thymopoietins I and II are distinct from the other thymic factors. At the present time there is no evidence of homology of thymopoietins I or II with any of the established structures of the polypeptides in calf thymosin fraction 5.

Schlessenger and colleagues also purified a third polypeptide which was initially felt to be a precursor of the thymopoietins. However, this molecule was subsequently found to have a wide distribution in nature in tissues other than the thymus and was termed ubiquitin (86). The sequence of ubiquitin has turned out to be identical to that of polypeptide $\beta_1$ isolated from thymosin fraction 5 (69).

Recently the synthesis of the entire 49 amino acid chain of thymopoietin II was achieved (104) and it was established that the product had biological activity similar to native thymopoietin II. A tridecapeptide fragment of thymopoietin, corresponding to residues 29 through 41, was synthesized by solid-phase methodology and was shown to have 3% of the biological activity of the entire molecule. In addition, a biologically active pentapeptide (Arg-Lys-Asp-Val-Tyr) corresponding to residues 32 through 36 of the 40 amino acid sequence of thymopoietin has been synthesized (99) and termed thymopentin (TP-5) (105). TP-5 has been the preparation that has been investigated clinically in immunodeficiency patients.

The cells of origin of thymopoietin appear to be the thymic epithelial cells. Using a heteroantiserum and immunofluorescent techniques, the peptide was shown to localize to thymic epithelial cells (106). In recent studies it has been demonstrated that both the subcapsular cortical as well as the medullary thymic epithelial cells react with antithymopoietin antibodies (52). A molecule that is indistinguishable from thymopoietin by immunoassay is also present in one major extra thymic site, the epidermis (79). Two to 15% of human epidermal cells appear to endogenously produce thymopoietin in tissue culture. These cells have been characterized as basal keratinocytes of the epidermis (79).

A radioimmunoassay for thymopoietin has been developed (107,108). However, the assay has not as yet been adapted to study serum levels of thymopoietin. A bioassay has been developed by Twomey and colleagues (109) which uses thymopoietin as a standard and measures the induction of a thymus-derived membrane surface antigen (Thy 1.2) on lymphocytes obtained from the spleens of nude (genetically thymus deficient) mice. This bioassay has been applied to evaluating serum thymic-hormone-like bioactivity in man and serum bioactivity has been shown to decrease significantly with age and following therapeutic thymectomy for myasthenia gravis (58).

## C.  Thymic Humoral Factor (THF)

The isolation of THF by Levey and colleagues was the culmination of studies to explain their observation that thymus tissue in millipore chambers implanted into neonatally thymectomized mice led to the restoration of specific immunologic competence in these animals (10). Subsequently, Umiel and Trainin pursued their observations by preparing cell-free extracts that conferred immune competence to spleen cells from neonatally thymectomized mice in vitro (110). The initial bioassay was an in vitro model of the graft versus host reaction. In this assay the immunocompetence of isolated lymphoid cell populations was assessed by the ability of these populations to induce an increase in weight or size of an allogeneic spleen explant. It was observed that spleen cells from neonatally thymectomized mice did not achieve this competence unless they were previously exposed to the thymic extracts.

The initial product was generally obtained from calf thymus, but syngeneic mouse extracts were also shown to be active in the assay. The method used for the isolation of purified THF involves prolonged dialysis of crude thymic homogenates against cold distilled water. More recently the further purification of THF to homogeneity has been achieved (111). The procedure involves successive chromatographic steps on Sephadex G-10 and G-25 and DEAE-Sephadex A-25. The homogeneity of THF has been established by isoelectric focusing on polyacrylamide gels. The isoelectric point of THF is 5.6. On the basis of leucine as unity, the minimal molecular weight is 3220 (112,113).

There is no apparent relationship between the amino acid composition of THF and other purified thymic factors. At the present time the primary amino acid sequence of THF has not been established, nor have the cells of origin of THF been identified.

### D.  Thymulin (Facteur Thymique Serique, FTS-Zn)

The isolation of FTS was the culmination of a number of studies by Bach, Dardenne, and colleagues, aimed at assessing the immunological status and likelihood of kidney rejection in patients with renal transplants. These investigators developed the azathioprine rosette bioassay that detected thymic hormone-like biological activity in the serum of animals and man (57,114-116). Although several different thymic extracts were active in their system (115), these investigators sought to isolate the active agents directly from pig serum (117-119). The active factor was initially termed facteur thymique serique or FTS because of its origin in serum. It has been characterized as a nonapeptide with a molecular weight of 847. The amino acid sequence of FTS is shown in Figure 2.

The extraction procedure employs large quantities of pig serum as starting material. Defibrinated serum is ultrafiltered on a hemodialyser, and concentrated on Amicon membranes. Amicon concentrates are then subjected to four consecutive chromatographic steps: Sephadex G-25, carboxymethyl cellulose, Sephadex G-25 in acetic acid medium, and Sephadex G-10. In every case, the active fractions are detected with the bioassay described above. From an initial 15 liters of normal pig serum containing 1200 g of total protein, the yield of FTS is about 3 $\mu$g, and the biological activity of the purified product is increased 100,000-fold.

There is no apparent species specificity, since the amino acid analysis of calf and human FTS is identical to that of porcine FTS. This sequence does not show any homology with any of the other thymic polypeptides (e.g., thymosin $\alpha_1$) that have been described. FTS has now been synthesized by both classical solution (110) and solid-phase (120) procedures. The synthetic material showed full biological activity and chromatographically displayed characteristics identical to those of natural FTS. Recently, it has been demonstrated that the biologically active form of FTS is coupled to zinc, whereas the inactive form lacks metal (121). After the presence of zinc in the molecule was revealed and when its production by thymic epithelial cells was directly demonstrated by immunofluorescence techniques (122) the name of the nonapeptide-Zn complex was changed to thymulin.

In detailed studies, thymulin has been shown to satisfy more criteria for categorization as a true thymic hormone, than any of the other well characterized thymic polypeptides. The physiology of thymulin production has been studied by several different methodologies including (i) measurement of serum levels using the murine rosette bioassay (57,61) and (ii) immunofluorescent studies using antithymulin antibodies produced in rabbits (123,124), and monoclonal antibodies produced in mice (122). In addition, a radioimmunoassay (RIA) using an antiserum raised in rabbits (123), as well as a RIA and an enzyme-linked immunosorbent assay (ELISA) using a monoclonal antibody (125,126) have been developed.

One of the requirements for establishing the thymic origin of any putative thymic hormone is to evaluate the effects of thymectomy and thymus grafting on circulating levels of the putative hormone. In a series of classic experiments, Bach, Dardenne, and colleagues demonstrated that circulating "FTS-like" bioactivity was absent in genetically athymic (nude) mice and disappeared following thymectomy in mice (31), pigs (127), and humans (61). Furthermore, serum "FTS-like" bioactivity reappeared in thymectomized mice after grafting of a thymus gland (31) or an epithelial thymoma (55), but not after thymocyte administration or lymph node grafting.

The murine rosette bioassay that has been utilized extensively to evaluate serum thymulin levels suffers from one major drawback, that is, it is a nonspecific assay and at least several of the other thymic peptides that have been described, thymosin $\alpha_1$ (128,129), and thymopoietin (130) exhibit activity in the assay in addition to thymulin. Thus, the active chemical species which produce "FTS-like" bioactivity in serum cannot be determined by utilizing the bioassay alone. The thymulin RIA and ELISA assay have been applied to studying both tissue extracts as well as serum in order to definitively establish the presence of FTS in both the thymus and blood. Significant amounts of thymulin have been detected using the RIA in thymic, but not splenic extracts (131). The presence of immunoreactive thymulin in normal serum and its absence in the serum of thymectomized animals has been demonstrated by RIA using Amicon filtration, concentration and G-25 Sephadex chromatography (132). Most recently, it has been demonstrated using the ELISA assay (125) that the monoclonal antibody against FTS could completely absorb the "FTS-like" bioactivity in human serum which is detected with the murine rosette bioassay. These results support the view that the "FTS-like" bioactivity in normal human serum is due solely to the activity of thymulin, or an "FTS-like" molecule which is immunologically indistinguishable from porcine FTS.

The most direct evidence for establishing the thymic origin of thymulin has come from immunofluorescence studies with antithymulin antibodies. Using conventional antithymulin rabbit antibodies, thymulin localization to thymic epithelial cells was independently obtained in several different laboratories (124, 133-135). These results were confirmed and expanded upon using a panel of antithymulin monoclonal antibodies (122). In each of these studies the fixation of anti-FTS antibodies to thymic epithelial cells was abolished by preincubation of the antibodies with synthetic FTS. Thymulin localization in the thymus was demonstrated both in human (133), and in mouse thymus (122,124,133,135), in frozen sections (124,134), and in thymic epithelial cell cultures (124). In general, the antithymulin antibodies appeared to be specific for epithelial cells of thymic origin, and although both medullary and cortical epithelial cells contained FTS, the overwhelming majority of FTS-containing cells were found in the thymic medulla. Nevertheless, only a minority of all thymic epithelial cells were found to contain FTS, amounting to approximately 1% of all medullary epithelial cells. In addition, thymus glands from old mice were almost totally devoid of thymulin-containing cells (56) which is consistent with the finding that serum FTS levels decline dramatically with age (31).

Recent studies have also suggested that thymulin may be carried in serum by carrier molecules, such as prealbumin (136,137) and that there may be a feedback mechanism by which thymulin secretion is regulated (138). As a result of studies which evaluated different fractions of serum in the murine bioassay, it was felt that inhibitors of thymulin activity are normally present in the circulation (31). It was also noted, however, that a second peak of biological activity analogous to native FTS was found in the region corresponding to that of pre-albumin. It has been previously reported that prealbumin isolated from serum was active in the murine rosette bioassay (139). However, since prealbumin levels are not altered in thymectomized or aged mice, when serum FTS levels are low, it has been postulated that this molecule serves as a carrier for FTS.

The initial insights into the mechanisms of feedback control of thymulin secretion resulted from experiments in which the grafting of thymuses into normal mice led to a transient increase in circulating FTS levels that were directly proportional to the number of thymic lobes grafted (140). However, several weeks after thymus grafting there was a diminution of serum FTS levels back to baseline. Conversely, depletion of serum thymulin levels by repeated injections of antithymulin monoclonal antibody or by immunization against thymulin induced an increase by five fold in the number of thymulin-containing cells (141). Thus, it has been postulated that feedback regulatory control mechanisms, based on circulating serum FTS levels control the number of thymic epithelial cells capable of producing the hormone.

## E. Thymostimulin (TS, TP-1)

Thymostimulin is an extract of calf thymus glands which has been partially purified by Falchetti and colleagues (142) in Italy. Calf thymus tissue is first minced and extracted with ammonium acetate and then fractionated with ammonium sulfate precipitation. The 0-25% ammonium sulfate cut is further purified by ultrafiltration on an Amicon PM-10 membrane, desalted on Sephadex G-25, and gel filtered on Sephadex G-50. The biologically active preparation consists of a group of polypeptides with molecular weights ranging from 1000-12,000 daltons and exhibits two predominant bands on polyacrylamide gels at pH 8.6. At the present time there have been no attempts to further define the constituents of this partially purified preparation. Although TP-1 is similar to TF5 in its purification schema, a 0-25% ammonium sulfate precipitation step is used whereas a 25-50% saturation fractionation cut is employed for the isolation of TF5. In addition, the purification procedure for TF5 includes an acetone precipitation step whereas this procedure is not included in the preparation of TP-1. Thus, there should be some differences in the components of TP-1, as compared to those isolated from TF5. In recent years many studies have been performed with TP-1 to characterize its biological activity as well as its possible therapeutic potential as an immune modifying agent for patients with primary immunodeficiency disorders and cancer.

## F.  Thymic Factor X (TFX)

The role of immunological mechanisms in the pathogenesis of leukemia and their effects on the course of the disease have been subject of study in Poland by Aleksandrowicz and colleagues since 1948. Between 1972 and 1974, this group of investigators focused its attention on assessing the clinical usefulness of thymus fragments taken from myasthenia gravis patients, and transplanted into selected patients with acute and chronic leukemia and Hodgkin's disease. With this treatment more than 50% of the patients exhibited some clinical improvement, although the effects tended to be transient, lasting usually only four to eight weeks. Nevertheless, the appearance of immunological enhancement a short time after thymus transplantation led the group in Krakow to begin work on isolating a calf thymus extract which was termed Thymic Factor X (TFX) (143).

In the early studies a crude aqueous extract of calf thymus tissue was employed. Evidence that the administration of TFX resulted in enhancement of humoral and cell-mediated immunity led to attempts to purify the crude aqueous extract. The purification procedure that was developed involves ammonium sulfate fractionation, desalting through a G-25 molecular sieve, and ion-exchange chromatography. FTX is a nucleotide and lipid-free polypeptide mixture, with a major component having a molecular weight of 4200, accompanied by traces of several other peptides with molecular weights ranging from 2000 to 18,000. The final purification of FTX has not yet been achieved. At the present time there is no information available concerning the relationship between TFX and any of the other purified or partially purified (e.g., thymosin fraction 5) thymic preparations. Many of the biological properties of TFX, both in vitro, as well as in vivo, are similar to those reported with other thymic preparations. The Polish group has had a broad experience in treating patients with a variety of primary and secondary immunodeficiencies with this preparation.

## G.  Other Thymic Factors

Many other extracts of both thymus tissue and blood have been described which exhibit thymic-hormone-like activity in various bioassays (5). These preparations include homeostatic thymic hormone (HTH) (144), lymphocytopoietic factors

(LSH) (145), hypocalcemic and lymphocytopoietic substances (TP) (146), thymic polypeptide preparation (147), thymosterin (148), prealbumin fraction of human plasma (139), and thymus-dependent human serum factor (SF) (149). Each of these preparations is described in a recent review (5). Several of the above mentioned products, in retrospect, are clearly not involved in the normal thymic physiological mechanisms. For example, the prealbumin fraction of human plasma probably exhibits biological activity in the murine bioassay of Bach and Dardenne because it contains the carrier molecule for FTS (31). On further biochemical analysis, SF was found to be identical with adenosine (150), so that its thymus dependency is unlikely, even though it does exhibit biological properties that are similar to other thymic preparations.

## IV. BIOLOGICAL ACTIVITIES OF WELL CHARACTERIZED THYMIC FACTORS

The in vitro biological activities attributed to TF can be divided into four major areas:

### A. Modulation of T-Cell Differentiation Antigens

Several TF are able to modulate the expression of a variety of T-cell antigen markers, including TL (T-cell leukemia markers), Thy 1 and the Lyt 1,2,3 phenotype, on bone marrow and spleen lymphocyte subpopulations derived from athymic and normal mice (151,152). Most of the classical bioassays employed to measure TF activity and the active fractions obtained after the purification procedures, are based on this property.

TF can either increase or decrease the expression of a particular phenotypic marker. For example, high concentrations of $T\alpha_1$ have been shown to increase (152) the expression of terminal deoxynucleotidyl transferase (TdT), a DNA polymerase found primarily in thymocytes (153), on bone marrow lymphocytes, whereas low concentrations reduced the TdT contents of murine thymocytes (151,154). This phenomenon has been interpreted as a shift toward a more "mature" population, and the same explanation has been applied to the TF-induced decrease in the percent of thymocytes which are agglutinated by peanut lectin agglutinin (PNA), another marker of differentiation exhibited in lesser amounts by medullary ("mature") than by cortical ("immature") thymocytes (151). Since the sequence of appearance and disappearance of phenotypic markers along the lymphocyte differentiation pathway has not been completely elucidated (151,155), it is very difficult to assess the precise role that TF play in lymphocyte maturation.

It is reasonable to hypothesize that the production of TF by several types of thymic epithelial cells might play a role in T-cell differentiation and maturation. This hypothesis is supported by recent reports (156) that showed the differentiation of a thymocyte population expressing dim Ly 1 antigen that appears to differentiate into Lyt 2,3+ L3T4+ thymocytes, which in turn lead to the appearance of Lyt 2+ and L3T4+ cells, the mature T lymphocyte subpopulations in the mouse. It was demonstrated that the expression of Lyt 2,3 antigens, and possibly L3T4, requires the presence of "cortical epithelial cells," since these cells appear at 15-17 days of gestation, immediately before thymocytes bearing the markers of the mature phenotype.

In humans, similar studies have yielded the same general conclusions. For example, in vitro incubation of TF with human bone marrow cells leads to the expression of E-rosette receptors and human T-lymphocyte antigen (HTLA), both expressed in 95-99% of peripheral blood lymphocytes (PBL), but absent in bone marrow cells. In this system, as it is also the case in murine systems, more than one TF is able to induce the same phenotypic changes. For example, the induction of E-rosettes and human T lymphocyte antigen (HTLA) were observed after incubation with thymulin, thymopoietin, and TP5 (reviewed in Ref. 157). Additionally, thymulin has recently been described to induce formation of E-rosettes and OKT3 antigen expression (present in 95-99% of normal PBL) in a PBL subpopulation which exhibit an "immature phenotype" (OKT3, E-rosettes) (158).

Since to date no well characterized TF has been shown to induce all the changes which characterize T-lymphocyte differentiation, it has been proposed that several TF may act sequentially to induce all the changes that occur in the normal maturational process (157). Further studies, both in the murine and human systems, will be necessary to accurately assess the relevance that the modulation by TF on the phenotypic expression of the different lymphocyte subpopulations have on T-cell differentiation.

## B. Modulation of T-Lymphocyte Biological Activities

The regulation of a broad spectrum of T-cell functions have been ascribed to TF (151,154,159). As previously described with regard to induction of T-cell markers, a number of well defined TF possess similar biological activities (160). However, it is well known that assays that measure T-cell function are readily susceptible to extrinsic perturbations. This makes it difficult at times to separate the so called "pleiotropic effects" of TF from their true inductive capabilities, resulting in confusing and sometimes controversial findings (155). However, well controlled studies and reproducible observations made in several laboratories have established a number of currently accepted TF activities, including:

1. Regulation of proliferation. Proliferative responses to mitogens such as phytohemagglutinin (PHA) and concanavalin A (Con A), can be either enhanced or depressed by incubation with TF, depending on the preparation tested, concentration, and culture conditions (157). In general, TF appear to act as modulatory agents, exerting positive effects when the immune responses of normal individuals are spontaneously depressed or when in vitro culture conditions are made suboptimal, for example, by suboptimizing mitogen or antigen concentrations.

In addition, TF have been shown to modulate the lymphoproliferative responses of T cells to foreign histocompatibility antigens in mixed leukocyte reactions (MLR) and in mixed lymphocyte tumor culture (MLTC). It is generally accepted that TF enhance the MLR and MLTC responses in mouse (161-163) and human (164-167) systems.

2. Increased development of cytotoxic effector cells. A number of TF, including TF5, TP-1, and TP5, have been shown to enhance specific cytotoxic T-cell activity (162,168-170). For example, incubation of normal human PBL with TP-1 resulted in an increase in the cytotoxic activity against allogeneic tumor cells (169). Similar results were observed in murine systems, in which TF5-mediated immunostimulation of T-cell activity in MLR and in the development of cytotoxic effector cells in MLTC assays was described (162,168).

3. Enhancement of helper T-cell activity. TF have been reported to enhance specific antibody responses in vivo and in vitro (171-174). Injection of immunodeficient old mice with $T \alpha_1$, shortly before antigen priming, enhanced the helper cell activity of their spleen cells (171). Injection of $T \alpha_1$ has been shown to augment antitetanus antibody production in response to tetanus toxoid immunization in young and old mice (172). TF5 and THF-mediated enhancement of anti-sheep red blood cell antibody production by spleen cells from nude mice has been also described (174).

4. Induction of T-cell differentiation. Although the phenotypic expression of specific antigens is largely employed as a measurement of how "mature" a lymphocyte subpopulation is, the response to immunoregulatory molecules can also be used as a marker of T-cell maturation. For example, the resistance to corticosteroids is one of the functional characteristics associated with a more mature thymocyte cell subpopulation (151). It has recently been shown that TF5 is able to reduce the steroid binding activity and increase the resistance to the cytolytic effect of dexamethasone of human infant thymocytes (175). These findings are compatible with a role of TF in the induction of changes associated with T-cell differentiation of human thymocytes.

5. Induction of suppressor T cells. Enhancement of suppressor T-cell activity by TF has been observed in MLTC (176), in T-cell-mediated cytotoxicity (177) and in T-helper-mediated plaque forming cell (152) systems. $T \alpha_7$ appears to be one of the TF mediating these activities (152).

6. Enhancement of lymphokine production. Although most of these effects have been known for almost a decade, only recently have the mechanisms by which TF may modulate this T-cell function been studied. Lymphokines are products of T cells produced during mitogenic or antigenic stimulation (including MLR) which play a pivotal role in the generation of normal immune responses (178). It has been demonstrated that TF are able to increase the production of a number of lymphokines, including migration inhibition factor (MIF) (179), interferon (180), colony-stimulating factor (161), and interleukin-2 (IL-2) (181-183). The latter lymphokine has been extensively studied since it plays a central role

in T-cell proliferation (184). It has recently been demonstrated that IL-2 production in response to PHA by normal PBL can be increased by TF5 (181). This activity could explain a number of the effects induced by TF on T-cell lymphoproliferative responses, including stimulation of PHA, MLR, and MLTC responses. In addition, stimulation of lymphokine release might be one of the mechanisms involved in the in vivo immunorestorative effects of TF in immunodeficiencies.

One of the critical steps leading to maturation and subsequent differentiation of mature T lymphocytes is the expression of receptors for interleukin-2 (IL-2R). In the thymus, the presence of IL-2R has been described on murine thymocytes expressing an immature phenotype (Lyt2⁻/L3T4⁻) (186,187), suggesting that the expression of IL-2R may play a role in T-cell development. It has recently been demonstrated that the active molecule in TF5 responsible for enhancement of PHA-induced IL-2 production and IL-2R expression is T $\alpha_1$ (187). TF5 is able to increase in vitro IL-2R expression in PHA-stimulated lymphocytes from normal individuals. Additionally, TF5 is able to increase the IL-2R expression of normal human lymphocytes stimulated with OKT3 monoclonal antibodies (187). These effects appear to be the direct effect of TF5, since abrogation of IL-2 production by cyclosporin A did not affect the response. These data, taken together with the fact that TF5 increases IL-2 production by normal human lymphocytes (181), point to a physiological role of thymic hormones in the maintenance of a competent immune system.

## C. Modulation of Natural Killer (NK) Cell Activity

Very recent evidence (188) appears to support the notion of a regulatory role of the thymus in NK activity. Furthermore, in vivo administration of TP-1 or T $\alpha_1$ has been shown to enhance NK activity in mice (189), while no effect has been observed with TF5 (162). In vitro, both enhancement and inhibition NK activity by TF have been reported, depending on the concentrations of TF used. These effects have been described for TP5 (190) and FTS (191).

## D. Effects on the Neuroendocrine System

TF5 has been found to increase in vitro luteinizing hormone releasing factor (LRF) and luteinizing hormone (LH) production by the hypothalamus and pituitary (192) and in vivo increase in adrenocorticotropin (ACTH), cortisone and beta-endorphin production in monkeys (193). Recently, evidence has been presented suggesting that the thymus is involved in the regulation of estrogen-induced suppression of bone marrow colony formation (CFU) leading to bone marrow hypocellularity, since thymectomy abolished the ability of estrogens to suppress CFU proliferation (194). It was hypothesized that these changes in CFU kinetics are due, at least in part, to abnormalities of regulatory factors produced by thymic epithelial cells in response to specific estrogen stimulus (194). On the other hand, it has also been shown that TF5 administration in vivo is able to advance vaginal opening and elevate estrogen levels (196), while estradiol injections decrease thymus weight and cause a transient decrease in T $\alpha_1$ levels in plasma (195).

All this information, together with the fact that certain molecules produced by the immune system (including T $\alpha_1$ and T $\beta_4$) are able to act on the central nervous system (196), strongly suggest a close relationship between the endocrine thymus and the neuroendocrine systems.

## V. THYMIC FACTORS AND AGING

The increase in the average life span of humans during the last century has been accompanied with a parallel increase of a number of diseases associated with aging, including cancer, and certain infectious and autoimmune diseases. The decline of immunocompetence with aging has been correlated with the increased incidence of the diseases (197-200) and extensive reviews describing the changes in the immune system during the ageing process have recently been published (198-200). Although the decline of the immune system is accompanied by alterations in all its compartments, the most affected appears to be the T-cell compartment. Decline in T-cell mitogen-induced proliferation, allogeneic MLR, cytotoxic T-lymphocyte responses (CTL), helper T-cell activity, IL-2 production, IL-2R expression, calcium uptake, PNP activity, adenylate cyclase activity, etc. have been observed in T cells from aging individuals and animals (199,200). These changes lead to an increased susceptibility to infections, decreased resistance to tumor growth and an increased incidence of autoimmune diseases, probably secondary to an immunological imbalance resulting in an increased response towards self-antigens (198), characterized by a rise in the frequency of autoantibodies observed in aged individuals (199).

The thymus gland controls the maturation and differentiation leading to normal T-cell function. The involution of the thymus, which starts at puberty, appears to precede a decline in thymic function and thymic-dependent immunity (198). This phenomenon is accompanied by a decline in the levels of TF (i.e., thymosin, TFS, and thymopoietin) detectable in serum after puberty. However, thymosin-like activity is demonstrable in serum with advancing age, but at reduced levels, probably due to the fact that some epithelial cells of the endocrine thymus remain functional (198) and the possible contribution of extrathymic sites of TF production.

Direct evidence of the involvement of the thymus in the aging of the immune system has been provided by experiments showing that adult thymectomy accelerates the age-related decline in the immune system, and that the success of a thymic transplant in reconstituting thymectomized mice is inversely proportional to the age of the adult thymus donor (198). Very recently, evidence was presented that sequential multiple grafting of syngeneic newborn thymus were able to partially restore immunocompetence in aging mice and extend their mean remaining life expectancy, without altering their maximal life-span (201).

The study of the number and distribution of thymus epithelial cells at different ages has demonstrated that there is a decrease in the number of TF-secreting cells, particularly after the third decade, which parallels the changes in thymus lymphoid volume and in blood levels of humoral factors (202). However, these studies demonstrated a biphasic age-dependency in thymosin positive cells, with the highest positive cell content found in the early postnatal period (2-4 months of age) and at 20-30 years, suggesting that the thymus humoral function is more complicated than suggested by the serum levels (202). It was hypothesized that feedback mechanisms, the existence of which have been already demonstrated for FTS (203), may play an important role in this phenomenon. A decrease in the thymic epithelial cells with age has also been documented for thymosin $\alpha_1$ (204) and FTS (205) -containing cells.

The in vitro and in vivo effects of TF on immune cells from aged animals and individuals have been studied in detail. Variable degrees of restoration of the immune response have been reported with several TF, including in vitro decrease in the formation of autologous rosette forming cells (ARFC) (which are increased in the spleen of aged mice), partial reconstitution of T-cell-mediated cytotoxicity and proliferative responses, increases in T-cell helper activity and MLR (198,200, 206,207). On the contrary, variable or no effects were observed on other immunological parameters like Con A-induced IL-2 production after in vitro preincubation with tertrahydrofuran (THF) (208) or the number of T-cells after in vitro incubation with TF5 (206). Finally, in vitro studies have demonstrated that supernatants from thymic adherent cells were able to augment the antigen/mitogen responses of thymocytes of 2-4-week-old mice if the donors of the thymic adherent cells were 2.5 months old (209). However, this augmenting factor was not present in the supernatant if the cells were obtained from 5-month-old donors. It was further shown that the supernatants from cells of 20-month-old donors contained an inhibitory factor (209).

Injection of old mice with thymosin $\alpha_1$, increased in vitro mitogen-induced IL-2 production (210) and specifically enhanced the in vitro T-cell-dependent activity of their spleen cells (211). These activities appear to be restricted to the N-terminal AA 1-14 (N-14) of the molecule, since the injection of N-14, but not C-14 (C-terminal AA 15-28), was as effective as the injection of the entire thymosin $\alpha_1$ molecule (210,211). Since cells from thymosin $\alpha_1$-injected old mice appeared to also display an enhanced response to exogenously added IL-2, it is postulated that thymosin $\alpha_1$ enhancement of T-cell helper activity by spleens of injected old mice is mediated by changes in both IL-2 production and responsiveness to IL-2 (211).

In another series of experiments, the effect of TF5 and thymosin $\alpha_1$ on the in vitro-specific antibody response by lymphoid cells from in vivo immunized young and old individuals with influenza and tetanous toxoid vaccines have been studied (212,213). It was demonstrated that TF5 and thymosin $\alpha_1$ were able to enhance the specific antibody responses to a trivalent influenza vaccine to a greater extent in cultures established from elderly volunteers (212), while TF5 was able to increase the antibody response against tetanus toxin of 7/10 individuals from the elderly group and of 3/12 volunteers from the younger group (213). Additionally, it was demonstrated that thymosin $\alpha_1$ injection was able to increase the specific antibody production against tetanus toxoid of inoculated young and old mice (214). Based on these studies, it has been suggested that thymosin may be useful as an adjuvant to active immunization for the elderly.

Compatible with these observations are the results of a clinical trial designed to study the immunoprophylactic effects of TP-1. In this study, 40 hospitalized aged individuals with no evidence of autoimmune, neoplastic or acute infectious diseases were divided in 2 groups: one received no therapy and the other was treated with TP-1 for 3 months. Individuals were followed for 180 days and several immune parameters, including Ig and complement levels, sheep rosette-forming cells, absolute lymphocyte numbers, and sedimentation rate were monitored. The incidence of infections was also determined. Results showed a significant reduction of infections and a decreased sedimentation rate in the TP-1-treated group, while the other parameters remained unchanged (215).

Although additional research is required to further determine the role of TF during the aging process, the studies completed to date would point to a potentially important use of TF as therapeutic modalities in the prevention and/or treatment of diseases associated with aging and the senescence of immune responses that occurs with the aging process.

## VI. THYMIC FACTORS AND INFECTIOUS DISEASES

Immunosuppressed animals have been used as models to study the role of TF in the protection against infectious agents in immunocompromised patients. Studies to date are very encouraging and suggest possible therapeutic applications. It has been demonstrated that administration of TF5 or thymosin $\alpha_1$-enhanced immunity and improved survival of immunosuppressed mice infected with BCG (216), candida, or cryptococcus, and also enhanced the production of interferon in mice infected with Newcastle disease virus (217). More recently, studies using nine inbred strains of mice with different degrees of susceptibility to infections with *Candida albicans* have demonstrated that the injection of TF5 increased resistance by some of the susceptible strains, but decreased the resistance of resistant strains (218). In contrast, TF5 enhanced delayed hypersensitivity reactions to specific antigen of the resistant-sensitized mice, while no effect was observed in the susceptible strains (218). Further experiments have shown that the capacity of a particular strain to increase its resistance to the infectious agent after in vivo administration of TF5 parallels its capacity to increase the in vivo release of MIF and gamma interferon (219). It was also demonstrated that TF5 increased in vivo delayed hypersensitivity responses, MIF production, and resistance to infections with an *Candida albicans* in mice treated with alloxan. Alloxan induces a diabetic state characterized by hyperglycemia and a marked decrease in the cellular immune responses to candida (220).

Other interesting observations reported recently involve the protection of 5-fluorouracil- (5-FU) immunosuppressed mice against opportunistic infections (i.e., *Candida albicans, Listeria monocytogenes, Pseudomonas aeruginosa,* and *Serratia marcescens*) by injection of TF5 and thymosin $\alpha_1$ (221). Finally, it has been shown that TP5 is able to greatly increase the survival rate and mean survival time of burned guinea pigs (20% of body surface) after being challenged with *P. aeruginosa* (222).

In humans, clinical studies using various TF preparations, including THF, TFX, and TP-1, have suggested that they can be of benefit to patients with viral infections (i.e., herpes zoster, herpes simplex, adenovirus, hepatitis, and cytomegalovirus), since the TF were able to shorten the course of viral infections and accelerate the restoration of T-cell immunity in such patients (223-227). Unfortunately, such studies were not randomized and therefore cannot be interpreted as conclusive evidence for the efficacy of TF in viral infections. More recently two randomized clinical trials involving control groups of patients have been reported. In one, TP-1 treatment successfully decreased the number or recurrences of herpes simplex labialis infection and improved several immunological parameters in immunosuppressed patients as compared to a placebo group (226). In the second study, TP-1 was found to decrease the incidence of respiratory infections and normalize T-cell subset proportions in children with recurrent respiratory infections as compared to a control group of untreated patients (227).

Thus, it appears that TF may be of therapeutic relevance in preventing or attenuating infectious diseases in immunocompromised hosts, although additional, well controlled clinical trials and the development of additional animal models are required.

## VII.  THYMIC FACTORS AND IMMUNODEFICIENCY DISEASES

The observations that TF are able to stimulate immune responses in immunocompromised animal models provided the rationale for the initiation of clinical trials with thymic preparations in patients with primary and secondary immunodeficiencies.

### A.  Primary Immunodeficiencies

Primary immunodeficiencies include a number of syndromes related to congenital defects of the immune system. They may involve B, T, or both lymphocyte populations. The in vitro effects of TF on PBL from these patients have been documented for TF5, THF, TP-1, thymopoietin, TP5, and thymulin (223). The most frequently observed change was an in vitro increase, although not a complete normalization, in the percentage and numbers of E-rosette-forming cells after incubation with TF.

Several TF preparations, including TF5, TP-1, TP5, thymulin, THF, and TFX, have already entered clinical trials (223,228-232). The administration of these preparations to children with primary immunodeficiencies is based on the effects observed in animals and on patient's PBL in vitro and is an attempt to replace the activity of the endocrine thymus. One of the problems involved in analyzing these trials has been the low incidence of these diseases which precludes randomized trials with placebo groups. However, immunoreconstitution has been achieved in a significant number of cases reported. The most consistent results were observed in children with the DiGeorge syndrome (228).

Improvement in T-cell function of these patients have been reported with TF5 (228), TP-1, and TP5 (229), and thymulin (230). In addition, improvements have been observed in patients with ataxia-telangiectasia (AT) treated with thymulin (230), or THF (233), in patients with Wiskott-Aldrich syndrome treated with TF5 (228), and occasionally in some combined immunodeficiency (CID) patients treated with TF5 (228). From reported studies it appears that the patients most likely to benefit from the TF therapy are those with the mildest immune defects. In contrast to the above mentioned trials, no beneficial effects have been observed in severe CID (SCID) or in most patients with chronic mucocutaneous candidiasis (228). It has been suggested that the lack of response in SCID patients is based on the fact that the defect appears to be at the stem cell level, and therefore these patients lack a population of TF-responsive pre-T cells.

In summary, clinical trials on the effects of TF in primary immunodeficient patients have suggested that TF are effective in reconstituting cellular immunity and improving the clinical status in some of these patients. Further trials involving increased patient numbers are warrant to conclusively establish the therapeutic value of TF in these syndromes.

## B. Secondary Immunodeficiencies

Secondary immunodeficiencies are usually associated with a number of clinical situations like severe burns, viral infections, and chronic renal failure. TF appear to be effective in improving the immune status in animals affected by several of these conditions. In vitro it has been demonstrated that TF are able to improve the percentage of E-rosette-forming cells from patients with severe burns, viral infections, and uremia (223). Furthermore, it has recently been reported that TF5 was able to increase in vitro to almost normal levels the percentage of helper T cells (OKT4+ cells) and all peripheral T cells (OKT3+ cells) without changing the percentage of suppressor T cells (OKT8+ cells) in patients with chronic renal failure (234).

A number of clinical trials have involved immunosuppressed patients with the acquired immunodeficiency syndrome (AIDS). AIDS is caused by a retrovirus termed HIV (human immunodeficiency virus) and is characterized by an increased incidence of opportunistic infections, unusual malignancies such as Kaposi's sarcoma, and a progressive crippling of the thymic-dependent immune system (235). A variety of immunological abnormalities have been described including an inversion of the T4/T8 ratio, a deficiency in helper T cells, decreased lymphoproliferative responses to mitogens and antigens, decreased MLR and decreased IL-2 production (235-238). Several clinical trials are in progress with TF (including TF5, T$\alpha_1$, TP5, THF, and TP-1) attempting to immunologically reconstitute patients at risk for developing AIDS. In a pilot clinical trial to evaluate the in vivo effects of TF5 and T$\alpha_1$, 42 male homosexuals and hemophiliacs received daily treatment for 10 weeks. A dose of 60 mg TF5 was found to transiently increase MLR and mitogen-induced IL-2 production (239). The patients who benefited the most were those with the least compromised immune system. None of the patients whose T-cell function improved have as yet developed frank AIDS with a 2 year minimal follow-up. Nevertheless, it has become apparent that combined modality approaches including antiviral drugs along with immunorestorative agents such as TF will be necessary to optimize treatment of HIV-infected patients at risk for developing AIDS.

## VIII. THYMIC FACTORS AND AUTOIMMUNE DISEASES

It is currently accepted that the emergence of autoimmunity is associated with an immunoregulatory T-cell imbalance, probably due to a decrease in T-lymphocyte suppressor cell activity, which leads to an uncontrolled antibody production by B lymphocytes and T-cell dyscrasias. Several animal models have been established as correlates of human autoimmune disorders. One that has been used extensively as a model of human systemic lupus erythematosus (SLE) is the NZB mice. Evidence obtained in the last few years supports the hypothesis that an abnormality of the endocrine thymus may be involved in the development of autoimmunity in NZB mouse (223). A decrease in FTS-like activity in the sera of these mice precedes the onset of the disease and grafting of a newborn thymus to adult NZB mice can correct some of the defects associated with the disease (i.e., autoimmune hemolytic anemia) (223). In addition, a number of the immune abnormalities associated with this disease can be partially corrected by the administration of several thymic preparations, including TF5, FTS, THF, TP5, and thymopoietin. For example, short-term administration of TF5 restored the capacity of lymph node lymphocytes to respond to PHA and Con A, increase MLR responses (240), and induced some reduction in the production of antinucleic acid antibodies (241). However, long-term administration of TF5 did appear to have no effect on overall survival (242). More recently it has been shown that FTS decreased the high NK activity observed in NZB mice (243), apparently through the activation of cells that suppress NK activity. The treatment of young female B/W ([NZB X NZW] $F_1$) mice with FTS retarded the appearance of Sjögren's syndrome (which is usually associated with the autoimmune disease in NZB mice) but led to an enhancement of anti-DNA autoantibody production and glomerulonephritis (228). Conversely, FTS treatment of aging B/W mice decreased anti-DNA antibody formation and improved glomerulonephritis (228).

Another animal model of autoimmune disease is experimental autoimmune thyroiditis (EAT), which is characterized by a lymphoid infiltration of the thyroid gland and the presence of antithyroglobulin antibodies. In this system TF5 was able to suppress the EAT development in a strain of guinea pig which is a high responder to thyroglobulin immunization, while no effect was observed in a low responder strain (244). On the other hand, TF5 has no suppressive effect on the incidence and severity of experimental allergic encephalomyelitis (EAE), an animal autoimmune disease used as a model for multiple sclerosis (MS) (245), whereas, thymulin has been shown to reduce EAE development (228).

In in vitro studies TF5, THF, thymulin, and TP-1 were able to increase one or more immune parameters, in vitro in PBL from patients with various autoimmune disease including E-rosette-forming cells (E-RFC), autologous MLR (A-MLR), production of lymphokines, and graft versus host responses (223). TF5 and FTS were able to modulate suppressor cell activity in autoimmune disorders, such as SLE (246), rheumatoid arthritis (RA) (247), chronic active hepatitis (CAH) (248), and autoimmune hemolytic anemia (AHA) (249), all associated with abnormal suppressor cell activity. In addition, FTS has been found to increase the percentage of autologous rosette-forming cells (Tar cells) in PBL of paients with SLE (250). Tar cells, considered to be postthymic T-cell precursors, are OKT3,4,8+ Dr− PBL which are able to generate cytotoxic effector cells against allogeneic target cells and TNP-labelled self-target cells provided they are activated by IL-2 or FTS (251). These observations suggest that TF exert a homeostatic role in diseases associated with an imbalanced immune system, and have provided a rationale basis for administering TF therapeutically in patients with autoimmune diseases.

Clinical trials are in progress in several autoimmune disorders, including SLE, RA, CHA, AHA, multiple sclerosis (MS), aplastic anemia (AA), and sarcoidosis. However, there are few published reports concerning the therapeutic efficacy of TF in patients with these disorders. Preliminary evidence indicated that some improvement in SLE and RA was obtained with TF5 (223), although there was no effect on the levels of antinuclear antibodies. TFX was found to induce clinical improvements, accompanied with a decrease in rheumatoid factor levels and normalization of the hypergammaglobulinemia in 16 of 20 RA patients (230). These studies have also shown an improvement in clinical and laboratory findings in 60-80% of CAH patients, while no promising results were observed in MS patients (230). Thymulin has shown promising preliminary results in the treatment of RA patients, since a clear improvement of the clinical signs, particularly those related to inflammation, has been observed (228). A recent report on 2 children with AHA suggested that TF5 may be of therapeutic value in the treatment of the T-suppressor-cell deficiency associated with this disease (249). Finally, hematological improvements have been reported in AA patients treated with TP-1 (253).

Although the clinical trials to date are encouraging, larger, placebo-controlled randomized studies will be necessary to provide definitive answers regarding the role of TF in the treatment of autoimmune disorders.

## IX. THYMIC FACTORS AND CANCER

A number of experiments in mice have clearly established that neonatal thymectomy increases the susceptibility to tumor transplantation and carcinogenesis, and that thymic grafts in diffusion chambers could restore normal antitumor responses (223). It has also been shown that TF5, FTS, and THF were able to accelerate the rejection of syngenic tumors in several immunosuppressed murine models (223). More recent animal studies have attempted to employ TF along with concurrent radiotherapy or chemotherapy as the primary antitumor treatment similar to that received by cancer patients. For example, it has been demonstrated that in vivo administration of TF5 or thymosin $\alpha_1$, in conjunction with cyclophosphamide (CY), can prevent reappearance of the MOPC-315 plasmacytoma resulting in increased survival compared to animals treated with CY alone (254). The combination of TF5 and bischloroethylnitrosourea (BCNU) was found to increase survival of mice with lymphocytic leukemia compared to mice treated with BCNU alone (255). The effect of thymosin $\alpha_1$ has been examined in mice immunosuppressed by cytostatics or x-ray irradiation (256). Such immunosuppressed mice died within a few days after challenge with P388 or L1210 leukemic cells. It was shown that thymosin $\alpha_1$ given concomitantly with cytostatics (5-FU or BCNU) or after irradiation prevented the decrease in resistance to tumors caused by those agents (256). These studies also demonstrated that thymosin $\alpha_1$ was able to restore NK activity in the spleens of mice treated with 5-FU or irradiation. Thymosin $\alpha_1$ also restored 5-FU-induced bone marrow cytotoxicity in mice, as measured by immune reconstitution of colony formation and lymphokine production (257). In addition, restoration of T-cell-mediated immune responses and induction of specific antitumor responses were obtained with TF5 in a fibrosarcoma model in spontaneously hypertensive rats with congenital T-cell depression (258). In other studies, TF5 was able to consistently immunostimulate T-cell responses against several tumors in vitro, as measured by enhanced MLR and the development of cytotoxic effector cells in mixed lymphocyte tumor response cell-mediated cytotoxicity assay (MLTC-CMC) (259). These studies also demonstrated that TF5 could act as an immunoadjuvant in vivo for the development of specific effector cells capable of rejecting a tumor challenge, as well as exhibit some therapeutic effects against pre-existing metastatic tumors (259).

Immunomodulatory effects of TF have also been observed in vitro in PBL obtained from cancer patients. For example, increased E-RFC formation has been described after incubation of lymphocytes from cancer patients with TF5, THF, TP-1, and TFX (223). Positive effects were seen only if preincubation E-rosette-forming colonies percentages were below normal levels. Additionally, enhanced LMIF production by TF5, increased proliferative responses by TF5 and TP-1, an increase in the percentage of Tar cells by thymosin $\alpha_1$, increased proliferative responses to allogeneic tumor cells by TP-1 and a decrease in the suppressor cell activity of cells from cancer patients with evidence of abnormally elevated suppressor activity have all been reported (223).

The clinical evaluation of thymic factors in cancer patients has been limited to five preparations, namely TF5, synthetic $T\alpha_1$, TP-1, THF, and TFX. THF (233) and TFX (232) have been employed predominantly in patients with infectious complications and such studies have been mostly anecdotal experiences involving relatively small patient numbers. In contrast, TF5, $T\alpha_1$, and TP-1 are currently being produced by pharmaceutical companies and relatively large quantities have been available for more extensive clinical trials.

The only reported classic phase I trials with TF have employed TF5 (260-268) or more recently $T\alpha_1$ (264-265). These preparations have been extremely well tolerated, even at high doses, so that the dose-limiting condition universally proved to be the maximal concentration of drug that could be prepared in solution for parenteral administration, rather than any specific systemic toxicity. Thus, it has not been possible to identify a maximal tolerated dose for thymic factors such as TF5 or $T\alpha_1$. Although one-third to one-half of patients exhibited varying degrees of immune reconstitution, no consistent immunorestorative effects were observed. With the exception of patients with renal cancer (266), there was no objective evidence of tumor regression. Several confirmatory phase II trials of TF5 in advanced renal cancer, have now been reported with response rates varying from 0-15% (268,269). Overall, only 8 of 73 patients (8%) with renal cancer treated with TF5 have exhibited objective tumor regression.

A number of clinical trials have now been reported in which the influence of TF on T-cell immunity was assessed as the primary study end point using fixed doses and schedule of administration. TP-1 has been evaluated in detail in patients with Hodgkin's disease (270-273). These trials were initiated after preliminary in vitro studies indicated that TP-1 could increase T-cell percentages and functions when incubated with peripheral blood lymphocytes (PBL) from untreated patients (273). In these studies TP-1 administration was associated with improvement in several immune parameters including T-cell numbers and to some degree T-cell function and delayed-type cutaneous skin reactions.

Randomized phase II/III trials have been reported with TF5 in patients with head and neck cancer receiving radiotherapy (274-277), with $T\alpha_1$ in patients with non-small cell lung cancer following radiotherapy (278-279), and with TP-1 in postsurgical patients with malignant melanoma (280). In each of these trials

TF administration was associated with improvements in T-cell immunity as well as disease-free survival. However, the relatively small numbers of patients involved in these studies preclude any definitive interpretation of the impact of TF therapy on overall survival. Several randomized multi-institutional phase III trials are currently in progress with T $\alpha_1$ in postradiotherapy patients with non-small cell lung cancer, and with TP-1 in postsurgical patients with malignant melanoma. These studies should provide definitive conclusions regarding the efficacy of TF administration in cancer patients.

TF have been administered in conjunction with a variety of chemotherapy regimens (281-288). Two trials have suggested that when administered concurrently with chemotherapy TP-1 (281) and TF5 (284,285), respectively, improved immunity and/or patient survival. However, other trials in patients with small cell lung cancer (287), and non-small cell lung cancer (286,288,289) have not shown any positive effects with a combination of chemotherapy + TF. Thus, at present there is no proven role in the administration of TF as adjuncts to cancer chemotherapy.

## X.  FUTURE PERSPECTIVES

In spite of the rapid progress that is being made, the current understanding of thymic physiology is far from complete. Although several thymic peptides have been isolated, sequenced, and synthesized, no specific biological assays for TF have yet been developed. It is anticipated that the development of such assays will contribute to a better understanding of the role of TF as they relate not only to the development and maturation of the T-cell-dependent immune system, but also to other components of the immune system as well as the autonomic, neuroendocrine, and endocrine systems.

The therapeutic potential of TF in aging and in a number of disease states, including infectious and autoimmune diseases, primary and secondary immunodeficiencies and cancer remains to be defined. The doses, schedules, and routes of administration all need further study. The large-scale phase III clinical trials employing T$\alpha_1$ in patients with non-small cell lung cancer, and TP-1 in patients with malignant melanoma, should provide the first definitive answers as to the potential role for TF in the treatment of human cancer.

## REFERENCES

1.  Stutman, O. Role of thymic hormones in T cell differentiation. Clin. Immunol. Allergy 3: 9, 1983.
2.  Bach, J.F., ed. Thymic hormones. Clin. Immunol. Allergy 3: 1983.
3.  Trainin, N., Rotter, V., and Yakir, Y. Biochemical and biological properties of THF in animal and human models. Annals NY Acad. Sci. 332: 9, 1979.

4. Goldstein, A.L., and White, A. The thymus gland: experimental and clinical studies of its role in the development and expression of immune functions. In *Advances In Metabolic Disorders,* Volume 5, Academic Press, Inc., New York, 1971, p. 149.

5. Goldstein, A.L., Low, T.L.K., Thurman, G.B., Zatz, M., Hall, N.R., McClure, J.E., Hun, S., and Schulof, R.S. Thymosins and other hormone-like factors of the thymus gland. In *Immunological Approaches to Cancer Therapeutics.* Edited by E. Mihich. John-Wiley & Sons, New York, 1982, p. 137.

6. Miller, J.F.A.P. Immunological function of the thymus. Lancet 2: 48, 1961.

7. Archer, O.K., and Pierce, J.C. Role of the thymus in development of the immune response. Fed. Proc. 20: 26, 1961.

8. Good, R.A., Dalmasso, A.P., Martinex, G., Archer, O.K., Pierre, J.C., and Papermaster, B.W. The role of the thymus in development of immunologic capacity in rabbits and mice. J. Exp. Med. 116: 773, 1962.

9. East, J., and Parrot, D.M.V. Prevention of wasting in mice thymectomized at birth and their subsequent rejection of allogeneic leukemia cells. J. Natl. Cancer Inst. 33: 673, 1964.

10. Levey, R.H., Trainin, N., and Law, L.W. Evidence for function of thymic tissue in diffusion chambers implanted in neonatally thymectomized mice, preliminary report. J. Natl. Cancer Inst. 31: 199, 1963.

11. Law, L.W., Dunn, T.B., Trainin, N., and Levey, R.H. Studies of thymic function. In *The Thymus.* Edited by V. Defendi and D. Metcalf. The Wistar Institute Press, Philadelphia, 1964, p. 105.

12. Osoba, D. The effects of thymus and other lymphoid organs enclosed in millipore chambers on neonatally thymectomized mice. J. Exp. Med. 122: 633, 1965.

13. Stutman, O., Yunis, E.J., and Good, R.A. Carcinogen-induced tumors of the thymus: restoration of neonatally thymectomized mice with thymomas in cell-impermeable chambers. J. Natl. Cancer Inst. 43: 499, 1969.

14. Osoba, D., and Miller, J.F.A.P. Evidence for a humoral thymus factor responsible for the maturation of immunological faculty. Nature 199: 653, 1963.

15. Gregoire, C. Reserches sur la symboise lymphoepitheliale au niveau du thymus de mannifere. Arch. Biol. Liege 46: 717, 1935.

16. Law, L.W., Goldstein, A.L., and White, A. Influence of thymosin on immunological competence of lymphoid cells from thymectomized mice. Nature 219: 1391, 1968.

17. Asanuma, T., Goldstein, A.L., and White, A. Reduction in the incidence of wasting disease in neonatally thymectomized CBA/W mice by the injection of thymosin. Endocrinology 86: 600, 1970.

18. Goldstein, A.L., Asanuma, Y., Battisto, J.R., Hardy, M.A., Quint, J., and White, A. Influence of thymosin on cell-mediated and humoral immune responses in normal and in immunologically deficient mice. J. Immunol. 104: 359, 1970.

19. Little, J.R., Brechen, G., Bradley, T.R., and Rose, S. Determination of lymphocyte turnover by continuous infusion of [3]H thymidine. Blood 19: 236, 1962.

20. Metcalf, D. Delayed effect of thymectomy in adult life on immunological competence. Nature 208: 1336, 1965.

21. Miller, J.F.A.P. Effect of thymectomy in adult mice on immunological responsiveness. Nature 208: 1337, 1965.

22. Johnston, J.M., and Wilson, D.B. Origins of immunoreactive lymphocytes in rats. Cell. Immunol. 1: 430, 1970.

23. Robson, L.C., and Schwarz, M.R. The influence of adult thymectomy on immunological competence as measured by the mixed lymphocyte reaction. Transplantation 11: 465, 1971.

24. Zatz, M.M., and Goldstein, A.L. Antigen-induced depression of DNA synthesis in mouse spleen. J. Immunol. 110: 1312, 1972.

25. Simpson, E., and Cantor, H. Regulation of the immune response by subclasses of T lymphocytes. II. The effect of adult thymectomy upon humoral and cellular responses in mice. Eur. J. Immunol. 5: 337, 1975.

26. Asherson, G.L., Zembala, M., Mayhew, B., and Goldstein, A. Adult thymectomy prevention of the appearance of suppressor T cells which depress contact sensitivity to picryl chloride and reversal of adult thymectomy effect by thymus extract. Eur. J. Immunol. 6: 699, 1976.

27. Reinisch, C.L., Andres, S.L., and Schlossman, S.F. Suppressor cell regulation of immune response to tumors: abrogation by adult thymectomy. Proc. Natl. Acad. Sci. (USA) 74: 2989, 1977.

28. Erard, D., Charreire, J., Auffredou, M.T., Galanaud, Pl., and Bach, J.F. Regulation of contact sensitivity to DNFB in the mouse. Effects of adult thymectomy and thymic factor. J. Immunol. 123: 1573, 1979.

29. Kappler, J.W., Hunter, P.C., Jacobs, D., and Lord, E. Functional heterogeneity among the T-derived lymphocytes of the mouse. J. Immunol. 113: 27, 1974.

30. Rocha, B., Freitas, A.A., and Coutinho, A.A. Population dynamics of T lymphocytes, renewal rate and expansion in the peripheral lymphoid organs. J. Immunol. 131: 2158, 1983.

31. Bach, J.F., and Dardenne, M. Studies on thymus products. II. Demonstration and characteristics of a circulating thymic hormone. Immunol. 25: 353, 1973.

32. Ito, T., and Hoshino, T. Fine structure of the epithelial reticular cells of the medulla of the thymus in the golden hamster. Z. Zellforsch. Mikrosk, Anat. 69: 311, 1966.

33. Goldstein, G., and MacKay, I.R. The Human Thymus. Green Publishing Co., St. Louis, Missouri, 1969.

34. Bearman, R.M., Levine, G.D., and Bensch, K.G. The ultrastructure of the normal human thymus: a study of 36 cases. Anat. Res. 190: 755, 1978.

35. Hirokawa, K., McClure, J.E., and Goldstein, A.L. Age-related changes in localization of thymosin in the human thymus. Thymus 4: 19, 1982.

36. Singh, J. The ultrastructure of epithelial reticular cells. In The Thymus Gland. Edited by M.F. Kendall. Academic Press, London, 1981, p. 133.

37. Frazier, J.A. Ultrastructure of the chick thymus. Z. Zellforsch. Mikrosk. Anat. 136: 191, 1973.

38. Hakanson, R., Larsson, L.I., and Sundler, F. Peptide and amine producing endocrine-like cells in the chicken thymus. Histochemistry 39: 25, 1974.
39. Kendall, M.D., and Frazier, J.A. Ultrastructure studies on erythropoiesis in the avian thymus. I. Description of cell types. Cell. Tiss. Res. 199: 37, 1979.
40. Kohnen, P., and Weiss, L. An electron microscopic study of thymic corpuscles in the guinea pig and the mouse. Anat. Res. 148: 29, 1964.
41. Weakley, B.S., Patt, D.I., and Shepro, D. Ultrastructure of the fetal thymus in the golden hamster. J. Morp. 115: 319, 1964.
42. Clark, S.L. In *The Thymus — Experimental and Clinical Studies.* Edited by G.E.W. Wolstenholme and R. Porter. CIBA Foundation Symposium, Little, Brown & Co., Boston, 1966, p. 3.
43. Chapman, W.L., and Allen, J.R. The fine structure of the thymus of the fetal and neonatal monkey (Macaca mulatta). Z. Zellforsch. Mikrosk. Anat. 114: 220, 1971.
44. Jordan, R.K. Ultrastructure studies on cells containing secretory granules in the early embryonic thymus. In *Biological Activity of Thymic Hormones.* Edited by D.W. van Bekkam. Kooykeu Scientific Publications, Rotterdam, 1975, p. 69.
45. Pinkel, D. Ultrastructure of human fetal thymus. Am. J. Dis. Child. 115: 222, 1968.
46. Vetters, J.M., and Macadam, R.F. Fine structural evidence for hormone secretion by the human thymus. J. Clin. Pathol. 26: 194, 1973.
47. Bloodworth, J.M.B., Hiratsuka, H., Hickey, R.C., and Wu, J. Ultrastructure of the human thymus, thymic tumors, and myasthenia gravis. In *Pathology Annual 10.* Appleton-Century Crafts, New York, 1975, p. 329.
48. Singh, J. The ultrastructure of thymic epithelial reticular cells. Ph.D. thesis, University of London, 1980.
49. Haynes, B.F., Warren, R.W., Buckley, R.H., McClure, J.E., Goldstein, A.L., Henderson, F.W., Hensley, L.L., and Eisenbarth, G.S. Demonstration of abnormalities of expression of thymic epithelial surface antigens in severe cellular immunodeficiency disease. J. Immunol. 130: 1182, 1983.
50. Haynes, B.F., Shimizu, K., and Eisenbarth, G.S. Identification of human and rodent thymic epithelium using tetanus toxin and monoclonal antibody $a_2B_5$. J. Clin. Invest. 71: 9, 1983.
51. Haynes, B.F. The human thymic microenvironment. Adv. Immunol. 36: 87, 1984.
52. Haynes, B.F., Scearce, R.M., Lobach, D.F., and Hensley, L.L. Phenotypic characterization and ontogeny of mesodermal-derived and endocrine epithelial components of the human thymic microenvironment. J. Exp. Med. 159: 1149, 1984.
53. Eisenbarth, G.S., Shimizu, K., Bowring, M.A., and Wells, S. Expression of receptors for tetanus toxin and monoclonal antibody $A_2B_5$ by pancreatic islet cells. Proc. Natl. Acad. Sci. (USA) 79: 5066, 1982.
54. Hammar, J.A. The new views as to the morphology of the thymus gland and their bearings on the problem of the function of the thymus. Endocrinology 5: 543 and 731, 1921.

55. Dardenne, M., Papiernik, M., and Bach, J.F. Studies on thymus products III epithelial origin of the serum thymic factor. J. Immunol. 27: 299, 1974.

56. Savino, W., Dardenne, M., and Bach, J.F. Thymic hormone containing cells. II. Evolution of cells containing the serum thymic factor (FTS or thymulin) in normal and autoimmune mice, as revealed by anti-FTS monoclonal antibodies. Relationship with Ia bearing cells. Clin. Exp. Immunol. 52: 1, 1983.

57. Bach, J.F., and Dardenne, M. Thymic dependency of rosette-forming cells. Evidence of a circulating thymic hormone. Transplant. Proc. 4: 345, 1972.

58. Twomey, J.J., Lewis, V.M., Patten, B.M., Goldstein, G., and Good, R.A. Myasthenia Gravis, thymectomy and serum thymic hormone activity. Am. J. Med. 66: 639, 1979.

59. Lewis, V., Twomey, J.J., and Bealmear, P.N. Age, thymic involution and circulating thymic hormone activity. J. Clin. Endocrinol. Metab. 47: 45, 1978.

60. Iwata, T., Incefy, G., and Cunningham-Rundles, S. Circulating thymic hormone activity in patients with primary and secondary immunodeficiency diseases. Am. J. Med. 71: 385, 1981.

61. Bach, J.F., Dardenne, M., and Papiernik, M. Evidence for a serum factor produced by the human thymus. Lancet 2: 1056, 1972.

62. Klein, J.J., Goldstein, A.L., and White, A. Enhancement of in vivo incorporation of labeled precursors into DNA and total protein of mouse lymph nodes after administration of thymic extracts. Proc. Natl. Acad. Sci. (USA) 53: 812, 1965.

63. Klein, J.J., Goldstein, A.L., and White, A. Effects of the thymus lymphocytopoietic factor. Annals NY Acad. Sci. 135: 485, 1966.

64. Goldstein, A.L., Slater, F.D., and White, A. Preparation, assay and partial purification of a thymic lymphocytopoietic factor (thymosin). Proc. Natl. Acad. Sci. (USA) 56: 1010, 1966.

65. Goldstein, A.L., and White, A. The thymus gland: experimental and clinical studies of its role in the development and expression of immune functions. Adv. Metabol. Disorders 5: 149, 1971.

66. Hooper, J.A., McDaniel, M.C., Thurman, G.B., Cohen, G.H., Schulof, R.S., and Goldstein, A.L. Purification and properties of bovine thymosin. Annals NY Acad. Sci. 249: 125, 1975.

67. Low, T.L.K., and Goldstein, A.L. The chemistry and biology of thymosin. II. Amino acid sequence analysis of thymosin $\alpha_1$ and polypeptide $\beta_1$. J. Biol. Chem. 254: 987, 1979.

68. Goldstein, A.L., Asanuma, Y., Battisto, J.R., Hardy, M., Quint, J., and White, A. Influence of thymosin on cell-mediated and humoral immune responses to normal and immunologically deficient mice. J. Immunol. 104: 359, 1970.

69. Low, T.L.K., Thurman, G.B., and McAdoo, M. The chemistry and biology of thymosin. I. isolation, characterization and biological activities of thymosin $\alpha_1$ and polypeptide $\beta_1$ from calf thymus. J. Biol. Chem. 254: 981, 1979.

70. Kater, L., Oosterom, R., McClure, J., and Goldstein, A.L. Presence of thymosin-like factors in human thymic epithelium conditioned medium. Int. J. Immunopharm. 1: 273, 1979.

71. Dalakas, M.C., engel, W.K., McClure, J.E., and Goldstein, A.L. Thymosin $\alpha_1$ in myasthenia gravis. N. Engl. J. Med. 302: 1092, 1980.

72. Haynes, B.F., Robert-Guroff, M., Metzgar, R.S., Franchini, G., Kalyanaraman, V.S., Palker, T.J., and Gallo, R.C. Monoclonal antibody against human T cell leukemia virus p19 defines a human thymic epithelial antigen acquired during ontogeny. J. Exp. Med. 157: 907, 1983.

73. Freire, M., Hannappel, E., and Rey, M. Purification of thymus RNA coding for a 16000 dalton polypeptide containing the thymosin alpha 1 sequence. Proc. Natl. Acad. Sci. (USA) 78: 192, 1981.

74. Low, T.L.K., McClure, J.E., Naylor, P.H., Spangelo, B.L., and Goldstein, A.L. Isolation of thymosin $\alpha_1$ from thymosin fraction 5 of different species by high-performance liquid chromatography. J. Chrom. 266: 533, 1983.

75. Haritos, A.A., Tsolus, O., and Horecker, B.L. Distribution of prothymosin $\alpha$ in rat tissues. Proc. Natl. Acad. Sci. (USA) 81: 1391, 1984.

76. McGillis, J.P., Hall, N.R., and Goldstein, A.L. Circadian rhythm of thymosin $\alpha_1$ in normal and thymectomized mice. J. Immunol. 131: 148, 1983.

77. Bershof, J.F., and Goldstein, A.L. Evidence for a circadian rhythm of thymosin alpha-1 in humans. Clin. Res. 31: 44, 1983.

78. Naylor, P.H., and Goldstein, A.L. unpublished observations, 1984.

79. Chu, A.C., Patterson, J.A.K., Goldstein, G., Berger, C.L., Takezaki, S., and Edelson, R.L. Thymopoietin-like substance in human skin. J. Invest. Dermatol. 81: 194, 1983.

80. Stahli, C., Takacs, B., and Kocyba, C. Monoclonal antibodies to thymosin $\alpha_1$. Molecular Immunol. 20: 1095, 1983.

81. Wang, S.S., Kulesha, I.D., and Winter, D.P. Synthesis of thymosin $\alpha_1$. J. Am. Chem. Soc. 101: 253, 1978.

82. Wang, S.S., Makofske, R., Bach, A.E., and Merrifield, R.B. Solid phase synthesis of thymosin $\alpha_1$. Int. J. Peptide Protein Res. 15: 1, 1980.

83. Wetzel, R., Heyneker, H.L., and Goeddel, D.V. Production of biologically active Na-desacetylthymosin $\alpha_1$ in Escherichia coli through expression of a chemically synthesized gene. Biochemistry 19: 6096, 1980.

84. Low, T.L.K., and Goldstein, A.L. Structure and function of thymosin factors. In *The Year in Hematology*. Edited by R. Silber, J. LaBue, and A.S. Gordon. Plenum Press, New York, 1978, p. 281.

85. Caldarella, J., Goodall, G.J., Felix, A.M., Heimer, E.P., Salvin, S.B., and Horecker, B.L. Thymosin $\alpha_{11}$: a peptide related to thymosin $\alpha_1$ isolated from calf thymosin fraction 5. Proc. Natl. Acad. Sci. (USA) 80: 7424, 1983.

86. Schlesinger, D.H., Goldstein, G., and Niall, H.D. The complete amino acid sequence of ubiquitin, and adenylate cyclase stimulating polypeptide probably universal in living cells. Biochemistry 14: 2214, 1975.

87. Olson, M.O.J., Goldsknopf, I.L., Guetzow, K.A., James, G.T., Hawkins, T.C., Mays-Rothberg, C.J., and Busch, H. The $NH_2$- and COOH-terminal amino acid sequence of nuclear protein A24. J. Biol. Chem. 251: 5901, 1976.

88. Hunt, L.T., and Dayhoff, M.O. Amino-terminal sequence identity of ubiquitin and the nonhistone component of nuclear protein A24. Biochem. Biophys. Res. Commun. 74: 650, 1977.

89. Wilkinson, K.D., and Rose, I.A. Glucose exchange and catalysis by two crystalline hexokinase glucose complexes. J. Biol. Chem. 255: 7569, 1980.

90. Low, T.L.K., Hu, S.K., and Goldstein, A.L. Complete amino acid sequence of bovine thymosin $\beta_4$: a thymic hormone that induces terminal deoxynucleotidyl transferase activity in thymolyte populations. Proc. Natl. Acad. Sci. (USA) 78: 1166, 1981.

91. Wang, S.S., Wang, B.S.H., Chang, J.K., Low, T.L.K., and Goldstein, A.L. Synthesis of thymosin $\beta_4$. In *Peptides, Synthesis-Structure-Functions*. Edited by D.H. Rich and E. Gross. *Proc. 7th Am. Peptide Symposium*. Pierce Chemical Co., Rockford, Illinois, 1981, p. 189.

92. Naylor, P.H., McClure, J.E., Spangelo, B.L., Low, T.L.K., and Goldstein, A.L. Immunochemical studies on thymosin: radioimmunoassay of thymosin $\beta_4$. Immunopharmacology 7: 9, 1984.

93. Xu, G.J., Hannappel, E., Morgan, J., Hempstead, J., and Horecker, B.L. Synthesis of thymosin $\beta_4$ by peritoneal macrophages and adherent spleen cells. Proc. Natl. Acad. Sci. (USA) 79: 4006, 1982.

94. Hanapell, E., Davoust, S., and Horecker, B.L. Thymosin beta 8 and beta 9: Two new peptides isolated from calf thymus homologous to beta 4. Proc. Natl. Acad. Sci. (USA) 79: 1708, 1982.

95. Erickson-Viitanen, S., Ruggieri, S., Natalini, P., and Horecker, B.L. Thymosin beta 10, a new analog of thymosin beta 4 in mammalian tissues. Arch Biochem. Biophys. 225: 407, 1983.

96. Erickson-Viitanen, S., and Horecker, B.L. Thymosin beta 11: A peptide from trout liver homologous to thymosin beta 4. Arch. Biochem. Biophys. 233: 815, 1984.

97. Goldstein, G., and Mananaro, A. Thymin: a thymic polypeptide causing the neuromuscular block of myasthenia gravis. Annals NY Acad. Sci. 183: 230, 1971.

98. Goldstein, G. Polypeptides regulating lymphocyte differentiation. Cold Spring Harbor Conf. on Cellular Proliferation 5: 455, 1978.

99. Goldstein, G., Scheid, M.P., Boyse, E.A., Schlesinger, D.H., and Van Waunue, J. A synthetic pentapeptide with biological activity characteristic of the thymic hormone thymopoietin. Science 204: 1399, 1979.

100. Basch, R.S., and Goldstein, G. Induction of T cell differentiation *in vitro* by thymin, a purified polypeptide hormone of the thymus. Proc. Natl. Acad. Sci. (USA) 71: 1474, 1974.

101. Goldstein, G. Isolation of bovine thymin: a polypeptide hormone of the thymus. Nature 247: 11, 1974.

102. Goldstein, G. The isolation of thymopoietin (thymin). Annals NY Acad. Sci. 249: 177, 1978.

103. Audhya, T., Schlesinger, D.H., and Goldstein, G. Complete amino acid sequences of bovine thymopoietin, I, II and III: Closely homologous polypeptides. Biochemistry 20: 6195, 1981.

104. Fugino, M., Shinagawa, S., Fukuda, T., Takaoki, M., Kawaji, H., and Sugino, Y. Synthesis of the nonatetracontrapeptide corresponding to the sequence proposed for thymopoietin II. Chem. Pharm. Bull. 23: 1486, 1977.

105. Zaruba, K., Rastorter, M., Grob, P.J., Joller-Jemelka, H., and Bolla, K. Thymopentin as adjuvant in non-responders or hyporesponders to hepatitis B vaccination. Lancet 1245, 1983.

106. Goldstein, G. What is a thymic hormone? In *Progress in Immunology III.* Edited by T.E. Mandel, C. Cheeus, C.S. Hosking, I.F.C. McKenzie, and G.J.V. Nossal. North Holland, Amsterdam, 1977, p. 390.

107. Goldstein, G. Radioimmunoassay for thymopoietin. J. Immunol. 117: 690, 1976.

108. Lisi, P.J., Teipel, J.W., Goldstein, G., and Schiffman, M. Improved radioimmunoassay technique for measuring serum thymopoietin. Clinica Chimica Acta 107: 111, 1980.

109. Twomey, J.J., Goldstein, G., Lewis, V.M., bealmear, and Good, R.A. Bioassay determinations of thymopoietin and thymic hormone levels in human plasma. Proc. Natl. Acad. Sci. (USA) 6: 2541, 1977.

110. Umiel, T., and Trainin, N. Increased reactivity of responding cells in mixed lymphocyte reaction by a thymic humoral factor. Eur. J. Immunol. 5: 85, 1975.

111. Shohat, B., Spitzer, S., Topilsky, M., and Trainin, N. Immunological profile in sarcoidosis patients. The in vitro and in vivo effect of thymic humoral factor. Biomedicine Experimentia 29: 91, 1978.

112. Kook, A.I., and Trainin, N. Hormone-like activity of a thymus humoral factor on the incubation of immune competence in lymphoid cells. J. Exp. Med. 139: 193, 1974.

113. Kook, A.I., Yakir, Y., and Trainin, N. Isolation and partial chemical characterization of THF, a thymus hormone involved in immune maturation of lymphoid cells. Cell. Immunol. 19: 151, 1975.

114. Bach, J.F., Dardenne, M., and Davis, A.J.S. Early effects of adults thymectomy. Nature (New Biology) 231: 100, 1971.

115. Dardenne, M., and Bach, J.F. Studies on thymus products: I modification of rosette-forming cells by thymic extracts determination of the target RFC subpopulation. Immunology 25: 343, 1973.

116. Bach, J.F., and Dardenne, M. antigen recognition by T lymphocytes. II. Similar effects of azathioprine, ALS and antitheta serum on rosette-forming lymphocytes in normals and neonatally thymectomized mice. Cell. Immunol. 3: 11, 1972.

117. Pleau, J.M., Dardenne, M., Blouquit, Y., and Bach, J.F. Structural study of circulating thymic factor: a peptide isolated from pig serum. II: Amino acid sequence. J. Biol. Chem. 252: 8045, 1977.

118. Dardenne, M., Pleau, J.M., Mann, N.K., and Bach, J.R. Structural study of circulating thymic factor: a peptide isolated from pig serum. I: Isolation and purification. J. Biol. Chem. 252: 8040, 1977.

119. Bricas, E., Martinez, T., and Blanot, D. The serum thymic factor and its synthesis. In *Proc. 5th Internatl. Peptide Symposium.* Edited by M. Goodman and Meienhofer. J. Wiley, New York, 1977, p. 564.

120. Strachan, R.G., Paleveda, W.J., Bergstrand, S.J., Nutt, R.F., Holly, F.W., and Verber, D.F. Synthesis of a proposed thymic factor. J. Med. Chem. 22: 586, 1979.

121. Dardenne, M., Nabarra, B., and Lefrancier, P. Contribution of zinc and other metals to the biological activity of the serum thymic factor (FTS). Proc. Natl. Acad. Sci. (USA) 79: 5370, 1982.

122. Savino, W., Dardenne, M., Papiernik, M., and Bach, J.F. Thymic hormone-containing cells. J. Exp. Med. 156: 628, 1982.

123. Pleau, J.M., Dardenne, M., Blouquit, Y., and Bach, J.F. In *Radioimmuno-assay and Related Procedures in Medicine.* Internatl. Atomic Energy Agency, Vienna, 1978, pp. 2, 505.

124. Monier, J.C., Dardenne, M., Pleau, J.M., Schmidt, D., Deschaux, P., and Bach, J.F. Characterization of facteur thymique serique (FTS) in the thymus. Clin. Exp. Immunol. 42: 470, 1980.

125. Ohga, K., Incefy, G.S., Wang, C.Y., and Good, R.A. Generation of a monoclonal antibody against facteur thymique serique (FTS). Clin. Exp. Immunol. 47: 725, 1982.

126. Ohga, D., Incefy, G.S., Folk, K.F., Erickson, B.W., and Good, R.A. Radioimmunoassays for the thymic hormone serum thymic factor (FTS). J. Immunol. Methods 57: 171, 1983.

127. Lacombe, M., Perner, F., Dardenne, M., and Bach, J.F. Thymectomy in the young pig: effects on the level of circulating thymic hormone. Surgery 76: 556, 1974.

128. Wong, T.W., and Merrifield, R.B. Solid-phase synthesis of thymoxin $\alpha_1$ using tert-butyloxycarbonylaminoacyl-4-(oxymethyl)phenylacetamidomethyl-resin. Biochemistry 19: 3238, 1980.

129. Ciardelli, T.L., Incefy, G.S., and Birr, C. Activity of synthetic thymosin $\alpha_1$ C-terminal peptides in the azathioprine E-rosette inhibition assay. Biochemistry 21: 4233, 1982.

130. Twomey, J.J., and Kouttab, N.M. Selected phenotypic induction of null lymphocytes from mice with thymic and nonthymic agents. Cell. Immunol. 72: 186, 1982.

131. Bach, J.F., Bach, M.A., and Blanot, D. Thymic serum factor. Bull. Inst. Past. 76: 325, 1973.

132. Bach, J.F., Dardenne, M., and Clot, J. Evaluation of serum thymic hormone and of circulating T cells in rheumatoid arthritis and in systemic lupus erythematosus. Rheumatology 6: 242, 1975.

133. Schmitt, D., Monier, J.C., Dardenne, M., Pleau, J.M., Deschaux, P., and Bach, J.F. Cytoplasmic localization of FTS (facteur thymique sterique) in thymic epithelial cells. An immunoelectronmicroscopical study. Thymus 2: 177, 1980.

134. Jambon, G., Montagne, P., Bene, M.C., Brager, M.P., Faure, G., and Duheille, J. Immunohistologic localization of facteur thymique serique' (FTS) in human thymic epithelium. J. Immunol. 127: 2055, 1981.

135. Kato, K., Ikeyama, S., Takaoki, M., Shino, A., Takeuchi, M., and Kakinuma, A. Epithelial cell components immunoreact with anti-serum thymic factor (FTS) antibodies: possible association with intermediate-sized filaments. Cell 24: 885, 1981.

136. Dardenne, M., Pleau, J.M., Blouquit, J.Y., and Bach, J.F. Characterization of facteur thymique serique (FTS) in the thymus. II. Direct demonstration

of the presence of FTS in thymosin fraction V. Clin. Exp. Immunol. 42: 477, 1980.

137. Dardenne, M., Pleau, J.M., and Bach, J.F. Evidence of the presence in normal serum of a carrier of the serum factor (FTS). Eur. J. Immunol. 10: 83, 1980.

138. Bach, J.F. Thymulin (FTS-Zn). In *Clinics in Immunology and Allergy.* Edited by J.F. Bach. Saunders and Co., London, 1983, pp. 3, 133.

139. Burton, P., Iden, S., Mitchell, K., and White, A. Thymic hormone-like restoration by human pre-albumin of azathioprine sensitivity of spleen cells from thymectomized mice. Proc. Natl. Acad. Sci. (USA) 75: 836, 1978.

140. Dardenne, M., and Tubiana, N. Neonatal thymus grafts. II. Cellular events. Immunology 36: 215, 1979.

141. Savino, W., Dardenne, M., and Bach, J.F. Thymic hormone containing cell. III. Evidence for a feed-back regulation of the secretion of the serum thymic factor (FTS) by thymic epithelial cells. Clin. Exp. Immunol. 52: 7, 1983.

142. Falchetti, R., Bergesi, G., Eishkof, A., Cafiero, G., Adorini, L., and Caprino, L. Pharmacological and biological properties of a calf thymus extract (TP-1). Drugs Exp. Clin. Res. 3: 39, 1977.

143. Skotnicki, A.B. Biologizcha okthwhosc i wlasciwosci fizykochmiczne wyciagu grascienzego TFX. Polski Tygodnik Lekarski 28: 1119, 1978.

144. Comsa, J. Thymus substitution and HTH, the homeostatic thymus hormone. In *Thymic Hormones.* Edited by T.D. Luckey. University Park Press, Baltimore, Maryland, 1973, p. 39.

145. Luckey, T.D., Robey, W.G., and Campbell, B.J. LSH, a lymphocyte-stimulating hormone. In *Thymic Hormones.* Edited by T.D. Luckey. University Park Press, Baltimore, Maryland, 1973, p. 167.

146. Mizutani, A. In *Thymic Hormones.* Edited by T.D. Luckey. University Park Press, Baltimore, Maryland, 1973, p. 193.

147. Milcu, S.M., and Potop, I. Biologic activity of thymic protein extracts. In *Thymic Hormones.* Edited by T.D. Luckey. University Park Press, Baltimore, Maryland, 1973, p. 97.

148. Potop, I., and Milcu, S.M. In *Thymic Hormones.* Edited by T.D. Luckey. University Park Press, Baltimore, Maryland, 1973, p. 205.

149. Astaldi, A., Astaldi, G.C.B., Schellekens, P. Th. A., and Eijsvoogel, U.P. Thymic factor in human sera demonstrable by a cyclic AMP assay. Nature 260: 713, 1976.

150. Astaldi, G.C.B., Astaldi, A., and Wijermans, P. A thymus-dependent serum factor induces maturation of thymocytes as evaluated by a graft-versus-host reaction. Cell. Immunol. 49: 202, 1980.

151. Zatz, M.M., Low, T.L.K., and Goldstein, A.L. Role of Thymosin and other thymic hormones in T-cell differentiation. In *Biological Responses in Cancer.* Edited by E. Mihicn. Plenum Press, New York, 1982, Vol. 1, p. 219.

152. Ahmed, A., Wong, D.M., Thurman, G.B., Low, T.L.K., Goldstein, A.L., Sharkis, S.J., and Goldschneider, I. T Lymphocyte maturation: cell surface markers and immune function induced by T lymphocyte cell-free

product and by thymosin polypeptides. Ann. NY Acad. Sci. 332: 81, 1979.

153. Pazmino, N.H., Ihle, J.N., and Goldstein, A.L. Induction in vivo and in vitro of terminal deoxinucleotidyl transferase by thymosin in bone marrow cells from athymic mice. J. Exp. Med. 147: 708, 1978.

154. Schulof, R.S., and Goldstein, A.L. Clinical applications of thymosin and other thymic hormones. In *Recent Advances in Clinical Immunology*. Edited by R.A. Thompson and N.R. Rose. Churchill Livingstone, New York, 1983, p. 243.

155. Mathieson, B.J. A re-viewing of thymocyte differentiation. In *Leukocyte Typing Human Leukocyte Differentiation Antigens Detected by Monoclonal Antibodies*. Edited by A. Bernard, L. Boumsell, J. Dausset, C. Milstein, and S.F. Schlossman. Springer Verlag, Berlin, 1984, p. 645.

156. Mathieson, B.J., and Fowlkes, B.J. Cell surface antigen expression on thymocytes: Differentiation of intrathymic subsets. Immunol. Rev. 82: 141, 1985.

157. Schulof, R.S. Thymic peptide hormones: Basic properties and clinical applications in cancer. In *CRC Critical Reviews in Oncology/Hematology*. Edited by S. Davis. CRC Press, Boca Raton, 1985, Vol. 3, p. 309.

158. Levai, J.S., and Utermohlen, V. The effect of a human plasma thymic factor on human peripheral blood mononuclear cells subpopulations. Clin. Immunol. Immunopathol. 27: 433, 1983.

159. Goldstein, A.L., Low, T.L.K., Thurman, G.B., Zatz, M.M., Hall, N.R., McClure, J.E., Hu, S., and Schulof, R.S. Thymosin and other hormone-like factors of the thymus gland. In *Immunological Approaches to Cancer Therapeutics*. Edited by E. Mihick. J. Wiley and Sons, New York, 1982, p. 137.

160. Kruisbeck, A.M. Summary of the results of the workshop. In *The Biological Activity of the Thymic Hormones*. Edited by D.W. Van Bekkum. Kooker Scientific Publications, Rotterdam, 1975, p. 209.

161. Zatz, M.M., and Goldstein, A.L. Mechanisms of action of Thymosin: I. Thymosin Fraction 5 increases lymphokine production by mature murine T cells responding in a mixed lymphocyte reaction. J. Immunol. 134: 1032, 1985.

162. Taldmadge, J.E., Uithoven, K.A., Lenz, B.F., and Chirigos, M.A. Immunomodulation and therapeutic characterization of thymosin fraction 5. Cancer Immunol. Immunother. 18: 185, 1984.

163. Cohen, G.H., Hooper, J.A., and Goldstein, A.L. Thymosin-induced differentiation of murine thymocytes in allogeneic mixed lymphocyte cultures. Ann. NY Acad. Sci. 249: 145, 1975.

164. Shoham, J., and Eshel, I. Thymic hormonal activity on human peripheral blood lymphocytes, in vitro. IV. Proliferative response to allogeneic tumor cells in healthy adults and cancer patients. Int. J. Immunopharmac. 5: 515, 1983.

165. Schafer, L.A., Goldstein, A.L., Gutterman, J.U., and Hersh, E.M. In vitro and in vivo studies with thymosin in cancer patients. Ann. NY Acad. Sci. 277: 609, 1976.

166. Wara, D.W., Barrett, D.J., Ammann, A.J., and Cowan, M.J. In vitro and in vivo enhancement of mixed lymphocyte culture reactivity by thymosin in patients with primary immunodeficiency disease. ann. NY Acad. Sci. 332: 128, 1979.

167. Shohan, J., and Eshel, I. Thymic hormonal effects on human peripheral blood lymphocytes in vitro. III. Conditions for mixed lymphocyte-tumor culture assay. J. Immunol. Methods 37: 261, 1980.

168. Zatz, M.M., and Goldstein, A.L. Enhancement of murine thymocyte cytotoxic T cell responses by thymosin. Immunopharmacology 6: 65, 1983.

169. Shoham, J., and Cohen, M. Thymic hormonal activity on human peripheral blood lymphocytes in vitro. V. Effect on induction of lymphocytotoxicity. Int. J. Immunopharmacol. 5: 523, 1983.

170. Lau, C., and Goldstein, G. Functional effects of thymopoietin 32-36 (TP-5) on cytotoxic lymphocyte precursor units (CLP-U). I. Enhancement of splenic CLP-U in vitro and in vivo after suboptimal antigenic stimulation. J. Immunol. 124: 1861, 1980.

171. Frasca, D., Garavini, M., and Doria, G. Recovery of T-cell functions in aged mice injected with synthetic thymosin alpha 1. Cell. Immunol. 72: 384, 1982.

172. D'Agostaro, G., Frasca, D., Garavini, M., and Doria, G. Immunorestoration of old mice by injection of thymus extract: enhancement of T-cell cooperation in the *in vitro* antibody response. Cell Immunol. 53: 207, 1980.

173. Weksler, M.E., Innes, J.B., and Goldstein, G. Immunological studies of aging. IV. The contribution of thymic involution to the immune deficiencies of aging mice and reversal with thymopoietin 32-36. J. Exp. Med. 148: 996, 1978.

174. Blankwater, M.J., Levert, L.A., Swart, A.C.W., and van Bekkum, D.W. Effect of various thymic and non-thymic factors on in vitro antibody formation by spleen cells from nude mice. Cell. Immunol. 35: 242, 1978.

175. Ma, D.D.F., Ho, A.H., and Hoffbrand, A.V. Effect of thymosin on glucocorticoid receptor activity and glucocorticoid sensitivity of human thymocytes. Clin. Exp. Immunol. 55: 273, 1984.

176. Marshall, G.D., Thurman, G.B., Rossio, J.L., and Goldstein, A.L. In vivo generation of suppressor T cells by thymosin in congenitally athymic nude mice. J. Immunol. 126: 741, 1981.

177. Marshall, G.D., Thurman, G.B., and Goldstein, A.L. Regulation of in vitro generation of cell-mediated cytotoxicity. I. In vitro induction of suppressor T lymphocytes by thymosin. J. Reticuloendothel. Soc. 28: 141, 1980.

178. Oppenheim, J.J., and Cohen, S. *Interleukins, Lymphokines and Cytokines*. Academic Press, San Francisco, 1983.

179. Thurman, G.B., Seals, C., Low, T.L.K., and Goldstein, A.L. Restorative effects of thymosin polypeptides on purified protein derivative-dependent migration inhibition factor production by the peripheral blood lymphocytes of adult thymectomized guinea pigs. J. Biol. Resp. Mod. 3: 160, 1984.

180. Shoham, J., Eshel, I., Aboud, M., and Salzberg, S. Thymic hormonal activity on human peripheral blood lymphocytes in vitro. II. Enhancement of

the production of immune interferon by activated T cells. J. Immunol. 125: 54, 1980.

181. Zatz, M.M., Oliver, J., Samuels, C., Skotnicki, A.B., Sztein, M.B., and Goldstein, A.L. Thymosin increases production of T-cell growth factor by normal peripheral blood lymphocytes. Proc. Natl. Acad. Sci. (USA) 81: 2882, 1984.

182. Umiel, T., Pecht, M., and Trainin, N. THF, a thymic hormone, promotes interleukin-2 production in intact and thymus-deprived mice. J. Biol. Resp. Mod. 3: 423, 1984.

183. Zatz, M.M., Oliver, J., Sztein, M.B., Skotnicki, A.B., and Goldstein, A.L. Comparison of the effects of thymosin and other thymic factors on modulation of interleukin-2 production. J. Biol. Resp. Mod. 4: 365, 1985.

184. Smith, K.A. Interleukin 2. Ann. Rev. Immunol. 2: 319, 1984.

185. Ceredig, R., Lowenthal, J.W., Nabholtz, M., and MacDonald, R. Expression of interleukin 2 receptors as a differentiation marker on intrathymic stem cells. Nature 314: 98, 1985.

186. Raulet. Expression and function of interleukin 2 receptors on immature thymocytes. Nature 314: 101, 1985.

187. Sztein, M.B., Serrate, S.A., and Goldstein, A.L. Modulation of interleukin 2 receptor expression in human lymphocytes by thymic hormones. Proc. Natl. Acad. Sci. (USA) 1986 (in press).

188. Flexman, J.P., Holt, P.G., Mayrhofer, G., Latham, B.I., and Shellam, G.R. The role of the thymus in the maintenance of natural killer cells in vivo. Cell. Immunol. 90: 366, 1985.

189. Bistoni, F., Baccarini, M., Puccetti, P., Marconi, P., and Garaci, E. Enhancement of natural killer cell activity in mice by treatment with a thymic factor. Cancer Immunol. Immunotherap. 17: 51, 1984.

190. Fiorilli, M., Sirianni, M.C., Sorrentino, V., Testi, R., Aiuti, F. In vitro enhancement of bone marrow natural killer cells after incubation with thymopoietin 32-36 (TP-5). Thymus 5: 375, 1983.

191. Dokhelar, M.C., Tursz, T., Dardenne, M., and Bach, J.F. Effect of a synthetic thymic factor (Facteur Thymique Serique) on natural killer cell activity in humans. Int. J. Immunopharmacol. 5: 277, 1983.

192. Rebar, R.W., Miyake, A., Low, T.L.K., and Goldstein, A.L. Thymosin stimulates secretion of luteinizing hormone-releasing factor. Science 214: 669, 1981.

193. Healy, D.L., Hodgen, G.D., Shulte, H.M., Chrousos, G.P., Loriaux, D.L., Hall, N.R., and Goldstein, A.L. The thymus-adrenal connection: Thymosin has corticotropin-releasing activity in primates.Science 222: 1353, 1983.

194. Luster, M.I., Boorman, G.A., Korach, K.S., Dieter, M.P., and Hong, L. Mechanisms of estrogen-induced myelocytotoxicity: Evidence of thymic regulation. Int. J. Immunopharmacol. 6: 287, 1984.

195. Allen, L.S., McClure, J.E., Goldstein, A.L., Barkley, M.S., and Michael, S.D. Estrogen and thymic hormone interactions in the female mouse. J. Reprod. Immunol. 6: 25, 1984.

196. Hall, N.R., McGillis, J.P., Spangelo, B.L., Goldstein, A.L. Evidence that thymosin and other biological response modifiers can function as neuroactive immunotransmitters. J. Immunol. 135: 806s, 1985.

197. De Weck, A.L., Kristensen, F., Joncourt, F., Bettens, F., Walker, C., Wang, Y. Lymphocyte proliferation, lymphokine production, and lymphocyte receptors in aging and various clinical conditions. Springer Semin. Immunopathol. 7: 273, 1984.

198. Goldstein, A.L., Low, T.L.K., Hall, N., Naylor, P.H., Zatz, M.M. Thymosin: Can it retard aging by boosting immune capacity? In *Intervention in the Aging Process, Part A: Quantitation, Epidemiology, and Clinical Research.* Edited by W. Regelson and F.M. Sinex. Alan R. Liss, Inc., New York, 1984, p. 169.

199. Makinodan, T., Jill James, S., Inamizu, T., and Chang, M.P. Immunological basis for susceptibility to infection in the aged. Gerontology 30: 279, 1984.

200. Wade, A.W., Szewczuk, M.R. Aging, idiotype repertoire shifts, and compartmentalization of the mucosal-associated lymphoid system. Adv. Immunol. 36: 143, 1981.

201. Hirokawa, K., Utsuyama, M. The effect of sequential multiple grafting of syngeneic newborn thymus on the immune functions and life expectancy of aging mice. Mech Aging Dev. 28: 111, 1984.

202. Schuurman, H.J., Van De Winjngaert, F.P., Delvoye, L., Broekhuizen, R., McClure, J.E., Goldstein, A.L., and Kater, L. Heterogeneity and age dependency of human thymus reticulo-epithelium in production of thymosin components. Thymus 7: 13, 1985.

203. Savino, W., Dardenne, M., and Bach, J.F. Thymic hormone containing cells III. evidence for a feed-back regulation of the secretion of the serum thymic factor (FTS) by thymic epithelial cells. Clin. Exp. Immunol. 52: 7, 1983.

204. Hirokawa, K., McClure, J.E., and Goldstein, A.L. Age-related changes in localization of thymosin in the human thymus. Thymus 4: 19, 1982.

205. Savino, W., Dardenne, M., and Bach, J.F. Thymic hormones containing cells. II. Evolution of cells containing the serum thymic factor (FTS or thymulin) in normal and autoimmune mice, as revealed by anti-FTS monoclonal antibodies. Relationship with $\alpha_1$ bearing cells. Clin. Exp. Immunol. 52: 1, 1983.

206. Cowan, M.J., Fujiwara, P., Wara, D.W., and Amman, A.J. Effect of thymosin on cellular immunity in old age. Mech. Aging Dev. 15: 29, 1981.

207. Ghanta, V.K., Noble, P.J., Brown, M.E., Cox, P.J., Hiramoto, N.S., and Hiramoto, R.N. Alloreactivity. I. Effects of age and thymic hormone treatment on cell-mediated immunity in C57B1/6NNia mice. Mech. Aging Dev. 22: 309, 1983.

208. Grimblat, S., Schauenstein, K., Saltz, E., and Trainin, N. Regulatory effects of thymic humoral factor on T-cell growth factor in aging mice. Mech. Aging Dev. 22: 209, 1983.

209. Sato, K., Chang, M.P., and Makinodan, T. Influence of age on the ability of thymic adherent cells to produce factors in vitro which modulate immune responses of thymocytes. Cell Immunol. 87: 473, 1984.

210. Frasca, D., Adorini, L., and Doria, G. Production of and response to inter-leukin-2 in aging mice. Modulation by thymosin $\alpha_1$. Symposium on Lymphokines. Edited by A. De Weck. Interlaken, 1984.

211. Doria, G., Adorini, L., and Frasca, D. Recovery of T cell functions in aged mice by injection of immunoregulatory molecules. Symposium on Lymphokines. Edited by A. De Weck. Interlaken June 14-15, 1984.

212. Ershler, W.B., Moore, A.L., and Socinski, M.A. Influenza and aging: Age-related changes and effects of thymosin on the antibody response to influenza vaccine. J. Clin. Immunol. 4: 445, 1984.

213. Ershler, W.B., Moore, A.L., Hacker, M.P., Ninomiya, J., Naylor, P., and Goldstein, A.L. Specific antibody synthesis in vitro. II. Age-associated thymosin enhancement of antitetanus antibody synthesis. Immunopharmacology 8: 69, 1984.

214. Ershler, W.B., Hebert, J.C., Blow, A.J., Granter, S.R., and Lynch, J. Effect of thymosin alpha one on specific antibody response and susceptibility to infection in young and aged mice. Int. J. Immunopharm. 7: 465, 1985.

215. Pandolfi, F., Quinti, I., Montella, F., Voci, M.C., Schipani, A., Urasia, G., and Aiuti, F. T-dependent immunity in aged humans. II. Clinical and immunological evaluation after three months of administering a thymic extract. Thymus 5: 235, 1983.

216. Collins, F.M., and Morrison, N.E. Restoration of T-cell responsiveness by thymosin: Expression of anti-tuberculous immunity in mouse lungs. Infec. Immun. 23: 330, 1979.

217. Huang, K., Kind, P.D., Jagoda, E.M., and Goldstein, A.L. Thymosin treatment modulates production of interferon. J. Interferon Res. 1: 411, 1981.

218. Salvin, S.B., and Neta, R. Resistance and susceptibility to infection in imbred murine strains. I. Variations in the response to thymic hormones in mice infected with *Candida albicans*. Cell Immunol. 75: 160, 1983.

219. Neta, R., and Salvin, S.B. Resistance and susceptibility to infections in imbred murine strains. II. Variations in the effect of treatment with thymosin fraction 5 on the release of lymphokines in vivo. Cell Immunol. 75: 173, 1983.

220. Salvin, S.B., and Tanner, E.P. Resistance and susceptibility to infections in imbred murine strains. III. Effect of thymosin on cellular immune responses of alloxan diabetic mice. Clin. Exp. Immunol. 54: 133, 1983.

221. Ishitsuka, A., Umeda, Y., Nakamura, J., and Yagi, Y. Protective activity of thymosin against opportunistic infections in animal models. Cancer Immunol. Immunother. 14: 145, 1983.

222. Stinnett, J.D., Loose, L.D., Miskell, P., Tenney, C.L., Gonce, S.J., and Alexander, J.W. Synthetic immunomodulators for prevention of fatal infections in a burned guinea pig model. Ann. Surg. 198: 53, 1983.

223. Schulof, R.S., and Goldstein, A.L. Clinical applications of thymosin and other thymic hormones. In *Recent Advances in Clinical Immunology*. Edited by R.A. Thompson and N.R. Rose. Churchill Livingstone, New York, 1983, p. 243.

224. Trainin, N., Handzel, Z.T., Pecht, M., Netzer, L., Elmalek, M., and Zaizov, R. The role of THF, a thymic hormone, as a regulator of T-cell differentiation in humans. In *Current Concepts in Human Immunology and Cancer*

*Immunomodulation*, volume 17. Edited by B. Serrou, C. Rosenfeld, J.C. Daniels, and J.P. Saunders. Elsevier Biomedical, New York, 1982, p. 85.

225. Businco, L., and Rezza, E. Therapy of viral disease in immunosuppressed patients with TP-1. In *Thymic Hormones and T-lymphocytes*. Edited by A.F. Wigzel. Academic Press, New York, 1981, p. 295.

226. Aiuti, F., Sirianni, M.C., Fiorilli, M., Paganelli, R., Stella, A., and Turbessi, G. A placebo-controlled trial of thymic hormone treatment of recurrent herpes simplex labialis infection in immunodeficient host: Results after a 1-year follow-up. Clin. Immunol. Immunopathol. 30: 11, 1984.

227. De Martino, M., Rossi, M.E., Muccioli, A.T., and Vierucci, A. T lymphocytes in children with respiratory infections: Effect of the use of thymostimulin on the alterations of T-cell subsets. Int. J. Tiss. Reac. VI: 223, 1984.

228. Wara, D.W., Cowan, M.J., and Ammann, A.J. Thymosin fraction 5 therapy in patients with primary immunodeficiency disorders. In *Thymic Factor Therapy*. Edited by N.A. Byrom and J.R. Hobbs. Serono Symposia Publications, Raven Press, New York, 1984, vol. 16, p. 123.

229. Aiuti, F., and Businco, L. Effects of thymic hormones on immunodeficiency. In *Clinics in Immunology and Allergy*. Edited by J.F. Bach. Saunders Co., Philadelphia, 1983, vol. 3, p. 187.

230. Bach, J.F., and Dardenne, M. Clinical aspects of thymulin (FTS). In *Thymic Hormones and Lymphokines*. Edited by A.L. Goldstein. Plenum Press, New York, 1984, p. 593.

231. Davies, E.G., and Levinsky, R.J. Experience in the use of thymic hormones for immunodeficiency disorders. In *Thymic Factor Therapy*. Edited by N.A. Byrom and J.R. Hobbs. Serono Symposium Publications, Raven Press, New York, 1984, vol. 16, p. 156.

232. Skotnicki, A.B., Dabrowska-Bernstein, B.K., Dabrowski, M.P., Gorsky, A.J., Czarnecki, J., and Aleksandrowicz, J. biological properties and clinical use of calf thymus extract TFX-Polfa. In *Thymic Hormones and Lymphokines*. Edited by A.L. Goldstein. Plenum Press, New York, 1984, p. 545.

233. Handzel, Z.T., Dolfin, Z., Levin, S., Altman, Y., Hahn, T., Trainin, N., and Gadot, N. Effect of thymic humoral factor on cellular immune functions of normal children and of pediatric patients with ataxia-telangiectasia and Down's syndrome. Pediatr. Res. 13: 803, 1979.

234. Abiko, T., and Sekino, H. Deacetyl-thymosin $\beta_4$: Synthesis and effect on the impaired peripheral T-cell subsets in patients with chronic renal failure. Chem. Pharm. Bull. 32: 4497, 1984.

235. Fauci, A.S., Macher, A.B., Longo, D.L., Lane, H.F., Rook, A.H., Masur, H., and Gelmann, E.P. Acquired immunodeficiency syndrome: Epidemiologic, clinical, immunologic and therapeutic considerations. Ann. Intern. Med. 100: 92, 1984.

236. Dwayer, J.M., McNamara, J.G., Sigal, L.H., and Wood, C.C. Immunological abnormalities in patients with the acquired immune deficiency syndrome (AIDS)-A Review. Clin. Immunol. Rev. 3: 25, 1984.

237. Goldstein, A.L., Naylor, P.H., Schulof, R.S., Simon, G.L., Sztein, M.B., Kessler, C.M., Robert-Guroff, M., and Gallo, M.C. Thymosin in the staging

and treatment of HTLV-III positive homosexuals and hemophiliacs with AIDS-related immune dysfunction. In *Proceedings on AIDS-Associated Syndromes.* Edited by S. Gupta. Plenum Press, New York, 1985, p. 129.

238. Naylor, P.H., Schulof, R.S., Sztein, M.B., Spira, T.J., McCurdy, P.R., Darr, F., Kessler, C.M., Simon, G., and Goldstein, A.L. Thymosin in the early diagnosis and treatment of high risk homosexuals and hemophiliacs with AIDS-like immune dysfunction. Ann. NY Acad. Sci. 437: 88, 1984.

239. Schulof, R.S., Simon, G.L., Sztein, M.B., Parenti, D.M., DiGioia, R.A., Courtless, J.W., Orenstein, J.M., Kessler, C.M., Kind, P.D., Schlesselman, S., Paxton, H.M., Robert-Guroff, M., Naylor, P.H., and Goldstein, A.L. Phase I/II trial of thymosin fraction 5 and thymosin alpha one in HTLV-III seropositive subjects. J. Biol. Resp. Mod. 1986 (in press).

240. Gershwin, M.E., Ahmed, A., Steinmberg, A.D., Thurman, G.B., and Goldstein, A.L. Correction of T cell function by thymosin in New Zealand mice. J. Immunol. 113: 1068, 1974.

241. Talal, N., Dauphinee, M., Pillarisetty, R., and Goldblum, R. Effects of thymosin on thymocyte proliferation and autoimmunity in NZB mice. Ann. NY Acad. Sci. 249: 438, 1975.

242. Gershwin, M.E., Steinberg, A.D., Ahmed, A., and Derkay, C. Studies of thymic factors. II. Failure of thymosin to alter the natural history of NZB and NZB/NZW mice. Arth. Rheum. 19: 862, 1976.

243. Bardos, P., Lebranchu, Y., and Bach, M.A. Thymic function in NZB mice. V. Decreased NK activity in NZB mice treated with circulating thymic factor. Clin. Immunol. Immunopathol. 23: 570, 1982.

244. Tomazik, V., Suter, C.M., and Chretien, P.B. Experimental autoimmune thyroiditis: modulation of the disease lel in high and low responder mice by thymosin. Clin. Exp. Immunol. 58: 83, 1984.

245. Woycienchowska, J., Goldstein, A.L., and Driscoll, B. Experimental allergic encephalomyelitis in guinea pigs. Influence of thymosin fraction V on the disease. J. Neuroimmunol. 7: 215, 1985.

246. Horowitz, S.D., Borcherding, W., Vishnu Moorthy, A., Chesney, R., Schulte-Wissermann, H., and Hong, R. Induction of suppressor T cells in systemic lupus erythematosus by thymosin and cultured thymic epithelium. Science 197: 999, 1977.

247. Zatz, M.M., Oliver, J., Goldstein, A.L., Novak, C., and Jacobs, R.P. Suppressor cell responses in patients with rheumatoid arthritis: The effect of thymosin. Thymus 6: 205, 1984.

248. Mutchnick, M.G., Schaffner, J.A., Prieto, J.A., Weller, F.E., and Goldstein, A.L. Increased thymic hormone responsive suppressor T lymphocyte function in chronic active hepatitis. Dig. Dis. Sci. 4: 328, 1983.

249. Horowitz, S.D., Borchending, W., and Hong, R. Autoimmune hemolytic anemia as a manifestation of T-suppressor-cell deficiency. Clin. Immunol. Immunopathol. 33: 313, 1984.

250. Palacios, R., Alarcon-Segovia, D., Llorente, L., Ruiz-Arguelles, A., and Diaz-Jocanen, E. Human post-thymic precursor cells in health and disease II. Their loss and dysfunction in systemic lupus erythematosus and their partial connection with serum thymic factor. J. Clin. Lab. Immunol. 5: 71, 1981.

251. Sugawara, I., and Palacios, R. Interleukin-2 and serum thymic factor enable autologous rosette-forming T lymphocytes to generate helper and cytotoxic functions. Scand. J. Immunol. 15: 233, 1982.

252. Veys, E.M., Mielants, H., Verbruggen, G., Spiro, T., Newdeck, E., Power, D., and Goldstein, G. Thymopoietin pentapeptide (thymopentin, TP5) in the treatment of rheumatoid arthritis. A compilation of several short- and long-term clinical studies. J. Rheumatol. 11: 462, 1984.

253. Giustolisi, R., Guglielmo, P., Caciola, E., and Cacciola, R.R. Thymostimulin in aplastic anemia. Acta Haematol. 69: 417, 1983.

254. Zatz, M.M., Low, T.L.K., and Goldstein, A.L. Role of thymosin and other thymic hormones in T-cell differentiation. In *Biological Responses in Cancer*. Edited by E. Mihicn. Plenum Publishing, New York, 1982, vol. 1, p. 219.

255. Chirigos, M.A. In vivo and in vitro studies with thymosin. In *Control of Neoplasia by Modulation of the Immune System*. Edited by M.A. Chirigos. Raven Press, New York, 1977, p. 241.

256. Umeda, Y., Sakamoto, A., Nakamura, J., Ishitsuka, H., and Yagi, Y. Thymosin $\alpha_1$ restores NK activity and prevents tumor progression in mice immunosuppressed by cytostatics or X-rays. Cancer Immunol. Immunother. 17: 78, 1983.

257. Ohta, Y., Tezuka, E., Tamura, S., and Yagi, Y. Protection of t-fluorouracil-induced bone marrow toxicity by thymosin $\alpha_1$. Int. J. Immunopharmacol. 7: 761, 1985.

258. Takeichi, N., Koga, Y., Fujii, T., and Kobayashi, H. Restoration of T-cell function and induction of anti-tumor immune response in T-cell depressed spontaneously hypertensive rats by treatment with thymosin fraction 5. Cancer Res. 45: 487, 1985.

259. Taldmadge, J.E., Uithoven, K.A., Lenz, B.F., and Chirigos, M. Immunomodulation and therapeutic characterization of thymosin fraction 5. Cancer Immunol. Immunother. 18: 185, 1984.

260. Schafer, L.A., Gutterman, J.U., Hersh, E.M., Mavligit, G.M., Dandridge, K., Cohen, G., and Goldstein, A.L. Partial restoration by in vivo thymosin of E-rosettes and delayed-type hypersensitivity reactions in immunodeficient cancer patients. Cancer Immunol. Immunother. 1: 259, 1976.

261. Costanzi, J.J., Gagliano, R.G., Delaney, F., Harris, N., Thurman, G.B., Sakai, H., Goldstein, A.L., Loukas, D., Cohen, G.B., and Thompson, P.B. The effect of thymosin on patients with disseminated malignancies. Cancer 40: 14, 1977.

262. Costanzi, J.J., Harris, N., and Goldstein, A.L. Thymosin in patients with disseminated solid tumors: Phase I and II results. In *Immune Modulation and Control of Neoplasia by Adjuvant Therapy*. Edited by M.A. Chirigos. Raven Press, New York, 1978, p. 373.

263. Costanzi, J., Daniels, J., Thurman, G., Goldstein, A.L., and Hokanson, J. Clinical trials with thymosin. Annals NY Acad. Sci. 332: 148, 1979.

264. Dillman, R.O., Beauregard, J.C., Mendelsohn, J., Green, M.R., Howell, S.B., and Royston, I. Phase I trials of thymosin fraction 5 and thymosin $\alpha_1$. J. Biol. Resp. Mod. 1: 35, 1982.

265. Dillman, R.O., Beauregard, J.C., Zavanelli, M.I., Halliburton, B.L., Worms-
     ley, S., and Royston, I. *In vivo* immune restoration in advanced cancer pa-
     tients after administration of thymosin fraction 5 or thymosin $\alpha_1$. J. Biol.
     Resp. Mod. 2: 139, 1983.
266. Wara, W.M., Neely, M.H., Flippin, L.J., and Wara, D.W. Phase I trial using
     thymosin fraction V in renal cancer—NCOG report. In *Thymic Hormones
     and Lymphokines*. Edited by A.L. Goldstein. Plenum Press, New York,
     1984, p. 587.
267. Fabrega, R., Pinsky, C., and Braun, D. Phase I trial of thymosin fraction 5
     in cancer patients. Proc. Am. Assoc. Cancer Res. 23: abstract 496, 126,
     1982.
268. Schulof, R.S., Lloyd, M.J., Ueno, W.M., Green, L.D., and Stallings, J.J.
     Phase II trial of thymosin fraction 5 in advanced renal cancer. J. Biol.
     Resp. Mod. 4: 147, 1985.
269. Dimitrov, N., Arnold, D., Manson, J., Singh, T., Borst, J., and Stott, P.
     Phase II study of thymosin fraction 5 in the treatment of metastatic renal
     cell carcinoma. Cancer Treat. Rep. 69: 137, 1985.
270. Martelli, M.F., Velardi, A., Rambotti, P., Cernetti, C., Bertotto, A., Spin-
     ozzi, F., Bracaglia, A.M., Falini, B., and Davis, S. The *in vivo* effect of a
     thymic factor (thymostimulin) on immunologic parameters of patients
     with untreated Hodgkin's disease. Cancer 50: 490, 1982.
271. Velardi, A., Spinozzi, F., Rambotti, P., Tabilio, A., Losito, A., Zampi, I.,
     Cernette, C., Martelli, M.F., Grignani, F., and Davis, S. The *in vivo* effect
     of thymic factor (thymostimulin) administration on circulating immune
     complexes and serum lysozyme levels in untreated Hodgkin's disease pa-
     tients. J. Clin. Oncol. 1: 117, 1983.
272. Liberati, A.M., Edwards, B.S., Brugia, M., Rambotti, P., and Grignani, F.
     *In vivo* immunorestorative properties of thymostimulin (TS) in patients
     with Hodgkin's disease. Proc. Am. Assoc. Cancer Res. 24: 194, 1983.
273. Martelli, M.F., Velardi, A., Rambotti, P., Cernetti, C., Bracaglia, A.M.,
     Ballatori, E., and Davis, S. The *in vitro* effect of calf thymus extract (thy-
     mostimulin) on the immunologic parameters of patients with untreated
     Hodgkin's disease. Cancer 49: 245, 1982.
274. Wara, W.M., Neely, M.H., Amman, A.J., and Wara, D.W. Thymosin adju-
     vant therapy. In *Advanced Head and Neck Cancer in Adjuvant Therapy of
     Cancer III*. Edited by S.D. Salmon and S.E. Jones. Grune and Stratton,
     New York, 1981, p. 169.
275. Wara, W.M., Neely, M.H., Ammann, A.J., and Wara, D.W. Biologic modifi-
     cation of immunologic parameters in head and neck cancer patients with
     thymosin fraction V. In *Lymphokines and Thymic Hormones: Their Po-
     tential Utilization In Cancer Therapeutics*. Edited by A.L. Goldstein and
     M.A. Chirigos. Raven Press, New York, 1981, p. 257.
276. Wara, W.M., Ammann, A.J., and Wara, D.W. Effect of thymosin and irra-
     diation on immune modulation in head and neck and esophageal cancer
     patients. Cancer Treat. Rep. 62: 1775, 1978.
277. Wara, W.M., Wara, D.W., Ammann, A.J., Bernard, J.L., and Phillips, T.L.
     Immunosuppression and reconstitution with thymosin after radiation ther-
     apy. Int. J. Radiat. Oncol. Biol. Phys. 5: 997, 1979.

278. Schulof, R.S., Chorba, T.L., Cleary, P.A., Palaszynski, S.R., Alabaster, O., and Goldstein, A.L. T-cell abnormalities after mediastinal irradiation for lung cancer: the *in vitro* influence of synthetic thymosin $\alpha_1$. Cancer 55: 974, 1985.

279. Schulof, R.S., Lloyd, M.J., Cleary, P.A., Palaszynski, S.R., Mai, D.A., Cox, J.W., Alabaster, O., and Goldstein, A.L. A randomized trial to evaluate the immunorestorative properties of synthetic thymosin $\alpha_1$ in patients with lung cancer. J. Biol. Resp. Mod. 4: 147, 1985.

280. Bernengo, M.G., Fra, P., Lisa, F., Meregalli, M., and Zina, G. Thymostimulin therapy in melanoma patients: correlation of immunologic effects with clinical course. Clin. Immunol. Immunopathol. 28: 311, 1983.

281. Shoham, J., Theodor, E., Brenner, H.J., Goldman, B., Lusky, A., and Chaitchick, S. Enhancement of the immune system of chemotherapy-treated cancer patients by simultaneous treatment with thymic extract, TP-1. Cancer Immunol. Immunother. 9: 173, 1980.

282. Patt, Y.Z., Hersh, E.M., Schafer, L.A., Heilbrun, L.K., Washington, M.L., Gutterman, J.U., Mavligit, G.M., and Goldstein, A.L. Clinical and immunological evaluation of the use of thymosin plus BCG ± DTIC in the adjuvant treatment of Stage 3B melanoma. In *Immune Modulation and Control of Neoplasia by Adjuvant Therapy*. Edited by M.A. Chirigos. Raven Press, New York, 1978, p. 357.

283. Patt, Y.Z., Hersh, E.M., Schafer, L.A., Smith, T.L., Burgess, M.A., Gutterman, J.U., Goldstein, A.L., and Mavligit, G.M. The need for immune evaluation prior to thymosin-containing chemoimmunotherapy for melanoma. Cancer Immunol. Immunother. 7: 131, 1979.

284. Cohen, M.H., Chretien, P.B., Ehde, D.C., Fossieck, B.E., Makuch, R., Bunn, P.A., Johnston, A.V., Shackney, S.E., Matthews, M.J., Lipson, S.D., Kenady, D.E., and Minna, J.D. Thymosin fraction V and intensive combination chemotherapy. J. Am. Med. Assoc. 241: 1813, 1979.

285. Chretien, P.B., Lipson, S.D., Makuch, R., Kenady, D.E., Cohen, M.H., and Minna, J.D. Thymosin in cancer patients: in vitro effects and correlations with clinical response to thymosin immunotherapy. Cancer Treat. Rep. 62: 1787, 1978.

286. Bedikian, A.Y., Patt, Y.Z., Murphy, W.K., Amsawasadi, T., Carr, D.T., Hersh, E.M., Bodey, G.P., and Valdivieso, M.V. Prospective evaluation of thymosin fraction V immunotherapy in patients with non-small cell lung cancer receiving vindesine, doxorubicin, and cisplatin (VAP) chemotherapy. Am. J. Clin. Oncol. 7: 399, 1984.

287. Shank, B., Scher, H., Hilaris, B., Pinsky, C., Marton, M., and Wittes, R.E. Increased survival with high-dose multifield radiotherapy and intensive chemotherapy in limited small cell carcinoma of the lung. Cancer 56: 2771, 1985.

288. Luzi, G., Tropea, F., Seminara, R., Tonachella, R.E., Palmisano, L., Abolito, M.S., LeMoli, S., Pontesilli, O., and Gallo Curcio, C. Clinical and immunological evaluation in non-resectable lung cancer patients treated with thymostimulin. In *Thymic Factor Therapy*. Edited by N.A. Byrom and J.R.

Hobbs. Serono Symposia Publications, Raven Press, New York, 1984, vol. 16, p. 309.

289. Del Glacco, G.S., Cenglarotti, L., Mantorani, G., Puxeddu, G., Di Tucci, A., Pischedda, A., and Vespa, F. Advanced lung cancer treated with combination chemotherapy with or without thymostimulin. In *Thymic Factor Therapy*. Edited by N.A. Byrom and T.R. Hobbs. Sereno Symposia Publications, Raven Press, New York, 1984, vol. 16, p. 321.

# 10

# Macrophage Migration Inhibitory Factor

Gary B. Thurman / Biotherapeutics Inc., Franklin, Tennessee

## I.  INTRODUCTION

The dictionary defines "miffed" as "offended or irritated." Certainly there is
nothing "offensive" about MIF (macrophage migration inhibitory factor), but
"irritating?"; that appears to be accurate. Those readers who have worked on
MIF research know the irritating difficulties inherent in working on a factor that
in reality may be several factors, the assays for which are difficult and tedious,
and the imitators of which may be many. This is evidenced by the substantial decline in the number of manuscripts on MIF being published over the last decade
(see Fig. 1).

Macrophage migration inhibitory factor probably was the first lymphokine
specifically described in the literature and has been the subject of many experiments, research papers, review articles, and grant proposals. It is the patriarch of
all lymphokines, and the discovery of its effects opened a new era of mediator
research. Yet, it has literally been left in the dust by relatively new factors on
the scene such as gamma interferon and interleukin-2 (IL-2), both of which have
been isolated, characterized, sequenced, cloned, mass produced in various forms
for various species, and are being tested with promising results in clinical trials
for diseases such as cancer. According to a Medline computer search of the literature, there have been 1780 papers published with MIF indicated in the title in
the last 20 years, with 1973 and 1974 being the peak years (see Fig. 1). Since
then, MIF research has been on a slow decline as evidenced by the declining
number of publications. During that same period the number of papers about
IL-2 or gamma-interferon has increased dramatically.

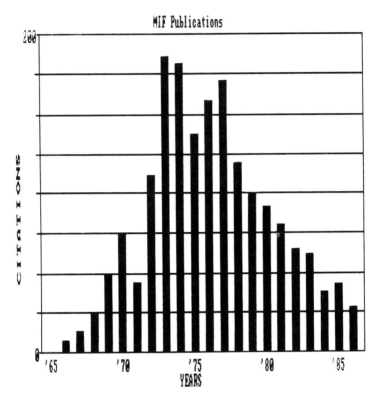

Figure 1   Results of a Medline computer search (10/86) on citations per year
that included the term MIF or migration inhibitory factor in their title. Although the search was not exhaustive, it is representative of the comparative
level of research activity on MIF over the last 20 years.

What are the "irritating" components of research on MIF that have left it
"withering in the dust" of the interferons and interleukins? They are severalfold
and will be covered in this chapter. The purpose of this chapter is not to summarize all existing information about MIF. That has been done reasonably well
on multiple occasions (1-10). The conflicting data and contrasting reports that
are still evident in the literature indicate that the status of research on MIF has
changed little in the last few years. Therefore, another extensive review about
MIF is not warranted at this time. What is warranted is a review of the concepts
and questions that motivate research on MIF so that new research initiatives can
be targeted more toward approaches that will answer important questions and
define the roles of MIF in biology and its potential roles for use in the treatment
of disease.

## II. PERTINENT QUESTIONS

1. Are there multiple MIFs?
2. What are the cellular sources of MIF?
3. What are the MIF imitators and how is their presence detected and their effect eliminated?
4. What is the best assay for measuring MIF, and what are the pitfalls and limitations of the assays used?
5. What is the biological role of MIF in immune reactivity?
6. Is there a relationship between MIF and other macrophage-active factors: e.g., macrophage activation factor, chemotactic factor, migration stimulatory factor, skin reactive factor, etc.?
7. Is MIF involved in diseases with immunological components?
8. Is there a role for MIF in the management of diseases with immunological components?

## III. PARTIAL ANSWERS

1. Multiple MIFs? If one defines macrophage migration inhibitory factor as a "lymphokine" (produced by lymphocytes, Ref. 11) that inhibits the migratory activity of monocytes/macrophages, then there have to be multiple MIFs since there are already several different lymphokines that have been reported to have MIF activity (12,13). Those working on the purification of human MIF from stimulated cell supernatants report finding multiple distinct MIF species that have MIF activity but do not have interferon (IFN) activity (12). Others have reported that human monocytes are extremely sensitive to migration inhibition by

Table 1 Comparison of Migration Inhibitory Activity of Natural and Recombinant Human Alpha IFN and Gamma IFN

| IFN | Source | Number of assays | Activity giving significant inhibition[a] Mean ± SE (range) |
|---|---|---|---|
| Alpha IFN | | | |
| Natural | Warner-Lambert Co. | 4 | 2225 ± 1057 (100-5000) |
| Recombinant | Hoffmann-La Roche | 4 | 2413 ± 1004 (200-5000) |
| Gamma IFN | | | |
| Natural | Meloy Labs., Inc. | 26 | 8 ± 2 (1-25) |
| Recombinant | Genentech, Inc. | 6 | 112 ± 51 (3-300) |

[a]Individual values obtained by plotting dose curves and determining the point (antiviral U/ml) where the curve crossed 20% migration inhibition.
*Source*: From Ref. 13.

human gamma IFN, both natural and recombinant, and, to a lesser extent, alpha
IFN (13) (see Table 1).

It was also recently reported that three of five purified natural human IL-2s
inhibited monocyte migration at 10-5000 reference units/ml and four of four recombinant IL-2s were also inhibitory to the migration of human monocytes at
50-500 reference units/ml (14). One could speculate that perhaps IFN and IL-2
caused contaminating lymphocytes within the purified monocyte population to
produce MIF, thereby inhibiting the monocytes from migrating. However, the
MIF activity of supernatants of Con A-stimulated lymphocytes was completely
eliminated by monoclonal antibody (MoAb) against gamma IFN (Table 2). Reports of partial separation of gamma IFN with no MIF activity (12,15,16) may
have been due to the use of xenogeneic target cells that are not very sensitive to
human gamma IFN, such as guinea pig peritoneal exudate cells (PEC) (Thurman,
G.B., unpublished observation). These results could also have been due to copur-
ification with gamma IFN of other factors which block the effect of gamma IFN
or augment the migration of the indicator cells, canceling out the inhibitory effect of the gamma IFN. Fractions that have MIF activity but no IFN activity may
indicate the existence of a MIF distinct from gamma IFN or may be due to loss

**Table 2**  Neutralization of Mitogen-Induced MIF Activity in Crude Supernatants
by MoAb to Human Gamma IFN

| MIF preparation[b] | MoAb anti-gamma[c] IFN | % MMI[a] | | | | |
|---|---|---|---|---|---|---|
| | | Dilution of culture supernatant | | | | |
| | | 1/2 | 1/4 | 1/8 | 1/16 | 1/32 |
| MIF-250 | − | 82.8 | 78.5 | 42.7 | 38.6 | ND[d] |
| | + | 8.5 | 0.3 | 3.7 | 0 | ND |
| MIF-268 | − | 69.3 | 55.1 | 23.6 | 14.6 | ND |
| | + | 8.8 | 18.5 | 17.8 | 0 | ND |
| MIF-343 | − | ND | 88.2 | 83.7 | 74.8 | 52.5 |
| | + | ND | 27.8 | −16.0 | 2.5 | −26.1 |

[a]Percent MMI was calculated by using the noninduced supernatants as the control. See Ref.
13 for further details.

[b]MIF preparations were made by inducing human mononuclear leukocytes to undergo blastogenesis with Con A-Sepharose. Parallel noninduced supernatants were also generated and
were used as controls.

[c]Meloy monoclonal anti-human gamma IFN antibody (clone 59) was used at a 1/1000 dilution.

[d]ND. Not done.

of the antiviral activity of the gamma IFN molecule without the loss of its MIF activity. The MIF activity of crude supernatants from stimulated lymphocytes probably represent the composite action of many factors, including factors that augment migration. This is consistent with the isolation of a number of MIFs with various molecular characteristics (8,12). Thus far, only a few of the multitude of lymphokines that have been identified have even been tested in purified form for MIF activity.

From the current data available, it is quite safe to conclude that there is a family of related factors that display MIF activity, as well as other factors that are not related that also have MIF activity. Therefore, the term MIF should be used to indicate a family of factors that inhibit monocyte/macrophage migration on plastic/glass in vitro. Herein lies some of the problem in conceptualizing MIF research. Researchers generally refer to MIF in their discussions as a single factor when in reality there are multiple factors involved. MIF has to be plural (MIFs), migration inhibitory factors, and scientists must adjust their thinking accordingly and determine ways to distinguish between the different MIFs.

2. Sources of MIF?  Since there are multiple MIFs, it is reasonable to assume that there may be multiple cellular sources. Experimental evidence supports this view. T cells (17,18), B cells (19,20), and a variety of cell lines (21,22), and hybridomas (23,24) have been shown to produce MIF. The relationship of these various MIFs remains to be determined. Does one cell type make multiple MIFs or are there multiple MIFs because there are multiple cell types making one or several MIFs? The characterization of the MIFs from each source will require extensive biochemical analysis and the production of anti-MIF MoAbs. Other questions, just as basic, remain to be answered, for example, do antigen-induced MIFs have the same composition as mitogen-induced MIFs?

One of the most intriguing aspects of MIF production by peripheral blood lymphocytes (PBL) is the report by Field and Shenton in 1973 (25) that thymectomy of guinea pigs during the development of an immune response to purified protein derivative (PPD) leads to the rapid loss of the ability of the PBL to make MIF in response to the antigen (see Fig. 2). They used a macrophage electrophoretic mobility assay (still somewhat controversial) and measured the % macrophage slowing in a electrical field. This observation has been confirmed utilizing the conventional capillary tube MIF assay (26) and the agarose droplet MIF assay (27). It has been utilized as a technique for assaying for thymosin polypeptide activity (27). Adding partially purified thymosin fraction 5 to the assay restored the ability of the PBLs to respond to PPD, as measured by macrophage migration inhibition activity. The assay was sufficiently sensitive to determine that thymosin alpha-1 was one of the polypeptide components of fraction 5 that contributed the T-cell maturational activity being measured. Further analysis using the MIF assay showed that the carboxy terminal end of that molecule contained the activity and that the C10-C14 region was necessary for the maturational activity to be displayed (Fig. 3). This indicates that even with the difficulties

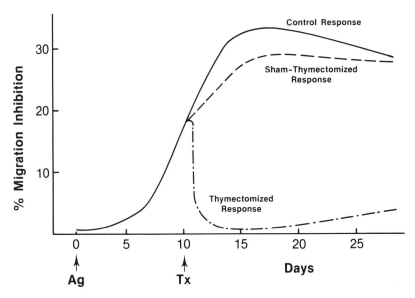

**Figure 2** Graphic presentation of the interpretation of the data of Field and Shenton (25). The peripheral blood lymphocytes of thymectomized guinea pigs rapidly lose their ability to produce MIF in response to an antigen (PPD) to which they have been sensitized.

inherent in the MIF assay, it still can be a powerful tool in unravelling some of the details of T-cell maturation and of molecular immunology.

This work indicates that the antigen-responsive circulating lymphocyte that makes MIF is a thymic-dependent cell—a T cell. Therefore, despite the observation that several non-T-cell cell lines can make MIF, it appears that the normal in vivo function of MIF is closely aligned with the function of thymic-dependent lymphocytes. This hypothesis is supported by the report that spleen cells of thymectomized chickens do not release MIF on exposure to antigen (28) and by the report that MIF-mediated macrophage disappearance reaction requires T lymphocytes (29).

3. MIF Imitators? If one is "miffed at MIF," as suggested in the Introduction, then one has to be "enraged" with endotoxin for its ability to mimic multiple cell mediators. Shands (30) stated that ". . . endotoxin is a marvelous substance for the experimentalist, . . ." and Bennett (31) illuminated the point well when he wrote, ". . . the spectrum of activities (of endotoxin) make possible at least one prediction: an investigator in almost any biological field is likely to obtain a positive result if he tries endotoxin in the experimental system he is using." MIF research is no exception. Human monocytes are exquisitely sensitive to a variety of endotoxins (unpublished data), and show significant inhibition

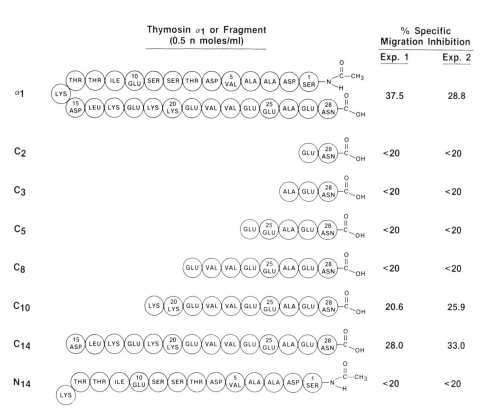

| | Thymosin $\alpha_1$ or Fragment (0.5 n moles/ml) | % Specific Migration Inhibition | |
|---|---|---|---|
| | | Exp. 1 | Exp. 2 |
| $\alpha_1$ | | 37.5 | 28.8 |
| $C_2$ | | <20 | <20 |
| $C_3$ | | <20 | <20 |
| $C_5$ | | <20 | <20 |
| $C_8$ | | <20 | <20 |
| $C_{10}$ | | 20.6 | 25.9 |
| $C_{14}$ | | 28.0 | 33.0 |
| $N_{14}$ | | <20 | <20 |

Figure 3 Use of the MIF assay to determine the restorative effects of thymosin alpha one on the peripheral blood lymphocytes of thymectomized guinea pigs (see Fig. 2). Data suggest a region of the peptide that is necessary for activity (C8-C10). Details of the assay are covered in Refs. 26 and 27.

of migration at concentrations of endotoxin that are beneath the detection level of the limulus lysate assay (32). Fortunately, most of the MIF activity of endotoxin is neutralized by polymixin B and routine inclusion of polymixin B in all solutions used in the MIF assay usually eliminates endotoxin false-positive readings in the MIF assay. Some of the research work on MIF needs repetition to eliminate the possibility that endotoxin affected the results. Other MIF imitators can be antigen-antibody complexes, cytophilic antibody, sea star protein, muramyl dipeptide, interferon inducers such as poly I:C, and mitogens, to name a few (see Ref. 33).

4. How to Assay for MIF. Most assays for MIF have been done with guinea pig mineral oil-induced peritoneal exudate cells (PEC) as indicator cells. The PEC are loaded into capillary tubes and packed into cell buttons by centrifugation.

The cell buttons are separated from the medium in the capillary tubes by breaking the glass at the cell-fluid interface. After cementing the glass capillary stub to a culture chamber and culturing for 18-24 hours, the area of migration of cells out from the tube is measured. There are many inherent disadvantages and pitfalls in this system. Most important are: (a) the variability in the animals themselves, (b) changes in their general health over time, and (c) the variability of the populations of cells found in the exudate. Even with inbred guinea pigs, heterogeneous cell populations are obtained from different individual animals and cell

Table 3  MIF Assay Comparison

|  | Capillary tube method | Agarose droplet method |
|---|---|---|
| 1. Macrophages used per determination | $2.5 \times 10^6$ | $.5 \times 10^6$ |
| 2. Culture volume per determination | 0.3 ml | 0.1 ml |
| 3. Average assay set up time per 100 determinants[a] | 3 hr | 1 hr |
| 4. Nutrient availability | Only through capillary tube orifice  Diffusion through cell pellet | Radial diffusion through agarose |
| 5. Culture time | 24 hr | 18 hr |
| 6. Migration of cells | Unidirectional until out of capillary tube | Radially out from agarose droplet |
| 7. Reading time per 100 determinants | 2 hr | 20 min[b] |
| 8. Pitfalls | Uniform loading of capillary tubes  Breaking capillary tubes exactly at cell-fluid interface  Placement of capillary tube so there is no interference with migration  Air bubbles in chamber | Agarose droplets smeared  Agarose droplets floating  Evaporation can cause problems unless environment is well humidified |

[a]After cells are available.
[b]Computer-assisted reading because of circular migration patterns.
*Sources*: Capillary tube method: Ref. 34; Agarose droplet method: Ref. 35.

yields are variable. Often cell yields are not high enough to do large assays using cells from individual animals. The considerable variability in the data necessitates the use of multiple determinations for each data point and greatly decreases the reproducibility of the assay from day to day (34).

The development of the agarose droplet method of Harrington and Stastny (35) was a major advance in MIF methodology. A comparison of the two methods is given in Table 3. There are multiple reasons why the agarose droplet technique is far superior to the capillary tube method. The paramount reasons are that five times the number of data points can be generated with the same number of cells, and that one-third the volume of test fluid is used per determinant. With restricted cell numbers and precious samples, these features can greatly assist research efforts.

It is evident that murine and guinea pig macrophages and human monocytes are good indicator cells for MIF assays. Guinea pig macrophages have been most commonly used because they are easy to obtain. Human monocytes can now be obtained in large numbers by cytapheresis and highly purified by countercurrent centrifugal elutriation (36). They can also be cryopreserved and used for MIF assays (37). Such cryopreserved cells from healthy adults are valuable indicator cells that allow repetition assays. There may be some major differences between the results obtained with different indicator cells. Since it is already evident that there are multiple factors involved in migration inhibition of macrophage/monocytes, species differences in responsivity for the indicator cells must be tested for each component of MIF.

Some of the work of the last two decades must be re-examined in light of the fact that migration enhancement factors are sometimes present in partially purified materials. These enhancement factors can mask the presence of MIF, creating spurious results and conclusions. MacSween et al. (38) called such activity MStF (migration stimulatory factor). However, there is no evidence to suggest that the migration stimulation observed was due to only one factor, and multiple factors may be involved. MStF was most frequently observed in the supernatant of stimulated lymphocytes when Con A was used as the inducing factor. MacSween et al. (38) used L-fucose to block the migration inhibitory effect of MIF, allowing the effects of MStF to be observed and measured. Negative results (without L-fucose) must be interpreted cautiously since they may indicate the absence of MIFs or the presence of both MIFs and MStF. To impart a degree of specificity to the MIF assay, MacSween et al. suggested that all negative fractions of an MIF purification scheme be tested with L-fucose since L-fucose invariably blocked the effects of MIF (38).

Migration stimulatory factors must be further explored and understood for the MIF assays to become more quantitatable and valid. It is quite conceivable that many of the reports of the absence of MIF activity in various biochemically purified fractions or from supernatants of various cell types may have been due to the presence of migration stimulatory factors copurifying with MIFs rather than the absence of MIFs.

A number of unique ideas for cellular migration assays have been reported. Brenan and Parish (39) reported the use of intracellular fluorochromes for measuring cellular migration in vitro and in vivo. McDaniel et al. (40) used a tritiated thymidine-labeled murine lymphoma cell line as target cells in an MIF assay. The level of radioactivity of the cells escaping the capillary tube was used as a measure of migration. Statistical analysis of MIF data has been extensively reviewed (41, 42). Even with these advances in technique and analysis, no assay has won unified acceptance in the scientific community and thus direct comparisons of results are limited. For rapid further progress a single assay must be agreed upon. Obviously, the vote of this author is for the universal acceptance and utilization of the agarose droplet MIF assay. A uniform indicator cell line for each species would also be important but the only likely candidate to emerge has been a murine macrophage cell line RAW 264-7 (38).

5. MIFs in Immune Response?   The physiological role of MIF in the immune response has not been fully delineated. Is MIF produced in vivo? The answer, most assuredly, is yes. The in vivo production of other lymphokines (IL-2, gamma IFN, etc.), for which suitable assays have been developed, has been shown. Salvin et al. (43) and Neta et al. (44) demonstrated MIF activity in the serum of mice undergoing a delayed hypersensitivity response to antigen. In a more recent review paper, Neta and Salvin (45) showed a distinct correlation between the in vivo production of MIF and gamma IFN. The time sequence of MIF production in vivo and the target cells, other than macrophages, it acts on are important questions that remain to be answered. Another difficult question is, "What are the roles of MIF in the involvement of macrophages in an immune response?" Sorg's work (reviewed in Ref. 8) with bone marrow macrophages undergoing maturational changes in vitro may give us a clue. He found that bone marrow macrophage precursors only express sensitivity to MIF between days 5 and 9 of culture and that as they are cultured longer they lose their MIF responsivity. If this in vitro observation can be extrapolated to the in vivo situation, one would hypothesize that monocytes are blood-borne macrophages from the bone marrow that will, upon appropriate signal, invade the site of immunoreactive tissue and undergo some maturational step. They then would become sensitive to MIF produced locally and remain localized until they become insensitive to MIF through further maturation. This is an attractive theory in that it suggests a routine ingress and egress of macrophages into and out from immunoreactive tissue while the immunoreaction is ongoing and would also help explain the marked invasion of reactive tissue by macrophages. However, in humans, blood monocytes are very migrationally active cells and their migration is readily inhibited by MIF and by human gamma IFN (13). That fact suggests that the monocytes are not only available for entry into an immunoreactive site but are probably the first cells to react with MIF in the initiation of an immune reaction. Lymphocytes would be assumed to enter the area of a cell-mediated response during normal

transit and due to a response to factors released by local cells, such as macrophages, reacting to the stimulus. Antigen-responsive lymphocytes then release MIF in response to the antigen to keep the macrophages that are in the area from leaving, allowing an accumulation of phagocytic cells. That would mean that areas of immunoreactivity would be populated mainly with immunoreactive lymphocytes and some macrophages. Macrophages would be inhibited from migrating into the area of highest reactivity for a period of time by the MIF being released by the reacting lymphocytes. the release of MIF by antigen-reacting lymphocytes may cause a lymphokine gradient effect in the reactive tissue where high levels of MIF at core of the reaction site inhibit the migration of invading macrophages into the area and very low concentrations of MIF at distant sites cause a stimulation of migrationary activity of macrophages. Enhancement of migration by very low MIF concentrations has been seen on occasion (Thurman, G.B., unpublished observation).

6. Relationship of MIFs to Other Factors? These questions cannot be answered until definitive progress has been made identifying the various component MIFs and purifying them. Monoclonal antibodies should be very helpful in sorting out the contribution of various factors with MIF activity. Neta and Salvin recently reviewed (33,45) the current knowledge in this area.

7. Are MIFs Involved in Disease? To my knowledge there has not been a description of a disease where a general inability of a patient to make MIF has been documented. Neither has there been an indication of an abnormal state where a person overproduces MIF. It is well known that some patients become immunologically anergic as their disease progresses (46) and thereby lose their ability to display normal immunoreactivity such as skin reactivity to antigen or MIF production. However, it is usually the disease which causes the inability to make MIF, not the inability to make MIF which causes the disease. MIF assays have been used in patients with chronic neutropenia to determine the patients' response to acute myeloblastic leukemia (AML) blasts (47). A positive MIF response was regarded as a warning sign of a preleukemic state to be closely followed for probable development of AML. Others have used the MIF assay for its predictive value of graft rejection in renal transplant patients (48). Production of MIF in response to Con A before and 3 days after transplantation correlated strongly with graft rejection. Production of migration stimulatory factors correlated with graft acceptance. Also, an initial vigorous MIF response to donor cell extract was associated with graft rejection. Hattler et al. (49) showed that lymphocytes obtained from a rejected kidney allograft produced MIF when put into culture.

It was shown by Ahmed et al. (50) using the MIF assay that patients with subacute sclerosing panencephalitis (SSPE) had a blocking factor in their serum and spinal fluid that prevented competent cells from interacting with the antigen and generating MIF.

It has been found that intravenous injection of MIF-containing supernatants of normal animals causes a dramatic reduction in the number of circulating monocytes (51). This observation suggests that the decrease in number of circulating monocytes that is evident after intravenous injection of antigen is caused by MIF production in vivo. Andreis et al. (52) showed that repeated injection of MIF-containing supernatants into the joints caused chronic synovitis, characterized by a mononuclear infiltrate. Stastny et al. (53) showed that rheumatoid synovial tissue with mononuclear cell infiltrates produced MIF when placed in culture.

It seems apparent that MIFs are involved in all diseases where immunological reactions with cell-mediated components are present. It would seem inevitable that there would be found in nature, aberrant conditions where an inability to produce MIF would lead to immunological anergy, or aberrant conditions where chronic production of MIF would lead to immunological paralysis or autoagressive immunological responses. Perhaps with better tools to measure MIFs and better identification of the components of MIF, such conditions will be identified. Once this is accomplished, intervention methods can be devised and implemented.

8. Clinical Role for MIF?  As mentioned above, diseases where a deficiency or overabundance of MIF production occurs represent unique possibilities for the clinical application of MIFs. However, as mediators of cellular immunity MIFs could also play an important role in clinical situations where cell-mediated immunity needs to be diminished or augmented. Bernstein et al. (54) made the intriguing observations that the growth of a syngeneic transplantable tumor in the skin of guinea pigs could be prevented by the local injection of partially purified MIF. However, the effect was only on the injected tumor nodule and did not affect distant sites with tumor involvement. Oldham (55) has reviewed the future perspectives of the clinical applications of lymphokines, and MIF may become a major biological "tool" in the "Fourth Modality of Cancer Treatment." A tremendous amount of basic research with highly purified MIFs will need to precede clinical intervention into immune responses, but the possibilities are certainly appealing.

## IV. CONCLUSION

It is the opinion of this author that the key for renewed progress with MIF research is the development and acceptance of a sensitive and reproducible assay utilizing techniques that will greatly reduce the variables in MIF research. Great strides in research on other lymphokines (interferons and IL-2 are the best examples) have followed development of assays that could be easily and consistently utilized in laboratories around the world with standards that are readily available to all. Although other opinions will undoubtedly vary, several suggestions for MIF researchers seem apparent:

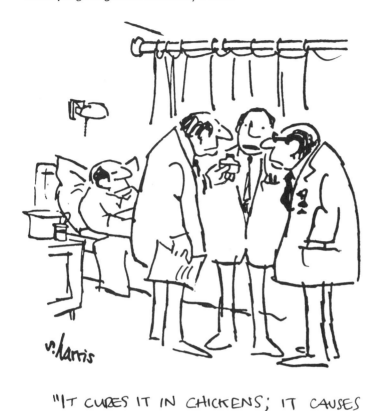

"IT CURES IT IN CHICKENS; IT CAUSES IT IN MICE."

Figure 4 © 1986 by Sidney Harris.

1. Work within one species for both MIF-producing cells and MIF-indicator cells. Species differences can be sorted out when substantial progress has been made in identifying the components of MIF, their receptors, and their modes of action (Fig. 4).
2. Standardize the indicator cells in the assay as much as possible by using highly purified cryopreserved cells or stable cell lines as indicator cells. Peritoneal exudate cells commonly contain a significant number of lymphocytes and granulocytes, both of which are migratory cells in the MIF assay. Lymphocytes greatly complicate the assay since they can be sources of in vitro-produced MIF under appropriate conditions. For example, an ongoing immunological reaction in the animals from which the PEC were obtained could greatly impact on the results of the assay using those PEC. Also, the presence of MIF

inducers in the fractions being tested could cause lymphocytes to produce MIF, giving a false positive for the presence of MIF.

3. Use a laboratory MIF standard in each assay until such time that defined MIF standards are available from the World Health Organization or the International Union of Immunological Societies.

4. Perform assays in such a manner that endotoxin cannot have a role in the effects observed. Be "endotoxin conscious" and use low-endotoxin media, serum (when used), additives, and reagents. Test all positive fractions in the presence of polymyxin B to assure effects observed are not caused by endotoxin. Macrophages/monocytes are sensitive to endotoxin (56), and in some cases, the sensitivity is even greater than that of the limulus lysate endotoxin assay (unpublished observation).

5. Determine if L-fucose blocks the activity of positive fractions containing MIF. Some MIFs are known to be blocked by L-fucose (57). This information will be important as the individual components of MIF (or the sequential MIFs released during a cell-mediated immune reaction) are identified and characterized.

6. Develop monoclonal antibodies against the MIFs when appropriate. Obviously, a rapid, reproducible assay is essential for screening the MoAbs for selection and this is not presently an easy task. Some have reported results in making MoAbs against MIF (24,58) but wide distribution and validation of the MoAbs have not been done. The degree of reactivity of various MoAbs with MIFs will provide clues into the relationship between the structures of different MIFs and may be the key to reducing the current complexity of MIF research.

7. Clone the genes for MIFs using the techniques mentioned above and molecular biology techniques so that genetic engineering can be used to mass produce adequate quantities of the MIFs to dissect their roles in the biology of the immune response.

Hopefully following these guidelines and suggestions will result in a targeted resurgence of research regarding this important family of mediators that play a central role in cell-mediated immune responses.

## ACKNOWLEDGMENTS

A great deal of thanks is due to several individuals who contributed to the completion of this review: my wife and family, who were patient with my prolonged absences while working on this manuscript; Jean Coats, whose subtle encouragement and skillful word processing helped to get this paper completed during an extremely busy period; Susan Pickeral, who was very supportive and helpful during a review of the MIF literature; and Dina Crumpacker, who helped bring my literature base up-to-date. Dr. Robert K. Oldham and Dr. William J. Hubbard were very helpful by reviewing the manuscript before publication.

## REFERENCES

1. Bloom, B.R. Adv. Immunol. 13: 101-208, 1971.
2. David, J.R., and David, R.A. Prog. Allergy 16: 300-449, 1972.
3. Remold, H.G. Clin. Immunol. Immunopathol. 4: 573-576, 1975.
5. Pick, E. In *Comprehensive Immunology*, Vol. 3. Edited by J.W. Hadden, R.G. Coffee, and F. Spreafico. Plenum Medical Book Co., New York, 1977, pp. 163-202.
5. Bergstrand, H. Allergy 34: 69-96, 1979.
6. Pick, E. In *Biology of Lymphokines.* Edited by S. Cohen, E. Pick, and J.J. Oppenheim. Academic Press, Inc., New York, 1979, pp. 60-120.
7. Rocklin, R.E., Bendtzen, K., and Greineder, D. Adv. Immunol. 29: 55-136, 1980.
8. Sorg, C. In *Lymphokines and Thymic Hormones.* Edited by A.L. Goldstein and M.A. Chirigos. Raven Press, New York, 1981, pp. 135-144.
9. Schwulera, U., Sonneborn, H.H., and Otz, U. In *Human Lymphokines.* Edited by A. Kahn and N.O. Hill. Academic Press, New York, 1982, pp. 33-38.
10. David, J.R., Remold, H.G., Liu, D.Y., Weiser, W.Y., and David, R.A. Cell. Immunol. 82: 75-81, 1983.
11. Dumonde, D.C., Woldstencroft, R.A., Panayi, G.S., Matthew, M., Morley, J., and Howson, W.T. Nature (London) 224: 38-42, 1969.
12. Weiser, W.Y., Greineder, D.K., Remold, H.G., and David, J.R. J. Immunol. 126: 1958-1962, 1981.
13. Thurman, G.B., Braude, I.A., Gray, P.W., Oldham, R.K., and Stevenson, H.C. J. Immunol. 134: 305-309, 1985.
14. Thurman, G.B., Maluish, A.E., Rossio, J.L., Schlick, E., Onozaki, K., Talmadge, J.E., Procopio, A.D.G., Ortaldo, J.R., Ruscetti, F.W., Stevenson, H.C., Cannon, G.B., Iyar, S., and Herberman, R.B. J. Biol. Resp. Mod. 5: 85-107, 1986.
15. Cohen, S., and Bigazzi, P. Lymphokines, cytokines, and interferon(s). In *Interferon*, Vol. 2, Edited by I. Gresser. Academic Press, New York, 1980, pp. 81-89.
16. Georgiades, J.A., Osborne, L.C., Moulton, R.G., and Johnson, H.M. Proc. Soc. Exp. Biol. Med. 161: 167-170, 1979.
17. Yoshida, T., Sonozaki, H., and Cohen, S. J. Exp. Med. 138: 784 797, 1973.
18. Kearns, R.J., and Campbell, P.A. Int. Arch. Allergy Appl. Immunol. 70: 59-64, 1983.
19. Bloom, B.R., Stoner, G., Gaffney, J., Shevach, E., and Green, I. Eur. J. Immunol. 5: 218-220, 1975.
20. Pick, E., Godny, Y., and Gold, E.F. Eur. J. Immunol. 5: 584-587, 1975.
21. Papermaster, B.W., Holtermann, O.A., Klein, E., Parmett, S., Dobkin, D., Laudico, R., and Djerassi, I. Clin. Immunol. Immunopathol. 5: 48-59, 1976.
22. Warrington, R.J., Rutherford, W.J., and Sauder, P.J. Cell. Immunol. 73: 159-168, 1982.
23. Kobayashi, Y., Asada, M., Higuchi, M., and Osawa, T. J. Immunol. 128: 2714-2718, 1982.

24. Weiser, W.Y., Remold, H.G., and David, J.R. Cell. Immunol. 90: 167-178, 1985.
25. Field, E.J., and Shenton, B.K. Lancet 1: 49, 1975.
26. Thurman, G.B., Rossio, J.L., and Goldstein, A.L. In *Regulatory Mechanisms of Lymphocyte Activation.* Edited by D.O. Lucas. Academic Press, New York, 1977, pp. 629-631.
27. Thurman, G.B., Low, T.L.K., Rossio, J.L., and Goldstein, A.L. In *Lymphokines and Thymic Hormones.* Edited by A.L. Goldstein and M.A. Chirigos. Raven Press, New York, 1981, pp. 145-157.
28. Morita, C., and Soekawa, M. Poult. Sci. 51: 1133-1136, 1972.
29. Sonoxaki, H., and Cohen, S. Cell. Immunol. 2: 341-352, 1971.
30. Shands, Jr., J.W. In *Microbiology.* Edited by D. Schlessinger. Am. Soc. for Microbiol., Washington, D.C., 1980, pp. 330-335.
31. Bennett, I.L. In *Bacterial Endotoxins.* Edited by M. Landy and W. Braun. Rutgers Univ. Press, New Brunswick, New Jersey, 1964, pp. 13-16.
32. Fumarola, D., and Jirillo, E. In *Biomedical Applications of the Horseshoe Crab (Limulidae).* Edited by E. Cohen. Liss, New York, 1979, pp. 379-385.
33. Neta, R., and Salvin, S.B. In *Lymphokines,* Vol. 7. Edited by E. Pick and M. Landy. Academic Press, New York, 1982, pp. 137-163.
34. Morris, J.A., Stevens, A.E., and Hebert, C.N. J. Immunol. Methods 12: 275-283, 1976.
35. Harrington, Jr., J.T., and Stastny, P. J. Immunol. 110: 752-759, 1973.
36. Stevenson, H.C., Miller, P.J., Akiyama, Y., Favilla, T., Beman, J.A., Herberman, R.B., Stull, H.B., Thurman, G.B., Maluish, A.E., and Oldham, R.K. J. Immunol. Methods 62: 353-363, 1983.
37. Thurman, G.B., Stull, H.B., Miller, P.J., Stevenson, H.C., and Oldham, R.K. J. Immunol. Methods 62: 353-363, 1983.
38. MacSween, J.M., Rajaraman, R., and Fox, R.A. J. Immunol. Methods 52: 127-136, 1982.
39. Brenan, M., and Parish, C.R. J. Immunol. Methods 74: 31-38, 1984.
40. McDaniel, M.C., Robbins, C.H., Hokanson, J.A., and Papermaster, B.W. J. Immunol. Methods 20: 225-239, 1978.
41. Bergstrand, H., and Kallen, B. Scand. J. Immunol. 2: 173-187, 1973.
42. den Hollander, F.C., van Lieshout, J.I., and Schuurs, A.H.W.M. Immunopharmacology 3: 161-178, 1981.
43. Salvin, S.B., Younger, J.S., and Lederer, W.H. Infect. Immun. 7: 68-75, 1973.
44. Neta, R., Salvin, S.B., and Sabaawi, M. Cell. Immunol. 64: 203-219, 1981.
45. Neta, R., and Salvin, S.B. Lymphokines Res. 1: 29-35, 1982.
46. Melief, C.J.M., and Schwartz, R.S. In *Cancer: A Comprehensive Treatise,* Vol. I. Edited by F.F. Becker. Plenum Press, New York, 1975, pp. 121-160.
47. Sidi, Y., Livni, E., Shaklai, M., and Pinkhas, J. Isr. J. Med. Sci. 17: 1119-1121, 1981.
48. MacSween, J.M., Cohen, A.D., Rajaraman, C.K., and Fox, R.A. Transplantation 34: 196-200, 1982.
49. Hattler, B.G., Rocklin, R., Ward, P.A., and Rickles, F.R. Cell. Immunol. 115: 914-921, 1973.

50. Ahmed, A., Strong, D.M., Sell, K.W., Thurman, G.B., Knudsen, R.C., Wistar, Jr., R., and Grace, W.R. J. Exp. Med. 139: 902-924, 1974.
51. Yoshida, T., and Cohen, S. J. Immunol. 112: 1540-1547, 1974.
52. Andreis, M., Stastny, P., and Ziff, M. Arthritis Rheum. 17: 537-551, 1974.
53. Stastny, P., Rosenthal, M., Andreis, M., and Ziff, M. Arthritis Rheum. 16: 572A, 1973.
54. Bernstein, I.D., Thor, D.E., Zbar, B., and Rapp, H.J. Science 172: 729-731, 1971.
55. Oldham, R.K. In *Cellular and Molecular Biology of Lymphokines.* Edited by C. Sorg and A. Schimple. Academic Press, New York, 1985, pp. 735-746.
56. Fox, R.A., and Rajaraman, K. Cell Immunol. 53: 333-346, 1980.
57. Remold, H.G. J. Exp. Med. 138: 1065-1076, 1973.
58. Burmeister, G., Sorg, C., and Tarcsay, L. In *Cellular and Molecular Biology of Lymphokines.* Edited by C. Sorg and A. Schimple. Academic Press, New York, 1985, pp. 315-320.

# 11

# Lymphokine Macrophage Activation Factors: Induction of Nonspecific, Macrophage-Mediated Cytotoxicity Against Tumor Cell and Microbial Targets

Monte S. Meltzer, Robert M. Crawford, David S. Finbloom, and Carol A. Nacy / Walter Reed Army Institute of Research, Washington, D.C.

## I. MACROPHAGE ACTIVATION FACTOR: A CHRONOLOGY

In 1966, David (1) and Bloom and Bennett (2) described a soluble factor released into culture fluids of specific antigen-stimulated immune lymphocytes that inhibited migration of normal peritoneal macrophages from capillary tubes: migration inhibition factor or MIF. These and other investigators postulated that this MIF might also activate macrophages for enhanced microbicidal activity. MIF was an obvious candidate for the soluble mediator of nonspecific resistance to *Listeria monocytogenes* in the model of Mackaness (3). This, in fact, was difficult to demonstrate. Assays for macrophage-mediated microbicidal activity against *L. monocytogenes* were not reproducible from lab to lab or even within a lab (4). The discovery of MIF, however, did introduce an era in which an ever increasing number of immunological activities were attributed to various nonantibody-soluble factors or lymphokines (LK) released by immune lymphoid cells (5). The term, macrophage activating factor (MAF), was first used to describe a LK activity that induced increased macrophage spreading on glass (6). At best this was an indirect measure of activated macrophage function, however, these authors felt that increased spreading by macrophages simulated changes that occurred during listeria infection. MIF was shown to induce cell spreading and also a broad range of other morphologic, functional, and biochemical changes in macrophages, including bacteriostasis perhaps but not microbicidal activity (4).

Measurement of macrophage-mediated tumor cytotoxicity induced in cells during in vivo immune reactions (allograft or tumor rejection, infection with *Mycobacterium bovis*, strain *Bacillus* Calmette Guerin, BCG) provided a quantitative and reproducible assay for study of both macrophage activation and MAF.

Tumor cytotoxicity was a welcome and useful alternative to the irreproducible microbicidal assays of that time. In 1972, Evans and Alexander and co-workers (7,8) identified a LK that apparently induced specific macrophage cytotoxicity. Macrophages from mice immune to tumor A and cultured with tumor A but not tumor B cells, released a specific macrophage arming factor or SMAF. This LK, in turn, activated normal macrophages to kill only tumor A and not tumor B target cells. SMAF functioned very much like antibody in antibody-mediated cell cytotoxicity (ADCC) and, in retrospect, probably was. It remained unclear what relation this phenomenon had to classical nonspecific macrophage activation in microbial systems. Subsequently, Churchill et al. (9), also using a tumoricidal assay for macrophage activation, demonstrated that culture fluids of antigen-stimulated lymphocytes activated macrophages to become nonspecifically cytotoxic. In these studies, the inducing antigen was completely unrelated to those of the tumor target cells and antigen was removed from "arming" LK without loss of activity. Whereas numerous laboratories subsequently repeated and expanded Churchill's studies, few investigators consistently reproduced the SMAF experiments.

As more and more LK (literally hundreds of activities) were described in crude culture fluids of antigen- or mitogen-stimulated lymphocytes, it became of obvious importance to purify and characterize the molecular entity associated with each of these activities to learn whether different biologic activities are induced by the same molecule or whether a separate molecule is responsible for each activity. Early studies failed to distinguish between MIF and MAF by molecular weight or isoelectric point. There was much overlap in both physicochemical and biologic activity (4). However, these LK continued to carry separate designations because biochemical characterization was not advanced enough to provide conclusive and direct evidence of their identity. In 1978, Ruco and Meltzer (10,11) reported physicochemical characteristics of MAF produced after purified protein derivative of tuberculin (PPD) stimulation of spleen cells from BCG-infected mice. Again, MAF for induction of macrophage tumoricidal activity and MIF activity eluted in overlapping fractions from Sephadex G-100. However, as the authors stated, the width of the MAF activity peak suggested that induction of macrophage-mediated tumor cytotoxicity may not be the effect of a single LK. Type II or gamma interferon (IFN), which then had a published relative molecular weight ($M_r$) of about 40,000 could certainly have fallen within the activity range for MAF.

During this time interval, Schultz and Chirigos reported striking functional similarities between MAF and fibroblast-derived, beta interferon (12). While MAF and beta interferon were soon shown to differ in many respects, an intense effort to determine the relationship between MAF and the various interferons followed. However, as long as purification and characterization of LK depended upon difficult assay methodology, only suggestive and often conflictive evidence about the identity of MAF was forthcoming. With the application of the various technological breakthroughs of the 1970s and 1980s, such as new molecular separation procedures or antibody, cell, and gene cloning, came rapid advances in LK research. Following reports that murine MAF and IFN, in contrast to type I interferons, share many physicochemical properties, numerous laboratories sought to prove identity between MAF and IFN (13). In 1983, Schultz and Kleinschmidt (14) published the first in a long series of reports that documented functional identity between recombinant IFN and MAF. However, as these authors pointed out, it was still not clear whether or not IFN is responsible for all the MAF activity produced by T cells. The availability of monoclonal antibody to IFN allowed selective depletion of IFN in LK with MAF activity. In most studies, this antibody treatment removed all MAF activity from conventional LK. These results led some investigators to propose IFN as the primary, if not only, MAF for induction of macrophage-mediated tumoricidal and microbicidal activities (15-19).

Scattered among reports of identity between IFN and MAF were several studies that challenged the concept of IFN as the only MAF. Many of these studies analyzed MAF from sources other than conventional LK: T-cell hybridomas, T-cell clones, or T-cell lines that produced either MAF but no IFN or MAF and IFN. In other studies, authors documented residual levels of MAF activity in culture fluids of antigen- or mitogen-stimulated T cells following treatment with anti-IFN antibodies. The first report of possible nonidentity between MAF and IFN appeared in 1981: Kniep et al. (20) used three sequential purification steps to separate MAF ($M_r$ 30,000; pI 7.4 and 8.4) from MIF and IFN in concanavalin A- (Con A) stimulated mouse spleen cell conditioned medium. Although the first, it was not the last of so-called "isolated" reports from laboratories purportedly identifying unique MAFs unrelated to IFN. In 1982, Erickson et al. (21) and Ratliff et al. (22) separately identified T-cell hybridomas and Meltzer et al. (23) a continuous T-cell line that produced MAF distinct from IFN. No further analysis has been published on the Erickson hybridoma. Ratliff's cell line subsequently proved unstable and was lost (22). Meltzer and co-workers continued their studies with the EL-4 T-cell line; these findings will be discussed in depth in subsequent sections. In 1983, Gemsa and co-workers (24) described isolation of separate T-cell clones that each secrete unique MAF for induction of different macrophage activities. Further work on MAF from these T-cell lines described synergy between two lymphokines: interferon, a priming LK and macrophage cytotoxicity inducing factor 2 (MCIF2), a trigger LK (25,26). While the priming and triggering phenomenon and numerous exogenous trigger signals, such as bacterial endotoxic lipopolysaccharides or LPS, were well established features of macrophage activation, this was the first report of actual physicochemical identification of an endogenous trigger signal. Unfortunately, the cell line source of MCIF2 was subsequently found to be infected with mycoplasma and thus these early findings now need to be re-evaluated (P.H. Krammer, personal communication).

The first evidence for a MAF distinct from IFN in humans was documented in systems that measured release of $H_2O_2$ from blood monocytes. Gately et al. described a human LK ($M_r$ 55,000; pI 5.5) that increased monocyte production of $H_2O_2$ in the absence of detectable IFN (27). Similar observations were made by Andrew and co-workers (28) who isolated T-cell clones that respond to purified *M. tuberculosis* antigen and produce LK able to activate both macrophages and macrophage-like cell lines (U937) for release of hydrogen peroxide. This activity had a $M_r$ of 25,000 and was not neutralized by monoclonal anti-IFN. Omata et al. described a MAF thought to be distinct from IFN in LK from specific antigen-stimulated spleen cells. Their conclusions were based on observations that specific antigen- but not Con A-stimulated spleen cells, produce LK that induce antitoxoplasma activity in mouse peritoneal macrophages. Although both LK had high titers of IFN, only the antigen-initiated LK induced macrophage microbicidal activity. The authors suggested that antimicrobial activity was mediated by interactions of two lymphokines: IFN and possibly granulocyte/macrophage colony-stimulating factor (GM-CSF) (29). Further reports of a human MAF unrelated to IFN were published in 1984 and directly examined macrophage-mediated tumor cytotoxicity rather than hydrogen peroxide secretion. Higuchi et al. (30) found MAF in a hybridoma prepared by somatic cell fusion of phytohemagglutinin-activated peripheral blood lymphocytes with a cloned T-cell leukemia cell line that produced no detectable IFN. Since this MAF only activated macrophages and not blood monocytes for tumor cytotoxicity, these authors reasoned that it might function as an endogenous trigger factor, similar to that described by Krammer et al. (26). Salahuddin et al. described secretion of MAF but not IFN by several human T-cell leukemia virus-I (HTLV-I)-infected T-cell lines (31). Kleinerman and colleagues (32) examined one of these HTLV-I-infected cell lines in detail: C10/MJ2-derived MAF was produced constitutively and its activity was not neutralized by monoclonal anti-IFN.

Nacy et al. (33) identified LK antigenically distinct from IFN that induced intracellular destruction of leishmania parasites within murine macrophages: several monoclonal anti-IFN failed to neutralize MAF activity in antigen- or mitogen-induced LK as well as LK from a cloned T-cell hybridoma reported earlier to contain only IFN as a MAF for induction of macrophage tumoricidal activity (34,35). Similar anti-IFN neutralization studies to separate MAF and IFN activities were also reported by Futch and Schook (36) in a macrophage-mediated amoebicidal system. Two T-cell hybridomas were constructed, one in which activity correlated with IFN and another in which it did not; monoclonal anti-IFN antibodies neutralized tumoricidal activity but not microbicidal activity in both supernatants. Rose et al. (37) demonstrated a MAF ($M_r$ 30-70,000; pI 2.2-3.3) from con A-stimulated human peripheral blood mononuclear cells that inhibited herpes simplex replication in human pulmonary macrophages, separated chromatographically and electrophoretically from IFN, and was not neutralized by monoclonal anti-IFN. Hoover et al. (38) identified factor(s) in a similar LK preparation that activated human monocytes to kill *Leishmania donovani*, an intracellular pathogen; these human MAFs ($M_r$ of 25,000 and 50,000, respectively) were physicochemically and antigenically distinct from IFN. Lee et al. (39) identified a HTLV-I-infected human T-cell line that constitutively produced MAF ($M_r$ 55,000; pI 5.5) but little or no IFN. Physicochemical and immunochemical studies confirmed that this MAF was not IFN. Finally, MAF activity was recently ascribed to another well characterized LK other than IFN: Grabstein et al. (40) demonstrated induction of macrophage activation for tumor cell killing when macrophages were incubated with recombinant GM-CSF.

By present day standards, nothing less than direct comparison of protein sequences of putative MAFs will unequivocally decide any question of their relatedness. Once IFN became established as a potent activator of macrophage cytotoxicity toward a broad range of tumor cell or microbial targets, differentiation between IFN and other MAFs became the foremost task confronting investigators studying macrophage activation signals. In the search for macrophage activation factors that may play a role in augmenting host resistance to infection or neoplasia, it is encouraging to note that the relatively sparse literature reports of MAF distinct from IFN emanate from an array of different laboratories; the disappointing aspect is the limited analysis done on any single factor. This limited analysis most certainly is due in part to the nature of macrophage activation assays which measure tumoricidal or microbicidal activity. These assays are cumbersome, time consuming, require stringent control of assay conditions, and may be affected by many seemingly uncontrollable variables.

Various criteria have been used in an effort to verify the existence of noninterferon MAF: (a) failure to demonstrate an effect of purified recombinant IFN in a MAF model system, (b) failure to demonstrate presence or effects of known exogenous activators such as LPS, (c) demonstration of disparate titers or activity patterns between IFN and MAF in LK, (d) demonstration of MAF activity in LK either when no IFN is detectable by viral or immunolgoical assay or following specific neutralization and/or removal of IFN by polyclonal or monoclonal antibody or following chromatographic separation from IFN. Most alleged noninterferon MAFs have not been characterized beyond this initial step, and have not been evaluated by *all* the above criteria. Moreover, any noninterferon MAFs that survive this initial analysis must now be subjected to the same standards for differentiation from GM-CSF (40).

## II. MACROPHAGE ACTIVATION FACTORS FROM EL-4: A LYMPHOKINE ODESSEY

A number of years ago, we screened more than 20 continuous murine T-cell lines for culture fluids that activated macrophages for tumor cytotoxicity (23). Most of these cell lines were inactive: culture fluids from unstimulated cells or cells treated with phytohemagglutinin, con A, or phorbol myristate acetate (PMA),

Table 1 Macrophage Activation Factor(s) in Culture Fluids of Continuous
Murine T-Cell Lines: MAF That Induce Macrophage-Mediated, Nonspecific
Tumor Cytotoxicity

| Cell line | | Induction of macrophage tumoricidal activity |
|---|---|---|
| BFS | (C57BL/6) | − |
| BW5147.G1.4 | (AKR/J) | − |
| P388 | (Balb/C) | − |
| R1.1 | (C58/J) | − |
| RLo-1 | (Balb/C) | − |
| WEHI 7.1 | (Balb/C) | − |
| YAC-1 | (A/SN) | − |
| EL-4$_{ATCC}$ | (C57BL/6) | − |
| EL-4$_{RALPH}$ | | − |
| EL-4$_{FARRAR}$ | | ++ |

alone or in combination, each failed to induce macrophage tumoricidal activity
(Table 1). One cell line, a variant of the C57BL/6N thymoma EL-4 (41), released
macrophage activation factor(s) in high titer. Interestingly, two other EL-4 variants (EL-4 ATCC TIB 39 and EL-4 RALPH) were inactivate. Culture fluids from
EL-4 cells treated with PMA induced significant macrophage cytotoxicity against
tumor target cells through a 1/40 dilution (Fig. 1). Active culture fluids were not
directly toxic to either tumor cells or macrophages. Macrophage activation fac-
tor(s) from EL-4 were not produced constitutively in medium or after stimulation with the T-cell mitogen, con A. Moreover, induction of macrophage tumor
cytotoxicity was not dependent upon PMA: titers of macrophage activation fac-
tor(s) in active culture fluids were unaffected by adsorption of PMA onto dex-
tran-coated charcoal.

Physicochemical characterization of the macrophage activation factor(s) in
EL-4 documented complete loss of activity after heating at 100°C for 15 min.
Most of the total activity remained stable to overnight dialysis against 0.15 M
NaCl buffered at pH 2.0 to 10.0. Similarly, the titer of activity in EL-4 culture
fluids for induction of macrophage-mediated tumor cytotoxicity remained unchanged after coincubation with 5 $\mu$g/ml polymyxin B. This antibiotic inhibits
the in vitro effects of lipopolysaccharides (LPS) on an equimolar basis (42). That
the titer of macrophage activation factor(s) in EL-4 were not reduced by polymyxin B and the total activity was abolished by heating at 100°C both suggest
little or no role for LPS under these assay conditions. To further characterize
the EL-4-derived LK, we applied active culture fluids to a preparative isoelectric

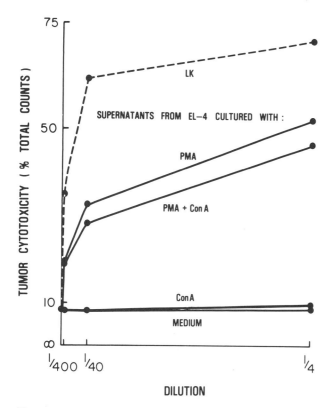

Figure 1  Induction of macrophage tumoricidal activity by supernatant fluids
from PMA- and con A-treated EL-4 cells (from Ref. 23). Adherent macrophages
from casein-treated mice were cultured in dilutions of con A-stimulated spleno-
cyte (LK) or PMA- and con A-treated EL-4 cell culture fluids with radiolabeled
tumor target cells. Cytotoxicity (% label release) was measured at 48 hr.

focusing column in pH 3.5 to 10.0 ampholines. Activity for induction of macrophage-mediated tumor cytotoxicity focused as a single but broad peak between
pH 4.1 and 5.7 (Fig. 2). The interferon activity (induction of antiviral activity in
vesicular stomatitis virus-infected L-929 cells) in this culture fluid focused between pH 5.2 and 5.6. Gel chromatography fractionation of the EL-4 culture
fluids on Sephadex G-100 or AcA-54 matrices documented two distinct areas of
activity: fractions that induced macrophage-mediated tumor cytotoxicity eluted
with apparent $M_r$ of 45,000 and 25,000 (Fig. 3). Interferon activity eluted as a single peak and cofractionated with the 45,000 $M_r$ macrophage activation factor(s).

As previously stated, culture fluids from PMA-stimulated EL-4 cells repro-
ducibly have detectable levels of interferon activity. The maximum concentration
of interferon activity released by EL-4 under a broad range of experimental con-

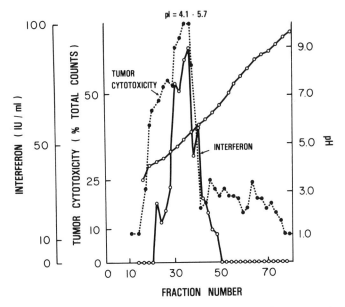

**Figure 2** Fractionation of MAF activity in PMA-stimulated EL-4 cell culture fluids by preparative isoelectric focusing (from Ref. 23). Culture fluids from PMA-stimulated EL-4 cells were applied to a preparative isoelectric focusing column in pH 3.5 to 10.0 ampholines. Eluted fractions were dialyzed against culture medium and assayed for induction of macrophage tumoricidal activity and fibroblast antiviral activity (interferon).

ditions, however, is $\leq 10$ IU/ml (43). This antiviral activity and activity for induction of macrophage-mediated tumor cytotoxicity in the 45,000 $M_r$ peak were both neutralized by 1/100 dilution of rabbit antimurine IFN antisera ($2 \times 10^4$ neutralizing units/ml). Thus, IFN is one of the macrophage activation factors produced by EL-4. Several investigators have now convincingly documented that all of the activity in conventional, spleen cell-derived lymphokines for induction of macrophage tumoricidal activity is IFN initiated and completely inhibited by anti-IFN sera (15-19). This is not the case with the EL-4 macrophage activation factors. Quantitatively, IFN represents $\leq 20\%$ of the total activity for induction of macrophage-mediated tumor cytotoxicity. Macrophage activation factor(s) that account for most of the activity from PMA-stimulated EL-4 cells elute in the 25,000 $M_r$ peak. These fractions, the 25K MAF, have no IFN detected either by antiviral activity or by ELISA (23).

But what is the 25K MAF? At first glance, it appeared likely that this macrophage activation factor was not IFN. However, this assumption was tenuous in light of recent experiments that document discrete functional domains within

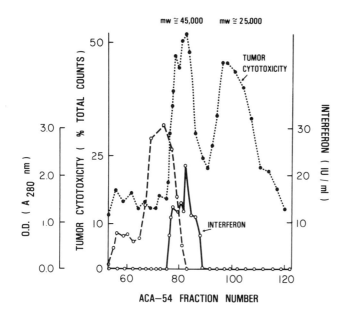

**Figure 3** Fractionation of MAF activity in PMA-stimulated EL-4 cell culture fluids by AcA 54 polyacrylamide gel chromatography (from Ref. 23). Culture fluids from PMA-stimulated EL-4 cells were concentrated 20x by ultrafiltration and applied to a calibrated AcA 54 column. Eluted fractions were assayed for induction of macrophage tumoricidal activity and fibroblast antiviral activity (interferon).

the murine IFN molecule. Molecular hybrids between murine and human IFN, derived from interchanged exons of the two genes and expressed in Cos cells, segregate the activity for induction of macrophage-mediated nonspecific tumor cytotoxicity and Ia antigen expression from that for induction of antiviral activity. This segregation is also documented through effects of monoclonal antibodies against different IFN epitopes: certain antibodies in the fluid-phase completely inhibit IFN-induced antiviral activity, yet do not affect induction of macrophage-mediated nonspecific tumoricidal activity; other antibodies inhibit both activities (44). Documentation of different functional domains within murine IFN raised the real question of whether or not the EL-4 derived 25K MAF is in fact a breakdown product or otherwise altered fragment of IFN. Indeed, a 25,000 $M_r$ factor from the 24/G1 T-cell hybridoma induces both antiviral activity and macrophage-mediated tumor cytotoxicity, both activities are completely inhibited by antiserum to recombinant murine IFN (45). We examined this question directly with a unique family of hamster monoclonal antimurine IFN antibodies and showed that the EL-4-derived MAF and IFN are antigenically unrelated (46).

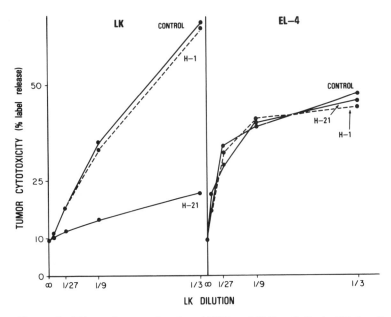

Figure 4   Effect of monoclonal anti-IFN on MAF activity in EL-4 culture fluids
(from Ref. 46). Adherent macrophages from starch-treated mice were cultured
in dilutions of conventional, spleen cell-derived LK or the 25K MAF partially
purified from culture fluids of PMA-stimulated EL-4 cells with and without H1
and H21 hamster monoclonal anti-IFN and radiolabeled tumor target cells. Cytotoxocity (% label release) was measured at 48 hr.

Hamster monoclonal antibodies H1 and H21 both inhibit IFN-induced fibroblast
antiviral activity. The H21 antibody, but *not* H1, also inhibits IFN-induction of
macrophage Ia antigen expression and nonspecific tumoricidal activity. The H1
epitope resides in or is dependent upon the aminoterminus of IFN; the H21 epitope is formed by the carboxy-terminal amino acid sequence (44). Fluid phase
H1 and H21 antibodies (0.7 $\mu$g protein/ml) were added to dilutions of spleen
cell-derived LK ($\sim$200 IU/ml IFN) or culture fluids from PMA-stimulated EL-4.
The mixtures were added to adherent macrophage cultures simultaneously with
radiolabeled tumor target cells. Cytotoxicity was estimated by radiolabel release
at 48 hr (Fig. 4). These antibody dilutions were sufficient to neutralize antiviral
activity of >20,000 IU/ml IFN for H1 and >500 IU/ml IFN for H21. Addition
of H1 anti-IFN monoclonal antibody had no effect on the LK dose-response for
induction of macrophage-mediated tumor cytotoxicity. In contrast, equal concentrations of H21 monoclonal antibody dramatically inhibited ($\geqslant$90% total
activity) LK-induced macrophage tumoricidal activity. These results confirmed
previous observations with IFN-induced nonspecific macrophage cytotoxicity

against another tumor target cell, the P815 mastocytoma. Effects of monoclonal anti-IFN on the 25K MAF from EL-4 were quite different from that of spleen cell-derived LK: neither H1 nor H21 antibodies affected the dose-response for induction of macrophage tumoricidal activity. Moreover, the ability of the 25K MAF to induce macrophage-mediated tumor cytotoxicity was also not affected by fluid-phase 1/100 dilution of polyclonal rabbit anti-IFN serum ($\sim$2 $\times$ 10$^4$ neutralizing units/ml) or a rat monoclonal anti-IFN ($\sim$4 $\times$ 10$^3$ neutralizing units/ml, kindly provided by Dr. George Spitalny) (17).

The preceding data convincingly show that a variety of monoclonal or polyclonal anti-IFN antibodies all fail to inhibit induction of macrophage-mediated tumor cytotoxicity by the 25K MAF. It was still possible, however, that any of these antibodies may have bound to the macrophage activation factor(s) and not neutralized their activity. This, in fact, is exactly what occurs with the H1 monoclonal antibody and IFN-induced macrophage tumor cytotoxicity. To examine this possibility, we constructed an H21 anti-IFN immunoaffinity chromatography column. H21 anti-IFN covalently coupled to polyacrylamide beads, removed all

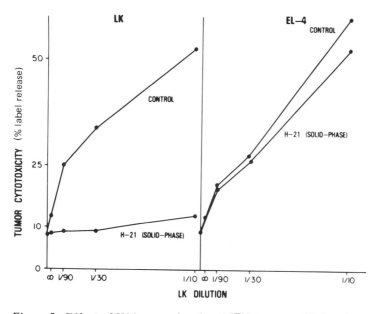

Figure 5  Effect of H21 monoclonal anti-IFN immunoaffinity chromatography on MAF activity in EL-4 culture fluids (from Ref. 46). Adherent macrophages from starch-treated mice were cultured in dilutions of conventional spleen cell-derived LK or the 25K MAF partially purified from culture fluids of PMA-stimulated EL-4 cells untreated or previously adsorbed by H21 monoclonal anti-IFN immunoaffinity chromatography and radiolabeled tumor target cells. Cytotoxocity (% label release) was measured at 48 hr.

IFN from spleen cell-derived LK by three different assays (antiviral activity, ELISA, or induction of macrophage Ia antigen expression). Equal volumes of culture fluids from PMA-stimulated EL-4 were applied to replicate columns: neither starting material nor column eluate demonstrated IFN activity. H21 antibody in solid-phase removed all activity in spleen cell-derived LK for induction of macrophage-mediated tumor cytotoxicity (Fig. 5). In striking contrast, treatment with an identical immunoaffinity column did not affect the dose-response of the 25K MAF. Equivalent results were also obtained with monoclonal H1 and H21 antibodies and rabbit polyclonal anti-IFN serum after passage through staphylococcal protein A-Sepharose beads: ability of spleen cell-derived LK to induce macrophage tumoricidal activity was completely inhibited by all antibodies and protein A-agarose; the 25K MAF in EL-4 were unaffected by these treatments (Table 2). Thus, by all of several experimental approaches, no antigenic relationship between IFN and the 25K MAF was evident.

It was clear from the preceding observations that the 25K MAF from EL-4 and IFN were both physicochemically and antigenically different. These separate macrophage activation factors, however, do share many common functional properties. In the tumor cytotoxicity assay we use, three features of conventional spleen-cell-derived LK- or IFN-activated macrophages are characteristic (47):

Table 2  MAF from Spleen Cell-Derived LK and EL-4: Effect of Anti-IFN Antibodies and Protein A-Agarose

| Antibody-protein A-agarose treatment | Macrophage tumoricidal activity induced by dilutions of: | | | |
| | Spleen cell-derived LK | | EL-4 | |
| | 1/10 | 1/50 | 1/10 | 1/50 |
|---|---|---|---|---|
| Control | 50%** | 36%** | 47%** | 31%** |
| Hamster monoclonal anti-IFN-gamma: | | | | |
| H1 | 8% | 7% | 52%** | 34%** |
| H21 | 8% | 8% | 45%** | 27%** |
| Rabbit polyclonal anti-IFN-gamma | 7% | 7% | 44%** | 30%** |

Spleen cell-derived LK or culture fluids from PMA-stimulated EL-4 were treated with hamster monoclonal (0.7 $\mu$g protein/ml) or rabbit polyclonal (1/100) anti-IFN-gamma then passed through staphylococcal protein-A Sepharose 4B chromatography columns. Column eluates concentrated back to original volumes were assayed for induction of macrophage tumoricidal activity. Cytotoxicity was estimated by measurement of tumor target radiolabel release at 48 hr in triplicate cultures and expressed as percent total counts. Tumor target cells cultured in medium alone released 8% of total counts.

**Significant toxicity.

1. The tumoricidal activity of macrophages and the capacity of macrophages to be activated for tumor cytotoxicity are both short-lived cell functions. In fact, the time course for acquisition and loss of macrophage tumoricidal activity is the single most distinctive feature of activation. Macrophage cytotoxic activity is evident within 4 hr of IFN treatment, reaches maximal levels by 6 to 12 hr, then progressively decreases to baseline by 24 hr (48,49). Loss of macrophage cytotoxic activity is not due to cell death (no change with time of vital dye uptake or in phagocytic capacity) or to depletion/destruction of IFN (rate of loss unaffected by replacement of IFN at any time through 24 hr). It should be noted that IFN-activated macrophages that lose nonspecific tumoricidal capacity with time in culture, retain capacity to kill the identical target through antibody-dependent cell cytotoxicity or through PMA-stimulated macrophage cytotoxicity. These latter cytotoxic reactions are most likely mediated through release of reactive toxic oxygen metabolites. Indeed, no difference in release of $O_2^-$ from IFN-activated macrophages was evident with cells cultured for 5, 10, or 24 hr (50). Thus, one distinctive subset of macrophage cytotoxic reactions, one apparently not mediated by toxic oxygen metabolites, is transiently induced by LK or IFN. The time courses for onset and loss of this transient, nonspecific tumoricidal activity with macrophages cultured continuously with LK or the 25K MAF were indistinguishable (Fig. 6).

2. Within the characteristic time course, LK or IFN induction of macrophage tumoricidal activity can be separated into two reaction stages: macrophages initially exposed to IFN enter into a receptive or primed state in which they are not yet cytotoxic, but can then respond to or be triggered by more IFN or any of certain other trigger signals unrelated to IFN (48). The prototypic trigger signal is the lipid A region of LPS, but several other bacterial cell wall components, heat-killed *Listeria monocytogenes*, or certain lectins also activate the IFN-primed macrophage to tumoricidal activity (51). Macrophage activation through priming and trigger reactions includes the following features: (a) Macrophage interaction with IFN as a priming stimulus to induce optimal responsiveness to trigger signals requires 4 hr continuous exposure at 37°C. This responsiveness, however, is short-lived and irreversibly decreases with time thereafter. (b) The interaction of IFN-primed macrophages with more IFN or other trigger signals requires less than 10 min exposure for maximal effects. Control macrophages treated with any of the trigger signals for this time interval do not develop cytotoxicity. (c) Treatment of macrophages with IFN and trigger signals must occur in a defined sequence. Cells treated with trigger signals before IFN priming are not cytotoxic. IFN and the 25K MAF function as both priming and trigger signals for induction of macrophage tumoricidal activity (Fig. 7). Tumor cytotoxicity induced by IFN or the 25K MAF are both increased about 5- to 10-fold across a wide range of concentrations by the simultaneous addition of small amounts (1 ng/ml) of LPS (52). IFN-primed but noncytotoxic macrophages respond to more IFN, LPS or the 25K MAF to develop potent cytotoxic activity. Similarly, macrophages primed

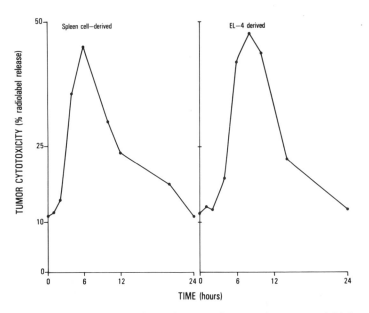

**Figure 6**  Time courses for induction of macrophage tumoricidal activity by conventional, spleen cell-derived LK and the 25K MAF (from Ref. 52). Adherent macrophages from casein-treated mice were cultured in dilutions of conventional, spleen cell-derived LK or the 25K MAF partially purified from culture fluids of PMA-stimulated EL-4 cells for different times before addition of radiolabeled tumor target cells. Cytotoxicity (% label release) was measured at 48 hr.

with the 25K MAF also respond to IFN, LPS, or more 25K MAF and develop equally strong tumoricidal activity.

3. Transient, nonspecific cytotoxic reactions by LK- or IFN-activated macrophages fails to develop with cells from certain strains of mice. Macrophages from mice with the *Lps*d gene (C3H/HeJ) for unresponsiveness to the lipid A region of LPS do not develop transient tumoricidal activity after in vivo treatment with *Mycobacterium bovis*, strain BCG or *Proprionobacterium acnes* or in vitro treatment with LK or IFN (53). Similar defects in the development of macrophage-mediated tumor cytotoxicity occurs with cells derived from mice of the A/J and P/J strain (54). The genetic basis for this macrophage defect in each of the three different mouse strains is distinct and complementary: cells from F1 progeny of any two of the three defective parental strains are fully responsive to in vivo and in vitro activation and develop significant tumoricidal activity (55). It is important to note that these genetic defects in macrophage function are quite selective: responses to phagocytic or chemotactic stimuli or production of toxic oxygen metabolites after secretagogue treatment are

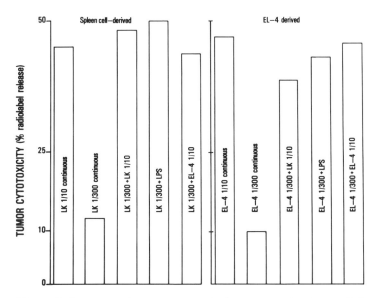

Figure 7 Priming and trigger signals by conventional, spleen cell-derived LK and the 25K MAF (from Ref. 52). Adherent macrophages from casein-treated mice were cultured in dilutions of conventional, spleen cell-derived LK or the 25K MAF partially purified from culture fluids of PMA-stimulated EL-4 cells for 4 hr, washed and then cultured for an additional 1 hr with LK, 25K MAF or LPS (1 ng/ml). Radiolabeled tumor targets were added to washed cultures. Cytotoxicity (% label release) was measured at 48 hr.

each intact. Macrophages from each of the three defective mouse strains also failed to develop tumoricidal activity after treatment with the 25K MAF (Fig. 8).

The preceding observations document many biologic similarities between IFN and the 25K MAF. There are, however, clear differences. The 25K MAF does not induce antiviral activity in fibroblasts, the major definition of an interferon. The EL-4-derived macrophage activation factor also does not induce Ia antigen expression on macrophage plasma membranes (56). Although IFN and the 25K MAF both induced macrophage microbicidal activity against extracellular skin-stage schistosomula of *Schistosoma mansoni*, only IFN induced microbicidal activity against intracellular amastigote forms of *Leishmania major* (56-58). Indeed, macrophage microbicidal activity against *L. major* is of special interest. This macrophage effector function documents the interactions of two distinct macrophage activation factors for optimal cytotoxic activity. Macrophages treated with recombinant IFN alone develop potent cytotoxic activity against intracellular amastigotes of *L. major* (33). In contrast, the 25K MAF failed to induce this

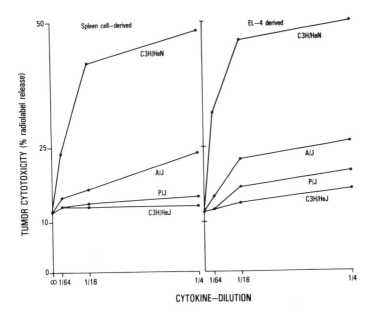

Figure 8   Genetic variation in development of activated, tumoricidal macrophages (from Ref. 52). Adherent macrophages from casein-treated C3H/HeN, C3H/HeJ, A/J or P/J mice were cultured in dilutions of conventional, spleen cell-derived LK or the 25K MAF partially purified from culture fluids of PMA-stimulated EL-4 cells with radiolabeled tumor targets. Cytotoxicity (% label release) was measured at 48 hr.

microbicidal activity throughout an extensive dose-response and time course. However, cells treated with IFN *and* the EL-4-derived MAF showed 5- to 10-fold more microbicidal activity than macrophages exposed to IFN alone (Fig. 9). The 25K MAF was not directly toxic to either leishmania or macrophages. In this system the 25K MAF did not act as a macrophage activation factor per se, but instead functioned as an accessory amplification factor to IFN for development of optimal cytotoxic effector function (59).

The precise molecular identity of the 25K MAF is not yet known. Culture fluids from PMA-stimulated EL-4 cells potentially have several known LK entities in this $M_r$ range: IL-2, IL-3, GM-CSF, and BSF-1 (B-cell stimulating factor). Each of these LK would be candidates for the 25K MAF. We addressed this issue directly by treating macrophages with murine IL-2, GM-CSF, and BSF-1 from recombinant DNA or highly purified IL-3 from a murine T-cell line (Fig. 10). Little or no tumoricidal activity was detected with macrophages treated with high concentrations ($\leqslant$250 units/ml) of IL-2 or IL-3. In contrast, both

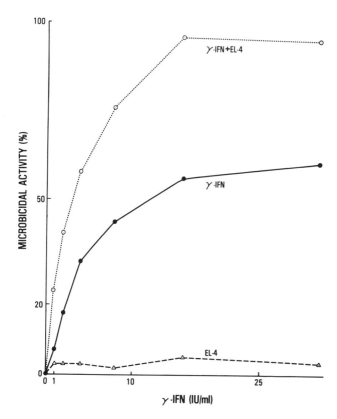

**Figure 9**  Synergistic interaction of IFN and the 25K MAF for induction of macrophage microbicidal activity against *L. major* (from Ref. 59). Resident peritoneal macrophages from untreated mice were cultured in dilutions of recombinant murine IFN with and without the 25K MAF and amastigotes of *L. major*. Microbicidal activity (% decrease in infected macrophages in infected compared to untreated control cultures) was estimated at 72 hr.

recombinant GM-CSF and BSF-1 induced significant macrophage-mediated tumor cytotoxicity. In these assays, BSF-1 was about 3- to 5-fold more active than equal concentrations of GM-CSF. The observation that GM-CSF activated murine macrophages for tumoricidal activity confirms similar reports with human monocytes (40). That BSF-1 is a macrophage activation factor was consistent with recent reports of BSF-1 receptors on murine macrophages (J. Ohara and W.E. Paul, NIH, Bethesda, Maryland, personal communication). In fact, BSF-1 has a broad range of activity in the regulation of macrophage function. Peritoneal macrophages treated with antibody-affinity-purified BSF-1 (60) developed potent tumoricidal

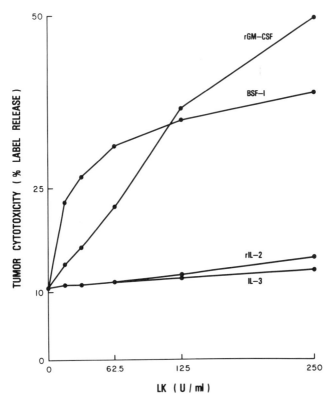

Figure 10  Induction of macrophage-mediated, nonspecific tumor cytotoxicity
by recombinant murine IL-2, GM-CSF, BSF-1 or highly purified IL-3 (from Ref.
61). Adherent macrophages from proteose peptone-treated mice were cultured
in dilutions IL-2, GM-CSF, BSF-2, or IL-3 with radiolabeled tumor targets. Cytotoxocity (% label release) was measured at 48 hr.

activity against several fibrosarcoma target cells. The concentration of BSF-1 that
induced 50% of maximal tumor cytotoxicity was 38 ± 6 units/ml for five separate
experiments; similar dose-responses were observed with recombinant BSF-1 (Fig.
11). BSF-1 alone was not directly toxic to tumor cells or macrophages through
500 units/ml. That BSF-1 dose-responses for induction of macrophage-mediated
tumor cytotoxicity were not affected by 5 µg/ml polymyxin B suggested that
contaminant LPS plays little or no role in cytotoxicity. However, addition of
exogenous LPS (1 ng/ml) synergistically increased (5- to 10-fold) the levels of
tumor cytotoxicity by BSF-1-activated macrophages. For example, low levels
of tumor cytotoxicity were induced in macrophages treated with 20 units/ml
BSF-1 (23% label release) or IFN (22% label release). Simultaneous treatment

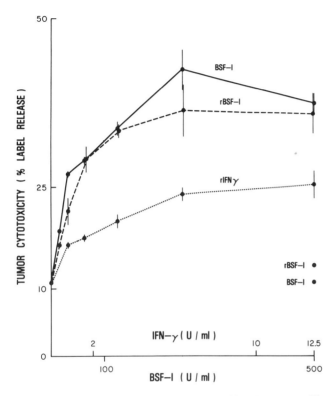

**Figure 11** Induction of macrophage-mediated, nonspecific tumor cytotoxicity by immunoaffinity-purified or recombinant murine BSF-1 (from Ref. 61). Adherent macrophages from proteose peptone-treated mice were cultured in dilutions of immunoaffinity purified or recombinant murine BSF-1 with radiolabeled tumor targets. Cytotoxicity (% label release) was measured at 48 hr.

of these activated macrophages with 1 ng/ml LPS dramatically increased macrophage-mediated tumor cytotoxicity to 54% (BSF-1) and 66% (IFN) label release. This low level of exogenous LPS had no direct effect on macrophage tumoricidal activity (8% label release). Macrophage tumoricidal activity induced by BSF-1 was inhibited ⩾ 90% by monoclonal anti-BSF-1 antibody; this antibody had no effect on macrophage-mediated tumor cytotoxicity induced by IFN. In other assays of macrophage function, BSF-1 and IFN induced expression of Ia antigen in more than 75% of peritoneal macrophages over 3 days in culture. Similarly, both BSF-1 and IFN increased (2- to 3-fold) the Fc-dependent binding of murine IgG immune complexes to bone marrow-derived macrophages. Thus by all of the preceding criteria, BSF-1 is certainly a macrophage activation factor (61).

Is either BSF-1 or GM-CSF the 25K (EL-4-derived) macrophage activation factor? Probably not! Culture fluids from PMA-stimulated EL-4 cells purified about 10,000-fold by sequential CM-Sepharose and G-100 Sephadex chromatography retained >80% of the starting activity for induction of macrophage-mediated tumor cytotoxicity. This partially purified 25K MAF had no GM-CSF activity (ability to support growth of bone marrow-derived granulocyte/macrophage stem cells) and no BSF-1 activity (ability to support growth of BSF-1-dependent T-cell lines). The ultimate answer to the preceding question, however, awaits final purification, amino acid sequence determination, and molecular cloning of this unique macrophage activation factor.

The complexity of macrophage activation just begins with the realization that multiple distinct LK signals interact to control macrophage effector function. Understanding the labyrinth of macrophage activation is made more difficult by the imprecision of the term "activated macrophage." Despite years of effort, there is still no one universally accepted biochemical marker for an activated macrophage. In fact, the unmodified term "activated macrophage" is now much too vague to be useful: activated macrophages should always be defined for the particular effector function at issue. A working definition of macrophage activation would include induction of specific cytotoxic effector functions not present in either resident tissue macrophages or in cells that accumulate at sites of sterile inflammation (Inflammatory macrophages). Analysis of this process must consider at least four interrelated variables: the cell that responds, the activation signal, the susceptible target, and the cytotoxic assay. Changes in any one of these variables markedly influences what one interprets as macrophage activation and, in turn, a macrophage activation factor. For example, macrophage response to a single, well defined activation signal for induction of cytotoxicity changes with cell maturation and/or differentiation (49,51). Although this concept seems eminently reasonable, the ultimate macrophage response may not be predictable (Fig. 12). For example, the level of tumoricidal activity induced by IFN-treated inflammatory macrophages is more than 10-fold greater than that induced by an equal number of resident peritoneal cells given identical treatment. Interestingly, differences in macrophage response are not related to number of IFN receptors: the number of IFN receptors/cell for inflammatory and resident macrophages are comparable. In the face of large differences in cell response for induction of tumoricidal activity, an entirely different phenomenon occurs with IFN-induced macrophage microbicidal activity (62,63). The number of macrophages infected with *Rickettsia tsutsugamushi* in resident and inflammatory cell populations are equal. Small amounts of IFN ($\leq$ 10 IU/ml) added to infected cell cultures activates macrophages to kill the intracellular bacteria. In contrast to tumoricidal activity, no difference in IFN dose-response was detected between resident and inflammatory cell populations for induction of microbicidal activity. Similarly, macrophages infected with amastigotes of *Leishmania major* also respond to IFN and develop microbicidal activity. In this case, microbicidal activity induced in

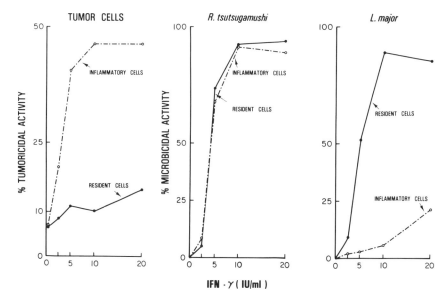

**Figure 12** Tumoricidal and microbicidal activities induced in resident or inflammatory peritoneal macrophages by recombinant IFN (from Ref. 49). Macrophages from casein-treated or untreated control mice were cultured in dilutions of IFN with radiolabeled tumor target cells, *R. tsutsugamushi* or *L. major*. Tumor cytotoxicity (% label release) was measured at 48 hr; microbicidal activity (% decrease in infected macrophages in infected compared to untreated control cultures) was estimated at 72 hr.

the resident macrophage population is more than 10-fold greater than that induced in inflammatory macrophages. Thus we easily document changes in macrophage response to activation stimuli with cell differentiation. We also document a striking system specificity: for any particular target, resident macrophages may be more, less, or equally responsive to an activation signal than equal numbers of inflammatory cells. Furthermore, superimposed upon differences in cell maturation are even greater changes in cell response that may occur with any of several other intrinsic or extrinsic factors: variation in macrophage activation among certain strains of mice (A/J, C3H/HeJ, P/J strains) or during certain viral and parasitic infections are examples that easily come to mind (51).

Target cell susceptibility to the cytotoxic reactions of an activated macrophage also determines the definition of a macrophage activation factor. One mechanism of macrophage-mediated cytotoxicity is through release of toxic oxygen metabolites including $H_2O_2$. For certain tumor cell and microbial targets (at least in certain assay systems) this is the predominant cytotoxic reaction. For these

systems, IFN is the only macrophage activation factor (16). However, susceptibility to macrophage-derived toxic oxygen metabolites or even reagent $H_2O_2$ is
certainly not uniform among either neoplastic or microbial targets. For example,
tumor cell susceptibility to lethal toxic effects of reagent $H_2O_2$ varies over a >10
fold concentration range; susceptibility of two leishmania species, *L. major* and
*L. donovani*, also varies over a 10-fold range (64). Similar target cell variation has
been documented for other macrophage-derived toxic effector molecules such as
prostaglandins and tumor necrosis factor. Not all cytotoxic mechanisms are induced in macrophages by each macrophage activation factor.

   Similarly, small changes in the actual mechanics of the cytotoxicity assay,
keeping macrophages, activation signal, and target otherwise constant, can profoundly affect induction of macrophage cytotoxic responses. As previously stated,
the ability of macrophages to respond to activation signals and kill neoplastic or
microbial targets changes with time in culture (Fig. 13). The time interval during
which macrophages are treated with macrophage activation factors determines

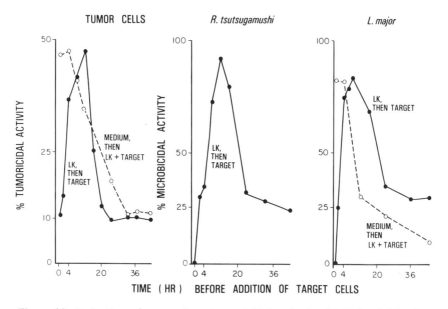

Figure 13  Induction of macrophage tumoricidal and microbicidal activities by
treatment with LK for various times before addition of target cells (from Ref.
49). Macrophages were cultured in 1/20 dilution of conventional, spleen cell-
derived LK for various times before addition of radiolabeled tumor target cells,
*R. tsutsugamushi* or *L. major*. Tumor cytotoxicity (% label release) was measured
at 48 hr; microbicidal activity (% decrease in infected macrophages in infected
compared to untreated control cultures) was estimated at 72 hr.

Table 3   Macrophage Microbicidal Activity Against *L. major*: Cell Pellet versus Adherent Monolayer Culture

| Macrophage culture | Macrophage microbicidal activity (% infected cells) of cultures treated with: | | |
|---|---|---|---|
| | Medium | LK | IFN |
| Cell pellet | 0% (62 ± 4) | 87% ( 8 ± 1)** | 90% ( 6 ± 2)** |
| Adherent monolayer | 0% (58 ± 3) | 7% (54 ± 3)** | 50% (29 ± 3)** |

Equal numbers of resident peritoneal macrophages were treated with culture medium, 1/20 spleen cell-derived LK or 20 IU/ml IFN as adherent cell monolayers or cell pellet cultures in polypropylene tubes and infected with amastigotes of *L. major*. Microbicidal activity is expressed as percentage decrease in infected macrophages in treated versus medium control cultures at 72 hr.
**Significant microbicidal activity.

the exact nature of the many cytotoxic effector reactions which are induced. The ability of macrophages to respond to activation signals and develop cytotoxic activity also differs between cells cultured as an adherent monolayer or as a cell pellet (Table 3). Macrophages cultured as a cell pellet respond to both LK and recombinant IFN to kill amastigotes of *L. major*. In contrast, macrophages cultured as an adherent monolayer, with or without the nonadherent peritoneal cells, respond less well to IFN and not at all to LK. Differences in macrophage response between adherent monolayer and cell pellet or suspension cultures are also documented for adenosine and lysine transport, glucose oxidation, procoagulant activity, and release of superoxide anion.

In many ways, regulation of nonspecific macrophage cytotoxicity is analogous to operation of a radio. The initial response is selection of an appropriate AM or FM radio. By analogy, the initial reaction in macrophage activation is accumulation of the appropriately responsive cell: for certain reactions, tissue macrophages are adequate or even optimal; other reactions are dependent upon inflammatory cells. The second response is turning the radio on. For the activated macrophage this is the priming reaction and for many cytotoxic effector functions the priming signal is IFN (65,66). Macrophages exposed to a priming signal enter into a receptive state in which they are not yet cytotoxic but are then able to respond to certain trigger signals and develop full tumoricidal or microbicidal activity. Trigger signals may be either endogenous (LK) or exogenous (LPS) stimuli. This trigger reaction is analogous to selection of an appropriate radio frequency or station. The final response for operation of the radio is volume control. The "volume" of the activated macrophage is regulated by certain accessory activation factors (Fig. 9). These signals either amplify or suppress cytotoxic reactions of activated macrophages. The interactions of each of the preceding signals form an integrated regulatory network for the initiation and fine control of macrophage effector function.

## REFERENCES

1. David, J.R. Delayed hypersensitivity in vitro: Its mediation by cell-free substances formed by lymphoid cell-antigen interaction. Proc. Natl. Acad. Sci. (USA) 56: 72, 1966.

2. Bloom, B.R., and Bennett, B. Mechanism of a reaction in vitro associated with delayed-type hypersensitivity. Science 153: 80, 1966.

3. Mackaness, G.B. The influence of immunologically committed lymphoid cells on macrophage activity *in vivo*. J. Exp. Med. 129: 973, 1969.

4. David, J.R., and Remold, H.G. Macrophage activation by lymphocyte mediators and studies on the interaction of macrophage inhibitory factor (MIF) with its target cell. In *Immunobiology of the Macrophage*. Edited by D.S. Nelson. Academic Press, New York, 1976, p. 401.

5. Waksman, B.H. Overview: biology of the lymphokines. In *Biology of the Lymphokines*. Edited by S. Cohen, E. Pick, and J.J. Oppenheim. Academic Press, New York, 1979, p. 585.

6. Mooney, J.J., and Waksman, B.H. Activation of normal rabbit macrophage monolayers by supernatants of antigen-stimulated lymphocytes. J. Immunol. 105: 1138, 1970.

7. Evans, R., and Alexander, P. Cooperation of immune lymphoid cells with macrophages in tumour immunity. Nature 228: 620, 1970.

8. Evans, R., Grant, C.K., Cox, H., Steele, K., and Alexander, P. Thymus-derived lymphocytes produce an immunologically specific macrophage-arming factor. J. Exp. Med. 136: 1318, 1972.

9. Churchill, W.H., Jr., Piessens, W.F., Sulis, C.A., and David, J.R. Macrophages activated as suspension cultures with lymphocyte mediators devoid of antigen become cytotoxic for tumor cells. J. Immunol. 115: 781, 1975.

10. Ruco, L.P., and Meltzer, M.S. Macrophage activation for tumor cytotoxicity: induction of tumoricidal macrophages by supernatants of PPD-stimulated Bacillus Calmette-Guerin-immune spleen cell cultures. J. Immunol. 119: 889, 1977.

11. Leonard, E.J., Ruco, L.P., and Meltzer, M.S. Characterization of macrophage activation factor, a lymphokine that causes macrophages to become cytotoxic for tumor cells. Cell. Immunol. 41: 347, 1978.

12. Schultz, R.M., and Chirigos, M.A. Similarities among factors that render macrophages tumoricidal in lymphokine and interferon preparations. Cancer Res. 38: 1003, 1978.

13. Roberts, W.K., and Vasil, A. Evidence for the identity of murine gamma interferon and macrophage activating factor. J. Interferon Res. 2: 519, 1982.

14. Schultz, R.M., and Kleinschmidt, W.J. Functional identity between murine gamma interferon and macrophage activating factor. Nature 305: 239, 1983.

15. Männel, D.N., and Falk, W. Interferon-gamma is required in activation of macrophages for tumor cytotoxicity. Cell. Immunol. 79: 396, 1983.

16. Nathan, C.F., Murray, H.W., Wiebe, M.E., and Rubin, B.Y. Identification of interferon-gamma as the lymphokine that activates human macrophage oxidative metabolism and antimicrobial activity. J. Exp. Med. 158: 670, 1983.

17. Spitalny, G.L., and Havell, E.A. Monoclonal antibody to murine gamma interferon inhibits lymphokine-induced antiviral and macrophage tumoricidal activities. J. Exp. Med. 159: 1560, 1984.

18. Svedersky, L.P., Benton, C.V., Berger, W.H., Rinderknecht, E., Harkins, R.N., and Palladino, M.A. Biological and antigenic similarities of murine interferon-gamma and macrophage activating factor. J. Exp. Med. 159: 812, 1984.

19. Le, J., and Vilcek, J. Lymphokine-mediated activation of human monocytes: neutralization by monoclonal antibody to interferon-gamma. Cell. Immunol. 85: 278, 1984.

20. Kniep, E.M., Domzig, W., Lohmann-Matthes, M.L., and Kickhöfen, B. Partial purification and chemical characterization of macrophage cytotoxicity factor (MCF, MAF) and its separation from migration inhibitory factor (MIF). J. Immunol. 127: 417, 1981.

21. Erickson, K.L., Circurel, L., Gruys, E., and Fidler, I.J. Murine T cell hybridomas that produce lymphokine with macrophage activating factor activity as a constitutive product. Cell. Immunol. 72: 195, 1982.

22. Ratliff, T.L., Thomasson, D.L., McCool, R.E., and Catalona, W.J. T-cell hybridoma production of macrophage activating factor (MAF). I. Separation of MAF from interferon gamma. J. Reticuloendothel. Soc. 31: 393, 1982.

23. Meltzer, M.S., Benjamin, W.R., and Farrar, J.J. Macrophage activation for tumor cytotoxicity: induction of macrophage tumoricidal activity by lymphokines from EL-4, a continuous T cell line. J. Immunol. 129: 2802, 1982.

24. Gemsa, D., Debatin, K-M., Kramer, W., Kubelka, C., Deimann, W., Kees, U., and Krammer, P.H. Macrophage-activating factors from different T cell clones induce distinct macrophage functions. J. Immunol. 131: 833, 1983.

25. Hamann, U., and Krammer, P.H. Activation of macrophage tumor cytotoxicity by the synergism of two T cell-derived lymphokines: immune interferon (IFN-gamma) and macrophage cytotoxicity-inducing factor 2 (MCIF2). Eur. J. Immunol. 15: 18, 1985.

26. Krammer, P.H., Kubelka, C.F., Falk, W., and Ruppel, A. Priming and triggering of tumoricidal and schistosomulicidal macrophages by two sequential lymphokine signals: interferon-gamma and macrophage cytotoxicity inducing factor 2. J. Immunol. 135: 3258, 1986.

27. Gately, C.L., Wahl, S.M., and Oppenheim, J.J. Characterization of hydrogen peroxide-potentiating factor, a lymphokine that increases the capacity of human monocytes and monocyte-like cell lines to produce hydrogen peroxide. J. Immunol. 131: 2853, 1983.

28. Andrew, P.W., Rees, A.D.M., Scoging, A., Dobson, N., Matthews, R., Whittal, J.T., Coates, A.R.M., and Lowrie, D.B. Secretion of a macrophage-activating factor distinct from interferon-gamma by human T cell clones. Eur. J. Immunol. 14: 962, 1984.

29. Omata, Y., Sethi, K.K., and Brandis, H. Analysis of the roles of immune interferon (IFN-gamma) and colony-stimulating factor(s) in the induction of macrophage anti-toxoplasma activity. Immunobiology 166: 146, 1984.

30. Higuchi, M., Nakamura, N., Tsuchiya, S.-I., Kobayashi, Y., and Osawa, T. Macrophage-activating factor for cytotoxicity produced by a human T-cell hybridoma. Cell. Immunol. 87: 626, 1984.

31. Salahuddin, S.Z., Markham, P.D., Linder, S.G., Gootenberg, J., Popoovic, M., Hemmi, H., Sarin, P.S., and Gallo, R.C. Lymphokine production by cultured human T cells transformed by human T-cell leukemia-lymphoma virus-I. Science 223: 703, 1984.

32. Kleinerman, E.S., Zicht, R., Sarin, P.S., Gallo, R.C., and Fidler, I.J. Constitutive production and release of a lymphokine with macrophage-activating factor activity distinct from gamma-interferon by a human T-cell leukemia virus-positive cell line. Cancer Res. 44: 4470, 1984.

33. Nacy, C.A., Fortier, A.H., Meltzer, M.S., Buchmeier, N.A., and Schreiber, R.D. Macrophage activation to kill *Leishmania major*: activation of macrophages for intracellular destruction of amastigotes can be induced by both recombinant interferon-gamma and non-interferon lymphokines. J. Immunol. 135: 3505, 1986.

34. Schreiber, R.D., Altman, A., and Katz, D.H. Identification of a T cell hybridoma which produces large quantities of macrophage activating factor. J. Exp. Med. 156: 677, 1982.

35. Schreiber, R.D., Pace, J.L., Russell, S.W., Altman, A., and Katz, D.H. Macrophage activating factor produced by a T cell hybridoma: physiochemical and biosynthetic resemblance to gamma-interferon. J. Immunol. 131: 826, 1983.

36. Futch, W.S., Jr., and Schook, L.B. Dissection of macrophage tumoricidal and protozoacidal activities using T-cell hybridomas and recombinant lymphokines. Infect. Immun. 50: 709, 1985.

37. Rose, R.M., Wasserman, A.S., Weiser, W.Y., and Remold, H.G. An acidic lymphokine distinct from interferon-gamma inhibits the replication of Herpes simplex virus in human pulmonary macrophages. Cell. Immunol. 97: 397, 1986.

38. Hoover, D.L., Finbloom, D.S., Crawford, R.M., Nacy, C.A., Gilbreath, M.G., and Meltzer, M.S. A lymphokine distinct from interferon-gamma that activates human monocytes to kill *Leishmania donovani* in vitro. J. Immunol. 136: 1329, 1986.

39. Lee, J.C., Rebar, L., Young, P., Ruscetti, F.W., Hanna, N., and Poste, G. Identification and characterization of a human T cell line-derived lymphokine with MAF-like activity distinct from interferon-gamma. J. Immunol. 136: 1322, 1986.

40. Grabstein, K.H., Urdal, D.L., Tushinshi, R.J., Mochizuki, D.Y., Price, V.L., Cantrell, M.A., Gillis, S., and Gonlon, P.J. Induction of macrophage tumoricidal activity by granulocyte-macrophage colony-stimulating factor. Science 232: 506, 1986.

41. Farrar, J.J., fuller-Farrar, J., Simon, P.L., Hilfiker, M.L., Stadler, B.M., and Farrar, W.L. Thymoma production of T cell growth factor (interleukin-2). J. Immunol. 125: 2555, 1980.

42. Ruco, L.P., Meltzer, M.S., and Rosenstreich, D.L. Macrophage activation for tumor cytotoxicity: control of macrophage tumoricidal activity by the *Lps* gene. J. Immunol. 121: 543, 1978.

43. Benjamin, W.R., Steeg, P.S., and Farrar, J.J. Production of immune interferon by an interleukin 2-independent murine T cell line. Proc. Natl. Acad. Sci. (USA) 79: 5379, 1982.
44. Schreiber, R.D., Hicks, L.J., Celada, A., Buchmeier, N.A., and Gray, P.W. Monoclonal antibodies to murine gamma-interferon which differentially modulate macrophage activation and antiviral activity. J. Immunol. 134: 1609, 1985.
45. Schreiber, R.D. Identification of gamma-interferon as a murine macrophage activating factor for tumor cytotoxicity. Contemp. Topics Immunobiol. 13: 171, 1984.
46. Meltzer, M.S., Gilbreath, M.O., Crawford, R.M., Schreiber, R.D., and Nacy, C.A. Macrophage activation factor from EL-4, a murine T cell line: antigenic characterization by hamster monoclonal antibodies to murine interferon-gamma. Cell. Immunol. 107: 340, 1987.
47. Meltzer, M.S. Tumor cytotoxicity by lymphokine-activated macrophages: development of macrophage tumoricidal activity requires a sequence of reactions. Lymphokines 3: 319, 1981.
48. Ruco, L.P., and Meltzer, M.S. Macrophage activation for tumor cytotoxicity: development of macrophage cytotoxic activity requires completion of a sequence of short-lived intermediatry reactions. J. Immunol. 121: 2035, 1978.
49. Nacy, C.A., Oster, C.N., James, S.L., and Meltzer, M.S. Microbicidal effector reactions of activated macrophages against intracellular and extracellular parasites. Contemp. Topics Immunobiol. 14: 147, 1984.
50. Meltzer, M.S., Lazdins, J.K., Occhionero, M., Nakamura, R.M., and Schlager, S.I. Tumor cytotoxicity by lymphokine-activated macrophages: characterization of macrophage, lymphokine and target cell interactions. In *Self-Defense Mechanisms: Role of Macrophages.* Edited by D. Mizuno, Z. Cohn, K. Takeya, and N. Ishida. University of Tokyo and Elsevier/North Holland Biomedical Press, Tokyo, 1982, p. 305.
51. Meltzer, M.S., Occhionero, M., and Ruco, L.P. Macrophage activation for tumor cytotoxicity: regulatory mechanisms for induction and control of cytotoxic activity. Fed. Proc. 41: 120, 1982.
52. Occhionero, M., Leonard, E.J., and Meltzer, M.S. Functional characterization of lymphokines from the EL-4 T cell line that activate macrophages for nonspecific tumor cytotoxicity. J. Leuk. Biol. 35: 405, 1984.
53. Ruco, L.P., and Meltzer, M.S. Defective tumoricidal capacity of macrophages from C3H/HeJ mice. J. Immunol. 120: 329, 1978.
54. Meltzer, M.S., Ruco, L.P., Boraschi, D., Mannel, D.N., and Edelstein, M.C. Macrophage activation for tumor cytotoxicity: genetic influences on development of macrophages with nonspecific tumoricidal activity. In *Genetic Control of Natural Resistance to Infection and Malignancy.* Edited by E. Skamene, P.A.L. Kongshavin, and M. Landy. Academic Press, New York, 1980, p. 537.
55. Meltzer, M.S., and Nacy, C.A. Macrophage cytotoxicity against tumor cell and microbial targets: genetic control of the activation network. Prog. Leuk. Biol. 3: 595, 1985.
56. Meltzer, M.S., Nacy, C.A., James, S.L., Benjamin, W.R., and Farrar, J.J. Transient cytotoxic responses of activated macrophages: characterization of signals that regulate cytotoxic activity. Adv. Immunopharm. 2: 229, 1983.

57. Nacy, C.A., James, S.L., Benjamin, W.R., Farrar, J.J., Hockmeyer, W.T., and Meltzer, M.S. Activation of macrophages for microbicidal and tumoricidal effector functions by soluble factors from EL-4, a continuous T cell line. Infect. Immun. 40: 820, 1983.

58. Nacy, C.A., Hockmeyer, W.T., Benjamin, W.R., Farrar, J.J., James, S.L., and Meltzer, M.S. Lymphokines from the EL-4 cell line induce macrophage microbicidal and tumoricidal activities. In *Interleukins, Lymphokines and Cytokines.* Edited by J.J. Oppenheim and S. Cohen. Academic Press, New York, 1983, p. 617.

59. Meltzer, M.S., Crawford, R.M., Gilbreath, M.J., Finbloom, D.S., Davis, C.E., Fortier, A.H., Schreiber, R.D., and Nacy, C.A. Lymphokine regulation of nonspecific macrophage cytotoxicity against neoplastic and microbial targets. Prog. Leuk. Biol. 6: 27, 1987.

60. Ohara, J., and Paul, W.E. Production of a monoclonal antibody to and molecular characterization of B-cell stimulatory factor-1. Nature 315: 333, 1985.

61. Crawford, R.M., Finbloom, D.S., Ohara, J., Paul, W.E., and Meltzer, M.S. B-cell stimulatory factor-1: a macrophage activation factor. J. Immunol. 139: 135, 1987.

62. Nacy, C.A., and Meltzer, M.S. Macrophages in resistance to rickettsial infection: macrophage activation in vitro for killing of *Rickettsia tsutsugamushi.* J. Immunol. 123: 2544, 1979.

63. Nacy, C.A., Meltzer, M.S., Leonard, E.J., and Wyler, D.J. Intracellular replication and lymphokine-induced destruction of *Leishmania tropica* in C3H/HeN mouse macrophages. J. Immunol. 127: 2381, 1981.

64. Nathan, C.F. Mechanisms of macrophage antimicrobial activity. Trans. Roy. Soc. Trop. Med. Hyg. 77: 620, 1983.

65. Pace, J.L., Russell, S.W., Torres, B.A., Johnson, H.M., and Gray, P.W. Recombinant mouse gamma-interferon induces the priming step in macrophage activation for tumor cell killing. J. Immunol. 130: 2011, 1983.

66. Buchmeier, N.A., and Schreiber, R.D. Requirement of endogenous interferon-gamma production for resolution of *Listeria monocytogenes* infection. Proc. Natl. Acad. Sci. (USA) 82: 7404, 1985.

# 12

# Differentiation and Maturation Inducer Factors for Leukemia Cells

J. W. Chiao and John Lutton / New York Medical College, Valhalla, New York

## I.  INTRODUCTION

### A.  Normal and Leukemic States

Many neoplastic cells are able to replicate but do not undergo appropriate differentiation and maturation, whereas normal cells may undergo the complete process of growth and differentiation into functional terminal cells that eventually die. Multiple examples can be seen in the hemopoietic system where strict regulation of growth and differentiation of red and white precursor cells lead to a fully differentiated cell which will be terminated after a specific time period. Normally, the immature hematopoietic cells are present in the bone marrow while their differentiated mature progenies are circulating in the blood. The more mature circulating cells are the predominant population and perform various functions. Leukemia cells of the hematopoietic compartment exemplify multiple growth and differentiation problems. In most leukemias, there are usually increased numbers of immature cells present in the bone marrow and peripheral blood. Furthermore, these immature leukemia cells resemble normal immature precursor cells present in normal bone marrow. They could be cells belonging to any lineage of the hematopoietic compartment, including erythroid, myeloid, lymphoid, or megakaryocytic lineages (Fig. 1). These leukemia cells are usually frozen at certain early stages of differentiation but retain the capacity to replicate. Thus, increased numbers of undifferentiated daughter cells are generated in the host. A number of hypotheses have been proposed to explain the etiology of leukemia. It is thought to be the consequence of disturbances in the hematopoietic equilibria which could be due to a deficiency of a maturation factor, a neoplastic process,

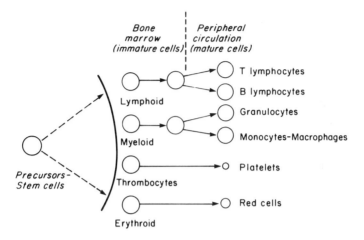

Figure 1   Developmental scheme of hematopoietic cell lineages.

or the inability of these cells to respond to forces which normally regulate their proliferation and maturation (1,2).

## B.  Proliferation and Differentiation

Although the cause of leukemogenesis and the mechanism of leukemia cell proliferation largely remains an enigma, considerable knowledge in this area has recently been gained. For example, the growth and differentiation of leukemia cells may in part be dependent on extrinsic molecules, provided by other cell types. These molecules, or factors, may also be an integral part of normal cellular development. Important in this regard are the mechanisms by which the process of cellular development takes place. This consists of an initial growth period, followed with the cessation of the replication process, and the parallel differentiation to more mature functional cells. This terminal differentiation process, complete from the birth of daughter cells to their termination, can be distinguished from a status referred to as partial differentiation. In this case, cells may have developed to certain stages while retaining their replication capacity. In other words, they can still produce daughter cells although they are more mature than their earlier precursor stages. Among cells of the hematopoietic system, analysis of the development or erythroid and myeloid lineages from normal and leukemic origin, have made the initial impacts for understanding the mechanism of leukemogenesis and the differentiation processes.

Recently, factors or cytokines capable of inducing differentiation and maturation of myeloid leukemia cells have been described (3,4). Upon differentiation induction, the leukemia cells cease their proliferation and a number of properties associated with the leukemic state are altered. With the accumulation of evidence that various leukemia cells can be induced to differentiate, scientists have attempted to understand the mechanism underlying the process of differentiation induction and to characterize the inducer molecules. Since some types of leukemic cells are frozen at specific differentiation stages of the hematopoietic process, the induction of terminal differentiation by certain inducers may be a viable approch to the therapy of the leukemias.

## II. PROCEDURES AND ASSAYS USED FOR ANALYZING GROWTH AND DIFFERENTIATION

Two types of tissue culture systems have been commonly used for analyzing growth and differentiation of hemopoietic cells and their regulator molecules (5-7). They are the classical liquid culture and the so called soft gel culture method. The liquid culture allows for mass growth of cells in a suspension or as adherence to a culture flask. The soft gel procedure allows for clonal growth of immobolized cells in a semisolid matrix, such as agar used at 0.3% which has a soft gel texture (Fig. 2).

In the mid-1960s, Pluznik and Sachs in Israel (8) and Bradley and Metcalf in Australia (9) reported the use of soft gel method for the growth of individual mouse bone marrow cells into colonies. These procedures employed a double layer or semisolid agar with the bone marrow cells seeded on the top layer while the

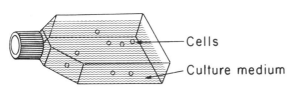

Cells

Culture medium

*LIQUID CULTURE*

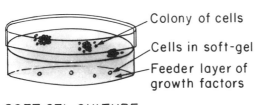

Colony of cells

Cells in soft-gel

Feeder layer of growth factors

*SOFT-GEL CULTURE*

Figure 2  Commonly used in vitro tissue culture techniques.

lower layer consisted of feeder leukocytes as the source of stimulants or growth factors for bone marrow cells. After a period of incubation, colonies or clusters of cells were found on the upper layer which, subsequently, were determined to be composed of granulocytes and macrophages. The colonies were derived from the bone marrow precursor cells with the colony-forming activity produced from the cells in the lower layer. In vitro generation of such colonies has been shown to be derived from precursor cells called colony-forming cells which are found in the bone marrow. These colony-forming cells are actually recognized as cells at a particular stage of differentiation and not the true stem cells. Both the liquid suspension culture and the soft gel method have been used as assay tools for the cells as well as the regulators. The liquid culture provides an advantage of assaying cells at any given time while the other technique is advantageous for observing clonal development of cells.

## A.  Target Cells

Blood cell types of normal or leukemic origin have been used as in vitro model systems that include human and various species of mammals. To investigate the controls of cell proliferation and differentiation of leukemia cells, various cell lines derived from the tumor cells have been established (10). These lines have specific characteristics at different stages of development and in some cases may be arrested at specific stages of the developmental process. Their growth characteristics and their development toward maturer stages can be monitored and the regulator molecules involved in this process can be studied. For example, the mouse Friend erythroleukemia cell line and the human HL-60 promyelocytic leukemia line have been employed extensively for the respective investigations relating to red blood cell and myeloid cell growth and differentiation.

## III.  MATURATION INDUCERS FOR MYELOID LEUKEMIA CELLS: A FAMILY OF FACTORS

### A.  Biological and Physiochemical Properties

Increasing evidence has demonstrated that myeloid leukemia cells can be manipulated to differentiate into terminal end-stage cells after exposure to biological inducers. Pioneers in the field of hematopoietic cell culture have clarified that growth and differentiation of normal and leukemic myeloid cells are controlled by a number of physiological protein factors, some of which control growth and others which control differentiation (11-13). Experiments with murine and human leukemia cells have indicated the presence of a family of cytokines, or physiological factors, that are capable of mediating myeloid leukemia cell differentiation and maturation. The identification of those cytokines and their specificities has pointed to the prospects of clinical trials for the therapy of leukemia and for other cancers.

Mouse Differentiation Factors

Identification of physiological protein factors capable of mediating myeloid leukemia cell differentiation have been reported since the early 1980s. These factors are distinct from the colony-stimulating factors (CSF). With the establishment of the mouse meyloid M1 leukemia blast cell line in 1969 (14). Ichikawa
initially reported that the conditioned media from mouse kidney cells, embryo
fibroblasts, splenic and peritoneal macrophages, and rat granulocytes could induce M1 cell differentiation as determined by morphological and functional
criteria (14). Yamamoto et al. (15) referred to the differentiation-inducing factor as D factor in their 1980 publication. Their assay was conducted in liquid
cultures of M1 cells containing conditioned medium from activated mouse spleen
cells. Various mitogens and copolymers of polyinosinic and polycytidylic acids
were shown to be effective in activating the splenic cells to produce D factor.
The differentiation was noted in the assays as the development of phagocytic-
macrophage-like cells. Initial reports showed that M1 cells were differentiated
into both granulocytes and macrophages (15), although later reports suggested
that primarily macrophages were developed (16). It was found that D-factor activities could be separated from the mouse colony-stimulating factor and interferons. Mitogen-stimulated splenic lymphocytes produce D factor(s) with a
molecular weight range of 40,000-50,000 while macrophage D factor(s) ranged
from 20,000 to 25,000 (15,16).

The differentiation-inducing properties of mouse D factor indicated that it
may be one of the mouse MGI-2 factors. MGI-2 is a general name used by Sachs
and colleagues initially for those murine factors inducing differentiation of normal myeloid cells, while MGI-1 refers to the growth-inducing substances. MGI-2
has also been called MGI-D or MGI-DF (17-19). It has been found that normal
hemopoietic cells endogenously generate MGI-2 after induction by MGI-1, whereas certain leukemia cells are able to generate MGI-2 only after exposure to an
agent such as endotoxin (20,21). Sachs and colleagues suggest that the induction
of MGI-2 by MGI-1 may serve as a regulatory mechanism that couples growth
and differentiation in normal cells (11).

There are clones of leukemia cells that are not dependent on MGI-1 for cellular viability and growth but can be induced to differentiate by MGI-2 (12). For
example, the murine myeloid leukemia MGI$^+$-D$^+$ cell line can undergo differentiation after exposure to exogenous MGI-2 (14-22). After differentiation, the
MGI$^{++}$-D cells now required MGI-1 for growth as do normal cells. The effects of
MGI-1 and MGI-2 are apparently specific since other growth and differentiation
factors could not substitute. In contrast to normals, MGI-1 was not able to induce endogenous production of MGI-2 in leukemia cells even though they again
required MGI-1 for growth.

Hozumi and collaborators have reported numerous biochemical changes that
occur when mouse myeloid leukemia cells (M1, WEHI-3B) are induced to differentiate by D factor (23). Following induction of differentiation of M1 leukemia

cells there was a marked increase in a specific cell surface glycoprotein called p180, which is thought to play a role in cell substrate adhesion. There were changes in phospholipid composition including an increase in methyl transferase activity and alterations in ganglioside composition. Various lysosomal enzymes were also noted to increase with lysozyme being the most predominant. The pattern of prostaglandin metabolism became altered so that differentiated M1 cells produced larger amounts of $PGE_2$. Finally, it was noted that the differentiated cells contained more mitochondria and expressed increments in cytochrome oxidase, glucose-6-phosphatase, and reverse transcriptase.

## Human Maturation Inducer, DIF, $\gamma$ Interferon, and TNF

Elias et al. (24), Lotem and Sachs (25), and Chiao et al. (26-27) were among the first to describe the presence of human differentiation- and maturation-inducing activities for myeloid leukemia cells in the early 1980s. These activities were initially found in the conditioned media of unseparated leukocyte cultures stimulated with 2-mercaptoethanal (24) or mitogen-stimulated peripheral blood lymphocytes. In their 1980 report, Chiao et al. (26) demonstrated that the activity present in mitogen- and antigen-stimulated lymphocyte-conditioned medium was derived primarily from T lymphocytes rather than B lymphocytes or monocytes (26). Helper T cells were later found to be the important producing cells (28). Employing a liquid differentiation assay system using human leukemic HL-60 promyelocytes, Chiao et al. have examined the relation of cellular proliferation to induced terminal differentiation (26-29). A reduction of proliferation occurred in parallel to a total RNA reduction along with the differentiation and maturation of HL-60 cells into monocytes and macrophages. During this development, differentiated and mature cells increased in number. This was evident since the mature cells possessed specific differentiation markers such as complement receptors, alpha-napthyl esterase activity, and phagocytic capacity. These leukemic cells died soon after terminal differentiation was accomplished. Greater than 90% cells were inducible to become monocytic cells (30) and cells of other lineages were not induced (26-30). Since the activity was distinct from colony-stimulating factors and there was no previous name for a human T-cell-produced mediator of monocyte development, Chiao et al. therefore, referred to this factor(s) as "maturation inducer" (26). At about the same time, Olsson et al. (31) reported that lymphocyte-conditioned medium contained activity inducing the differentiation of HL-60 cells into granulocytic or myelomonocytic cells. They called the activity differentiation-inducing factor(s) (DIF). Later publications by the same authors showed that DIF primarily induced monocyte differentiation (32).

The maturation inducer activity produced by activated normal human lymphocytes has been shown to be a protein lymphokine and multiple biochemical procedures were used for isolation from a serum-free lymphocyte-conditioned medium (33). Multiple species of molecules were detected and a major activity was originally shown to range from 36,000 to 58,000 in molecular weight. Further biochemical isolation as well as analysis by use of an affinity column with antibody against maturation inducer has resolved a purified protein of approximately 50,000 m.w. as determined by sodium dodecyl sulfate (SDS) gel electrophoresis (34). According to Olsson et al. (31), a smaller molecular weight of approximately 25,000 was also present in the lymphocyte-conditioned media.

The maturation inducer of 50,000 m.w. was demonstrated not to have antiviral activity and was distinct from interferons, macrophage-activating factor, colony-stimulating factor, and interleukins I, II, and III, as reported by a number of laboratories (32-35). A similar interpretation has been reported for murine D factor (23). Its biological activities indicate it as a physiological mediator for human monocytic cell development since it can induce the terminal differentiation and maturation of normal and leukemic myeloid cells to monocytic cells. It is also capable of inducing mouse M1 cells to differentiate into monocytic cells while mouse D factor could not induce differentiation in human leukemia cells. The maturation inducer activity from normal lymphocytes was effective for inducing patient leukemia cells to differentiate. In 1982, Chiao et al. (29) demonstrated that myeloid leukemia cells with a genetic defect could be induced to differentiate by the maturation inducer activity. The hyperdiploid DNA defect was found in the differentiated mature monocytic cells in the same manner as that in the undifferentiated leukemia cells. These observations indicate that differentiation induction may overcome the tumor state, despite certain genetic defects. Leukemia cells from most of the myeloid and nonlymphoid cases including acute myeloblastic leukemia (AML) and blastic chronic myeloblastic leukemia (CML), have been shown to be inducible in vitro. Similar data has since been reported by Lotem et al. using lymphocyte-conditioned medium. They estimate that the maturation inducer is approximately 55,000 in molecular weight (36).

Perussia et al. reported that human gamma interferon could induce patient myeloid leukemia cells to differentiate into mature monocytes (37). They suggested that gamma interferon could account for all of the activity in lymphocyte-conditioned medium. A later report by Takei et al. (38) demonstrated that gamma interferon activity could be depleted from lymphocyte-conditioned media by affinity column chromatography, whereas the maturation inducer activity was not removed and was thus distinct from gamma interferon. Similar results have been reported by others (35). Gamma interferon has been reported to induce either monocytic cells (37,38) or granulocytic development (39). Whether gamma interferon mediates terminal differentiation of myeloid cells has not yet been fully clarified. It is thought, but not confirmed, that gamma interferon may activate cells in general and therefore play a role in partial differentiation induction.

In 1983, Chiao and Minowada reported that human T-cell line HUT-102 constitutively produces a maturation inducer activity (28). It was suggested that the activity was identical to the maturation inducer derived from normal peripheral blood T cells. Olsson et al. (32) subsequently attempted isolation of the activity from HUT-102 culture supernatants. Their final DIF preparation was estimated to be a molecule of approximately 46,000 in molecular weight as determined by SDS gel electrophoresis, whereas gel filtration yielded a molecule of approximately 55,000. DIF was found to induce HL-60 cells but not U937 cells to differentiate. Chiao et al. have recently compared the isolated maturation inducers from normal lymphocyte conditioned media and that from HUT-102 and found that they were similar and identical in biological activities and molecular weight.

Recently Takeda et al. (40) Reported identical molecular characteristics between DIF and recombinant human tumor necrosis factor (TNF) (TNF, see separate review chapter). Human myeloblastic leukemia cells (ML-1) were used as target cells and DIF was obtained from lymphocyte-conditioned medium. Results demonstrated that purified DIF had a molecular weight of approximately 17,000 with $NH_2$-terminal sequences identical to that for human TNF. Differentiation was measured by nitrotetrazolium dye reduction and morphology of the ML-1 cells. However, there was no conclusion drawn as to whether differentiation into monocytic or granulocytic cells occurred, nor was there any reference made to cellular proliferation which would allow one to distinguish terminal and partial differentiation.

TNF could be the smaller molecular weight species of (25,000 m.w.) which had been identified in both murine and human lymphocyte-conditioned media (15,31). This smaller molecular species was shown to be produced by macrophages (15,31). TNF is likely to be distinct from the 50,000 m.w. maturation inducer. Our laboratory found that antibodies against the 50,000 m.w. maturation inducer blocked the differentiation induction activity mediated by isolated maturation inducer, but not that by genetically cloned TNF. The maturation inducer antibodies were found to block greater than 85% of the differentiation inducer activity in lymphocyte-conditioned medium, indicating that the 50,000 m.w. maturation inducer accounts for a major activity (41,42). The maturation inducer, TNF, gamma interferon, and possibly others may be a family of physiological factors important in normal monocytic cell and leukemia cell development.

## B. Differentiation Process and Mechanism

The differentiation of myeloid leukemia cells and the regulation by physiological factors has been analyzed mainly with mouse and human cell models. The process of terminal differentiation of leukemia cells into monocytic cells has been shown to be similar in murine and human systems and consists of multiple changes in cellular characteristics (23,24,29). The initiation of differentiation and maturation is dependent on the interaction of the cells with the physiological inducers, such as the human maturation inducer or the mouse D factor. The degree of differentiation and maturation is related to the dosage of the inducer. Within an effective dose range, the two are in direct proportion. Within a given dosage, the degree of differentiation is also time dependent, and more mature cells develop with a longer exposure time (33). These two facts were taken into consideration in the initial quantitation of the maturation inducer activity. It is defined as the minimal amount required in a given unit volume of culture to induce a certain number of mature cells within a given time period (33).

Figure 3 shows schematically the major events in the differentiation induction of myeloid leukemia cells to monocytic cells. Yen and Chiao (43) have quantitatively correlated the degree to which cellular proliferation is connected to differentiation. Analyzing cell cycle distribution during differentiation, they showed that the relative inhibition of population growth and differentiation into monocytic cells was associated with increased relative numbers of cells with $G_1$ DNA content. These data were directly attributable to the increased number of terminally arrested macrophages in $G_1$. In addition, the kinetic data indicated that most of the cells which differentiated became macrophages after one cell

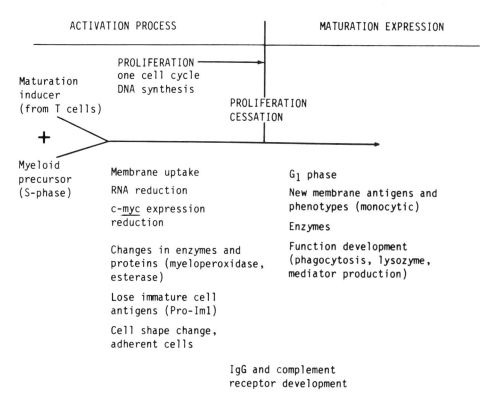

**Figure 3** Schematic diagram of the process of induced terminal differentiation of myeloid cells.

division. Approximately 21% of the cell population required a subsequent entire cell cycle before differentiating. The data suggest a model in which cells exposed to maturation inducer must undergo an S-phase differentiation control point in order to differentiate into the subsequent $G_1$ phase.

The relationship between the induction of differentiation and the cell cycle kinetics of murine M1 cells has been examined by Hayashi et al. (44). The kinetics of the decrease in proliferative capacity of M1 cells after induction are similar to that of the human cells. When M1 cells are treated with a differentiation inducer found in embryo-conditioned media, the cells traverse the S-phase of the cell cycle at least once. The cells then lose their ability to enter S phase and accumulate in $G_1$ phase. Tritiated thymidine incorporation into induced cells decreased after 12-18 hr, and the morphology of the cells changed in association with significant decrease in the nuclear cell ratio. These results suggest that M1 cells in any phase of the cell cycle can respond to the protein inducer and can be initiated to differentiate.

Within one day of exposure to an inducer, adherent monocytic cells were developed. The proportions of monocytes and macrophages increase with the induction period, concomitant with a decrease of cells with immature morphology. The increase of monocytes and macrophages is relatively linear with time, as is the increase of mature cells with functions such as phagocytosis. The acquisition of membrane receptors for IgG, Fc, complement components, and alpha-napthyl esterase enzyme is in parallel with the decrease of a total cellular RNA content (26). The differentiated cells become nonreplicating and the events of proliferation of some immature cells and the concurrent growth cessation of maturing cells appear to be intertwined. Later in the culture period, the nonreplicating cells become predominant, leading to termination of the culture (26,29). Leukemic HL-60 promyelocytes have also been shown to lose the Pro-Im1 antigen (86,000 m.w.) as detected by a monoclonal antibody (30). Grahmberg et al. (45) have shown the loss of a major 160,000 m.w. surface glycoprotein on HL-60 cells during induced differentiation. Associated with the maturation is the acquisition of new cellular antigen expression. They include antigen Leu M3, which is expressed on normal monocytes but not granulocytes, and other antigens such as GA2, GA11, H121 (46), and OKM1 (26). Knowledge about detailed mechanisms of myeloid cell differentiation wll lead to further understanding of the controls of differentiation induction. The interaction of factors with cells, as well as cellular genetic and enzymatic events have been areas of analysis. Weisinger and Sachs (47) showed that the mouse MGI-2 differentiation inducer is a DNA-binding protein. Lieberman et al. reported that differentiation programs for granulocytes or monocytic cells involve different cellular protein changes (48). It was shown that those protein changes could be due to the induction of new mRNA synthesis. This could take place by increasing or decreasing the amount of preexisting mRNA or by modulating the translation of a constant amount of mRNA (49). Induction of leukemic HL-60 and U937 cells to differentiate into monocytic cells has been shown to involve an increase in the level of pp60 [c-src]kinase activity (50). The induction of the kinase activity becomes apparent 14 to 72 hr after induction and this was correlated with elevated levels of c-src protein in the differentiated cells. The activation of the kinase activity has also been found to become elevated during normal bone marrow monocytic cell differentiation. It was suggested that activation of this kinase is a normal physiological event associated with myeloid cell differentiation.

One of the early events in monocytic differentiation is a rapid decrease in the phosphorylation of a 75 kD cytosol protein. This occurs shortly after a cell-factor interaction event takes place (51). Torelli et al. (52) analyzed kinetic data and the composition of polyadenylated RNAs during differentiation. Their studies suggested that during myeloid differentiation, possible transcriptional and regulatory mechanism of gene expression are active long after the commitment of events in the undifferentiated cell.

It is clear that differentiation processes involve metabolic and enzymatic changes. An alteration in purine metabolism was found to occur within 24 hours of differentiation induction, and the synthesis of purine nucleotides decreased in cells induced to mature (53). A decreased activity of both hypoxanthine phosphoribosyltransferase and inosine monophosphate (IMP) dehydrogenase was also suggested. In other experiments, manipulation of membrane phospholipid composition by choline analogues was found to induce differentiation and maturation of murine M1 leukemia cells (54). These studies suggested that phospholipid metabolism is involved in the mechanisms of differentiation.

Factors Influencing Maturation Inducer Activity

There are physiological factors and chemicals capable of augmenting or regulating the differentiation activity of the maturation inducers. Together they comprise a family of regulatory factors. The combined use of these factors and chemicals has helped form new approaches in leukemia treatment strategies. The human $\beta$ interferon has been shown to augment the degree of differentiation of leukemic cells into monocytic cells in the presence of reduced amounts of maturation inducer (55). The augmentation effect was not apparent when a sufficient quantity of maturation inducer was used. Recently $\beta$ interferon has also been found to be capable of augmenting granulocyte differentiation (56). Combined addition of retinoic acid with DIF isolated from HUT-102-conditioned media was shown to increase the spectrum of DIF activity (32).

Kasukabe et al. reported inhibition of differentiation of mouse myeloid leukemia cells by a heat-stable calf serum component of very high molecular weight (57). In other experiments, differentiation of mouse myeloid leukemia cells by D factor was shown to be inhibited by a factor from nondifferentiating leukemia cells (58). An inhibitory activity was detected only in the lysate of M1 leukemia cells that were resistent to the D factor induction.

Heteroantisera have been obtained for murine D factor and human maturation inducer. Tomida and colleagues have demonstrated that rabbit antiserum
against mouse D factor would effectively block the maturation-inductive activity
for mouse M1 leukemia cells (59). Antisera to D factor was prepared by immunizing rabbits with D factor partially purified from conditioned medium of mouse
L929 cells. The antiserum suppressed almost completely the activities of various
D stimulating factor. Chiao and Leung reported the effect of rat antisera against
human maturation inducer activity (41,42). A maturation inducer preparation
isolated from normal lymphocytic-conditioned medium was used as immunogen.
Treatment of lymphocyte-conditioned medium with 0.3% antisera resulted in
the reduction of approximately 85% of the mature cell development, indicating
that the maturation inducer molecules were responsible for the major activity in
the conditioned medium. Rat monoclonal antibodies against the 50,000 m.w. of
maturation inducer have since been obtained (60). Those antibodies were demonstrated to block the activity of maturation inducer in leukemia cell differentiation inductions. The antibodies showed no effects on the antiviral activities
of interferons and on tumor necrosis factor- (TNF) mediated differentiation (60).

## IV.  NONMYELOID LEUKEMIA DIFFERENTIATION

A considerable amount of work has been done utilizing Friend erythroleukemia
cells to study the induction of erythroid differentiation in leukemia. Carnot and
DeFlandre (61) were the first to suggest a humoral mechanism for the regulation
of erythropoiesis. It has been almost 82 years since Carnot and DeFlandre first
described what they called "Hemopoietine" and what we now call erythropoietin (Epo). Epo is the natural regulator of erythroid differentiation in humans
and animals. We will not attempt to review erythropoiesis and erythroleukemia
in this report, however, numerous review articles are available (62-67). It is of
concern only to draw an analogy between the myeloid and erythroid leukemic
states and their potential for induced differentiation.

Murine erythroleukemia cells, which are obtained from mice infected with
Friend virus complex, appear to be arrested at the proerythroblastic stage of development (68). The cells can be induced in vitro to undergo erythroid differentiation by the addition of various chemical agents (68). Under basal conditions,
less than 1% of the erythroleukemia cells spontaneously differentiate along the
erythroid pathway, a process which occurs independently of Epo (68). When
these cells are cultured in the presence of dimethyl sulfoxide (DMSO) for 4
days, the percentage of differentiated cells increased to 40-60%. This is accompanied by the development of responsiveness to Epo and the cells become capable of erythroid colony (CFU-E) formation in plasma clots (69,70). When erythroid differentiation of the cells was induced with DMSO prior to culture in
agar, there appeared to be a decline in agar colony-forming ability. The decline
in clonogenicity in agar occurred while the cell numbers in DMSO-containing

suspension cultures increased exponentially. This was further evidenced by the fact that more than 90% of the cells were synthesizing DNA (71). These results suggested that the progressive decline in agar colony-forming ability by DMSO-exposed cells is a reflection of the increasing proportion of differentiating cells in culture. Sassa (72) has demonstrated changes in the heme biosynthetic enzyme activities and heme concentration during DMSO-induced differentiation of Friend erythroleukemia cells. These enzymatic events are very significant to the differentiation process since heme synthesis plays a pivotal event during erythroid maturation.

In contrast to the murine erythroleukemia model, there is less information available concerning the induction of differentiation in human erythroleukemia cells. Human K562 and HEL erythroleukemia-like cell lines have been established and these cells can be induced to undergo erythroid differentiation after exposure to various agents such as hemin. HEL cells were originally derived from a patient with erythroleukemia or DiGuglielomo's disease (73). The cells are arrested in the erythroblast stage, apparently are biopotential, and can be triggered to differentiate into more mature erythroid cells and or macrophages. The K562 cells were originally derived from a patient with chronic granulocytic leukemia in terminal blast crisis (74). The cell line has been reported to carry the Philadelphia chromosome and it was originally thought that the K562 cell was a primitive granulocytic cell. However, it is known that the cell line may consist of early myeloid blasts, early erythroblasts, or a combination of both. Hoffman et al. (75) have characterized the heme biosynthetic and degradative enzymatic events in K562 cells after DMSO-induced differentiation. These studies clearly indicate that the enzymatic events of heme metabolism during differentiation of K562 are similar to that for normal bone marrow erythropoiesis (75).

In other studies, Hoffman et al. (76) characterized the ability of K562 cells to generate erythroid colonies in plasma clot cultures. Rare benzidine-positive colonies formed spontaneously when cloned in plasma clots ($3/10^4$ cells), and their number was not substantially increased by the addition of Epo ($9.5/10^4$ cells). However, addition of sodium butyrate markedly enhanced the number of colonies ($10/10^4$) while the combination of butyrate plus Epo exerted a synergistic effect on colony formation ($57/10^4$ cells).

The ability of bone marrow cells from patients with erythroleukemia to form, in vitro, erythroid colonies (CFU-E) in response to Epo appears to be quite variable. Early studies by Hoffman et al. (77) revealed that bone marrow cells from patients with erythroleukemia failed to generate CFU-E in plasma clots, whereas one patient in remission grew small numbers of CFU-E. Spontaneous endogenous CFU-E growth has also been reported for bone marrow cells from a patient with erythroleukemia, whereas 3 other patients demonstrated little or no CFU-E growth in the presence of Epo (78).

In summary, studies with murine and human erythroleukemia cell lines demonstrate that otherwise undifferentiated leukemia cells may become responsive to a cytokine-like growth substance (Epo), which then allows erythroid differentiation to ensue. However, the responsiveness to Epo appears to be dependent upon prior exposure or priming of the cells by various chemical agents such as DMSO, butyric acid, or hemin. Therefore, the erythroleukemia model may in some ways be analogous to the induction of differentiation in the myeloid leukemias by lymphokines.

Although induction of differentiation of human leukemia cells has been investigated mainly with myeloid leukemia cells, induction of differentiation of several human lymphoid leukemia cell lines into mature lymphoid cells has also recently been demonstrated (79-85). Most of these studies employ nonphysiological agents such as the phorbol esters TPA or PDB, and these agents are able to induce differentiation in several lymphoid leukemia cell lines such as MOLT-3, Jurkat, CCRF-CEM, HPB-ALL, and RPMI 8402. Little information is available concerning the role of natural lymphokines in the induction of differentiation in lymphoid leukemia cells, however, the thymus may contain factors which play a role in this process.

Previous studies have shown that thymic factors play an essential role in the maturation of normal T cells (82). Of the thymic factors and hormones, thymosin fraction 5 has been extensively studied. It is known to induce prothymocytes from bone marrow and spleen to express terminal deoxynucleotidyl transferase (TdT), Lyt 1, 2, and 3 antigens on mouse cells, and other properties that characterize mature lymphocytes. Ho et al. (82) reported that 5-ectonucleotidase (a differentiation marker) and certain surface characteristics were induced in malignant MOLT-3 cells exposed to thymosin, and this was followed by a decrease in proliferation and the percentage of cells positive from a primitive T-cell antigen. These findings suggested that thymosin stimulated biochemical and antigenic changes in malignant cells that are consistent with normal differentiation of T cells.

It is generally known that lymphokines of T-cell origin are required for the optimal differentiation of B cells (86-88). In addition, bone marrow stromal cells have been reported to produce a factor(s) which potentiates the differentiation of pre-B cells from a hemopoietic progenitor population (89). We will not attempt to review the process of B-cell differentiation in this report.

## V.  COLONY-STIMULATING FACTORS AND OTHER CYTOKINES

### A.  Nomenclature and History

Little was known about the physiological regulation of growth of bone marrow cells until the development of clonal culture techniques in the 1960s. In such cultures, individual progenitor cells of a particular lineage are able to proliferate and generate a clone of mature cells providing the proper conditions and growth substances are present (1,2,64-66,90). Clonal culture permitted the growth of bone marrow myeloid, erythroid, and lymphoid cells and the colony of cells is referred to as the colony-forming unit (CFU). Since cell proliferation and colony formation are dependent upon specific regulatory molecules, these molecules have been referred to as colony-stimulating factors (CSF) or colony-stimulating activity (CSA). Regulatory molecules that are mediated by cells have also been referred to as "cytokines," and those of lymphocyte origin have been termed "lymphokines." Colony-stimulating factors can be found circulating in many biological fluids, however, the number of cells in humans that produce and release CSF is rather limited. Basically the CSFs are named so as to designate the hemopoietic cell lineage they stimulate in an in vitro clonogenic assay. Thus, granulocytic colonies are stimulated by granulocyte CSF (G-CSF), macrophage clonal growth by macrophage CSF (M-CSF), and mixed colonies of granulocytes and macrophages by GM-CSF. In some instances, different nomenclature has been ascribed such as CSF $\alpha$, $\beta$, 1, 2, etc.

Recently it has been demonstrated that mononuclear phagocytes recruit stromal cells of the marrow to produce multilineage growth factors in vitro (91). It was also found that phagocytes consitutively produce soluble factor(s) that stimulate T lymphocytes, fibroblasts, and endothelial cells to produce colony-stimulating activity in vitro (92-96). Additionally, monocytes produce a factor that stimulates the production of burst-promoting activity (BPA) and megakaryocyte colony-stimulating activity (meg-CSA) by endothelial cells (97,98). Activation of specific genes through cellular interactions may result in specific production of a CSF or lymphokine. For example, the gene for human GM-CSF resides on the long arm of chromosome 5 (99). The locus of the gene is near the position of genes for other growth hormones and hormone receptors. Stimulation of the gene may occur by agents that activate macrophages, and activated macrophages may then induce resting T lymphocytes to express the GM-CSF gene. Thus, these studies emphasize the importance of complex cell-cell interactions in the regulation of hemopoiesis-lymphopoiesis.

The majority of the CSFs are acidic glycoproteins which may exist as monomeres consisting of a molecular weight (m.w.) range of 21-28,000, of which approximately 40% is carbohydrate (100). They also exist as dimers (m.w. = 70,000) of several polypeptide subunits each with a m.w. of approximately 14,000. Deglycosylation experiments have suggested that the carbohydrate portion is not of major importance for the in vitro growth-stimulating activity (100). Several types of CSFs controlling the production of hemopoietic cells in animals and humans have now been isolated, purified, and cloned by recombinant DNA technology.

Clinical Applications

There are many potential clinical applications for the use of recombinant forms of CSF. These molecules may be used in situations where there is a granulocytic deficit. For example, chemotherapy is frequently associated with leukopenia, and

CSFs could be administered before and after chemotherapy to accelerate leukocyte regeneration. Preliminary studies in Japan suggest that therapeutic administration of CSF has potential for improving the engraftment of transplanted bone
marrow cells. It has also been suggested that CSFs could be useful for differentiation therapy. In this respect, treatment of chronic myeloid leukemia with CSF
could induce the leukemia cells to differentiate rather than replicate, and differentiated macrophages could possess direct antitumor activity (2,101,102).

Current studies underway at UCLA Medical Center are aimed at determining
the potential usefulness of CSF therapy in patients with acquired immune deficiencies such as AIDS (101,102). It is thought that CSFs may increase the host
defenses and possibly enhance antibody-dependent cell-mediated cytotoxicity
(ADCC) against viral infected cells.

### B.  Granulocyte Macrophage Colony-Stimulating Factors

Granulocyte-macrophage-CSF (GM-CSF) has been isolated and has been referred
to as CSF-$\alpha$ or CSF-2 (100). It is a glycoprotein with a m.w. of approximately
23,000, and the murine form has been purified from endotoxin-treated mouse
lung (103). Elution studies from hydrophobic columns have identified at least
two separable forms of human CSF that can stimulate human granulocyte-
macrophage colony formation (104,105). These have been designated as CSF-$\alpha$
(nonbinding) and CSF-$\beta$ (binding). CSF-$\alpha$ has been purified to homogeneity and
may represent the natural form of GM-CSF. CSF-$\beta$ has not been fully purified,
but is able to stimulate differentiation of murine WEHI 3 leukemia cells, and
may be a close analogue of murine G-CSF (106).

Human GM-CSF has been obtained from medium conditioned by the Mo
hairy T-cell leukemia line (107-109). It was purified to homogeneity and found
to have a m.w. of approximately 20-23,000. Clones of cDNA were then isolated
by direct expression screening of cDNA libraries from Mo leukemic cell mRNA
(110) or a human T-cell line (111). Transfection of these clones to monkey COS
cells produced a GM-CSF that was active on human cells. Sequencing studies indicated that the polypeptide contains 127 amino acids (m.w. = 14,000) with four
cysteine residues. the recombinant GM-CSF produced by transfected COS cells
had a m.w. of 19,000 and a specific activity of $4 \times 10^7$ U/g protein (110-112).

The cellular receptor for GM-CSF has been isolated and its m.w. is approximately 52,000 (113). It has been estimated that resting noninduced HL-60 cells
have about 50 high affinity receptors/cell (113,114), whereas DMSO-induced
HL-60 cells may have more than 1000 receptors/cell. All normal granulocytes
and monocytes bear receptors for GM-CSF and the numbers decrease with increasing cellular maturation.

GM-CSF has now been cloned from three species including mouse, gibbon
ape, and human (114-117). Both human and ape GM-CSF cDNA clones revealed
substantial sequence homology of the amino acid sequence as compared with

human material. GM-CSF has also been shown to stimulate eosinophil colony formation (118) to initiate multipotential erythroid and megakaryocyte colony formation (119,120).

Production of recombinant human GM-CSF has permitted the evaluation of its in vivo effects in primates (121). Continuous infusion of human recombinant GM-CSF into healthy monkeys elicited a dramatic leukocytosis and substantial reticulocytosis. A similar effect was observed in one pancytopenic immunodeficient monkey. These studies provide the opportunity to test the potential clinical use of GM-CSF in various disorders such as in the treatment of some types of cytopenias. Thus, clinical trials on monkeys demonstrate that GM-CSF is a potent stimulator of primate hematopoiesis in vivo.

Recent evidence suggests that GM-CSF is probably not the single in vivo systemic hemopoietic regulator of granulopoiesis as is Epo for erythropoiesis. Instead, GM-CSF may function in collaboration with a variety of cellular interactions and the resultant combination of cytokines-lymphokines may then regulate a more localized hematopoiesis. The biological activity of GM-CSF in humans is not clearly defined and may overlap into several compartments. For example it will stimulate the limited proliferation of some multipotent colonies (CFU-Mix) and the proliferation and development of eosinophil colonies (CFU-Eos) (2).

## C.  Macrophage Colony-Stimulating Factor

Macrophage CSF (M-CSF, CSF-1) is a glycoprotein that stimulates growth and differentiation of cells from the mononuclear phagocyte lineage. CSF-1 has been purified to homogeneity from mouse L-cells (122) and a radioimmunoassay has been developed (123,124). The CSF-1 molecule is a 65-80,000 m.w. sialoglycoprotein composed of two similar chains lined by disulfide bonds (72). Recently, a human CSF-1 analogous to murine CSF-1 has been cloned (125,126). Sequence studies of the cDNA clone indicates the existence of a pre-pro CSF-1 of 252 residues which is then further processed to a more active form. In other experiments it has been reported that the product of the c-Fms proto-oncogene is identical to the receptor for CSF-1 (127,128). It is significant that the c-Fms gene is located on human chromosome 5 (129) and that a deletion in this chromosome (5q) in bone marrow cells is frequently associated with a syndrome that may develop into myeloid leukemia (99) or polycythemia Vera (130). It is known that the CSF-1 receptor is similar to the epidermal growth factor (EGF) receptor and c-Fms proto-oncogene product. These receptors possess tyrosine kinase activities, and antibodies to Fms protein will precipitate the CSF-1 receptor complex (128,131,132). Binding of CSF-1 with its surface receptor has been noted to initiate a series of cellular events. Within 1-2 minutes, membrane ruffling takes place, protein synthesis is stimulated by 30 minutes, and DNA synthesis is initiated by 12 hours. After 12 hours, CSF-1 becomes degraded, the cells then undergo proliferation and finally differentiation takes place (128). CSF-1 is known to have other biological effects on monocyte-macrophage cells that are distinct from growth and differentiation. For example, CSF-1 promotes the production of prostaglandin E (133), IL-1 (134), plasminogen activator (135,136), interferons (137), acidic isoferritins (138), peroxide formation (139), phagocytosis, tumor cytostasis (140), and tumor necrosis factor (141).

## D. Granulocytic Colony-Stimulating Factor

Murine granulocytic CSF (G-CSF), which has been isolated and purified from mouse lung-conditioned media, stimulates the production of granulocytic colonies in vitro (142,143). Polyacrylamide gel electrophoresis revealed that G-CSF is a distinct molecular species different than GM-CSF and separated as one band with a m.w. of 25,000. The human analogue of murine G-CSF has also been isolated from human placental-conditioned media and was referred to as CSF-$\beta$ (144). The murine and human G-CSF molecules demonstrated almost complete biological and receptor-binding cross-reactivities to normal and leukemic murine or human cells (144). Both G-CSFs were able to induce the production of terminally differentiated cells from WEHI 3B and other myeloid leukemia cell lines (145-152) and to suppress renewal and leukemogenicity of leukemia cells (153-158).

Iodinated forms of murine G-CSF and human CSF-$\beta$ were found to bind specific bone marrow target cells and cells from several forms of human leukemia such as acute myeloblastic leukemia, chronic myeloid leukemia, acute promyelocytic leukemia, preleukemia, and the cell line HL60 (145-145). Acute myelomonocytic leukemias showed little binding and unlabeled G-CSF could competitively inhibit the binding of the iodinated CSF in a dose-dependent manner whereas unlabeled M-CSF, GM-CSF, or multi-CSF were without effect (144, 145).

Recently a human pluripoietin growth factor with G-CSF growth- and differentiation-like activities has been isolated from conditioned media produced by a human bladder carcinoma cell line 5637 (159,160). In addition, the gene for human pluripoietin CSF was cloned and a recombinant form of the growth factor was produced (161). Because of the similarities to murine G-CSF, the factor was referred to as human G-CSF or hG-CSF. The similarities to murine G-CSF include the ability to stimulate growth and development of granulocytic colonies in vitro and to induce terminal differentiation of WEHI 3B (D+) cells. However, unlike murine G-CSF, recombinant hG-CSF supported early erythroid and mixed colony formation. The secreted form of the protein produced by the cell line was found to be O-glycosylated, had an isoelectric point of 5.5, and a m.w. of 19,600. It is important to note that the G-CSF-like molecules described above have a differentiation-inducing activity which was consistently found to copurify or be associated with an activity-stimulating growth. In addition, h-CSF had pluripoietin-like activity on erythroid and multiple lineages. It remains possible

Table 1  Comparison of Granulopoietic CSFs

| | G-CSF (Murine) | CSF-β (Human) | G-CSF (Human) | Pluripoietin (β) (Human) |
|---|---|---|---|---|
| Colony (CFU) progeny stimulation | Granulocyte | Granulocyte | Granulocyte | Granulocyte, some macrophage, BFU-E (erythroid) |
| Differentiation induction | + WEHI – 3β | + WEHI – 3β | None | CFU-GEMM (mixed), +WEHI – 3β, +HL-60 |
| Molecular characteristics | glycoprotein 25,000 m.w. SH groups necessary | glycoprotein 25,000 m.w. | O-linked glycosides m.w. = 14,000 IP = 6.1 | O-glycosylated m.w. = 18,000 IP = 5.5 |
| Specific activity (50%) | $5 \times 10^{-12}$ M | | $2.37 \times 10^{-11}$ M | $\sim 2 \times 10^{-11}$ M |
| Comments | $^{125}$I G-CSF specifically competes for CSF-β binding | | Not induce differentiation | α Form stimulates leukemic cell divisions, β-not stimulate |
| References | 142,143 | 144,145 | 161 | 159,160,171 |

that a true biological G-CSF may be specific only for the granulopoietic lineage. However, others distinguish that differentiation-inducing activity is due to a separate molecule and have subsequently purified it to homogeneity (162). In fact, two different cDNAs and mRNAs for human G-CSF have recently been isolated and could account for differences in growth and differentiating activities (163-165). Table 1 compares the different types of granulopoietic CSF.

A human squamous cell line, CHU-2, was found to produce large amounts of G-CSF that were very specific for the human and murine granulocytic lineage (163). Purification of the factor to homogeneity revealed that the factor did not stimulate other types of colony growth nor did it induce differentiation in leukemia cells such as $KG_1$ or HL60. It was found that the concentration of the factor required to obtain one half maximum colony formation $(2.37 \times 10^{-11}$ M) was equivalent to the value reported for pluripoietin. The molecule is a hydrophobic glycoprotein, m.w. 19,000, isoelectric point 6.1, with possible O-linked glycosides. Amino acid sequence determination of the molecule gave a single $NH_2$ terminal sequence which had no homology to corresponding sequences of other CSFs previously reported (164,165). Utilizing oligonucleotides as probes, two clones were isolated containing G-CSF-complementary DNA from the cDNA library prepared with mRNA from CHU-2 cells. Complete nucleotide sequences of the cDNAs were determined and hybridization analysis with monkey cells suggested that the human genome contains only one gene for G-CSF. This gene is interrupted by four introns and a comparison of the cDNAs structures indicated that two mRNAs are generated by alternative use of the sequences in the second intron of the gene. The finding of two mRNAs for the G-CSF polypeptide suggests that specific functional differences exist. Therefore, it will be necessary to produce each G-CSF molecule on a large scale by recombinant DNA technology, and study the function of each in vitro and in vivo.

### E.  Other Factors

Finally, other murine and human growth factors called multi-CSFs or interleukin 3s (IL-3) have been purified and genetically cloned (166,167). The cDNAs and gene sequences for human and murine forms appear to have significant sequence homology and the factors appear to be functionally related. IL-3 supports the growth of multilineage colonies and in this respect, human GM-CSF does exhibit some multilineage activity that is similar to IL-3. Thus, IL-3 and GM-CSF are two separate molecules with some overlapping biological activities. Both IL-3 and GM-CSF often show coordinate expression which suggests that the gene may be transcriptionally linked in some T cells and expressed in response to the appropriate stimulus (2,168-170).

Recently, a human pluripotent CSF has been prepared and apparently has properties that encompass the activities of IL-3 and G-CSF (159-171). Another area of overlap in growth-stimulating activity is seen with IL-3 and GM-CSF, so that at least three molecules influence CFU-Eos (172). Bartelmez et al. (173) have isolated a small molecular weight peptide (m.w. 5000) capable of stimulating eosinophil colony growth in vitro (Eos-CSF). Others have described eosinophil-differentiating factor(s), however, the relationship of differentiating factor to colony-stimulating factor has not yet been clarified (174,175).

The primary growth factors for lymphoid growth are B-cell growth factor (BCGF) and T-cell growth factor (TCGF, IL-2). These factors will not be discussed in detail here since they are reviewed in another chapter of this book.

In brief, it is now possible to grow T-cell clones with purified TCGF and B-cell clones using partly purified BCGF. The response of T lymphocytes to IL-2 depends on both the TCGF concentration, and the number of TCGF receptors. There is no apparent structural relationship between TCGF and BCGF. Continuous B-cell clones have been derived in the presence of BCGF and monoclonal antibodies have been made specific for the clones.

The production of immunoglobulin by B cells is also influenced by factors elaborated by T cells (87,88), in particular, B-cell-differentiating factors (BCDF), which stimulate IgM secretion and the release of another differentiating factor, BCDF, which induces a type of IgG class switching rather than a new clone of cells. Thus, growth, differentiation, and functions of lymphocytes themselves depend upon the complex production and interaction of regulatory molecules.

Not included in this review are the growth and differentiation regulators for erythropoiesis and thrombopoiesis. Erythropoietin (Epo) is the major regulator for erythropoiesis and there is considerable information on the physiology and biochemistry of this hormone. Less information is available regarding thrombopoietin, the presumed regulator of thrombopoiesis.

## REFERENCES

1. Goustin, A.S., Leof, E.B., Shipley, G.D., and Moses, H.L. Growth factors and cancer. Cancer Res. 46: 1015-1029, 1986.
2. Dexter, T.M., and Moore, M. Growth and development in the haemopoietic system: the role of lymphokines and their possible therapeutic potential in disease and malignancy. Carcinogenesis 7 (4): 509-516, 1986.
3. Hozumi, M. Fundamentals of chemotherapy of myeloid leukemia by induction of leukemia cell differentiation. Adv. Cancer Res. 38: 121-169, 1983.
4. Hozumi, M. Established leukemia cell lines: their role in the understanding and control of leukemia proliferation. CRC Crit. Rev. Oncol./Hematol. 3 (3): 235-277, 1985.
5. Kurland, J.I. Granulocyte-monocyte progenitor cells. In *Hematopoiesis*. Edited by D. Golde. Churchill Livingstone, New York, 1984, pp. 87-122.
6. Rozenszain, L.A., Radnay, J., Nussenblatt, R., and Sredni, B. Human lymphoid cells and their progenitors: isolation, identification and colony growth. In *Hematopoiesis*. Edited by D. Golde. Churchill Livingstone, New York, 1984, p. 150.

7. Preisler, H., Kirshner, J., and Early, A.P. Leukemia cell cultures. In *Hematopoiesis*. Edited by D. Golde. Churchill Livingstone, New York, 1984, p. 243.

8. Pluznik, D.H., and Sachs, L. The cloning of normal mast cells in tissue culture. J. Cell Comp. Physiol. 66: 319, 1965.

9. Bradley, T.R., and Metcalf, D. The growth of mouse bone marrow cells in vitro. Aust. J. Exp. Biol. Med. Sci. 44: 287, 1966.

10. Harris, P., and Ralph, P. Human leukemia models of myelomonocytic development: a review of the HL60 and U937 cell lines. J. Leuk. Bio. 37: 407, 1985.

11. Sachs, L. Regulation of membrane changes, differentiation, and malignancy in carcinogenesis. Harvey Lectures 68: 1, 1974.

12. Sachs, L. Control of normal cell differentiation and the phenotypic reversion of malignancy in myeloid leukemia. Nature 274: 535, 1978.

13. Sachs, L. Constitutive uncoupling of pathways of gene expression that control growth and differentiation in myeloid leukemia. Proc. Natl. Acad. Sci. (USA) 77: 6512, 1980.

14. Ichikawa, Y. Differentiation of a cell line of myeloid leukemia. J. Cell. Physiol. 74: 223, 1969.

15. Yamamoto, Y., Tomida, M., and Hozumi, M. Production by mouse spleen cells of factors stimulating differentiation of mouse myeloid leukemic cells that differ from the colony-stimulating factor. Cancer Res. 40: 4804, 1980.

16. Tomida, M., Yamamoto, Y., and Hozumi, M. Characterization of a factor inducing differentiation of mouse myeloid leukemic cells purified from conditioned medium of mouse Ehrlich ascites tumor cells. Fed. Eur. Biochem. Soc. 178: 291, 1984.

17. Maeda, M., Huriuchi, M., Numa, S., and Ichikawa, Y. Characterization of a differentiation stimulating factor for mouse myeloid leukemia cells. Gann 68: 435, 1977.

18. Hozumi, M., Umezawa, T., Takenaga, K., Ohno, T., Shikita, M., and Yamane, I. Characterization of factors stimulating differentiation of mouse myeloid leukemia cells from Yoshida sarcoma cell line cultured in serum-free medium. Cancer Res. 39: 5127, 1979.

19. Burgess, A., and Metcalf, D. Characterization of a serum factor stimulating the differentiation of myelo monocytic leukemic cells. Int. J. Cancer 26: 647, 1980.

20. Falk, A., and Sachs, L. Clonal regulation of the induction of macrophage and granulocyte inducing proteins from normal leukemic myeloid cells. Int. J. Cancer 26: 595-601, 1980.

21. Weiss, B., and Sachs, L. Indirect induction of differentiation in myeloid leukemic cells by lipid A. Proc. Natl. Acad. Sci. (USA) 75: 1374-1378, 1978.

22. Fibach, E., Hayashi, M., and Sachs, L. Control of normal differentiation of myeloid leukemic cells to macrophages and granulocytes. Proc. Natl. Acad. Sci. (USA) 70: 343-346, 1973.

23. Hozumi, M. Fundamentals of chemotherapy of myeloid leukemia by induction of leukemia cell differentiation. Adv. Cancer Res. 38: 121, 1983.

24. Elias, L., Wagenrich, F.J., Wallace, J.M., and Longonire, J. Altered pattern of differentiation and proliferation of HL-60 promyelocytic leukemia cells in the presence of leukocytes conditioned medium. Leukemia Res. 4: 301, 1980.

25. Lotem, J., and Sachs, L. Regulation of normal differentiation in mouse and human myeloid leukemic cells by phorbal esters and the mechanism of tumor promotion. Proc. Natl. Acad. Sci. (USA) 76: 5158, 1979.

26. Chiao, J.W., Freitag, W.F., Steinmetz, J.C., and Andreeff, M. Changes of cellular markers during differentiation of HL-60 promyelocytes to macrophages as induced by T lymphocyte conditioned medium. Leukemia Res. 5: 477, 1981.

27. Chiao, J.W., Freitag, W.B., and Andreeff, M. Changes in cellular markers and functions accompanying differentiation in HL-60 promyelocytes by lymphocyte conditioned medium. In *Leukemia Markers*. Edited by W. Knapp. Academic Press, New York, 1981, p. 305.

28. Chiao, J.W., and Minowada, J. Regulation of leukemic cell differentiation by lymphokines from T cell subclasses and a T cell line. Fed. Proc. 42: 681, 1983.

29. Chiao, J.W., Andreeff, M., Freitag, W.B., and Arlin, Z. Induction of in vitro proliferation and maturation of human aneuploid myelogenous leukemic cells. J. Exp. Med. 155: 1357, 1982.

30. Chiao, J.W., and Wang, C.Y. Differentiation antigens of HL-60 promyelocytes during induced maturation. Cancer Res. 44: 1031, 1984.

31. Olsson, I., Olofsson, T., and Mauritzon, N. Characterization of mononuclear blood cell-derived differentiation inducing factor for the human promyelocytic leukemia cell line HL-60. J. Natl. Cancer Inst. 67: 1225, 1981.

32. Olsson, I., Sarngadharan, M.G., Breitman, T.R., and Gallo, R.C. Isolation and characterization of a T lymphocyte-derived differentiation inducing factor for the myeloid leukemic cell line HL-60. Blood 63: 510, 1984.

33. Leung, K., and Chiao, J.W. Human leukemia cell maturation induced by a T cell lymphokine isolated from medium conditioned by normal lymphocytes. Proc. Natl. Acad. Sci. (USA) 82: 1209, 1985.

34. Chiao, J.W. Maturation inducer and the process of differentiation induction of human myeloid leukemia cells. Blood Cells 13: 111, 1987.

35. Harris, P.E., Ralph, P., Litcofsky, P., and Moore, M.A.S. Distinct activities of interferon-gamma, lymphokine and cytokine differentiation-inducing factors acting on the monoblastic leukemia cell line U937. Cancer Res. 45: 9, 1985.

36. Lotem, J., Berrebi, H., and Sachs, L. Screening for induction of differentiation and toxicity to blast cells by chemotherapeutic compounds in human myeloid leukemia. Leukemia Res. 9: 249, 1985.

37. Perussia, B., Dayton, E.T., Fanning, V., Thiagarajan, P., Hoxie, J., and Trinchieri, G. Immune interferon and leukocyte-conditioned medium induced normal and leukemic myeloid cells to differentiate along the monocytic pathway. J. Exp. Med. 158: 2058, 1983.

38. Takei, M., Takeda, K., and Konno, K. The rate of interferon gamma in induction of differentiation of human myeloid leukemia cell lines, ML-1 and HL-60. Biochem. Biophys. Res. Comm. 124: 100, 1984.

39. Buessow, S., Mahaley, M.S., and Gillespie, G.Y. Interferon promotes myeloid differentiation and augments cytotoxicity of a human promyelocytic leukemia line. Fed. Proc. 43: 1986, 1984.

40. Takeda, K., Iwamoto, S., Sugimoto, H., Tetsuo, T., Kawatani, N., Noda, M., Masaki, A., Marise, H., Arimura, H., and Kinno, K. Identity of differentiation inducing factor and tumor necrosis factor. Nature 323: 338, 1986.

41. Chiao, J.W., and Leung, K. Antibodies suppress the maturation inducer (a T cell lymphokine) mediated differentiation of human leukemic cells. Fed. Proc. 44: 1686, 1985.

42. Chiao, J.W., and Leung, K. Antisera suppressing the maturation inducer mediated differentiation of human leukemia cells. Submitted 1988.

43. Yen, A., and Chiao, J.W. Control of cell differentiation during proliferation. Exp. Cell Res. 146: 87, 1983.

44. Hayashi, M., Okabe-Kado, J., and Hozumi, M. Flow cytometric analysis of unbalanced control of protein accumulation and DNA synthesis in differentiating mouse myeloid leukemia cells. Exp. Cell Res. 146: 109, 1983.

45. Grahmberg, C.G., Neilson, K., and Anderson, L.C. Specific changes in the surface glycoprotein pattern of human promyelocytic leukemic cell line HL-60 during morphologic and functional differentiation. Proc. Natl. Acad. Sci. (USA) 76: 4087, 1979.

46. Hayashi, K., Hiraiwa, A., Namikawa, R., Shika, H., and Chiao, J.W. Human myeloid cell antigens during differentiation. Fed. Proc. 44: 1689, 1985.

47. Weisinger, G., and Sachs, L. DNA-binding protein that induces cell differentiation. EMBO J. 2: 2103, 1983.

48. Lieberman, D., Hoffman-Lieberman, B., and Sachs, L. Regulation of gene expression by tumor promoters. Int. J. Cancer 28: 285, 1981.

49. Hoffman-Lieberman, B., Lieberman, D., and Sachs, L. Regulation of gene expression by tumor promoters. Int. J. Cancer 28: 615, 1981.

50. Gee, G.E., Griffin, J., Sastre, L., Miller, L.J., Springer, T.A., Piwnica-Worms, H., and Roberts, T.M. Differentiation of myeloid cells is accompanied by increased levels of $pp^{60}$ c-SRC protein and kinase activity. Proc. Natl. Acad. Sci. (USA) 83: 5131, 1986.

51. Mita, S., Nakaki, T., Yamamoto, S., and Kato, R. Phosphorylation and dephosphorylation of human promyelocytic leukemia cell (HL-60) proteins by tumor promoter. Exp. Cell Res. 154: 492, 1984.

52. Torelli, G., Donelli, A., Ferrari, S., Moretti, L., Cadossi, R., Cecherelli, G., Ferrari, S., and Torelli, U. Sequence complexity and diversity of polyadenylated RNA molecules transcribed in human myeloid cells. Differentiation 27: 133, 1984.

53. Lucas, D.L., Webster, H.K., and Wright, D.G. Purine metabolism in myeloid precursor cells during maturation. J. Clin. Invest. 72: 1889, 1983.

54. Honma, Y., Kasukabe, T., and Hozumi, M. Modification of membrane phospholipid composition by chaline analogues induces differentiation of cultured mouse myeloid leukemia cells. Biochem. Biophys. Acta 721: 83, 1982.

55. Chiao, J.W., Heil, M.F., and Wa, J. Enhancing effect of interferon on leukemic cell differentiation. Fed. Proc. 43: 1929, 1984.

56. Saguston, J., and Chiao, J.W. The enhancing role of interferon on human leukemia cell differentiation. Fed. Proc. 46: 1511, 1987.

57. Kasukabe, T., Honma, Y., and Hozumi, M. Inhibition of differentiation of

mouse myeloid leukemia cells by heat-stable calf serum components of very high molecular weight. Leukemia Res. 6: 695, 1982.

58. Okabe, J., Hayashi, M., Honma, Y., and Hozumi, M. Differentiation of mouse myeloid leukemia cells is inhibited by a factor from non-differentiating leukemia cells. Int. J. Cancer 22: 570, 1978.

59. Tomida, M., Yamamoto-Yamaguchi, Y., and Hozumi, M. Preparation and neutralization characteristics of an antibody to the factor inducing differentiation of mouse myeloid leukemic cells. FEBS Letters 151: 281, 1983.

60. Leung, K., and Chiao, J.W. Monoclonal antibodies neutralizing the maturation inducer activity for myeloid leukemia cells. Fed. Proc. 46: 785, 1987.

61. Carnot, P., DeFlandre, C. Sur/activite hemopoietique du serum un couis de la regeneration du sugn. Comptes. Rend. Acad. Sci. 143: 1906.

62. Izak, G. Erythroid cell differentiation and maturation. Prog. Heamtol. 10: 1-41, 1977.

63. Ogawa, M., and Leury, A.G. Erythroid progenitors. In *Hematopoiesis*. Edited by D. Golde. Churchill Livingston, New York, 1984, p. 123.

64. Quesenberry, P., and Levitt, L. Hematopoietic stem cells I, N. Engl. J. Med. 301 (14): 755, 1979.

65. Quensenberry, P.L., and Levitt, L. Hematopoietic stem cells II. N. Engl. J. Med. 301 (15): 8193, 1979.

66. Quensenberry, P., and Levitt, L. Hematopoietic stem cells III. N. Engl. J. Med. 301 (16): 868, 1979.

67. Rifkind, R.A., Sheffery, M., and Marks, P.A. Induced differentiation of murine erythroleukemia cells: cellular and molecular mechanisms. Adv. Cancer Res. 42: 149-166, 1984.

68. Friend, C., Scher, W., Holland, J.G., and Sato, T. Hemoglobin Synthesis in murine virus induced leukemic cells in vitro. Stimulation of erythroid differentiation by dimethylsulfoxide. Proc. Natl. Acad. Sci. (USA) 68: 378, 1971.

69. Goldshein, K., Preisler, H.D., Lutton, J.D., and Zanjani, E.D. Erythroid colony formation in vitro by dimethylsulfoxide-treated erythroleukemic cells. Blood 44 (6): 831, 1974.

70. Mishina, Y., and Ofinata, M. Induction of commitment of murine erythroleukemia cells (TSA8) to CFU-E with DMSO. Exp. Cell Res. 162: 319, 1985.

71. Preisler, H.D., Lutton, J.D., Giladi, M., Goldstein, K., and Zanjani, E.D. Loss of clonogenicity in agar by differentiating erythroleukemia cells. Life Sci. 16: 1241, 1975.

72. Sassa, S. Sequential induction of heme pathway enzymes during erythroid differentiation of mouse friend leukemia virus infected cells. J. Exp. Med. 143: 305, 1976.

73. Martin, P., and Papayannopoulou, T. HEL cells, a new human erythroleukemia cell line with spontaneous and induced globin expression. Science 216: 1233, 1982.

74. Lozzio, C.B., and Lozzio, B.B. Human chronic myelogenous leukemia cell line with positive Philadelphia chromosome. Blood 45: 321, 1975.

75. Hoffman, R., Ibraham, N.G., Diamond, A., Bruno, E., Levere, R.D., Forget, G.B., and Benz, E.J. Characterization of a human leukemia cell line. In *Hemoglobins in Development and Differentiation*. Edited by G. Stamatoyannopoulos. A.R. Liss Inc., New York, 1981, p. 487.

76. Hoffman, R., Murrane, M.J., Benz, E.J., Prohaska, R., Floyd, V., Dainiak, N., Forget, B.G., and Furthmayr, H. Induction of erythropoietic colonies in a human chronic myelogenous leukemia cell line. Blood 54 (5): 1182, 1979.

77. Hoffman, R., Zanjani, E.D., Lutton, J.D., Zalasky, R., and Waserman, L.R. Erythroid colony growth in disorders of erythropoiesis. Blood 46 (6): 1023, 1975.

78. Anderson, W.F., Beckman, B., Beltran, G., Fisher, J.W., and Stuckey, W.J. Erythropoietin independent erythroid colony formation in patients with erythroleukemia and related disorders. Br. J. Hematol. 52: 311, 1982.

79. Nagasawa, K., Howatson, A., and Mak, T.W. Induction of human malignant T-lymphoblastic cell lines MOLT-3 and Jurkat by 12-0-tetradecanoylphorbol-13-acetate: biochemical, physical, and morphological characterization. J. Cell Physiol. 109: 181, 1981.

80. Nagasawa, K., and Mak, T.W. Induction of differentiation in human T-lymphoblastic leukemia cell lines by 12-0-tetradecanoylphorbol 13-acetate (TPA): studies with monoclonal antibodies to T cells. Cell Immunol. 71: 396, 1982.

81. Cassel, D.L., Hoxie, J.A., and Cooper, R.A. Phorbol ester modulation of T-cell antigens in the Jurkat lymphoblastic leukemia cell line. Cancer Res. 43: 4582, 1983.

82. Ho, A.D., Ma, D.D.F., Price, G., and Hoffbrand, A.V. Effect of thymosin and phorbol ester on purine metabolic enzymes and cell surface phenotype in a malignant T-cell line (MOLT-3). Leuk. Res. 7: 779, 1983.

83. Rvffel, B., Henning, C.B., and Huberman, E. Differentiation of human T-lymphoid leukemia cells into cells that have a suppressor phenotype is induced by phorbol 12-myristate 13-acetate. Proc. Natl. Acad. Sci. (USA) 79: 7336, 1982.

84. Nakao, Y., Matsuda, S., Fujita, T., Watanabe, S., Morikawa, S., Saida, T., and Ito, Y. Phorbol ester-induced differentiation of human T-lymphoblastic cell line HPB-ALL. Cancer Res. 42: 3843, 1982.

85. Sacchi, M., Fiorini, G., Plevani, P., Badaracco, G., Breviario, D., and Ginelli, E. Acquisition of deoxyguanosine resistance by TPA-induced T lymphoid lines. J. Immunol. 130: 1622, 1983.

86. Vasquez, A., Gerard, J.P., Delfraissy, J.F., Dugas, B., Auffredou, M.T., Crevon, M.C., Fradelizi, D., and Galanaud, P. Differentiation factors for human specific B cell response. J. Immunol. 16: 803, 1986.

87. Noell, R.J., Snow, E.C., Uhr, J.W., and Vitetta, E.S. Activation of antigen specific B cells: role of T cells, cytokines and antigens in induction of growth and differentiation. Proc. Natl. Acad. Sci. (USA) 80: 6628, 1983.

88. Howard, M., and Paul, W.E. Regulation of B cell growth and differentiation by soluble factors. Ann. Rev. Immunol. 1: 307, 1983.

89. Landreth, V.S., Witt, P., Woodward, T., Buber, G., and Quesenberry, P.J. A bone marrow stromal cell line produces growth factors which synergize

with known hemopoietic regulatory molecules and potentiate the generation of pre-B cells. Submitted 1988.

90. Metcalf, D. The molecular biology and functions of the granulocyte-macrophage colony stimulating factors. Blood 67 (2): 2577, 1986.

91. Broudy, V.C., Zuckerman, K.S., J.S., Jetmalani, S., Fitchen, J.H., and Bagby, G.C. Monocytes stimulate fibroblastoid bone marrow stromal cells to produce multilineage hematopoietic growth factors. Blood 68 (2): 530-534, 1986.

92. Bagby, G.C., Rigas, V.D., Bennett, R.M., Vanenbark, A.A., and Gared, H.S. Interaction of lactoferrin, monocytes and T-lymphocyte subsets in the regulation of steady-state granulopoiesis in vitro. J. Clin. Invest. 68: 56, 1981.

93. Bagby, G.C., McCall, E., and Layman, D.L. Regulation of colony-stimulating activity production. Interactions of fibroblasts, mononuclear phagocytes and lactoferrin. J. Clin. Invest. 71: 340, 1983.

94. Bagby, G.C., McCall, E., Bergstrom, K.A., and Burger, D. A monokine regulates colony-stimulating activity production by vacular endothelial cells. Blood 62: 663, 1983.

95. Geson, S.L., Friedman, H.M., and Clines, D.B. Viral infection of vascular endothelial cells alters production of colony-stimulating activity. J. Clin. Invest. 76: 1382, 1985.

96. McCall, E., and Bagby, G.C. Monocyte-derives recruiting activity: kinetics of production and effects of endotoxin. Blood 65: 689, 1985.

97. Zuckerman, K.S., Bagby, G.C., McCall, E., Sparks, B., Wells, J., Phatei, V., and Goodrum, D. A monokine stimulates production of human erythroid burst-promoting activity by endothelial cells in vitro. J. Clin. Invest. 75: 722, 1985.

98. Segal, G.M., McCall, E., Stueve, T., and Bagby, G.C. Monokine-stimulated endothelial cells promote human megakaryocyte and mixed-cell colony growth. Blood 66: 464a, 1985.

99. Sokal, G., Michaux, J.L., van den Berghe, H., Corbier, A., Rodhain, J., Ferrant, A., Moriam, M., deBruyere, M., and Sonnet, J. A new hematopoietic syndrome with a distinct karyotype: the 5q chromosome. Blood 46: 519-533, 1975.

100. Metcalf, D. The granulocyte macrophage colony stimulating factor. Science 229: 16-22, 1985.

101. Golde, D. Clinical role, therapeutic promise of CSF's. Oncology Times October: 3, 1986.

102. Platzer, E., Gramatzki, M., Rollinghoff, M., and Kalden, J.R. Lymphokines and monokines in the clinic. Immunol. Today 7 (7): 185-187, 1986.

103. Burgess, A.W., Camakaris, J., and Metcalf, D. Purification and properties of colony-stimulating factor from mouse lung conditioned medium. J. Biol. Chem. 252: 1998, 1977.

104. Begley, C.G., Metcalf, D., Lopez, A.F., and Nicola, N.A. Fractionated populations of normal human marrow cells respond to both colony-stimulating factors with granulocyte-macrophage activity. Exp. Hematol. 13: 956-962, 1985.

105. Nicola, N.A., Metcalf, D., Johnson, G.R., and Burgess, A.W. Separation of functionally dinstinct human granulocyte macrophage colony stimulating factors. Blood 54: 614, 1979.
106. Nicola, N.A., Begley, C.G., and Metcalf, D. Identification of the human analogue of a regulator that induces differentiation in murine leukemic cells. Nature 314: 625, 1985.
107. Gasson, J.C., Weisbart, R.H., Kaufman, S.E., Clark, S.C., Hewick, R.M., Wong, G.G., and Golde, D.W. Purified human granulocyte macrophage colony stimulating factor: direct action on neutrophils. Science 226: 1339, 1984.
108. Golde, D.W., Quan, S.G., and Cline, M.J. Human T-lymphocyte cell line producing colony stimulating activity. Blood 52 (5): 1068, 1978.
109. Hesketch, P.J., Sullivan, R., Valeri, R., and McCarroll, L.A. The production of granulocyte-monocyte colony stimulating activity by isolated human T-lymphocyte subpopulations. Blood 63 (5): 1141, 1984.
110. Wong, G.G., Witek, J., Temple, P.A., Wilkens, K.M., Leary, A.C., Luxenberg, D.P., Jones, S.S., Brown, E.C., Kay, R.M., Orr, E.C., Shoemaker, C., Golde, D.W., Kaufman, R.J., Hewick, R.M., Wang, E.A., and Clark, S.C. Human GM-CSF: Molecular cloning of the complementary DNA and purification of the natural and recombinant proteins. Science 228: 810, 1985.
111. Lee, F., Yokota, T., Otsuka, T., Gemmell, L., Larson, N., Luh, J., Arai, K.I., and Rennick, D. Isolation of cDNA for a human granulocyte-macrophage colony-stimulating factor by functional expression in mammalian cells. Proc. Natl. Acad. Sci. (USA) 82: 4360, 1985.
112. Metcalf, D., Begley, C.G., Johnson, G.R., Nicola, N.A., Vadas, M., Lopez, A., Williamson, D.J., Wang, E.A., Wang, C.G., and Clark, S.C. Biologic properties in vitro of recombinant human granulocyte-macrophage colony-stimulating factor. Blood 67: 37, 1986.
113. Walker, F., and Burgess, A.W. Specific binding of radioiodinated granulocyte-macrophage colony-stimulating factor to hemopoietic cells. EMBO J. 4: 933, 1985.
114. Park, L.S., Friend, D., Gillis, S., and Urdal, D.L. Characterization of the cell surface receptors for human granulocyte/macrophage colony stimulating factors. J. Exp. Med. 164: 251, 1986.
115. Koeffler, H.P., and Golde, D.W. Human meyloid leukemia cell lines: A review. Blood 56 (3): 344, 1980.
116. Gough, N.M., Gough, J., Metcalf, D., Kelso, A., Grail, D., Nicola, N.A., Burgess, A.W., and Dunn, A.R. Molecular cloning of cDNA encoding a murine haematopoietic growth regulator, granulocyte-macrophage colony stimulating factor. Nature (Lond.) 309: 763, 1984.
117. Cantrell, M.A., Anderson, D., Cerretti, D.P., Price, V., McKereghan, K., Tushinski, R.J., Mochizuki, D.Y., Larsen, A., Grabstein, K., Gillis, S., and Cosman, D. Cloning, sequence and expression of a human granulocyte macrophage colony-stimulating factor. Proc. Natl. Acad. Sci. (USA) 82: 6250, 1985.

118. Kaushansky, K., Ohara, P.J., Berkner, K., Segal, G.M., Hagen, F.S., and Addamson, J.W. Genomic cloning characterization and multilineage growth-promoting activity of human granulocyte-macrophage colony stimulating factor. Proc. Natl. Acad. Sci. (USA) 83: 3101, 1986.

119. Metcalf, D., and Johnson, G.R. Interactions between purified GM-CSF, purified erythropoietin and spleen conditioned medium on hemapoietic colony formation in vitro. J. Cell. Physiol. 99: 159, 1979.

120. Metcalf, D., Johnson, G.R., and Burgess, A.W. Direct stimulation by purified GM-CSF of the proliferation of multipotential and erythroid precursor cells. Blood 55: 138, 1980.

121. Donahue, R.E., Wang, E.A., Stone, D.K., Kamen, R., Wong, G.G., Sehgal, P.K., Mather, D.G., and Clark, S.C. Stimulation of hematopoiesis in primates by continuous infusion of recombinant human GM-CSF. Nature 3231 (6073): 872, 1986.

122. Stanley, E.R., and Heard, P.M. Factors regulating macrophage production and growth. Purification and some properties of the colony stimulating factor from medium conditioned by mouse L cells. J. Biol. Chem. 252: 4305, 1977.

123. Stanely, E.R., and Guilbert, L.J. Methods for the purifications, assay, characterization and target cell binding of a colony stimulating factor (CSF-1). J. Immunol. Methods 42: 253, 1981.

124. Das, S.K., and Stanley, E.R. Structure-function studies of a colony stimulating factor (CSF-1). J. Biol. Chem. 257: 13679, 1982.

125. Kawasaki, E.S., Ladner, M.B., Wang, A.M., Van Arsdell, J., and Warren, M.K. Cloning of a cDNA encoding human macrophage-specific colony stimulating factor (CSF-1). Science 230: 291, 1985.

126. Ralph, P., Warren, M.K., Lee, M.T., Csejtey, J., Weaver, J.F., Broxmeyer, H.E., Williams, D.E., Stanley, E.R., and Kawaski, E.S. Inducible production of human macrophage growth factor, CSF-1. Blood 68 (3): 633, 1986.

127. Sherr, C.J., Rettenmier, C.W., Sacca, R., Roussel, M.F., Look, A.T., and Stanley, E.R. The c-fms proto-oncogene product is related to the receptor for the mononuclear phagocyte growth factor, CSF-1. Cell 41: 665, 1985.

128. Sacca, R., Stanley, E.R., Sherr, C.J., and Rettenmier, C.W. Specific binding of the mononuclear phagocyte colony-stimulating factor CSF-1 to the product of the v-fms oncogene. Proc. Natl. Acad. Sci. (USA) 83: 3331, 1986.

129. Heisterkamp, N., Groffen, J., and Stephenson, J.R. Isolation of v-fms and its human cellular homolog. Virology 126: 248, 1983.

130. Wisniewski, L.P., and Hirschhorn, K. Acquired partial deletions of the long arm of chromosome 5 in hematologic disorders. Am. J. Hematol. 15: 295, 1983.

131. Rettenmier, C.W., Chen, J.H., Roussel, M.F., and Sherr, C.J. The product of the c-fms proto-oncogene: a glycoprotein with associated tyrosinekinase activity. Science 228: 320, 1985.

132. Sherr, C.J., Rettenmier, C.W., Sacca, R., Roussel, M.F., Look, A.T., and Stanley, E.R. The c-fms proto-oncogene product is related to the receptor for the mononuclear phagocyte growth factor, CSF-1. Cell 41: 665, 1985.

133. Kurland, J.I., Pelus, L.M., Ralph, P., Bockman, R.S., and Moore, M.A.S. Induction of prostaglandin E synthesis in normal and neoplastic macrophages: Role for colony stimulating factor(s) distinct from effects on myeloid progenitor cell proliferation. Proc. Natl. Sci. (USA) 76: 2326, 1979.

134. Moore, R.N., Oppenheim, J.J., Farrar, J.J., Carter, C.S., Jr., Waheed, A., and Shadduck, R.K. Production of lymphocyte-activating factors (interleukin 1) by macrophages activated with colony-stimulating factors. J. Immunol. 125: 1302, 1980.

135. Lin, H.S., and Gordon, S. Secretion of plasminogen activator by bone-marrow-derived mononuclear phagocytes and its enhancement by colony-stimulating factor. J. Exp. Med. 150: 231, 1979.

136. Hamilton, J.A., Stanley, E.R., Burgess, A.W., and Shadduck, R.K. Stimulation of macrophage plasminogen activator activity by colony-stimulating factors. J. Cell Physiol. 103: 435, 1980.

137. Fleit, H.B., and Rabinovitch, M. Interferon induction in marrow-derived macrophages: Regulation by L cell conditioned medium. J. Cell Physiol. 108: 347, 1981.

138. Broxmeyer, H.E., Juliano, L., Waheed, A., and Shadduck, R.K. Release from mouse macrophages of acidic isoferritins that suppress hematopoietic progenitor cells is induced by purified L cell colony stimulating factor and suppressed by human lactoferrin. J. Immunol. 135: 3223, 1985.

139. Wing, E.J., Ampel, N.M., Waheed, A., and Shadduck, R.K. Macrophage colony-stimulating factor (M-CSF) enhances the capacity of murine macrophages to secrete oxygen reduction products. J. Immunol. 135: 2052, 1985.

140. Wing, E.J., Waheed, A., Shadduck, R.K., Nagle, L.S., and Stephenson, K. Effect of colony-stimulating factor on murine macrophages: Induction of antitumor activity. J. Clin. Invest. 69: 270, 1982.

141. Warren, M.K., and Ralph, P. Macrophage growth factor CSF-1 stimulates human monocyte production of interferon, tumor necrosis factor, and myeloid CSF. J. Immunol. 138: 3019, 1987.

142. Nicola, A., Metcalf, D., Matsumoto, M., and Johnson, G.R. Purification of a factor inducing differentiation in murine myelomonocytic leukemia cells: Identification as granulocyte colony-stimulating factor (G-CSF). J. Biol. Chem. 258: 9017, 1983.

143. Metcalf, D., and Nicola, N.A. Proliferative effects of purified granulocyte colony-stimulating factor (G-CSF) on normal mouse hemopoietic cells. J. Cell Physiol. 116: 198, 1983.

144. Nicola, N.A., Metcalf, D., Johnson, G.R., and Burgess, A.W. Separation of functionally distinct human granulocyte-macrophage colony stimulating factors. Blood 54 (3): 614, 1979.

145. Nicola, N.A., Begley, C.G., and Metcalf, D. Identification of the human analogue of a regulator that induces differentiation in murine leukemic cells. Nature 314 (6012): 625, 1985.

146. Lotem, L., Lipton, J.M., and Sachs, L. Separation of different molecular forms of macrophage- and granulocyte-inducing proteins for normal and leukemic myeloid cells. Int. J. Cancer 25: 763, 1980.

147. Burgess, A.W., and Metcalf, D. Characterization of a serum factor stimulating the differentiation of myelomonocytic leukemic cells. Int. J. Cancer 26: 647, 1980.
148. Metcalf, D. Clonal extinction of myelomonocytic leukemic cells by serum from mice injected with endotoxin. Int. J. Cancer 25: 225, 1980.
149. Nicola, N.A., and Metcalf, D. Binding of the differentiation-inducer, granulocyte-colony stimulating factor, to responsive but not unreponsive leukemic cell lines. Proc. Natl. Acad. Sci. (USA) 81: 3765, 1984.
150. Metcalf, D. clonal analysis of the response of HL60 human myeloid leukemia cells to biological response modifiers. Leuk. Res. 7: 117, 1983.
151. Metcalf, D. Regulatory control of the proliferation and differentiation of normal and leukemic cells. J. Natl. Cancer Inst. Monogr. 60: 123, 1982.
152. Ichikawa, Y. Further studies on the differentiation of a cell line and myeloid leukemia. J. Cell Physiol. 76: 175, 1970.
153. Fibach, E., and Sachs, L. Control of normal differentiation of myeloid leukemic cells, VIII. Induction of differentiation to mature granulocytes in mass culture. J. Cell Physiol. 86: 221, 1975.
154. Honma, J., Kasukabe, T., Okabe, J., and Hozumi, M. Prolongation of survival time of mice innoculated with myeloid leukemia cells by inducers of normal differentiation. Cancer Res. 39: 3167, 1979.
155. Metcalf, D. Clonal extinction of myelomonocytic leukemic cells by serum from mice injected with endotoxin. Int. J. Cancer 25: 225, 1980.
156. Metcalf, D. Regulator-induced suppression of myelomonocytic leukemic cells: clonal analysis of early events. Int. J. Cancer 30: 203, 1982.
157. Lotem, J., and Sachs, L. Mechanisms that uncouple growth and differentiation in myeloid leukemia cells: restoration of requirement for normal growth inducing protein without restoring induction of differentiation-inducing protein. Proc. Natl. Acad. Sci. (USA) 79: 4347, 1982.
158. Lotem, J., and Sachs, L. In vivo inhibition of the development of myeloid leukemia by injection of macrophage and granulocyte inducing protein. Int. J. Cancer 28: 375, 1981.
159. Welte, K., Platzer, E., Lu, L., Gabrilove, J.L., Levi, E., Mertelsmann, R., and Moore, M.A.S. Purification and biochemical characterization of human pluripotent hematopoietic colony-stimulating factor. Proc. Natl. Acad. Sci. (USA) 82: 1526, 1985.
160. Svet-Moldavsky, G.J., Zinzar, S., Svet-Moldavsky, I.A., Mann, P.E., Holland, J.F., Fogh, J., Arlin, Z., and Clarkson, B.D. CSF-producing human tumor cell lines: lack of CSF-activity of human stromal bone marrow fibroblasts. Exptl. Hematol. 8 (suppl. 7): 76, 1980.
161. Souza, L.M., Boone, C., Gabrilove, G., Lai, H., Zsebo, M., Murdock, C., Chazin, R., Bruszewski, J., Lu, H., Chen, K., Barendt, J., Platzer, E., Moore, M.A.S., Mertelsmann, R., and Welte, K. Recombinant human granulocyte colony-stimulating factor: Effects on normal and leukemic myeloid cells. Science 232: 61, 1986.
162. Tomida, M., Yamato-Yamaguchi, Y., and Hozumi, M. Purification of a factor inducing differentiation of mouse myeloid leukemic M1 cells from conditioned medium of mouse fibroblast L929 cells. J. Biol. Chem. 259: 10978, 1982.

163. Nomura, H., Imazeki, I., Oheda, M., Kubota, N., Tamura, M., Ono, M., Ueyama, Y., and Asano, S. Purification and characterization of human granulocyte colony stimulating factor (G-CSF). EMBO J. 5 (5): 871, 1986.

164. Nagata, S., Tsuchiya, M., Asano, S., Kuziro, Y., Yamazuki, T., Yamamoto, D., Hirata, Y., Kubota, N., Oheda, M., Nomura, H., and Ono, M. Molecular cloning and expression of cDNA for human granulocyte colony stimulating factor. Nature 319: 415, 1986.

165. Nagata, S., Tsuchiya, M., Asano, S., Yamamoto, O., Hirata, Y., Kubota, N., Oheda, M., Nomura, H., and Yamazaki, T. The chromosomal gene structure and two m-RNAs for human granulocyte colony stimulating factor. EMBO J. 5 (3): 575, 1986.

166. Yokota, T., Lee, F., Rennick, D., Hall, C., Arai, N., Mosmann, T., Nagel, G., Cantor, H., and Arai, K. Isolation and characterization of a mouse cDNA clone that expresses mast cell growth factor activity in monkey cells. Proc. Natl. Acad. Sci. (USA) 81: 1070, 1984.

167. Fung, M.C., Hapel, A.J., Ymer, S., Cohen, D.R., Johnson, R.M., Campbell, H.D., and Young, I.G. Molecular cloning of cDNA for murine interleukin-3. Nature 307: 233, 1984.

168. Howard, M., Burgess, A.W., McPhee, D., and Metcalf, D. T-cell hybridoma secreting hemopoietic regulatory molecules: granulocyte-macrophage and eosinophil colony-stimulating factors. Cell 18: 993, 1979.

169. Nabel, G., Greenberger, J.S., Sakakeeny, M.A., and Cantor, H. Multiple biologic activities of a cloned inducer T-cell population. Proc. Natl. Acad. Sci. (USA) 78: 1157, 1981.

170. Watson, J.D. Biology and biochemistry of T-cell derived lymphokines. I. The co-ordinate synthesis of interleukin-2 and colony-stimulating factors in a murine T-cell lymphoma. J. Immunol. 131: 293, 1983.

171. Platzer, E., Welte, K., Gabrilove, J.L., Lu, L., Harris, P., Mortelsmann, R., and Moore, M.A.S. Biological activities of a human pluripotent hemopoietic colony stimulating factor on normal and leukemic cells. J. Exp. Med. 162: 1788, 1985.

172. Warren, D.J., and Sanderson, C.J. Production of a T-cell hybrid producing a lymphokine stimulating eosinophil differentiation. Immunology 54: 615, 1985.

173. Bartelmez, S.H., Dodge, W.H., Mahmound, A.A.F., and Bass, D.A. Stimulation of eosinophil production in vitro by eosinophilopoietin and spleen cell derived eosinophil growth stimulating factor. Blood 56: 706, 1980.

174. Enokihara, A., Hamaguchi, H., Sakamaki, H., Sukae, H., Saito, K., Furusawa, S., and Shishido, H. Specific production of eosinophil colony stimulating factor from sensitized T-cells from a patient with allergic eosinophilia. Br. J. Hematol. 59: 85, 1985.

175. Strath, M., and Sanderson, C.J. Detection of eosinophil differentiation factor and its relationship to eosinophilia in mesocestodes corti infected mice. Exp. Hematol. 14: 16, 1986.

# 13

# Transfer Factor: Past, Present, and Future

W. Borkowsky / New York University Medical Center, New York, New York

## I. EARLY HISTORY AND DEFINITION

The history of cellular immunology began with the classic experiments of Landsteiner and Chase from 1942-1945 when they successfully transferred delayed-type cutaneous hypersensitivity (DTH) to contact chemicals and tuberculin among outbred guinea pigs (1). Following this lead, Lawrence was able to duplicate the passive transfer of specific local and generalized DTH to tuberculin in humans, employing intradermal injection of viable leukocytes isolated from the peripheral blood of tuberculin-sensitive humans (2). Three years later, in 1952, that study was extended to additionally demonstrate the passive transfer of streptococcal DTH in 14 consecutive instances to streptococcus in nonimmune human recipients by means of viable leukocytes from streptococcal-immune individuals (3).

The phenomenon of "transfer factor" (TF) was established firmly in 1955 when Lawrence described the successful passive transfer of DTH to streptococcal M and tuberculin antigens using only disrupted leukocytes (4). Although Jeter and colleagues had reported on the transfer of DTH to 2,4-dinitrochlorobenzene (DNCB) in guinea pigs with disrupted leukocytes, attempts by his and other labs to repeat this with tuberculin were unsuccessful (5). In addition, whereas the passive transfer of DTH with viable leukocytes was short-lived in the guinea pig and assumed to be due to the effects of the viable transferred cells, the DTH reaction in the recipients of the disrupted leukocytes was relatively long-lasting, exceeding 10 months in 2 of the recipients. In addition, treatment of the leukocyte lysates with the enzymes DNAse and RNAse did not diminish their capacity to transfer DTH. This series of experiments suggested that neither viable donor cells nor their nucleic acids were responsible for the transfer and persistence of the recipient's DTH response and implied that the recipient's cells had acquired the immunologic memory present in the donor.

In 1956 Lawrence and Pappenheimer further elaborated the uniqueness of transfer factor (TF) when, using purified diphtheria toxoid as the test antigen, they demonstrated that the transfer of DTH to nonimmune recipients was not accompanied by the acquisition of circulating antibody to the toxin (6). Furthermore, they were able to transfer DTH not only with disrupted leukocytes but also with the physiologic buffer that the immune viable leukocytes had bathed in for one hour at 37°C. The addition of antigen to the incubating cells increased the release of TF from the immune cells into the surrounding medium, suggesting an interaction between TF and antigen. Since immunoglobulins were then recognized as the smallest antigen recognition units, and DTH was now dissociated from antibody, TF was thrust into the role of a substance whose effects could not be explained by the conventional immunologic dogma.

In 1960, the immunologic consequences of TF administration were extended to include the acquisition of the ability of unimmunized recipients to demonstrate accelerated skin homograft rejection (7). These reactions were antigenically specific in that accelerated rejection was only evident toward skin grafts that the TF donor was sensitized to and not toward other skin grafts. In addition to adding evidence that TF transferred specific immunologic memory from donor to recipient, it established the potential of TF to transfer antigen reactivity produced in the donor by immunization and the ability of the recipient to acquire a reactivity to an antigen never seen before by that recipient. Thus TF did not simply amplify a pre-existent yet subliminally disguised latent hypersensitivity but actually induced DTH de novo. This concept was reinforced by Maurer when he successfully transferred DTH from donors sensitized with a neoantigen, ethylene-oxide-treated human serum albumin to nonimmune individuals using leukocyte extracts (8).

Eichberg et al. designed a very convincing experiment to eliminate the possibility that the ability of TF to transfer DTH required pre-exposure to antigen (9). This group had previously shown the suitability of primates as an animal model of DTH as well as responding to primate TF and human TF activity. Human TF was given to 2 baboons and a chimpanzee who were raised in a germ-free environment. No prior skin tests were performed to avoid sensitization, however, in vitro blastogenic assays confirmed their nonreactivity to multiple antigens. Subsequent skin test and blastogenic responses were strongly positive for the antigens the donor was sensitive to. This experiment strongly supports the above results showing that de novo sensitivity to antigens is induced by TF.

## II. SPECIFICITY

A continuing source of controversy relates to whether TF: (a) is antigen specific in its mode of action; (b) is only an antigen-dependent amplifier molecule; or (c) is an antigen-independent adjuvant. The early work of Lawrence and colleagues suggested that TF transferred antigen-specific immunologic memory de novo to nonimmune recipients. The strongest evidence for this was the appearance of coccidioidin DTH in lifetime East Coast dwelling (coccidioidin-naive) TF recipients and the transfer of accelerated specific skin homograft rejection by TF from highly immunized donors (requiring 4 successive skin grafts) to unsensitized recipients (10). However, Lawrence's experiments involving microbial antigens (i.e., tuberculin, streptococcal antigens, diphtheria toxoid, and coccidioidin) required preliminary skin testing of potential TF recipients to document their nonreactivity to the respective antigens. In addition to this "priming," subsequent skin testing was performed to document the onset and persistence of DTH in TF recipients. Critics argued that repeated skin testing of an immunologically naive recipient could sensitize such an individual to a state of immunologic reactivity by itself. Burger et al. compiled the retrospective experience of collective investigators' skin test experiments where unreactive recipients of either TF or no TF were often repeatedly skin tested (11). The antigens tested ranged from bacterial, fungal, viral, and allogeneic skin grafts to ethylene-oxide-treated serum. Skin test conversion occurred in 67% (330/492) of the TF recipients and in only 5% (5/93) of individuals not receiving TF. These data suggest that repeated skin testing alone cannot induce the appearance of DTH in nonimmune individuals.

Other critics have argued that the experiments accounting for the data presented above do not prove that TF is antigen specific, but only suggest that TF is an antigen-dependent amplification factor or simply an adjuvant. However, Burger has further summarized the skin transfer attempts where TF derived from immune and nonimmune donors has been tested for its ability to transfer DTH. "Immune" TF induced skin test conversion in 78% (157/200) of tests recorded. "Nonimmune" TF was successful in only 8% (12/151) of attempts to transfer DTH. While these results speak strongly for the antigen specificity of TF effects, they also reflect potential biases inherent in retrospective studies where skin test results were evaluated in a nonblinded fashion.

Burger has recently conducted prospective experiments evaluating the specificity of human TF derived from individuals immunized with: (a) keyhole lympet hemocyanin (KLH); or (b) horseshoe crab hemocyanin (HCH); or (c) both KLH and HCH. Preimmunization TF served as the negative control (12). Dermal reactivity to KLH (100 $\mu$g/0.1 ml) and HCH (95 $\mu$g/0.1 ml) was evaluated in nonimmune TF recipients. Significant DTH responses to KLH were seen only in recipients of KLH(+) HCH(−) TF or KLH(+) HCH(+) TF. Significant HCH reactivity was only seen in recipients of HCH(+) KLH(−) TF or HCH(+) KLH(+) TF. These results would appear to suggest that TF functions in an antigen-specific manner to transfer DTH to antigens not commonly experienced among humans. However, Ashorn et al., using both identical lots of TF and an identical experimental protocol, were unable to confirm the specificity seen by Burger (13). DTH responses of KLH were seen in recipients of KLH(−) TF as well as KLH(+) TF. In addition, DTH responses of HCH were seen in HCH(−) TF recipients and not in those receiving HCH(+) KLH(+) TF preparations. Thus, 20-year-old Finnish recipients of TF appeared to acquire nonspecific reactivity to those antigens whereas 40-year-old inhabitants of Portland, Oregon acquired only specific dermal reactivity. This discrepancy has failed to resolve the controversy over specificity of TF.

Although KHL and HCH were chosen as test neoantigens to determine if TF could transfer DTH de novo, it is now believed that subliminal sensitization to these antigens could occur by way of dietary indulgences among seafood lovers. The transfer of DTH to ethylene-oxide-treated serum reported by Maurer using immune TF would appear to qualify as a true de novo transfer. However, attempts to transfer cell-mediated immunity (CMI) to contact allergens have been less than encouraging. Brandriss used dialyzable TF from dinitrochlorobenzene- (DNCB) sensitized donors, who were also purified protein derivative- (PPD) sensitive, to attempt to transfer contact allergy. While 4 of 7 TF recipients developed DTH to PPD, only 2 of 7 recipients developed reactions to DNCB (14). Arala-Chaves and Pinto also attempted to transfer reactivity to DNCB but used immune leukocyte lysates rather than a dialysate. Only 3 of 19 (16%) recipients of TF concurrent with either a 10 or 20 μg challenge of DNCB reacted to the antigen, whereas 0 of 21 control subjects acquired any skin reactivity (15). Epstein and Byers attempted to transfer reactivity to beryllium salts while attempting to investigate whether antigen priming was a prerequisite for such a dermal reaction (16). None of 20 controls repeatedly patch tested with beryllium acquired dermal reactivity, whereas 14 of 39 (37%) of TF recipients who were repeatedly skin tested developed dermal reactivity. However, none of 14 TF recipients reacted to beryllium in the absence of "priming" exposures. Unfortunately, only TF derived from immunized individuals was tested in these experiments and the question of the importance of antigen specificity was not addressed along with the question of "priming" antigenic exposures.

Although these studies with contact antigens suggest that antigen pretreatment is required for the successful transfer of CMI, experiments by Steele would appear to contradict such a conclusion (17). Using leukemic children in hematologic remission who were never previously exposed to the varicella zoster (VZ) virus as TF recipients, he was able to document that 10 of 12 recipients of TF prepared from donors recently recuperated from chicken pox acquired reactivity to 1 of 3 in vitro parameters of VZ specific CMI (lymphocyte blastogenesis, cytotoxicity, and leukocyte inhibitory factor production). Although only 3 of 12 TF recipients became positive to all three parameters, 8 of 12 became positive to 2 of 3 in vitro tests. No skin test evaluation was attempted in this group. In a subsequent clinical trial, 11 of 15 TF recipients acquired DTH responses to a VZ skin test antigen (18).

## III. COMPONENTS OF LEUKOCYTE DIALYSATES

The term transfer factor (TF) was coined originally (6) to designate the material or materials in extracts of blood leukocytes obtained from immune human donors responsible for the transfer of cutaneous delayed type hypersensitivity (DTH) to nonimmune recipients. It was a convenient shorthand, operational description which recognized the need for further purification and characterization of the active moiety present in leukocyte extracts which was resistant to enzymatic treatment with DNAse, RNAse (4), and trypsin (19,20).

Our subsequent findings revealed that this biological activity was dialyzable and could be separated from all of the macromolecules present in the leukocyte extract by dialysis through a Visking cellophane sac of nominal pore size of 40,000 D. To purify the material in the dialysate further we employed Sephadex chromatography and found that activity could be recovered from the eluate of Sephadex G-25 in a broad region where molecules of <10,000 D appear (21).

The dialyzable nature of the activity, its low molecular weight, polypeptide-polynucleotide composition, and the application of Sephadex chromatography for further purification was confirmed rapidly and adopted by several groups of investigators (22-25). However, it soon became apparent that the active moiety bound to Sephadex and as a result of smearing, was reported to appear in different void volumes in various publications (26-28) rather than emerging consistently as a single molecular species.

To complicate matters further it became clear that dialysates containing the antigen-specific moiety, transfer factor, also contained a family of other small, pharmacologically active molecules with adjuvant-like properties. These contaminating molecules consisted of histamine, nicotinamide, ascorbate, serotonin, bradykinin, prostaglandin, cyclic nucleotides (29-31), and most recently, thymosin alpha 1 (32,33).

Thus the search to purify and characterize transfer factor was impeded by the lack of adequate technology available at that time to separate one small molecule from a plethora of other small biologically active molecules (18). This impasse was subsequently ameliorated to a great extent with the introduction and availability of high pressure reverse phase liquid chromatography (HPLC). This technique has been most effectively applied to the purification and characterization of transfer factor by two groups of investigators, Burger et al. (34) and Wilson and Fudenberg (35). Their findings are discussed in detail below.

Our own recent investigations in this area (36-40) have employed the leukocyte migration inhibition (LMI) test, introduced by Wilson and Fudenberg (35) as a reproducible in vitro assay for the antigen-specific activity (transfer factor) present in dialysates of human leukocyte extracts (DLE). Using this assay we have found that dialysates prepared from immune donors contain two opposing antigen-specific activities—an inducer/helper activity which we have termed inducer factor and a suppressor activity which we have termed suppressor factor (36,41).

Inducer factor binds to the related antigen and the activity can be recovered from the antigen immunoadsorbant following treatment with 8 M urea (38,39); it is a product of donor $T_H$ cells which binds to recipient $T_S$ cells and macrophages (40). Inducer factor functions thus to convert nonimmune cell populations to an antigen-specific state of reactivity in a dose-dependent fashion by virtue of its capacity to bind antigen. This results in inhibition of migration of the cells when exposed to the related antigen.

Suppressor factor binds to the related IgG and the activity can be recovered from the antibody-immunoadsorbant following treatment with glycine-HCl; it is a product of donor $T_S$ cells and binds to recipient $T_H$ cells and macrophages (41). Suppressor factor blocks the response of *immune* cell populations in vitro, resulting in a failure to be inhibited in their migration when exposed to the related antigen; it also functions as an anti-transfer (inducer) factor in that it blocks the response of nonimmune cells to inducer factor in a dose-dependent fashion (41).

The inducer factor and the suppressor factor can be separated from contaminating molecules of lower molecular weight by redialysis of the <12,000 D dialysate at a nominal 3500 D cutoff. The antigen-specific inducer factor and suppressor factor appear in the >3500 D dialysis fraction and the smaller molecules asso-

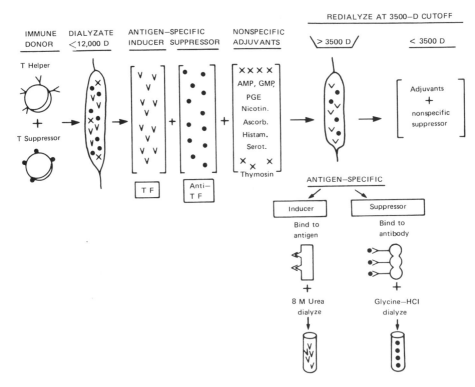

Figure 1  Qualitative analysis of leukocyte dialysates containing inducer factors and suppressor factors of varying specificities—isolation and purification by differential dialysis and affinity immunoadsorption. (From Ref. 95.)

ciated with adjuvant-like activity appear in the <3500 D dialysis fraction. Also detected in the <3500 D dialysis fraction is a nonspecific suppressor activity.

The qualitative analysis of leukocyte dialysates containing inducer and suppressor factors is schematically outlined in Figure 1.

As may be seen in Figure 1, the <120,000 D dialysate prepared from Ficoll-Hypaque-purified human lymphocytes contains a mixture of inducer and suppressor factors of varying antigenic specificities determined by the immunological profile of the donor. The antigen-specific activities are contaminated by an array of smaller molecules with nonspecific adjuvant-like activities (e.g., serotonin, histamine, bradykinin, ascorbate, nicotinimide, prostaglandins, cyclic nucleotides, chemotactic peptides, and thymosin alpha 1). When the <12,000 D dialysate is redialyzed at a 3500 D cutoff, the >3500 D dialysis fraction contains the smaller contaminating molecules. When either the <12,000 or the >3500 D fraction are exposed sequentially to specific antigens, the inducer factor of the related specificity binds to its antigen, is removed from the dialysate, and can be recovered from the immunoadsorbant following treatment with 8 M urea (38, 42). The eluates recovered from such inducer factor depleted dialysates contain suppressor factors of the related specificities which can be removed subsequently by sequential binding to the respective IgG immunoadsorbant and recovered following treatment with glycine-HCl (42).

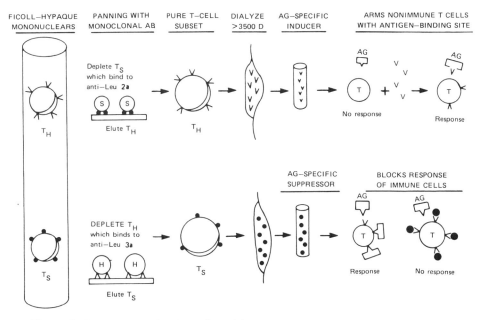

**Figure 2** Preparation of inducer factof from enriched $T_H$ cell populations and suppressor factor from enriched $T_S$ cell populations. (From Ref. 95.)

Since we had observed that the inducer factor is a product of $T_H$ cells (25) and the suppressor factor is a product of $T_S$ cells (26), we have prepared purified $T_H$ and $T_S$ cells using negative selection panning techniques and the respective monoclonal anti-$T_H$ or anti-$T_S$ antibody. The preparation of dialysates from such enriched $T_H$ and $T_S$ cell populations allows one to prepare a more concentrated starting material for subsequent affinity immunoadsorption purification. This approach is diagrammatically outlined in Figure 2.

## IV. IMMUNOCHEMICAL PROPERTIES

Burger et al. have supplied most of the information pertaining to the biochemical properties of human TF as assayed in vivo in their KLH skin transfer system (43). TF activity was found to elute at 2-3 $V_o$ on Sephadex G25 as had been previously suggested by other investigators. TF had an isoelectric point below 2, a finding similar to that of Foster et al., using a murine skin transfer model to measure TF activity (44). TF activity was found in two chromatographic regions by HPLC using octadecyl silane resin with 1% acetic acid or 5% methanol as solvents. These fractions (R1,2 and R 4,5) comigrated with 5' inosine monophosphate (IMP) and inosine, respectively.

The treatment of TF with a variety of enzymes interacting with peptides and nucleic acids resulted in a loss of activity following some treatments but not others. These are summarized in Table 1.

The results of enzyme action on the in vivo effects of TF agree in large part with those effects on TF measured in vitro by Wilson and Fudenberg (45) except for the susceptibility of the HPLC late elution fractions (H4 and R4,5) to alkaline phosphatase (see Table 1). This has resulted in a somewhat different structural model proposed by Wilson with a suggested molecular weight of 2-3000.

Applying the LMI assay in vitro and using a variety of peptide and nucleotide separation techniques, Wilson et al. (47) have recovered human TF activity from Sephadex G25 columns in fractions eluting at 2-3 $V_o$ (Fraction 4b eluting just pre-$V_T$ and fraction 5 eluting at 5/4 $V_T$). Burro TF was only found in fraction 4b. When the active Sephadex fractions were further separated in Biogel P2 columns, TF activity could be recovered in a fraction ($T_X$) which eluted as the smaller of two absorption peaks at approximately twice the void volume using an ammonium bicarbonate buffer (pH 7.8). It is claimed that this represented a 2500-fold purification of TF activity with the fraction consisting of 30% RNA and 70% protein. Subsequent separation of this fraction using HPLC containing an octadecyl silane resin and an acetic acid solvent resulted in the isolation of activity in two components (H5 and H7) with distinct retention times of 10-30 minutes and 45-60 minutes, respectively. Fraction 5 had a mobility close to that of guanosine while fraction 7 had a mobility similar to that of uridine monophosphate (UMP).

Table 1 Enzymatic Treatment of TF

| Enzyme | In vivo DTH induction | | In vitro LIF production | |
|---|---|---|---|---|
| | Humans | Mice | Fr 5 | Fr 7 |
| Pronase | + | + | + | + |
| Proteinase K | + | NT | NT | NT |
| Carboxypeptidase A | + | NT | + | + |
| Trypsin | − | − | − | NT |
| Chymotrypsin | − | NT | − | NT |
| Leucine aminopeptidase | − | NT | − | − |
| Dimerized ribonuclease A | NT | + | NT | NT |
| Deoxyribonuclease | − | − | − | − |
| Ribonuclease A | − | − | − | + |
| T1 ribonuclease | − | NT | + | − |
| P1 nuclease | NT | NT | + | + |
| Phosphodiesterase I | + | + | − | + |
| Phosphodiesterase II | − | NT | + | − |
| Alkaline phosphatase | − | NT | − | + |
| NADase | − | NT | NT | NT |
| Ribosyl transferase A | − | NT | NT | NT |
| Ribosyl transferase B | + | NT | NT | NT |

Key: + = sensitive; − = resistant; NT = not tested.

Wilson et al. (47) have also subjected their HPLC-separated fractions with a variety of chemical and enzymatic treatments. Based on the results summarized in Table 1, they have proposed a model for the nucleopeptide structures of TF fractions 5 and 7. They postulate that TF-5 may be secreted by antigen-activated T cells and become part of a T-cell receptor, while TF-7 is proposed as an intracellular product which may function as a gene regulator.

Burger also found that an n-aminophenyl boronic acid adsorbent with a coplanar cis-diol (ribose) binding capacity bound TF activity. Since Basten et al. (46) had suggested the presence of carbohydrate-determined Ia-like molecules in murine TF, Burger attempted to remove activity with a combination lectin immunoadsorbant with specificities for galactose, glucose, mannose, fucose, sialic acid, N-acetyl glucosamine, and D-glucopyranoside. TF activity was not removed by this lectin nor by a conventional anti-DR immunoadsorbant with specificity for the DR determinants possessed by the TF donor. It should be noted that Borkowsky and Lawrence have demonstrated the removal of TF activity as assayed in the LMI assay by adsorption of the dialysate with polyclonal rabbit and monoclonal murine anti-DR antibodies directed at the public specificities of the Ia structure (40). Thus, the presence of Ia-like molecules in TF remains controversial. Burger has also confirmed the findings of Borkowsky and Lawrence whereby specific TF activity is depleted after absorption with an antigen immunoadsorbant. KLH-specific activity could not be adsorbed by anti-KLH immunoadsorbants but was depleted by a mixture of anti-idiotypic KLH (anti-anti KLH) monoclonal antibodies.

The work has suggested a TF model structure shown below with a possible $V_H$ region present in the peptide moiety. Borkowsky and Lawrence have described the ability of TF "inducer" factor to interact with anti-$V_H$ antibodies produced by Givol and Eisen and directed at framework residues in murine and human immunoglobulin. In addition, they have also described the interaction of the "inducer" factor with antibodies prepared by Marchalonis against T-cell leukemic cells with specificity for human $V_H$ determinants (40).

Very little work has been published on the chemical properties of the suppressor moiety in leukocyte dialysates, by us (36,41) although Wilson and Fudenberg have also described antigen-dependent activity in TF which enhances rather than inhibits leukocyte migration (45). They currently believe that this suppressor-like substance is an enzymatically modified TF with exposed phosphate groups. The relationship between this factor and the one described by Borkowsky and Lawrence remains to be determined.

Both findings, however, suggest that a given TF may be inactive biologically because of the existence of moieties which may compete with or inactivate TF.

## V. ANIMAL MODELS OF INDUCER ACTIVITY

It is of some historical interest that following the demonstration of transfer of cutaneous DTH in humans (2) and in guinea pigs (5) with extracts of leukocytes, early attempts to confirm this observation using leukocyte extracts in laboratory animals, particularly the guinea pig, have been fraught with difficulties. However, more recent work with murine models and the cow suggest that technical problems may have been responsible for these difficulties. The references listed in Table 2 show that TF is not only unrestricted by histocompatibility major histocompatibility complex (MHC) boundaries, but it is also functional across species boundaries.

Basten et al. (46) have demonstrated transfer of immunologically specific CMI responses to DNFB or to PPD between Balb/c mice with TF using macrophage migration inhibition and lymphocyte transformation as in vitro endpoints. These studies have provided clues that may help understand the origins of and avoid the difficulties previously encountered in the detection of TF activity in other laboratory rodents: (a) TF was not present in draining lymph nodes of the

Table 2  Animal Recipient

| TF animal donor | G.P. | Mouse | Rabbit | Monkey | Cow | Dog | Sheep | Chicken | Others | In vitro |
|---|---|---|---|---|---|---|---|---|---|---|
| Guinea pig | 5,48-52 | | | | | | | | | 53-56 |
| Mouse | | 46,57-63 | | | | | | | Human 64 | 65,66 |
| Rabbit | | | 67 | | | | | | Hamster 68 | |
| Monkey | | | | 69,70 | | | | | | |
| Cow | 77 | 71 | 72,73 | | 72-74 | | | | Human 75,76,78 | 79 |
| Dog | | | | | | 80,81 | | | | |
| Sheep | | | | | | | 82-85 | | | |
| Chicken | | | | | | | | 86 | | |
| Burro | | | | | | | | | | 79 |
| Human | 87-88 | 89,90 | | 9,70 | | | | | | See Text |

405

donors at the height of sensitization and appeared only after one month had elapsed; (b) when TF did appear it was detected only in preparations made from lymph node cells but not in preparations made from spleen cells (possibly due to the presence of a suppressor effect); and (c) the activity in the lymph node cell dialysate was separated in a purified Sephadex fraction and its chromatographic pattern resembled that of human TF.

Rifkind et al. (57,58) have also reported on the transfer of footpad DTH reactions and antigen-induced lymphocyte transformation using TF from human donors as well as TF from murine donors administered to CF1 mice. The reactivity transferred was antigen-specific and concordant with the DTH reactions expressed by the donor for coccidioidin, candida, or PPD, respectively. This group repeated these studies using TF prepared from spleen cells of CF1 mice inoculated with *Coccidioides immitis, Candida albicans,* or BCG and confirmed the transfer of antigen-specific CMI to naive mice as measured by cutaneous DTH and footpad swelling. They also found the coccidioidin-specific TF was inactivated by pretreatment with pronase in vitro and the BCG-specific TF was inactivated by pretreatment with snake venom phosphodiesterase (phosphodiesterase I) enzymes which Berger et al. have shown to inactivate human TF (43).

Further enzymatic studies were undertaken by these authors to block the capacity of murine TF to transfer antigen-specific coccidioides or candida DTH and revealed the pretreatment of TF in vitro with dimerized ribonuclease A abolished this activity, whereas pretreatment with monomeric ribonuclease A was without effect on the capacity to transfer DTH. The authors interpret their data to suggest that murine TF contains ribonucleotides complexed to pronase-sensitive peptides and that the ribonucleotide component is as essential as the peptide component for the biological activity of this complex. Thus, murine TF expresses identical susceptibility and resistance to treatment with specific enzymes as has been reported for human TF by Burger et al. Additionally, the same stringent requirement of a peptide-ribonucleotide complex for the expression of the biological activity of murine TF suggests a structural similarity to human TF.

These findings are of interest in relation to the evidence that TF prepared from other species is capable of transferring antigen-specific DTH and CMI responses to various inbred lines of mice. We have discussed above the cross-species transfer of antigen-specific footpad DTH and lymphocyte transformation to PPD and oocyst antigen to C57 BL/6 mice by means of bovine TF. The additional test of specificity in this system was the demonstration of resistance to infectious challenge with oocysts in the TF-treated animals and the subsequent serial transfer of both CMI and resistance to infectious challenge from immune cattle to naive mice and then serially to secondary naive mice recipients (see Ref. 106).

Olson and Drube (see Ref. 107) have reported on the antigen specificity and suvival from lethal challenge with influenza virus (Az Japan 305) in Swiss-Webster mice treated with TF prepared from the peritoneal exudate cells of immunized guinea pigs. In preliminary studies the influenza-specific guinea pig TF also was shown to transfer antigen-specific cutaneous DTH in vivo to influenza virus but not to candida to other guinea pigs. Groups of naive mice were next given influenza immune guinea pig TF and 3 days before, at 0 time, and 3 days after intranasal challenge with 1 $LD_{50}$ of virus and observed 10 days for death or survival. By the 10th day only 40-55% of untreated mice were alive compared to 80-100% survivors in the group treated with TF 3 days before virus challenge. Unprotected mice started to die on day 6 and reached the maximum of 60% by the 10th day, while 100% of the group that received TF 3 days before challenge survived through the 14th day. In addition to significantly improved survival, the lungs of the TF-treated mice exhibited less cellular infiltration, consolidation, and epithelial stripping on histological examination, did not exhibit viral-induced leukopenia, and exhibited reduced viral replication by 1-2 logs with more rapid clearance of virus from their lungs compared to the untreated control groups of mice.

In additional tests of the specificity of protection, the authors compared the protective effects of guinea pig TF of different antigenic specificities on survival of mice challenged with candida infection. The survival at 31 days of untreated control mice was 0% compared to 50% survival of mice treated with candida-immune guinea pig TF 3 days before challenge with candida infection. Of additional interest were the relative rates of survival from candida infection in groups of mice treated with guinea pig TF of unrelated specificities: influenza-immune TF resulted in 10% survival; klebsiella-immune TF resulted in 20% survival; and nonimmune TF resulted in a 30% survival.

Recent studies done in our laboratories have explored the mouse as an in vivo animal assay system to study the activities of both human TF and murine TF. We find, as have others, that human TF is capable of transferring antigen-specific DTH to naive Balb/c mice (44,59). In these studies SKSD-positive-BSA-negative human TF transferred cutaneous DTH to SKSD (streptokinase-streptodornase) but not to BSA (bovine serum albumin) in Balb/c mice as determined by induration in flank skin and by quantitative uptake of radiolabel ($[^{125}I]UdR$) at skin sites tested with alum-precipitated antigen. Preliminary attempts at partial purification of the components of SKSD-positive human TF responsible for this activity suggest that it resides in the >3500 m.w. dialysis fraction and not in the <3500 m.w. fraction when the <12,000 m.w. crude TF is redialyzed through cellophane with a nominal 3500 m.w. cutoff. Further purification of the >3500 m.w. fraction by ion-exchange chromatography in DEAE Sephadex revealed this biological activity to segregate in fractions II and III.

We have obtained similar results using murine TF in the transfer of antigen-specific cutaneous DTH between Balb/c mice as determined by induration and $[^{125}I]UdR$ uptake at skin test sites in naive recipients (44). In these studies reciprocal tests for specificity were done using SKSD and tetanus toxoid as antigens and lymph node cells or spleen cells from immunized mice as the source of TF. It was found that SKSD-positive-toxoid-negative TF transferred cutaneous DTH to SKSD but not to tetanus toxoid and conversely toxoid-positive-SKSD-negative TF transferred cutaneous DTH to tetanus toxoid but not to SKSD. Additionally, lymph node cells proved to be a more potent source of TF than spleen cells and larger skin reactions were transferred to tetanus toxoid than to SKSD corresponding to the degree of reactivity achieved in the respective TF donor.

To delineate the cell type responsible for this murine TF activity, lymph node cells obtained from immunized mice were fractionated on a nylon wool column into a nonadherent fraction enriched in T cells (95% T cells, <2% B cells) and an adherent fraction enriched in B cells (86% B cells, 20-25% T cells) (see Ref. 139).

The activity of TF prepared from nonadherent and from adherent nylon-wool cell fractions, respectively, was compared to that of TF prepared from unseparated lymph node cells. It was found that the TF preparation with the capacity to transfer antigen-specific cutaneous DTH resided in the nonadherent T-cell-enriched fraction and not in the adherent B-cell-enriched fraction of lymph node cells. This finding agrees with identical results which we have obtained using nylon-wool separated viable lymph node lymphocytes in an adoptive cellular transfer system, where the capacity to transfer with viable lymphocytes was also found to reside in the nonadherent fraction and not in the adherent fraction.

Kirkpatrick et al. (62) have recently described the transfer of delayed hypersensitivity with spleen cell dialysates in mice using synthetic polyaminoacid antigens. Dialysates from $GAT^{10}$-sensitized donors sensitized recipients to $GAT^{10}$, but not to $GLA^{5}$ or cytochrome c, whereas dialysates from $GLA^{5}$-sensitized donors sensitized recipients to $GLA^{5}$, but not to $GAT^{10}$ or cytochrome c. They subsequently confirmed the ability of TF to bind antigen using this murine model (63). The incubation of TF-containing dialysates from ferritin-sensitized mice on ferritin-coated plastic surfaces removed the antigen-sensitizing activity whereas incubation of the same preparation on cytochrome c-coated surfaces did not deplete this activity. In contrast, cytochrome c-specific TF activity was removed upon incubation on cytochrome c-coated surfaces but not with incubation on ferritin-coated surfaces. As we had shown using the LMI assay system (38), they were also capable of recovering TF activity from the antigen absorbant with 8 M urea and additionally with acetonitrile. These experiments using in vivo footpad swelling as an endpoint also confirm the validity of the human LMI assay as a parallel model of in vitro effects of TF since results obtained in both models are in agreement with respect to the activities in TF and the antigen binding by TF.

An additional animal model for studies using TF has been reported by Liburd et al. in the rat (92). The endpoint measured in the rat following transfer was not cutaneous DTH, but immunity to infection with an intracellular protozoan parasite (*Eimeria neisulzi*). These investigators prepared TF from the lymphoid tissues of rats that had experienced coccidiosis infection and were immune to the parasite. Immune TF was given to nonimmune rate 48 hours before challenge with the infectious agent and the number of oocysts excreted in the stool was measured as an index of immunity. Rats given immune TF experienced a

7-fold reduction of oocyst excretion (ca. $5 \times 10^6$) compared either to untreated control animals (ca. $35 \times 10^6$) or controls that had received nonimmune TF. The rats treated with immune TF before the primary challenge with *Eimeria* were completely immune to a second challenge with the parasite. As indicated above similar protective effects versus infectious challenge with *Eimeria* oocysts subsequently have been confirmed both in cattle (73) and in mice (106) using bovine TF prepared from immunized calves.

Most recently, crude leukocyte lysates from immune sheep have transferred CMI to nonimmune sheep as measured by resistance to infectious challenge with gastrointestinal nematode parasites (82). On challenge with the respective worm (*T. axei, O. circumcineta,* or *T. colubriformis*) the recipients of immune leukocyte lysate responded with a decreased worm burden compared to controls (e.g., 7720 vs. 12,690). Similarly, the pretreatment of lambs with specifically immune leukocyte lysates before infectious challenge resulted in a decreased worm burden of such recipients (5949) which was similar to the response of actively immunized animals (4447) and differed from the response of the unimmunized control group (12,937).

Klesius et al. (72) prepared TF from the lymph nodes of calves immunized with oocysts of *Eimeria bovis* and transferred cutaneous DTH to oocyst antigen which was comparable to that achieved in control animals receiving viable immune lymphocytes. They next examined the effectiveness of pretreatment of 5 calves with oocyst-specific immune TF 7 days before challenge with *E. bovis* infection. The TF-treated calves responded like actively immunized control calves with mean oocyst excretion per gram of 3.6 compared to 47.6 of 5 control calves. These authors also showed that TF prepared from calves with cutaneous DTH to oocyst antigen and to diphtheria toxoid could transfer both reactivities across species to rabbits, dogs, and rhesus monkeys.

Subsequent studies by this group showed a 39.8% reduction of oocyst excretion in 9 additional calves treated with oocyst-specific TF before challenge when compared to 11 untreated control calves among whom 3 deaths occurred (93). Sephadex G-25 chromatography yielded bovine TF activity in a purified fraction which eluted at $2.6 \times V_0$ under a peak with ultraviolet absorption 254/280 similar to human TF fractionated by this means. In more recent reports the above studies have been extended to include use of ethanol-precipitated bovine TF fractions (74). The TF had been prepared by leeching TF from cells by incubation of lymphocytes for 4 hours at $37^\circ$C in Hanks' solution and dialyzing the culture supernatant. It is of interest that the ethanol-precipitated bovine TF, when reconstituted, transferred cutaneous DTH and lymphocyte blastogenesis to *E. bovis* oocyst antigen and to PPD to 6 calves, while the supernatant from which the TF was precipitated failed to do so in 4 calves.

Evaluation of prior skin testing as a requirement to prime the calves for expression of TF activity revealed no difference in the results achieved. An additional group of 6 calves that had no prior skin tests responded to *E. bovis*-positive-PPD-positive TF administration with acquisition of significant cutaneous DTH reactivity and lymphocyte transformation to each antigen. To evaluate further the specificity of TF as well as the role of prior skin testing in priming the recipient, 5 additional calves were skin tested with PPD but not KLH and then given PPD-positive-KLH-negative TF. This resulted in conversion of cutaneous DTH and lymphocyte transformation to PPD. The skin test to KLH was withheld and lymphocyte transformation test with KLH in vitro revealed no reactivity had been transferred. Subsequent administration of KLH-positive TF to the same calves resulted in the conversion of cutaneous DTH reactivity in 4 of 5 and lymphocyte transformation in 5 of 5 to KLH. The cutaneous reactivity and lymphocyte responses to PPD remained unchanged. The authors interpret their findings to support evidence for the specificity of TF and that prior exposure to antigen via skin test is not obligatory for its activity to be expressed.

The most recent extension of this work on bovine TF has been the transfer of resistance to infection to C57 BL/6 mice subsequently challenged with *E. ferrisi* (71). The TF was prepared from lymph nodes of cattle immune to *E. bovis* and reactive to PPD and transferred CMI responses to PPD and to oocyst antigen as judged by DTH footpad reactions and lymphocyte transformation tests. Prior treatment with the same *E. bovis*-immune TF conferred protection on a group of 10 nonimmune mice when subsequently challenged with *E. ferrisi* infection. This immunity resulted in a decrease of oocyst excretion by 68% over control nonimmune mice.

Of further interest are experiments designed to evaluate the capacity of TF to effect a serial transfer of CMI from calf to mouse to mouse. For this purpose, a group of naive mice that had developed footpad DTH responses and lymphocyte transformation to oocyst antigen as a result of administration of immune bovine TF served in turn as secondary donors. TF prepared from spleen lymphocytes from such mice made immune by TF also transferred resistance to infectious challenge to a group of 10 nonimmune mice. The immunity induced by TF resulted in a decrease of oocyst excretion by 79% over control nonimmune mice. Additionally, in this system Klesius et al. (94) compared the efficacy of active immunization with infectious oocysts to immunization with immune bovine TF in the protection achieved in C57 BL/6 mice upon infectious challenge. It was found that a single dose of oocysts failed to confer protection and several consecutive, large doses were required to induce resistance which was comparable to that produced by a single dose of immune bovine TF.

Of great interest was the finding that immune bovine TF given orally to mice in their drinking water was equally effective in inducing resistance to infectious challenge with oocysts. This finding is consonant with Mohr's (95) suggestion that TF released from degenerate mononuclear cells in the colostrum of nursing mothers may be responsible for transfer of DTH and CMI which has been demonstrated in human infants following breast feeding. In other studies Jeter et al. (96) have reported on the capacity of coccidioidin-positive and tuberculin-

positive bovine TF as well as tuberculin-positive human TF to confer specific cu-
utaneous DTH responses following oral administration to human subjects.

Most recently Berger et al. (91,97) have reported on the transfer of KLH-
specific cutaneous DTH to humans following the injection of bovine TF prepared
from cattle immunized with KLH. This observation paves the way for the use of
bovine TF in the treatment of human disease and should lead to virtually unlimited supplies of a well standardized, highly purified preparation of TF of desired
antigenic specificity that is readily available for clinical trials.

## A. Nonhuman Primates

Transfer factor has proved as consistently successful in the transfer of DTH and
CMI between nonhuman primates as well as from human to primate and the results have been as predictable and repetitive as transfers achieved between humans. The species include monkey (rhesus, macaca, cebus), baboon, marmoset,
and chimpanzee. The antigens used covered a broad range of specificities including
keyhole limpet hemocyanin (KLH), tuberculin (PPD), streptokinase-streptodornase (SKSD), schistosomal antigen, herpes simplex virus 1 (HSV-1), hepatitis-B
surface antigen (HBsAg), candida, tetanus toxoid, and coccidioidin. The recurrent
conclusion derived from studies detailed below is that recipient animals acquired
only DTH and CMI responses to those antigens to which the human or nonhuman
primate donor was reactive and not to control antigens to which the donor was
unreactive. A more stringent test of the antigenic specificity of TF was also evident when gnotobiotic (germ-free) animals were shown to respond to TF administration the same as normal controls. This unique demonstration excludes any
possible contribution of prior antigenic exposure to the effects of TF observed.

Perhaps the most convincing test of the specificity of TF derives from Pas-
teurian experiments demonstrating that prior administration of HSV-1-immune
TF prevented infection and death in marmosets upon lethal challenge with HSV-1
but had no effect on the responses to lethal challenge with *Herpes saimiri*.

To summarize the data on primates: Maddison et al. (98) prepared TF by the
usual method from blood leukocytes of macaca mulatta monkeys sensitive to
mycobacterial antigens and transferred cutaneous reactivity to PPD but not to
schistosomal antigens to nonimmune monkeys, and conversely, TF prepared from
blood or lymph nodes of infected monkeys reactive to schistosomal antigens,
transferred cutaneous DTH to schistosomal antigens but not to PPD. Lymphocytes taken from two animals of the latter group following in vivo transfer, responded to schistosomal antigen in vitro with transformation and proliferation.
These investigators also prepared TF from tuberculin-positive human donors who
were unreactive to schistosomal antigens. The nonimmune monkey recipients of
such human TF developed biopsy-positive cutaneous DTH to PPD but not to
schistosomal antigen controls in vivo, and their lymphocytes also responded to
PPD in vitro with transformation and proliferation. These in vitro and in vivo
effects of TF are similar to those described following human-to-human transfer.

In subsequent studies Maddison et al. (99) evaluated the protective effect of administering TF to monkeys (rhesus) which were subsequently challenged by infection with 1000 cercariae of *Schistosoma mansoni*. It was found that administration of TF prepared from either immune or nonimmune monkeys had no effect on the worm burden of the experimental group compared to untreated controls. However when hyperimmune antiserum was administered along with either normal or immune TF, significant protection and decreased worm burden resulted following infectious challenge. This result is of interest in relation to the reported failure of TF alone to alter the course of human schistosomiasis (139).

Gallin and Kirkpatrick (100) have also reported on successful transfer in vivo of cutaneous DTH to monkeys (rhesus) using human TF and determined by skin biopsy. These authors used human donors who expressed different patterns of cutaneous reactivity to mumps, SKSD, candida, and PPD and found the monkey recipients acquired cutaneous reactivity only to those antigens to which the donor was reactive, not to those to which he was unreactive. They also showed that this activity could be segregated in purified fractions of TF isolated by chromatography on Sephadex G-25.

Zanelli and Adler (101) also have successively transferred cutaneous DTH to monkeys (rhesus) using TF from human donors reactive to tuberculin (PPD), to keyhole limpet homocyanin (KLH), or to both antigens. The results were assessed by gross appearance and confirmed by biopsy of skin test reactions. The transferred state of sensitivity was detectable within 48 hours after administration of TF and endured for at least 3 months with diminishing intensity of cutaneous DTH reactions upon retesting. The results of transfer with human TF were immunologically specific, and recipient monkeys developed reactivity only to PPD but not to KLH when the donor was reactive to PPD only, and conversely only to KLH but not to PPD when tuberculin-negative donors reactive to KLH were used to prepare TF.

Steele et al. (102) using human TF or baboon TF transferred antigen-specific cutaneous DTH in vivo and lymphocyte proliferation in vitro to baboons, cebus monkeys, and marmosets. The antigenic specificity of TF was confirmed by the failure to transfer either cutaneous DTH or lymphocyte proliferation to antigens towhich the donors were unreactive. The antigen-specific reactivities transferred by immune TF were candida, mumps, tetanus, coccidioidin, and HSV-1. The negative control antigens to which reactivity was not transferred were PPD, histoplasmin, and HSV-2. The cumulative conversion rate following administration of human TF was 45% for cutaneous DTH and 75% for the antigen-induced lymphocyte transformation test, while the conversion rate following administration of baboon TF was 17% for cutaneous DTH and 33% for the lymphocyte transformation test.

Steele et al. (103) went on to evaluate the protective effect of human TF prepared from donors immune to herpes simplex (HSV-1) and administered to marmosets before lethal challenge with HSV-1 virus infection. Of the 15 marmosets challenged with HSV-1 only the 2 animals that were pretreated 32 weeks before virus challenge with specific TF ($1 \times 10^8$ lymphocyte equivalents) survived and only 1 of 2 animals that were pretreated with TF 3 days before virus challenge survived. The remaining 8 animals that received specific TF at the time of challenge or 1, 3, and 7 days after virus challenge died as did the 3 untreated control animals.

The human donor of TF used in the above experiments had a positive lymphocyte transformation response to HSV-1 but a negative response to HSV-2 and *H. saimiri*. The specificity of TF was supported by the failure of other marmosets given this TF to develop blastogenic response to HSV-2 or to *H. saimiri* in the face of developing CMI responses to HSV-1. Additionally, 3 of 3 marmosets pretreated with this same HSV-1-specific TF died of malignant lymphoproliferative disease following challenge with *H. saimiri* virus.

This group has also studied the effects of human TF administration to gnotobiotic (germ-free) primates (chimpanzee, baboon) in the absence of exposure to prior skin tests (104). Lymphocyte transformation responses to antigen were determined pre- and post-TF administration while skin tests were withheld for 2 days after TF administration. The recipients only developed lymphocyte transformation responses and cutaneous DTH reactivities to antigens to which the donor was reactive (mumps, HSV-1, tetanus, candida, coccidioidin) and not to antigens to which the donor was unreactive (HSV-2, PPD, histoplasmin). The transfer efficiency was 73% for in vitro and 67% for in vivo tests. The results achieved in such germ-free primates indicate that TF is able to induce CMI responses both in vivo and in vitro in the absence of a "priming" exposure to antigen in the environment or by skin tests with antigens, and that the transfers achieved are immunologically specific.

Trepo and Prince have also reported on the transfer of antigen-specific leukocyte migration inhibition and cutaneous DTH to hepatitis B surface antigen (HBsAg) to 3 chimpanzees who were chronic asymptomatic carriers of HBsAg for more than 2 years (105). In one set of experiments TF was prepared from a human donor reactive to PPD and to HBsAg and both reactivities transferred to the chimpanzee recipient. Conversely, TF prepared from a chimpanzee donor reactive to HBsAg and unreactive to PPD transferred reactivity to HBsAg but not to PPD to the chimpanzee recipient.

## VII.  ANIMAL MODELS OF SUPPRESSOR ACTIVITY

In vivo experimentation with suppressor factors in leukocyte dialysates are in their infancy. The first studies have utilized murine models to demonstrate a suppression of cell-mediated immunity. Borkowsky and Lawrence were able to demonstrate that inoculation of crude dialysates from diphtheria and tetanus toxoid immune mice were able to cause a 40% diminution of specific footpad swelling when given to immune mice simultaneously with footpad antigen inoculation. This suppression was largely depleted when the animals were retested 2 months later. However mice treated with the same dialysates depleted of inducer activity by preabsorption on antigen absorbants continued to be suppressed in their delayed type hypersensitivity responses 2 months after a single inoculation of dialysate. Mice treated with a sham dialysate such as purified inducer factor (eluted from the antigen immunoabsorbant) and mice treated with suppressor-depleted dialysates (by virtue of immunoabsorption with antitoxoid antibody) demonstrated no evidence of suppression (41).

We have extended these studies (108) using a murine model of type 1 diabetes mellitus which requires that a disease-susceptible strain of mice (CD-1) receive multiple low doses of the pancreatic beta-cell toxin, streptozotocin (STZ). These mice become progressively diabetic beginning one week after such treatment with histologic evidence of an autoimmune insulitis. When these mice are given crude dialysate derived from an STZ-resistant strain of mice (Balb/c) simultaneously with the STZ, the onset of diabetes is delayed for several months. More impressively, CD-1 mice treated with such dialysate early in their disease do not demonstrate any further progression with a stabilization of their plasma glucose values and their insulitis with a resultant preservation of islets as detected by histologic examination. This effect perseveres for over 3 months after therapy with the dialysates. Such dialysates are even more effective in suppressing autoimmune diabetes after they have been preabsorbed on a rat insulinoma cell line which may be eliminating any inducer activity which may abrogate suppressor activity (unpublished observations).

The presence of an antigen-specific suppressor factor with in vivo long-lasting activity in crude lymphocyte dialysates may prove to be a potent immunotherapeutic modality for the treatment of known or suspected autoimmune diseases. It also may be a contributor to some of the inconsistencies encountered by investigators attempting to produce immunopotentiation in certain disease states.

## VII.  CLINICAL TRIALS

Since the mid-1960s TF has been used to treat a variety of diseases which responded poorly to available therapies. Unfortunately, the serious nature of many of these diseases has precluded the design of randomized clinical trials. Nevertheless, it is worth reviewing some of these experiences.

### A.  Treatment of Congenital Immunodeficiency States

The Wiskott-Aldrich syndrome is characterized by severe recurrent infections, related to diminished cell-mediated immunity, eczema, thrombocytopenia, hemolytic anemia, and lymphoma. Spitler (109-111) have treated 32 such patients with TF. Forty-four percent of treated patients appeared to benefit from therapy.

Conversion of immunologic reactivity correlated with clinical benefit. The median survival was greater than 5 years in the patients who responded to TF whereas it was only 18 months in those who showed no clinical benefit. Since the mechanisms causing this disease are unknown, one cannot speculate why some patients responded to TF while others did not. However, any therapeutic successes of TF in this disease as well as in other congenital immunodeficiencies without any obvious isolated immunodeficiencies such as the hyperimmunoglobulinemia E syndrome (112,113) are likely to result from the nonspecific adjuvant-like molecules present in crude dialysates as well as the antigen-specific ones.

## B. Fungal Disease

In contrast to the previously mentioned immunodeficiencies, chronic mucocutaneous candidiasis (CMC) appears to represent a disease with a specific lacunar defect in immunity, the inability to mount a cell-mediated response to candida. Several investigators have documented the efficacy of TF in the therapy of this disease (114-117). However, these investigators failed to evaluate the role of specific inducer factors on the success of these responses. David et al. treated one such patient with active disease and no candida-specific release of migration inhibition factor (MIF) with TF prepared from an individual with strong reactivity to candida. This resulted in a clinical remission and the restoration of MIF production. In time, this patient relapsed and was treated with TF prepared from an individual responsive to streptococcal antigens but unresponsive to candida. Neither a clinical remission nor MIF production was seen following this therapy. Subsequent treatment with candida-immune TF, however, resulted in another clinical remission and immunologic recovery (118). This suggests the requirement for treatment with TF derived from individuals strongly immune to the antigen to which the patient is unreactive and which results in the disease state. Kirkpatrick has also reviewed the therapy of 12 patients with CMC. All were anergic to candida. Five patients received TF from individuals not immune to candida. Seven patients were treated with candida-immune TF. Only those patients who acquired skin test reactivity to candida achieved clinical remissions. This was most commonly achieved with candida-immune TF (119).

## C. Mycobacterial Disease

Although most individuals with mycobacterial disease are capable of eradicating these bacteria, particularly in the presence of effective chemotherapy, occasional patients fail to do so. These patients always have an associated anergy to mycobacterial antigens. Rubinstein et al. treated one such patient suffering from progressive tuberculosis with tuberculin-immune TF. Within 2 weeks of initiation of TF therapy, improvement in both pulmonary and bone disease was noted objectively and the patient continued to a cure over the ensuing weeks (120). Zielenski et al. have recently reported their findings of TF therapy of 11 patients with fistulating tuberculosis of bones and joints whose diseases had persisted for a mean of 20 years and had proved to be resistant to antibiotics and tuberculostatic drugs. After 2 years of pooled TF therapy derived from individuals that are largely responsive to tuberculin, a closure of the fistulae was achieved in 9 of the 11 patients with a concomitant decrease in symptoms (121). Other investigators have successfully treated disseminated atypical mycobacterial infections such as *M. avium-intracellulare, M. fortuitum,* and *M. xenopi* with antigen-specific TF. In each case therapy with nonspecific TF was unsuccessful (122-124). In addition, Sharma et al. have reported their successful treatment of progressive BCG infection in an immunodeficient child with TF from a tuberculin-positive donor (125).

## D. Parasitic Infections

Cutaneous leishmania infection in humans is usually a self-limited disease. In rare cases persistent infection in an otherwise normal individual occurs. Sharma et al. used TF to treat individuals with disease who failed to respond to antiprotozoal therapy. Therapy was given in a blinded protocol as either no TF, leishmanin-immune TF, or nonimmune TF. Healing of cutaneous lesions was most apt to occur in those receiving immune TF and least likely to occur in those not receiving TF (126). These results again suggest the need to select donors of TF with antigenic specificity related to the infectious agent.

Cryptosporidiosis is usually a self-limited gastrointestinal infection caused by the coccidian parasitic cryptosporidium, a relative of the *Eimeria* species treated in animals by Klesius et al. (72-74). However this parasite produces an unrelenting gastroenteritis in individuals suffering from the acquired immunodeficiency syndrome (AIDS). This disease appears unresponsive to any chemotherapy and frequently causes the death of the host. Louie et al. (127) have recently treated 8 AIDS patients suffering from unresponsive cryptosporidiosis with bovine TF delivered orally at weekly intervals for 3 months. The bovine donors of the TF had recently survived challenge with the parasite. Five of 8 patients experienced a clinical improvement to therapy and of these 3 individuals completely cleared their stool of oocysts for some period of time.

## E. Viral Infections

Herpes virus infections have been the subject of extensive TF immunotherapy trials. They have responded well as a group to such therapy. As mentioned earlier, Steele et al. have successfully transferred both cell-mediated immune responses and protection from infection to varicella zoster virus infection in susceptible children suffering from acute lymphoblastic leukemia (17,18). Two studies have shown a clear cut decrease in recurrences of herpes simplex (HSV-1 or HSV-2) in patients who were experiencing unusually frequent reactional disease after treatment was initiated with HSV-specific TF (128,129). Chronic cytomegalovirus (CMV) infection in infants has also been treated with CMV-specific TF. In one study viruria ceased after treatment with human TF (130). In another study viremia and viruria ceased and was accompanied by clinical improvement after oral bovine TF therapy. The donor of the TF had been immunized with bovine rhinotracheitis virus, a herpes virus which is antigenically cross-reactive with human CMV (131).

Shulman et al. have conducted a controlled prospective double blinded trial of TF in the treatment of hepatitis B-associated chronic active hepatitis (132). TF was prepared from adults who had recovered from acute hepatitis B and was given to 5 patients. Placebo was given to 4 patients. Four of the TF-treated patients showed clinical, biochemical, and histologic improvements. None of the placebo-treated group showed improvement.

## F.  Tumor Immunotherapy

Osteogenic sarcoma is a malignancy of young adults which in 1971 was amenable only to surgical excision and radiotherapy. The 3-year survival rate after such therapy was about 10-20% because the majority of patients have subclinical pulmonary metastases at the time of diagnosis. Levin et al. initiated studies at that time with TF immunotherapy (133). The group had noted that household contacts of patients had significantly higher levels of cellular cytotoxicity against an osteogenic sarcoma cell line than did noncontacts and these served as TF donors. Phase I studies were performed with patients bearing nonresectable primary or metastatic tumors. This group showed no increase in survival as compared to historical controls. Phase II trials were initiated in 7 clinically disease-free patients. Injections of TF were begun shortly after surgery and were continued at 2-week intervals for 2 years. One patient died at 33 months while the others are disease free 5-7 years after surgery. This survival was significantly longer ($p<.01$) compared to historic controls (133-135).

Blume et al. treated 100 patients with stage 1 malignant melanoma with TF prepared from unselected blood donors. The actuarial nonfailure rate was 90% with a survival rate of 99% at 5 years. A nonrandomized control group treated with surgery alone was found to have a nonfailure rate of 63% and a survival rate of 69%. This study thus suggested a successful adjuvant effect in early melanoma (136).

Fujisawa et al. randomized 149 patients with primary resected lung cancers to receive TF prepared from household contacts or a placebo. The overall survial rates of the TF-treated group at 2 and 4 years postoperatively were 69% and 53%, respectively. Although these were 15% better than the placebo-treated group, only the stage I and II patients treated with TF survived significantly longer than controls (90% vs. 60%, $p<.05$). There was no significant effect apparent in patients with more advanced disease (137).

In summary, TF tumor immunotherapy may prove efficacious in the treatment of early stage solid tumors. It is not apparent if the donor source of the TF is important to achieve this effect.

## IX. PROSPECTS FOR THE FUTURE

Advances in molecular biology and other technologies offer the possibility of removing the mystery that has always shrouded TF. The ability to purify, sequence, and clone the molecules in dialysates responsible for antigen-specific inducer and suppressor activity will allow comparisons to other T-lymphocyte-derived molecules such as the antigen receptor. We have taken steps toward this goal by creating human T-cell hybridomas which produce dialyzable molecules containing antigen-specific inducer activity (138). Unfortunately, human T-cell hybrids are very unstable, as compared to murine T-cell hybrids. In addition, mere fentamoles of TF produce biologic activity while nano- to micromoles of material are required for sequencing. Thus the development of better suited T-cell lymphoma parental cells for the production of human hybrids or more stable human murine hybridomas will be needed for the production of sufficient quantities of material for sequencing.

The discovery of bovine TF which can protect cattle and mice from coccidiosis and which is also effective in man promises to provide a potent, well standardized, virtually unlimited source of material of desired antigenic specificity for human use. Hormonal peptides of bovine origin have been administered to humans for decades with safety and efficacy. It would only require immunization of cattle with the infectious agent or tumor cell line required to produce a TF of desired specificity. Moreover, the availability of large amounts of TF prepared in cattle would allow sequencing of this low molecular weight peptide-ribonucleotide complex, which in turn may be amenable to biosynthetic approaches.

Our discovery of suppressor activity in dialysates (36,41,108) opens up the prospect for possible effective therapy of a variety of human autoimmune diseases where the antigen target is known or suspected such as autoimmune thyroiditis, type 1 diabetes mellitus, rheumatoid arthritis, multiple sclerosis, and chronic active hepatitis. The suppressor factor may also allow for specific allograft suppression required in transplants. Current therapies aim at global suppression of immunity while antigen-specific suppression is undoubtedly preferable.

Whether either antigen-specific augmentation or suppression of immune responses are desired, the presence of both moieties in crude lymphocyte dialysates will necessitate "purification" of these substances prior to initiation of therapy. This can be accomplished by selection of appropriate T cells prior to processing into a dialysate or, alternatively, by appropriate absorption of the crude dialysates on antigen or antibody. These precautions may eliminate the inconsistencies previously encountered in clinical trials using different lots of TF prepared from different sources.

## REFERENCES

1. Chase, M.W. Proc. Soc. Exp. Biol. Med. 59: 135, 1945.
2. Lawrence, H.S. Proc. Soc. Exp. Biol. Med. 71: 516, 1949.
3. Lawrence, H.S. J. Immunol. 68: 159, 1952.
4. Lawrence, H.S. J. Clin. Invest. 34: 219, 1955.
5. Jeter, W.S., Tremaine, M.M., and Seebohm, P.M. Proc. Soc. Exper. Biol. Med. 86: 251, 1954.
6. Lawrence, H.S., and Pappenheimer, Jr., A.M. J. Exp. Med. 104: 321, 1956.
7. Lawrence, H.S., Rappaport, F.T., Converse, J.M., and Tillett, W.S. J. Clin. Invest. 39: 185, 1960.
8. Maurer, P.H. J. Exp. Med. 113: 1029, 1961.
9. Eichberg, J.W., Steele, R.W., Kalter, S.S., Kniker, W.T., Heberling, R.L., Eller, J.J., and Rodriguez, A.R. Cell. Immunol. 26: 114, 1976.
10. Rappaport, F.T., Lawrence, H.S., Miller, J.W., Pappagianis, D., and Smith, C.E. J. Immunol. 84: 358, 1960.
11. Burger, D.R., Vandenbark, A.A., Dunnick, W., Kraybill, W.G., and Vetto, R.M. J. Reticuloendothel. Soc. 24: 385, 1978.
12. Burger, D.R. et al. In *Lymphokines and Thymic Hormones: Their Potential Utilization in Cancer Therapeutics.* Edited by A.L. Goldstein and M.A. Chirigos. Raven Press, New York, 1981, p. 121.
13. Ashorn, R.G.I., Krohn, K.J.E., Vandenbark, A.A., and Acott, K. In *Immunobiology of Transfer Factor.* Edited by C.H. Kirkpatrick, D.R. Burger, and H.S. Lawrence. Academic Press, New York, 1983, p. 311.
14. Brandriss, M.W. J. Clin. Invest. 47: 2152, 1968.
15. Arala-Chaves, M.P., and Pinto, A.S. Int. Arch. Allergy Appl. Immunol. 43: 410, 1972.
16. Epstein, W.L., and Byers, V.S. J. Allerg. Clin. Immunol. 63: 115, 1979.
17. Steele, R.W. Cell. Immunol. 50: 282, 1980.
18. Steele, R.W., Myers, M.G., and Vincent, M.M. N. Engl. J. Med. 303: 355, 1980.
19. Lawrence, H.S. In *Cellular and Humoral Aspects of the Hypersensitive States.* Edited by H.S. Lawrence. Hoeber, New York, 1959, p. 279.
20. Lawrence, H.S. In *Advances in Immunology,* vol. II. Edited by F.J. Dixon and H.G. Kunkel. Academic Press, New York, 1969, p. 195.
21. Lawrence, H.S., Al-Askari, S., David, J., Franklin, E.C., and Zweiman, B. Trans. Assoc. Am. Physicians 79: 84, 1963.
22. Baram, P., and Mosko, M.M. Immunology 8: 461, 1965.
23. Baram, P., Yuan, L., and Mosko, M.M. J. Immunol. 97: 407, 1966.
24. Avala-Chaves, M.P., Lebacq, E.G., and Heremans, J.F. Int. Arch. Allergy Appl. Immunol. 31: 353, 1967.
25. Brandriss, M.W. J. Clin. Invest. 47: 2152, 1968.
26. Neidhart, J.A., Schwartz, R.S., Hurtubise, P.E., Murphy, S.G., Metz, E.N., Balcerzak, S.P., and LoBuglio, A.F. Cell. Immunol. 9: 919, 1973.
27. Zuckerman, K.S., Neidhart, J.A., Balcerzak, S.P., and LoBuglio, A.F. J. Clin. Invest. 54: 997, 1974.
28. Gottlieb, A.A., Foster, L.G., Waldman, S.R., and Lopez, M. Lancet 2: 822, 1973.

29. Gallin, J.S., and Kirkpatrick, CH. Proc. Natl. Acad. Sci. (USA) 71: 498, 1974.
30. Lawrence, H.S. Summation. In *Transfer Factor—Basic Properties and Clinical Applications*. Edited by M.S. Ascher, A.A. Gottlieb, and C.H. Kirkpatrick. Academic Press, New York, 1976, p. 741.
31. Burger, D.R., Vandenbark, A.A., Daves, D., Anderson, W.A., Vetto, R.M., and Finke, P. J. Immunol. 117: 797, 1976.
32. Wilson, G.B., Paddock, G.V., Floyd, E., Newell, R.T., Dopson, M.H. In *Immunobiology of Transfer Factor*. Edited by C.H. Kirkpatrick, D.R. Burger, and H.S. Lawrence. Academic Press, New York, 1983, p. 395.
33. Kirkpatrick, D.H., Khan, A., and McClure, J.E. In *Immunobiology of Transfer Factor*. Edited by C.H. Kirkpatrick, D.R. Burger, and H.S. Lawrence. Academic Press, New York, p. 413.
34. Burger, D., Vandenbark, A., Vetto, R.M. In *Immunobiology of Transfer Factor*. Edited by E.H. Kirkpatrick, D.R. Burger, and H.S. Lawrence. Academic Press, New York, 1983, p. 33.
35. Wilson, G.B., and Fudenberg, H.H. In *Lymphokines*, Vol. 4. Edited by E. Pick and M. Landy. Academic Press, New York, 1981, p. 107.
36. Borkowsky, W., and Lawrence, H.S. J. Immunol. 123: 1741, 1979.
37. Borkowsky, W., Suleski, P., Bhardwaj, N., and Lawrence, H.S. J. Immunol. 126: 80, 1981.
38. Borkowsky, W., and Lawrence, H.S. J. Immunol. 126: 486, 1981.
39. Lawrence, H.S., and Borkowsky, W. Cell. Immunol. 62: 301, 1981.
40. Borkowsky, W., and Lawrence, H.S. In *Immunobiology of Transfer Factor*. Edited by C.H. Kirkpatrick, D.R. Burger, and H.S. Lawrence. Academic Press, New York, 1983, p. 75.
41. Borkowsky, W., Berger, J., Pilson, R., and Lawrence, H.S. In *Immunobiology of Transfer Factor*. Edited by C.H. Kirkpatrick, D.R. Burger, and H.S. Lawrence. Academic Press, New York, 1983, p. 91.
42. Holzman, R., Borkowsky, W., Pilson, R., and Lawrence. H.S. In *Immunobiology of Transfer Factor*. Edited by C.H. Kirkpatrick, D.R. Burger, and H.S. Lawrence. Academic Press, New York, p. 117.
43. Burger, D., Vandenbark, A., Betto, R.M., and Klesius, P. In *Immunobiology of Transfer Factor*. Edited by C.H. Kirkpatrick, D.R. Burger, and H.S. Lawrence. Academic Press, New York, 1983, p. 33.
44. Foster, L.G., Brummer, E., Bhardwaj, N., and Lawrence, H.S. In *Transfer Factor—Basic Properties and Clinical Applications*. Edited by M.S. Ascher, A.A. Gottlieb, and C.H. Kirkpatrick. Academic Press, New York, 1976, p. 397.
45. Wilson, G.B., and Fudenberg, H.H. In *Lymphokines*, Vol. 4. Edited by E. Pick and M. Landy. Academic Press, New York, 1981, p. 107.
46. Basten, A., Croft, A., and Edwards, J. In *Transfer Factor: Basic Properties and Clinical Applications*. Edited by M.S. Ascher, A.A. Gottlieb, and C.H. Kirkpatrick. Academic Press, New York, 1976, p. 75.
47. Wilson, G.B., Paddock, G.V., and Fudenberg, H.H. Thymus 2: 257, 1981.
48. Jeter, W.S., Laurence, K.A., and Seebohm, P.M. J. Bact. 74: 680, 1957.

49. Cummings, M.M., Patnode, R.A., and Hudgins, P.C. Am. Rev. Tuber. Pulm. Dis. 73: 246, 1981.

50. Kochan, I., and Bandel, W.L. J. Allergy 37: 284, 1966.

51. Dunn, D.J., and Patnode, R.A. J. Immunol. 99: 467, 1976.

52. Burger, D.R., and Jeter, W.S. Infect. Immun. 3: 575, 1971.

53. Dunnick, W., and Bach, F.H. Proc. Natl. Acad. Sci. (USA) 72: 4573, 1975.

54. Whitacre, C.C., and Paterson, P.Y. Cell. Immunol. Immunopathol. 13: 287, 1979.

55. Dunnick, W., Burger, D.R., and Vandenbark, A.A. Clin. Immunol. Immunopathol. 17: 55, 1980.

56. Philp, J.R., McCormack, J.G., Moore, A.L., and Johnson, J.E. J. Immunol. 126: 1469, 1981.

57. Rifkind, D., Frey, J.A., Peterson, E.A., and Dinowitz, M. Infect. Immun. 16: 258, 1977.

58. Rifkind, D., Frey, J.A., Davis, J.R., Peterson, E.A., and Dinowitz, M. J. Infect. Dis. 133: 533, 1976.

59. Bhardwaj, N., Brummer, E., Foster, L.G., and Lawrence, H.S. In *Immune Regulators in Transfer Factor*. Edited by A. Khan, C.H. Kirkpatrick, and N.O. Hill. Academic Press, New York, 1979, p. 285.

60. Williams, M.E., and Kauffman, C.A. Infect. Immun. 27: 187, 1980.

61. Petersen, E.A., Greenberg, L.E., Manzara, T., and Kirkpatrick, C.H. J. Immunol. 126: 2480, 1981.

62. Kirkpatrick, C.H., Rozzo, S.J., Mascali, J.J., and Merryman, C.F. J. Immunol. 134: 1723, 1985.

63. Kirkpatrick, C.H., Rozzo, S.J., and Mascali, J.J. J. Immunol. 135: 4027, 1985.

64. Vich, J.M., Garcia, J.U., Engel, P., and Garcia, P.A. Lancet i: 265, 1978.

65. Borkowsky, W., Suleski, P., Bhardwaj, N., and Lawrence, H.S. J. Immunol. 126: 80, 1981.

66. Mayer, V., Gajdosova, E., and Oravec, C. Acta Virol. 24: 459, 1980.

67. Burger, D.R., Cozine, W.S., and Hinrichs, D.J. Proc. Soc. Exp. Biol. Med. 136: 1385, 1971.

68. Tsang, K.Y., Fudenberg, H.H., Wilson, G. In *Immunobiology of Transfer Factor*. Edited by C.H. Kirkpatrick, D.R. Burger, and H.S. Lawrence. Academic Press, New York, 1983. p. 157.

69. Maddison, S.E., Hicklin, M.D., and Kagan, I.G. Exp. Parasitol. 39: 29, 1976.

70. Steele, R.M., Eichberg, J.W., Heberling, R.L., Eller, J.J., Kalter, S.S., and Kniker, W.T. Cell. Immunol. 22: 110, 1976.

71. Klesius, P.H., Qualls, D.F., Elston, A.L., and Fudenberg, H.H. Clin. Immunol. Immunopathol. 10: 214, 1978.

72. Klesius, P.H., Kramer, T., Burger, D., and Malley, A. Transplant. Proc. 7: 449, 1975.

73. Klesius, P.H., and Kristensen, F. Clin. Immunol. Immunopathol. 7: 240, 1977.

74. Klesius, P.H., and Fudenberg, H.H. Clin. Immunol. Immunopathol. 8: 238, 1977.

75. Jeter, W.S., Kibler, R., Soli, T.C., and Stephens, C.A.L. In *Immune Regulators in Transfer Factor*. Edited by A. Khan, C.H. Kirkpatrick, and N.O. Hill. Academic Press, New York, 1979, p. 451.

76. Jones, J.F., Minnich, L.L., Jeter, W.S., Pritchett, R.F., Fulgeniti, V.A., and Wedgewood, R.J. Lancet ii: 122, 1981.

77. LeSourd, B., Marescot, M.R., Doumerc, S., Thiollet, M., Moulias, R., Person, J.F., Ederlenis, A., and Pilet, C.L. In *Immunobiology of Transfer Factor* (see ref. 32) p. 203.

78. Viza, D., Rosenfeld, F., Phillips, J., Vich, J.M., Denis, J., Bonissent, J.F., and Dogbe, K. In *Immunobiology of Transfer Factor* (see ref. 32) p. 245.

79. Wilson, G.B., Newell, R.T., and Burdash, N.M. Cell. Immunol. 47: 1, 1979.

80. Simon, M.R., Silva, J., Freier, D., Bruner, J., and Williams, R. Infect. Immun. 18: 73, 1977.

81. Shifrine, M., Thilsted, J., and Pappagianis, D. In *Transfer Factor: Basic Properties and Clinical Applications.* (see ref. 30) p. 349.

82. Ross, J.G., Duncan, J.L., and Halliday, W.G. Res. Vet. Sci. 26: 258, 1978.

83. Ross, J.G., and Halliday, W.G. Res. Vet. Sci. 27: 41, 1979.

84. Ross, J.G., and Halliday, W.G. Int. J. Parasitol. 9: 281, 1979.

85. Ross, J.G., and Halliday, W.G. Vet. Res. Comm. 4: 287, 1981.

86. Klesius, P.H., and Kirkpatrick, C.H. In *Immunobiology of Transfer Factor* (see ref. 32) p. 129.

87. Welch, T.M., Wilson, G.B., and Fudenberg, H.H. In *Transfer Factor: Basic Properties and Clinical Applications* (see ref. 30) p. 399.

88. Vandenbark, A., Burger, D.R., and Vetto, R.M. (see ref. 30) p. 425.

89. Petersen, E.A., Frey, J.A., Dinowitz, M., and Rifkind, D. (see ref. 30) p. 387.

90. Brummer, E., Foster, L.G., Bhardwaj, N., and Lawrence, H.S. (see ref. 30) p. 27.

91. Burger, D.R., Klesius, P.H., Vandenbark, A.A., Vetto, R.M., and Swann, I.A. Cell. Immunol. 43: 192, 1979.

92. Liburd, E.M., Pabst, H.F., and Armstrong, W.D. Cell. Immunol. 5: 487, 1972.

93. Klesius, P.H., Kristensen, F., Ernst, J.V., and Kramer, T. In *Transfer Factor: Basic Properties and Clinical Applications*. Edited by M.A.S. Ascher, A.A. Gottlieb, and C.H. Kirkpatrick. Academic Press, New York, 1976, p. 311.

94. Klesius, P.H., Elston, A.L., Chambers, W.H., and Fudenberg, H.H. *Transfer Factor: Basic Properties and Clinical Applications.* Edited by M.A.S. Ascher, A.A. Gottlieb, and C.H. Kirkpatrick. Academic Press, New York, pp. 143-149.

95. Mohr, J.A. J. Pediatr. 82: 1062, 1973.

96. Jeter, W.S., Kibler, R., Soli, T.C., and Stephens, C.A.L. In *Immune Modulators* pp. 451-458 (see ref. 75).

97. Burger, D.R., Klesius, P.H., Vandenbark, A.A., Vetto, R.M., and Swann, A.I. Cell. Immunol. 43: 192, 1979.

98. Maddison, S.E., Hicklin, M.D., and Kagan, I.G. Science 178: 757, 1972.

99. Maddison, S.E., Hicklin, M.D., and Kagan, I.G. Exp. Parasitol. 39: 29, 1976.

100. Gallin, J.J., and Kirkpatrick, C.H. Proc. Natl. Acad. Sci. (USA) 71: 498, 1974.

101. Zanelli, J., and Adler, W.H. Cell. Immunol. 15: 475, 1975.
102. Steele, R.W., Eichberg, J.W., Heberling, R.L., Eller, J.J., Katler, S.S., and Kniker, W.T. Cell. Immunol. 22: 110, 1976.
103. Steele, R.W., Heberling, R.L., Eichberg, J.W., Eller, J.J., Katler, S.S., and Kniker, W. In *Transfer Factor: Basic Properties and Clinical Applications.* Edited by M.S. Ascher, A.A. Gottlieb, and C.H. Kirkpatrick. Academic Press, New York, 1976, p. 381.
104. Eichberg, J.W., Steele, R.W., Katler, S.S., Kniker, W.T., Heberling, R.L., Eller, J.J., and Rodriguez, A.R. Cell. Immunol. 26: 114, 1976.
105. Trepo, C.G., and Prince, A.M. In *Transfer Factor: Basic Properties and Clinical Applications.* Edited by M.S. Ascher, A.A. Gottlieb, and C.H. Kirkpatrick. Academic Press, New York, 1976, p. 449.
106. Klesius, P.H., Qualls, D.F., Elston, A.L., and Fudenberg, H.H. Clin. Immunol. Immunopathol. 10: 214, 1978.
107. Olson, G.B., and Drube, C.G. J. Reticuloendothel. Soc. 24: 589, 1978.
108. Borkowsky, W., Pilson, R., and Lawrence, H.S. Pediatr. Res. 20: 1000A, 1986.
109. Levin, A.S., Spitler, L.E., Stites, D.P., et al. Proc. Natl. Acad. Sci. (USA) 67: 821, 1970.
110. Spitler, L.E., Levin, A.S., Stites, D.P., et al. J. Clin. Invest. 51: 3216, 1972.
111. Spitler, L.E. Am. J. Med. 67: 59, 1979.
112. Kesarwala, H.H., Prasad, R.V.S.K., Szep, R., et al. Clin. Exp. Immunol. 36: 465, 1979.
113. Friedenberg, W.R., Marx, Jr. J.J., Hansen, R.L., and Haselby, R.C. Clin. Immunol. Immunopathol. 12: 132, 1979.
114. Kirkpatrick, C.H., Chandler, J.W., and Schimke, R.N. Chronic mucocutaneous moniliasis with impaired delayed hypersensitivity. Clin. Exp. Immunol. 6: 375-385, 1970.
115. Pabst, H.F., and Swanson, R. Successful treatment of candidiasis with transfer factor. Br. Med. J. 2: 442-443, 1972.
116. Schulkind, M.L., Adler, III, W.H., Altemeier, III, W.A., and Ayoub, E.M. Transfer factor in the treatment of a case of chronic mucocutaneous candidiasis. Cell. Immunol. 3: 606-615, 1972.
117. Schulkind, M.L., and Ayoub, E.M. Transfer factor as an approach to the treatment of immune deficiency disease. In *Immunodeficiency in Man and Animals, Birth Defects: Original Article Series, 11*: 436-440, 1975.
118. Littman, B.H., Rocklin, R.E., Parkman, R., and David, J.R. In *Transfer Factor: Basic Properties and Clinical Applications.* Edited by M.S. Ascher, A.A. Gottlieb, and C.H. Kirkpatrick. Academic Press, New York, 1976, p. 495.
119. Kirkpatrick, C.H. Cell. Immunol. 41: 62, 1978.
120. Rubinstein, A., Melamed, J., and Rodescu, D. Clin. Immunol. Immunopathol. 8: 39, 1977.
121. Zielenski, C.C., Savioni, E., Ciotti, M., et al. Cell. Immunol. 84: 200, 1984.
122. Simon, M.R., Salberg, D.J., Silva, Jr., J., et al. Clin. Immunol. Immunopathol. 20: 123, 1981.

123. Wilson, G.B., Metcalf, J.F., and Fudenberg, H.H. Clin. Immunol. Immunopathol. 23: 478, 1982.

124. Dwyer, J.M., Gerstenhaber, B.J., and Dobuler, K.J. Am. J. Med. 74: 161, 1983.

125. Sharma, M.K., Foroozanfar, N., and Ala, F.A. Clin. Immunol. Immunopathol. 10: 369, 1978.

126. Sharma, M., Firouz, R., Ala, F., and Momtaz, A. In *Immune Regulators in Transfer Factor.* Edited by A. Kahn, C.H. Kirkpatrick, and N.O. Hill. Academic Press, New York, 1979, p. 563.

127. Louie, E., Borkowsky, W., Klesius, P. et al. Clin. Immunol. Immunopathol. 44: 329, 1987.

128. Dwyer, J.M. In *Immunobiology of Transfer Factor.* Edited by C.H. Kirkpatrick, D.R. Burger, and H.S. Lawrence. Academic Press, New York, 1983, p. 233.

129. Viza, D., Vich, J.M., Phillips, J., and Rosenfeld, F. Lymphokine Res. 4: 27, 1985.

130. Thomas, I.T., Soothill, J.F., Hawkins, G.T., and Marshall, W.C. Lancet ii: 1056, 1977.

131. Jones, J. et al. Lancet ii, 122, 1981.

132. Shulman, S.T., et al. Cell. Immunol. 43: 352, 1979.

133. Levin, A.S. et al. J. Clin. Invest. 55: 487, 1975.

134. Spitler, L.E. et al. J. Clin. Invest. 52: 3216, 1972.

135. Byers, V.S. et al. Cancer Immunol. Immunother. 6: 253, 1979.

136. Blume, M.R. et al. Cancer 47: 887, 1981.

137. Fujisawa, T. et al. Cancer 54: 663, 1984.

138. Borkowsky, W., and Lawrence, H.S. Pediatr. Res. 18: 945A, 1984.

139. Warren, K.S., Cook, J.A., David, J.R., and Jordan, P. Trans. R. Soc. Trop. Med. Hyg. 69: 488, 1975.

# Part IV
**Chemicals that Influence the Activities of Biological Response Modifiers**

# 14

## Chemotherapy and the Immune Compartments: Interactions with Other Biological Response Modifiers

Abraham Mittelman / New York Medical College, Valhalla, New York

Since the introduction of chemotherapeutic agents the notion that they are immunosuppressive has been widely accepted (1,2). Despite the observation that cancer patients are immunosuppressed in the first place, the standard approach to therapy has been to achieve myelosuppression and thereby one may obtain a higher response rate. The dissection of the exact nature of the suppression induced by chemotherapy has not been clearly defined. But this suppression has generally been accepted as inhibition of all cellular compartments.

The understanding about tumor immunology and host immune reactions to a variety of antigens has led investigators to explore the possibility of using cytotoxic agents as possible immunoaugmenting agents in a complex regulatory immune system. An important aspect of immunosuppression is the association with cytotoxic agents that is attributed to the high doses that were administered in the treatment of cancer patients. The use of select cytotoxic agents at lower doses has recently been explored in the role of immune potentiation.

Most chemotherapeutic agents have been evaluated for their effect on the immune system. However, currently available literature has not precisely defined the role of these agents as immune modulators. The chemotherapeutic agents which have been extensively studied in their role as immunomodulators have been cyclophosphamide (CY) and its derivatives, less extensively 6-mercaptopurines, adriamycin, melphelan, and cis-diamine dichlorplatinum.

With the development of bone marrow transplantation, it has been observed that the depletion of T cells from the graft might aid in avoiding graft vs. host disease. The search for agents that will be specific for T-cell depletion has been extensive because these agents had to be cytotoxic and specific, therefore many chemotherapy agents have been tested in this aspect. A number of agents that recently have been evaluated as part of the CTEP program at the NCI have demonstrated the ability to deplete the marrow selectively of T cells (cyclophosphamide, fludarabine phosphate, and didemenin B). The implication of such specific immunosuppression may be important in the future when cytotoxic agents are combined with biologic response modifiers, in the hope that these combinations will lead to a more potent antitumor response.

## I. CYCLOPHOSPHAMIDE (CY)

The most widely studied agent as immunomodulator has been cyclophosphamide (CY). Its interaction with all the subcomponents of the immune system demonstrated that at low doses CY may affect the cellular as well as the humoral immunity.

It appears that at low dose (50 mg/kg) in mice CY augmented antibody response (3,4) while at higher doses in mice there was suppression of antibody formation (5,6). Furthermore, the dose-dependent activity of CY and its ability to modulate specific antibody formation suggests this agent's ability to modulate B-cell activity as well as T cell in the delayed hypersensitivity (DTH) reaction.

The ability of CY to augment the induction of contact dermatitis in guinea pigs (7,8) demonstrated its ability to modulate T-cell function. In mice it has been shown that pretreatment with low dose CY DTH can be selectively augmented without affecting antibody response (9). Other components of the immune system have also been affected by alkylating agents, specifically CY. The decrease of peritoneal macrophages as well as the decrease of phagocytic activity against bacterial and viral antigens has been related to CY exposure (10,11). The role of macrophages in immune modulation is still to be defined but it has been shown that the induction of cytotoxic lymphocytes require the presence of monocytic/macrophage cells, which by secretion of different monokines may stimulate lymphokine-activated killer cells (LAK). Other cellular compartments affected by CY are the lymphocytes. Their development is antigen dependent and are stimulated by a number of lymphokines. CY at doses of 300 mg/$\mu$g depleted lymphocytes from dependent areas in the lymph nodes and spleen without substantially affecting lymphocytes in T-dependent tissues (12). In comparative studies there has been a greater relative sensitivity of B cells compared to T cells following exposure to CY in peripheral blood, lymph nodes, spleen, and bone marrow (13). Studies involved transfer of lymphoid cells from drug-treated donors to anergic recipients, followed by challenge with antigens has been observed in mice treated with CY on different days; this demonstrated that the transfers were unable to restore immunoresponsiveness for antibody synthesis to anergic mice, although partial restoration was achieved with drug-treated donor spleen cells in combination with normal bone marrow cells indicating the relative sensitivity of cells to CY (14).

While extensive literature exists to demonstrate CY's ability to increase anti-tumor immunomodulation in animal tumor systems its role appears to be two-fold. A cytotoxic agent against a number of different tumor systems and is an immunomodulator in combination with biological response modifiers (BRMs) (15).

While CY may enhance or suppress both T- and B-cell-mediated immune responses, a synthetic alkylating agent, 4-hydroperoxycyclophosphamide (4-HC), is spontaneously hydrolyzed in aqueous solution to 4-hydroxycychophosphamide which is the initial metabolite formed by microsomal activation. In murine tumor systems there is selective enhancement of immune response to sheep erythrocytes by 4-HC by selective inactivation of suppressor T cells or their precursors at low concentrations (16,17). In addition, the use of 4-HC at low doses selectively appears to inhibit the differentiation of presuppressors to suppressor-effector cells (18).

The use of selective inhibition of T cells have led investigators to use 4-HC in bone marrow transplants when lectin separation is required, to reduce graft versus host disease (19).

Based on CY effect on the immune system, it appears that CY augments cell-mediated immunity by inhibition of what appears to be suppressor B cells and inhibition of immunoglobulin secretion (20,21). Therefore, current belief in CY ability to augment immunity by selective toxicity for suppressor T cells and their precursors have led use of CY in combinations with BRMs in low doses as well as high doses. In addition, the use of CY and 4-HC in bone marrow transplantation has grown in importance. Two mechanisms appear to have major impact on CY use in clinical medicine. (a) Its direct cytotoxicity to achieve marrow aplasia. (b) CY can be used in establishing marrow T-cell depletion. Both mechanisms have clearly demonstrated the importance of CY's immunoaugmentative and directly cytotoxic effects.

## II. ADRIAMYCIN

Adriamycin is one of the most commonly used cytotoxic chemotherapeutic agents in medical oncology. It has been demonstrated that adriamycin exerts direct cytotoxicity as a DNA intercalating agent. Its use as a possible immune modulator has not been defined at this time. However, in addition to being immunode-pressive, adriamycin can lead to reduction of both T and B cells, and a smaller reduction in the macrophage cell line (23,24). In 1977, preliminary observations that adriamycin augmented cellular cytotoxicity developed in cultures following pretreatment of splenic cells from mice (22).

Additional studies demonstrated that a single intraperitoneal administration of adriamycin resulted in an increase in cytotoxic activity of peritoneal cells in various mouse strains (25). As with CY the immunoaugmentative ability of adriamycin was achieved at low dose. In [51]chromium release assays adriamycin, administered as a single dose of 25 mg/m$^2$ in inducing cytotoxicity against Raji cell lines, was evaluated on days 5, 7, 10, and 26. The peak level of cytotoxicity was observed on day 7. There was a significant increase in the percentage of OKT8-positive cells, resulting in marked increase of interleukin-2 (IL-2) production (26). Modulating cytotoxic response against allogeneic tumor cells has been demonstrated utilizing low-dose adriamycin in combination of splenic cells when cultured with allogeneic tumor cells, the effector population appears to be related to possible T-cell subsets (27). With the addition of activation of monocytic cytotoxic cell population (22), the mechanism by which adriamycin may act as an immunoaugmentative agent is still difficult to define. These results suggest that adriamycin may enhance monocyte-macrophage cell-mediated immunity, and in addition possibly increase OKT8-positive T cells, and increase the production of IL-2. These various responses suggest that adriamycin may act on multiple immune compartments. While the full range of adriamycin's immune potentiation is unknown it will be determined by future trials. With increased interest in IL-2 the combination of low-dose adriamycin and IL-2 may provide additional possibilities of future combination of BRMs and cytotoxic agents.

## III. 6-MERCAPTOPURINE

Of the antimetabolites, 6-mercaptopurine (6-MP) has been used extensively in the treatment of acute and chronic leukemias. 6-MP is a potent immunosuppressor, affecting all levels of cellular and humoral immunity. It inhibits antibody synthesis and DTH, and retards the rejection of allografts (28-30). A number of experiments have demonstrated that the administration of 6-MP in low dose to rabbits caused a lymphoid hyperplasia and enlargement of the spleen (31). Evaluation of the dose and schedule of administration of 6-MP demonstrated an increase in antibody synthesis, suggesting modulation through the B-cell compartment (32). While 6-MP is being used as a cytotoxic agent in therapy of acute leukemia, its unique property of increasing antibody synthesis and B-lymphocyte stimulation may play an important role in immune modulation which when combined with other agents such as monoclonal antibodies may lead to synergism and increased antitumor activity.

## IV. MELPHELAN

The use of melphelan in the therapy of leukemias and ovarian tumors has been well established. But as with other cytotoxic agents, melphelan is immunosuppressive when used in current therapy and frequently leads to prolonged myelosuppression. Recently melphelan underwent evaluation for its ability to induce synthesis of immunoglobulins by B cells in normal healthy donors (33). Human blood B cells were cultured in the presence of autologous T cells which were treated with melphelan or adriamycin in the presence of pokeweed mitogen (PWM) at three different concentrations. It appeared that melphelan-treated cells (at low dosages of 0.04-4 $\mu$g/ml) produced increased secretions of IgG and IgM, while adriamycin was more suppressive to B cells (33). The full extent of melphelan use as an immune modulator has just begun to be explored its full implication will be determined by future trials.

## V.  BIOLOGIC RESPONSE MODIFIERS AND CHEMOTHERAPY

The availability of interleukin-2 in its natural form and the recombinant type has made it possible to carry out large-scale preclinical evaluations and multiple clinical trials to determine this agent's activity against different tumor systems. Similar trials have been carried out with interferon and other lymphokines (34-37). There have been numerous trials evaluating the efficacy of interleukin-2 in animals specifically in mice bearing tumors such as B16 melanoma and lewis lung tumors (38,39). In order to determine the activity of adoptive immunotherapy, extensive work was carried out to evaluate the mechanism by which autologous LAK cells (lymphokine-activated killer cells) maintain and develop their activity against host tumors; but even more important was the ability to sustain the antitumor activity of LAK cells once they have been stimulated ex vivo and reinfused into the animals (40,41). An important concept developed from these experiments was the determination that inducing antitumor activity, LAK cells maintained their ability to recognize tumor-related antigens and thereby induce cell-mediated cytotoxicity.

The milestone in immunotherapy was established when Rosenberg et al. (42) published their paper on adoptive immunotherapy in patients with advanced cancer, overcoming a number of potential difficulties. Their studies showed a possible dose-response relationship of LAK and IL-2 infusions, with high-dose rIL-2 (recombinant interleukin-2) such as 100,000 units/kg. There have been several preclinical studies combining adoptive immunotherapy CY and rIL-2. The presumptions were that since CY was able to suppress or eradicate suppressor T lymphocytes which are tumor induced, rIL-2's activity may be augmented and combined, higher levels of cell-mediated toxicity can be achieved (43-47).

The combination of IL-2 and CY in animals recently demonstrated the augmentative effects of CY to rIL-2. Syngeneic BC mice were inoculated by $B_5{}^9$ melanoma cells as well as sarcoma cells. CY was administered ip (intraperitoneally) and was followed by IL-2 administration near the tumor inoculation site. In all groups of mice the combination of CY and rIL-2 achieved cures; but most important, this combination successfully achieved regression in $B_5{}^9$ melanoma-bearing mice. This work demonstrated that 60-80% mice treated in combination with CY and rIL-2 achieved cures without the use of autologous LAK cell infusion and without the toxicity that is attributed to the adoptive rIL-2 and LAK cell therapy (48). The mechanism by which rIL-2 and CY achieved antitumor effect has not been fully determined at this time. But a number of other mediators have been known to be involved when rIL-2 is infused. These are lymphokine, interferon, and possibly tumor necrosis factor (49,50).

These therapeutic modalities have been further developed in a recent study which demonstrated that the use of tumor-infiltrating lymphocytes (TIL) have greater specific antitumor activity than LAK cells. It has long been shown that tumors evaluated under a phase contrast microscope are known to have mononuclear cell infiltrates which are presumed to be of monocytic, macrophage, or lymphocytes cell lineages. These cells potentially are exposed to tumor-specific antigens and thereby develop specific antitumor cell cytotoxicity. Therefore when these cells are combined with rIL-2 they appear to show greater antitumor effects. The combination of rIL-2, TIL, and CY has recently been evaluated as well. These results showed that the combination of these agents induced a greater antitumor response than their use as single agents in mice (51). The full clinical impact of this combination is still to be determined.

## VI. CONCLUSION

The role of chemotherapy in immunomodulation on a large scale has only recently begun to undergo extensive evolution. It appears that many cytotoxic medications have a role in immunomodulation and may act at different compartments of this system (Table 1). The recent demonstration of the use of CY in combination with rIL-2 and TIL has defined a possible role for cytotoxic drugs as immune modulators. The complete implication of their use and the possible use of combinations of chemotherapeutic agents and BRMs is yet to be fully explored.

Even more important, the possible determination of the molecules that induce the killing may ultimately play a major additional role in the therapy of

Table 1  The Role of Cytotoxic Medications in Immunomodulation

| Delayed hypersensitivity reaction | T Cell | B Cell | Macrophage/Monocyte |
|---|---|---|---|
| CY ↑ | CY ↓ | CY ↓ | CY ↑ |
| Thiotepa ↑ | Fludarabine ↓ | Adriamycin ↓ | |
| Adriamycin ↑ | Didemnin B ↓ | 6-MP ↑ | Adriamycin ↑ |
| Mitomycin ↑ | Adriamycin ↑ | Melphelan ↑ | |
| 5FU ↑ | | | |
| Vincristine ↑ | | | |
| Methotrexate ↑ | | | |

DTH = delayed hypersensitivity; ↓ = decreased activity; ↑ = increased activity.

malignancy. The development of recombinant DNA technology cloning these proteins may become a reality and their use in combination of BRMs, cytotoxic chemotherapy, and ex vivo expansion of different cellular killer cells such as LAK, NK, and TIL cells will offer a diversified approach to the treatment of human malignancy.

The role of chemotherapy has been to induce direct cell killing by administering massive doses of a variety of agents, thereby inducing increased toxicity and morbidity from therapy. While the role of chemotherapy as an immune modulator has been in existence for many years, its use has only recently gained interest. Rather than administering massive doses of drugs, in light of their toxicity, an alternative use of these agents is in combination with BRMs may lead to a more rational therapeutic approach to the treatment of cancer patients.

# REFERENCES

1. Bodey, G.P., Hersh, E.H., Valdivieso, M., Feld, R., and Rodrequez, V. Effects of cytotoxic and immunosuppressive agents on the immune system. Postgrad. Med. 58: 67-74, 1975.
2. Harris, J., Sengar, D., stewart, T., and Myslop, D. The effect of immunosuppressive chemotherapy on immune functions in patients with malignant disease. Cancer 37: 1058-1069, 1976.
3. Kerckaert, J.A., Hofhuis, F.M., and Willers, J.M. Effects of variation in time and dose of cyclophosphamide on delayed hypersensitivity and antibody formation. Cell Immunol. 29: 232-237, 1977.
4. Berd, D., Maguire, H.C., and Mastroangelo, M.J. Potentiation of human cell-mediated and humeral immunity by low dose cyclophosphamide. Cancer Res. 44: 5439-5443, 1984.
5. Chiorazzi, N., Fox, D.A., and Katz, D.H. Hapten-specific IgE antibody response in mice. VI. Selective enhancement of IgE antibody production by low doses x-irradiation and by cyclophosphamide. J. Immunol. 117: 1629-1637, 1976.
6. Glaser, M. Regulation of specific cell-mediated cytotoxic response against SV 40-induced tumor associated antigens by depletion of suppressor T cells with cyclophosphamide in mice. J. Exp. Med. 149: 774-779, 1979.
7. Maguire, Jr., H.C., and Ettore, V.L. Enhancement of dinitrochlorobenzene (DNCB) contact sensitization by cyclophosphamide in the guinea pig. J. Invest. Dermatol. 48: 39-43, 1967.
8. Hunziker, N. Effects of cyclophosphamide on the contact eczema in guinea pigs. Dermatologica 136: 187-191, 1968.
9. Askenase, P.W., Hayden, B.J., and Gershon, R.K. Augmentation of delayed-type hypersensitivity by doses of cyclophosphamide which do not affect antibody responses. J. Exp. Med. 141: 697-702, 1975.
10. Gadeberg, O.V., Rhodes, J.M., and Larsen, S.O. The effect of venous immunosuppressive agents on mouse peritoneal macrophages and on the *in vitro* phagocytosis of escharichia coli 04:HS and degredation of 125 I-labeled HSA-antibody. Immunology 28: 59-70, 1975.

11. Kabiri, M., and Hadulgh, M.D. Interaction of Coxsackievirus B-3 and peritoneal exudate cells of adult mice treated with cyclophosphamide. J. Med. Virol. 1(3): 183-191, 1977.

12. Turk, J.L., and Poulter, L.W. Selective depletion of lymphoid tissue by cyclophosphamide. Clin. Exp. Immun. 10: 285-296, 1972.

13. Johansen, R.S., Johansen, T.S., and Talmage, D.W. T-cell rosette formation in primates, pigs and guinea pigs. J. Allergy Clin. Immunol. 54: 86-93, 1974.

14. Willers, J.M., and Sluis, E. The influence of cyclophosphamide on antibody formation in the mouse. Ann. Immunol. (Inst Posteur) 126C: 267-279, 1975.

15. Rosenberg, S.A., Spiess, P., and Lafreniere, R. A new approach to the adoptive immunotherapy of cancer with tumor-infiltrating lymphocytes. Science 233: 1318, 1986.

16. Kaufman, S.H., Hahn, H.W., and Diamantstein, T. Relative susceptabilities of T cell subsets involved in delayed type hypersensitivity to sheep red blood cells to the in vitro action of 4-hydroperoxycyclophosphamide. J. Immunol. 125: 1104, 1980.

17. Kiamantstein, T., Klos, M., Hahn, H., and Kaufman, S.H. Direct in vitro evidence for different susceptibilities to 4-hydroxyperoxycyclophosphamide of antigen-primed T cells regulating humeral and cell-mediated immune responses to sheep erythrocytes: a possible explanation for the inverse action of cyclophosphamide on humorel and cell mediated immune response. J. Immunol. 126: 1717, 1981.

18. Ozer, H.T., Cowens, W., Colvin, M., Nussbaum-Blumenson, A., and Sheedy, D. In vitro effects of 4-hydroxyperoxycyclophosphamide on human immunoregulatory T subset function. I. selective effects on lymphocytes function in T-B cell collaboration. J. Exp. Med. 155: 276, 1982.

19. Yeager, A.M., Kaizer, H., Santos, G.W., Saral, R., et al. Autologous Bone Marrow Transplantation in patients with acute nonlymphocytic leukemia, using ex vivo marrow treated with 4-hydroperoxycyclophosphamide. N. Engl. J. Med. 315: 141, 1986.

20. Kutz, S.I., Parker, D., and Turk, J.L. B-cell suppression of delayed hypersensitivity reactions. Nature 251: 550-551, 1974.

21. Lagrange, P.H., Mackaness, G.B., and Miller, T.E. Potentiation of T cell mediated immunity by selective suppression of antibody formation with cyclophosphamide. J. Exp. Med. 139: 1529-1539, 1974.

22. Orsini, F., Pavclia, Z., and Mihick, E. Increased primary cell-mediated immunity in culture subsequent to adriamycin or daunorubicin treatment of spleen donor mice. Cancer Res. 37: 1719-1726, 1977.

23. Mantovani, A. In vivo and in vitro cytotoxicity of adriamycin and daunorubicin for murine macrophages. Cancer Res. 37: 815-820, 1977.

24. Mantovani, A., Tagliabue, A., Vecchi, A., and Spreafico, F. Effects of adriamycin and daunomycin on spleen cell population in normal and tumor allografted mice. Eur. J. Cancer 2: 381-387, 1976.

25. Santori, A., Riccardi, C., Sorce, V., and Hersherman, R.B. Effects of adriamycin on the activity of mouse natural killer cells. J. Immunol. 124: 2329-2335, 1980.

26. Arinaga, S., Akiyoshi, T., and Tsuji, H. Augmentation of the generation of cell-mediated cytotoxicity after a single dose of adriamycin in cancer patients. Cancer Res. 46: 4213-4216, 1986.
27. Tomazic, V., Ehrke, M.J., and Mihich, E. Modulation of the cytotoxic response against allogeneic tumor cells in culture by adriamycin. Cancer Res. 40: 2748-2755, 1980.
28. Schwartz, R., Eisner, A., and Dameshek, W. The effect of 6-mercaptopurine on primary and secondary immune responses. J. Clin. Invest. 38: 1394, 1959.
29. Hoyer, J.R., Hoyer, L.W., Good, R.A., and Condie, R.M. The effect of 6-mercaptopurine on delayed hypersensitivity in guinea pigs. J. Exp. Med. 116: 679, 1962.
30. Schwartz, R., and Dameshek, W. The effect of 6-mercaptopurine on homograft reactions. J. Clin. Invest. 39: 956, 1960.
31. Sahiar, K., and Schwartz, R. The immunoglobulin sequence. II. Histoligical effects of the suppression of $\gamma$M and $\gamma$G antibody synthesis. Intern. Arch. Allergy Appl. Immunol. 29: 52, 1960.
32. Devendrathan, C., and Schwartz, R. Enhancement of antibody synthesis by 6-mercaptopurine. J. Exp. Med. 124: 363, 1966.
33. Baral, E., Blomgren, H., Wasserman, J., Von Stedingk, L.V., Rotstein, S., and Vivving, L. Melphelan treatment of human peripheral T cells promotes Ig production by B cells *in vitro*. Eur. J. Cancer Clin. Oncol. 21: 81, 1985.
34. Doyle, M.V., Lee, M.T., and Fong, S. Comparison of the biological activities of human recombinant interleukin-2 and native interleukin-2. J. Biol. Resp. Mod. 4: 96, 1985.
35. Roifman, C.M., Mills, G.B., Chu, M., and Gelfand, E.W. Functional comparison of recombinant interleukin-2 (IL-2) with IL-2 containing preparations derived from cultured cells. Cell Immunol. 95: 146, 1985.
36. Rosenberg, S.A. Lymphokine activated killer cells: A new approach to immunotherapy of cancer. J. Natl. Cancer Inst. 75: 595, 1985.
37. Lotze, M.T., Grimm, E.A., Mazumder, A., Strausser, J.L., and Rosenberg, S.A. In vitro of cytotoxic human lymphocytes IV. Lysis of fresh and cultured autologous tumor by lymphocytes cultured in T cell growth factor (TCGF). Cancer Res. 41: 4420-4425, 1981.
38. Mule, J.J., Shu, S., Schwartz, S.L., and Rosenberg, S.A. Adoptive immunotherapy of established pulmonary metastases with LAK cells and recombinant interleukin 2. Science 225: 1487, 1984.
39. Lafranziere, R., and Rosenberg, S.A. Successful immunotherapy of murine experimental hepatic metastases with lymphokine activated killer cells and recombinant interleukin 2. Cancer Res. 45: 3735, 1985.
40. Ettinghausen, S.E., Lipford, E.A., Mule, J.J., et al. Systemic administration of recombinant interleukin 2 stimulates in vivo lymphoid cell proliferation in tissues. J. Immunol. 135: 1488, 1985.
41. Ettinghausen, S.E., Lipford, E.H., Mule, J.J., et al. Recombinant interleukin 2, stimulates in vivo prolification of adoptively transferred lymphokine activated killer (LAK) cells. J. Immunol. 135: 3623, 1985.

42. Rosenberg, S.A., Lotze, M.T., Muul, L.M., et al. Observation on the systemic administration of autologous lymphokine activated killer cells and recombinant interleukin-2 to patients with metastatic cancer. N. Engl. J. Med. 313: 1485, 1985.

43. North, R.J. Cyclophosphamide-facilitated adoptive immunotherapy of an established tumor depends upon elimination of tumor-induced suppressor T cells. J. Exp. Med. 55: 1063, 1982.

44. Evans, R. Combination therapy by using cyclophosphamide and tumor sensitized lymphocytes: a possible mechanism of action. J. Immunol. 130: 2511, 1983.

45. Greenberg, P.D., Kern, D.E., and Cheever, M.A. Therapy of dissiminated murine leukemia with cyclophosphamide and immune lyt-1+, 2- T cells. J. Exp. Med. 161: 1122, 1985.

46. Cheever, M.A., Greenberg, P.D., and Fefer, A. Specificity of adoptive chemoimmunotherapy of established syngenic tumors. J. Immunol. 125: 711, 1980.

47. Bosberg, H., Oettgen, H.F., Choudry, K., and Beattre, Jr., E.J. Inhibition of established transplants of chemically induced sarcomas in syngenic mice by lymphocytes from immunized donors. Int. J. Cancer 10: 539, 1972.

48. Silagi, S., and Schaefer, A.E. Successful immunotherapy of mouse melanoma and sarcoma with recombinant interleukin-2 and cyclophosphamide. J. Biol. Res. Mod. 5: 411, 1986.

49. Kosahora, T., Hoole, J.J., Dougherty, S.F., and Oppenheim, J.J. Interleukin-2 mediated immune interferon (IFN-$\gamma$) production by human T cells and T cells subsets. J. Immunol. 130: 1784, 1983.

50. Svedersky, L.P., Nedwin, G.E., Goeddel, D.V., and Palladino, M.A. Interferon-$\gamma$ enhances induction of lymphotoxin is recombinant interleukin-2 stimulated peripheral blood mononuclear cells. J. Immunol. 134: 1604, 1958.

51. Rosenberg, S.A., Spiess, P., and Lafraniere, R. A new approach to the adoptive immunotherapy of cancer with tumor infiltrating lymphocytes. Science 233: 1318, 1986.

# Index

437